Cellular and Molecular Aspects of Cirrhosis

Aspects cellulaires et moléculaires de la cirrhose

***Colloques* INSERM**
ISSN 0768-3154

Other *Colloques* published as co-editions by John Libbey Eurotext and INSERM

133 Cardiovascular and Respiratory Physiology in the Fetus and Neonate. *Physiologie Cardiovasculaire et Respiratoire du Fœtus et du Nouveau-né.*
Scientific Committee : P. Karlberg, A. Minkowski, W. Oh and L. Stern;
Managing Editor : M. Monset-Couchard.
ISBN : John Libbey Eurotext 0 86196 086 6
INSERM 2 85598 282 0

134 Porphyrins and Porphyrias. *Porphyrines et Porphyries.*
Edited by Y. Nordmann.
ISBN : John Libbey Eurotext 0 86196 087 4
INSERM 2 85598 281 2

137 Neo-Adjuvant Chemotherapy. *Chimiothérapie Néo-Adjuvante.*
Edited by C. Jacquillat, M. Weil and D. Khayat.
ISBN : John Libbey Eurotext 0 86196 077 7
INSERM 2 85598 283 7

139 Hormones and Cell Regulation (10th European Symposium). *Hormones et Régulation Cellulaire (10e Symposium Européen).*
Edited by J. Nunez, J.E. Dumont and R.J.B. King.
ISBN : John Libbey Eurotext 0 86196 084 X
INSERM 2 85598 284 7

147 Modern Trends in Aging Research. *Nouvelles Perspectives de la Recherche sur le Vieillissement.*
Edited by Y. Courtois, B. Faucheux, B. Forette, D.L. Knook and J.A. Tréton.
ISBN : John Libbey Eurotext 0 86196 103 X
INSERM 2 85598 309 6

149 Binding Proteins of Steroid Hormones. *Protéines de liaison des Hormones Stéroïdes.*
Edited by M.G. Forest and M. Pugeat.
ISBN : John Libbey Eurotext 0 86196 125 0
INSERM 2 85598 310 X

151 Control and Management of Parturition. *La Maîtrise de la Parturition.*
Edited by C. Sureau, P. Blot, D. Cabrol, F. Cavaillé and G. Germain.
ISBN : John Libbey Eurotext 0 86196 096 3
INSERM 2 85598 311 8

Suite page 377
(Continued p. 377)

Cellular and Molecular Aspects of Cirrhosis

Aspects cellulaires et moléculaires de la cirrhose

Proceedings of the International Conference on "Cellular and Molecular Bases of Liver Cirrhosis" held in Rennes (France) on July 3-5, 1991

Sponsored by the Institut National de la Santé et de la Recherche Médicale (INSERM)

Edited by

Bruno Clément
André Guillouzo

John Libbey EUROTEXT

LES EDITIONS INSERM

British Library Cataloguing in Publication Data
Cellular and molecular aspects
of cirrhosis
I. Clément, Bruno
II. Guillouzo, André

ISBN 0 86196 342 3
ISSN 0768-3154

First published in 1992 by

Editions John Libbey Eurotext
6 rue Blanche, 92120 Montrouge, France. (33) (1) 47 35 85 52
ISBN 0 86196 342 3

John Libbey and Company Ltd
13 Smiths Yard, Summerley Street, London SW18 4HR, England.
(44) (81) 947 27 77

Institut National de la Santé et de la Recherche Médicale
101 rue de Tolbiac, 75654 Paris Cedex 13, France.
(33) (1) 44 23 60 00
ISBN 2 85 598 483 1

ISSN 0768-3154

Preface

This book contains 43 lectures and poster communications presented at the international conference on the "Cellular and Molecular Bases of Liver Cirrhosis" held in Rennes on July 3-5, 1991 and chaired by Professor Michel Bourel, member of the French Academy of Medicine, under the patronage of the French Association for the Study of the Liver. Only lectures placed in the first part of each section, have both English and French abstracts.

This conference was sponsored by the Institut National de la Santé et de la Recherche Médicale (INSERM). We would like to thank for their invaluable help : the city of Rennes, and particularly the Major, Mr Edmond Hervé ; the Ecole Nationale de la Santé Publique and its Director, Mr Christian Rollet, and the following companies : Biologie Servier, Biopredic, Crédit Mutuel de Bretagne, Ferring S.A., Hoechst AG, Hoechst-Société Française, Laboratoires Duphar et Cie, Laboratoires Meram, Rhone-Poulenc Rorer, Servier Medical and Smithkline Beecham.

A special note of gratitude should be given to Mrs Maryvonne André and Annie Vannier for their constant and efficient assistance in both the organization of the conference and the preparation of the book.

Bruno Clément
André Guillouzo

Scientific committee
Comité scientifique

Charles Balabaud *(Bordeaux)*
Pierre Berthelot *(Paris)*
Michel Bourel *(Rennes)*
Pierre Brissot *(Rennes)*
Bruno Clément *(Rennes)*
Daniel Dhumeaux *(Paris)*
Serge Erlinger *(Clichy)*
Jean-Alexis Grimaud *(Lyon)*
André Guillouzo *(Rennes)*
Dominique Pessayre *(Clichy)*
Raoul Poupon *(Paris)*

Local organizing committee
Comité d'organisation local

Michel Bourel (Président / *Chairman)*
Pierre Brissot
Jean-Pierre Campion
Bruno Clément
Yves Deugnier
Philippe Gripon
Christiane Guguen-Guillouzo
André Guillouzo
Gérard Lescoat
Damrong Ratanasavanh

Programme coordinators
Coordinateurs du programme

Bruno Clément
André Guillouzo

Secretary
Secrétariat

Maryvonne André
Annie Vannier

Préface

Ce livre contient 43 conférences et communications par affiche présentées à Rennes du 3 au 5 Juillet 1991 dans le cadre du colloque international sur les “Bases Cellulaires et Moléculaires de la Cirrhose du Foie” présidé par le Professeur Michel Bourel, membre de l’Académie de Médecine, et placé sous les auspices de l’Association Française pour l’Etude du Foie. Seules les conférences placées en début de partie ont un résumé en français et en anglais.

Ce colloque a bénéficié de l’aide de l’Institut National de la Santé et de la Recherche Médicale (INSERM). Nous tenons également à remercier pour leur soutien : la mairie de Rennes, et plus particulièrement Monsieur le député-maire Edmond Hervé ; l’Ecole Nationale de la Santé Publique et son Directeur, Monsieur Christian Rollet, ainsi que les sociétés suivantes : Biologie Servier, Biopredic, Crédit Mutuel de Bretagne, Ferring S.A., Hoechst AG, Hoechst-Société Française, Laboratoires Duphar et Cie, Laboratoires Meram, Rhone-Poulenc Rorer, Servier Medical et Smithkline Beecham.

Nous tenons à exprimer notre gratitude à Mmes Maryvonne André et Annie Vannier pour leur aide constante et efficace à l’organisation du colloque et à la réalisation de ce livre.

Bruno Clément
André Guillouzo

Contents
Sommaire

FIBROGENESIS
FIBROGENÈSE

DYNAMICS IN CIRRHOSIS : REMODELING, REGENERATION, HEPATOCARCINOGENESIS
DYNAMIQUE DE LA CIRRHOSE : REMODELAGE, RÉGÉNÉRATION, HÉPATOCARCINOGENÈSE

Cellular and Molecular Aspects of Cirrhosis. Eds B. Clément, A. Guillouzo. Colloque INSERM/John Libbey Eurotext Ltd. © 1992, Vol. 216, pp. 1-9

Liver cirrhosis : evolving aspects of an old problem

Valeer Desmet

University Hospital Sint Rafaël, Laboratory of Histochemistry and Cytochemistry, K.U. Leuven, Leuven, Belgium

SUMMARY

An overview is given of some of the salient points in the evolving aspects of cirrhosis from antiquity till today. For centuries, the problem was slow progress and scarcity of scientific data.

Known since Hippocrates, cirrhosis of the liver was only better defined after the introduction of anatomy by Vesalius (16th century) and pathology by Morgagni (18th century), ending with a confusing diversity in classification in the early 20th century.

Most of what is know about cirrhosis stems from the eclosion of "the youngest science" (L. Thomas) in this century : recognition of liver cell damage, fibroplasia and regeneration as the main driving forces in morphogenesis; delineation of cirrhosis from mimicking conditions; identification of several aetiologies; advances in diagnostic strategies and in therapy of complications; and studies on mechanisms of cell death, inflammation, fibrosis and repair.

The recent powerful techniques of molecular biology have focussed new research on basic mechanisms of cells and molecules : the fascinating interplay of various cell types in the liver, constituting a harmonious ecosystem within the supersystem of the living organism, and its disturbance by disease. Problems of today become the speed of progress, the divergence of techniques, and the wealth of information.

FROM ANTIQUITY TO THE 20TH CENTURY

The early history of cirrhosis was recently reviewed by Schaffner and Sieratzki (1987); they describe it as "a fascinating saga of the slowness in the development of knowledge and the contribution of a few imaginative and far sighted thinkers and observers".

Hippocrates was probably the first to recognize "hardening of the liver" which he regarded as a bad sign if it was accompanied by jaundice. Erasistratos, a Greek physician active in Alexandria around 300 BC, recognized a relation between hardening of the liver and ascites. In the second century AD, Aretaeus of Cappadocia suggested that non-suppurative inflammations of the liver may lead to hardening of the organ or scirrhus and incurable dropsy or ascites. However, he did not distinguish scirrhus from hepatic induration due to tumour; he related various pathological conditions, including fever and mental disorders, to contamination of blood with bile.

The concept of a psychopathologic significance of bile apparently had its roots in the early observations of depression and encephalopathy in association with jaundice. The famous book of Aretaeus was translated from Greek into Latin by Boerhaave in 1735 (Schaffner & Sieratzki, 1987).

In ancient Rome, Celsus believed that ascites caused cirrhosis. In the late second century AD, the most prominent Roman physician Galen described the liver as the site of blood formation and heat production. His physiologic theory persisted for centuries throughout the Middle Ages until the 17th century. Dogmatic belief rendered progress of science impossible, and nothing was learned about cirrhosis for more than 1000 years.

With the Renaissance and the revival of science, anatomy became the most important foundation of medicine. Andreas Vesalius published his famous and masterfully illustrated anatomic atlas 'De humani Corporis Fabrica" in 1543. He mentioned the shrunken liver and enlarged spleen in alcoholics. The 16th century surgeon Ambroise Paré discussed ascites and techniques and complications of paracentesis.

In 1684 Bonet collected some cases of scirrhus and ascites, some also associated with jaundice, epistaxis and portal vein thrombosis, as related to alcohol abuse. Harvey thought that scirrhus was caused by ascites, itself resulting from excessive consumption of plain water. According to Sydenham, ascites resulted from weakness of the blood debilitated by bleeding, chronic disease and from drinking spirit liquors in excess.

The first illustration of a micronodular cirrhotic liver was presented in a short case report in 1685 by John Brown(e), who ascribed the disease to drinking too much water.

The first extensive discussion on scirrhus of the liver was by G.B. Morgagni, in the letters 36, 37, 38 of his "De Sedibus et Causis Morborum" in 1761.

He did not distinguish scirrhus from cancer, but thought that constriction of blood vessels and the appearance of granulations were typical features. In line with the ancient concept, he maintained that jaundice ("morbus regius" because of the gold-like colour) was due to the constriction of the liver by hepatic nerves, caused by passion and emotional disturbances.

In 1795, Baillie was the first to differentiate scirrhus from carcinoma and other hardening or granulated liver diseases; he also established a link between alcohol abuse and scirrhus, "the gin-drinker's liver".

In 1837 Laennec introduced the term, CIRRHOSIS in a footnote to this text "Traité de l'Auscultation" (Laënnec, 1837).

The first semi-microscopic examination of the cirrhotic liver was described by Cruveilhier about 1830; he stated that the granulations contained normal spongious liver tissue and that the space between was occupied by fibrous tissue; the difference in size of the granulations was ascribed to atrophy and compensatory hypertrophy. Hallmann provided the first relatively precise microscopic description of cirrhosis in 1839. In 1842, Rokitansky produced an excellent macroscopic, but relatively simple microscopic description, and still adhered to the concepts of humoral pathology.

The revolution to cellular pathology came with the work of R. Virchow "Cellular Pathologie" in 1858.

Studies on pathophysiology started in the middle of the 19th century with the demonstration by Claude Bernard of the role of the liver in glucose production and other physiologic discoveries. Frerichs in 1858 added new clinical aspects to those already described by Budd in 1846; most important was his description of hepatic coma. In 1885, Murchison was apparently the first to recognize fatal gastrointestinal hemorrhage in pre-ascitic stages, and to note cerebral symptoms, jaundice and hemorrhage as frequent complications in advanced cirrhosis (Schaffner & Sieratzki, 1987).

Towards the end of the 19th century, Victor Hanot (1876) had described a hypertrophic form of cirrhosis and emphasized bile duct lesions. Charcot and Gombault (1876) demonstrated a relationship between bile duct obstruction and liver damage, and described obstructive biliary cirrhosis.

Around the turn of the century, there was debate about hypertrophic and atrophic, portal, biliary, and other forms of cirrhosis, resulting in a flood of types and classifications of cirrhosis. "Chaque auteur arrive à avoir sa cirrhose : c'est l'anarchie" (Desoil, 1897). The debate went on until well into the 20th century.

FROM 1900 TO 1990

Definition and classification of cirrhosis

The term "cirrhosis" coined by Laënnec in 1837 was rapidly accepted all over the world despite criticism by Rokitansky and other morphologists, who suggested designations like "granular atrophy" or "tuberculization" (Schaffner & Sieratzki, 1987)

There remained problems with the definition of cirrhosis. The term cirrhosis was often wrongly implied to mean hardening of the liver. Even in 1947, Himsworth wanted to discard the term "cirrhosis" and to use simply the term "fibrosis", because of the disagreement in defining the lesion (Popper & Schaffner, 1957).

It took a conference in Havannah in 1955 (Report of the Board of Classiciation and Nomenclature of Cirrhosis of the Liver, 1956) and a meeting of a committee of the World Health Organization (Anthony et al., 1977) to arrive at the present definition of cirrhosis : "a diffuse process characterized by fibrosis and a conversion of normal architecture into structurally abnormal nodules".

It has been argued that this definition is incomplete because it does not include reference to the important vascular changes present in cirrhosis : the establishment of intrahepatic porto-hepatic shunts (Rappaport et al., 1983).

If definition of cirrhosis is a problem, attempts at classification have given rise to even greater taxonomic exercises, reflected in some of the synonyms mentioned in the table below.

The present **morphological** classification of cirrhosis distinguishes (Anthony et al., 1977):

1. Micronodular cirrhosis (or monolobular or regular cirrhosis, Gall type II, diffuse septal, portal, nutritional, alcoholic, or Laënnec's cirrhosis).
2. Macronodular cirrhosis (or multilobular, irregular or variform cirrhosis), which comprises two subtypes :
   a) postnecrotic type (Nagayo type A, Gall type I, post collapse cirrhosis, subacute or healed yellow atrophy, toxic cirrhosis, coarsely nodular cirrhosis, multiple nodular hyperplasia, Kartoffelleber, lobar form of cirrhosis)
   b) incomplete septal type (posthepatitic, cirrhosis Gall type II, Nagayo type B, coarse nodular cirrhosis)
3. Mixed macro-micronodular cirrhosis.

Cirrhosis is most satisfactorily classified by its aetiology; however, aetiological and macroscopical classifications are not mutually exclusive.

Aetiologically, cirrhosis is now recognized as a late stage of the most diverse liver diseases of various aetiology (see further).

Morphogenesis of cirrhosis

The main morphogenetic components in the evolution towards cirrhosis are parenchymal damage and atrophy, active fibroplasia and nodular parenchymal regeneration (Rössle, 1930).

For several decades the discussion went on whether the primary lesion was active mesenchymal proliferation (Rössle, 1930) or parenchymal damage followed by reparative scarring (Moon, 1932) and compensatory parenchymal regeneration. The prevailing theory became that parenchymal damage was the primary lesion, although recent studies indicating the direct stimulating effect on collagen synthesis, by metabolites of alcohol (acetaldehyde) may again give credit to Rössle's concept (Savolainen et al., 1984).

Part of the discussion also focussed on the starting point of the fibrosis : portal or central. It was the merit of Popper's group to demonstrate that in late stage human cirrhosis the intraseptal vessels could be injected from both the hepatic and the portal vein : end stage human cirrhosis was both portal and central : portal-central cirrhosis (Popper et al., 1952) (la cirrhose biveineuse de Charcot).

This study further emphasized the portal-hepatic shunting nature of a large number of the blood vessels in the fibrous septa, and indicated pre-existing sinusoids as the origin of these intrahepatic vascular shunts.

The intrahepatic vascular shunt abnormality of the liver circulation in cirrhosis was recognized as a key feature of cirrhosis, and its development as the stage of irreversibility (the point of no return).

Development of regenerative nodules or pseudolobules was to be explained by parenchymal regeneration within the framework of an altered or altering connective tissue stroma.

Three-dimensional reconstruction studies indicated that cirrhotic nodules are not completely isolated by fibrous septa, but constitute an interconnected nodular network (Takahashi, 1978), with a pattern corresponding to a scarring of liver acini (Rappaport et al., 1983). Small (micronodular) nodules correspond to regenerated simple or complex acini, whereas larger (macronodular) nodules are derived from acinar agglomerates or develop through "relobulisation" of growing nodules which originally were smaller in size (Smetana, 1956). Cirrhotic nodules were shown to be preferentially vascularized by the hepatic artery (Yamamoto et al., 1984), which may explain, at least in part, the adenoma-like hyperplastic regeneration in cirrhotic nodules.

Liver fibrosis

Although the detailed mechanisms involved in the progression from normal liver into cirrhosis remain largely unknown, a predominant role has been ascribed to piecemeal necrosis and confluent (bridging) necrosis in the cirrhogenic evolution of chronic hepatitis. Piecemeal necrosis appears to be a cell mediated immunological mechanism of liver cell destruction (Desmet, 1985), whereas "bridging hepatic necrosis" may rather result from humoral immune effects (Desmet, 1990; Desmet, 1991). Piecemeal necrosis gives rise to inflammatory, "active" septa, whereas confluent necrosis results in paucicellular, "passive" septa (Bianchi et al., 1971).

Research on hepatic fibrosis during this century passed through three periods (Popper, 1982). The first was a descriptive period, dealing with morphological and biochemical observations, during which the increase in connective tissue in the liver was considered stable and inert.

The second period, starting in the mid-sixties, might be designated as the physiologic period which recognized, under the influence of basic research on connective tissue, that hepatic fibrosis is a dynamic process of formation and degradation of connective tissue components.

The third period followed in the eighties with quantitation of cellular and molecular events in fibrosis, characterizing it as the kinetic period (Popper, 1982).

In accelerating speed, investigations of the last ten years have led to the program of the present symposium in Rennes.

Experimental models of cirrhosis

Several animal models for experimental production of liver fibrosis and cirrhosis have been studied. These include : 1. high-fat/low protein (choline-deficient) diets in rats and primates; 2. carbon tetrachloride in rodents; 3. thioacetamide in rodents; 4. galactosamine in rodents; 5. dimethylnitrosamine in rodents and dogs; 6. ethionine in rodents; 7. ligation of the common bile duct in rodents; 8. foreign protein administration in rodents; 9. alpha-naphtyl isothiocyanate producing biliary fibrosis; 10. prolonged ethanol administration to baboons; and 11. Schistosomiasis in mice and rabbits (Popper, 1982; Tsukamoto et al., 1990).

Differentiation between cirrhosis and conditions resembling cirrhosis

In the second half of this century, a number of conditions have been identified which clinically or morphologically may be confused with cirrhosis (Desmet et al., 1990).

Idiopathic portal hypertension (or hepatoportal sclerosis) refers to patients with portal hypertension, in whom all other known causes of portal hypertension, including cirrhosis, have been excluded.

The incomplete septal type of cirrhosis appears to be on the borderline between cirrhosis and non-cirrhotic portal hypertension (Sciot et al., 1988).

Nodular regenerative hyperplasia is characterized by diffuse, regular nodularity of the liver without real septal fibrosis.

Partial nodular transformation can be considered a focal and macronodular analogue of the previous entity.

Focal nodular hyperplasia resembles biliary cirrhosis microscopically, but is a focal lesion.

All these entities seem to be caused by some form or another of intrahepatic portal venopathy, and to result from inhomogeneous distribution of blood flow through the liver (Wanless, 1990).

Congenital hepatic fibrosis resembles a biliary fibrosis, with intrahepatic bile ducts in immature, embryologic shapes, and causes portal hypertension in children and young adults (Desmet et al., 1990).

Identification of the aetiology of cirrhosis

In the fifties, several etiologic factors in cirrhosis were already recognized: malnutrition (including alcoholism), viral hepatitis, intoxications, intrahepatic and extrahepatic cholestasis, granulomatous diseases, parasitic infestations, metabolic disorders, and chronic passive congestion (Popper & Schaffner, 1957).

After World war II, the broader application of liver biopsy allowed the histopathologic study of liver disease before the end stage of cirrhosis; one of the major acquisitions was the recognition of chronic hepatitis, and subsequently identification of its various aetiologies by progress in virology and immunology.

During the last forty years, an impressive expansion of knowledge took place : the identification of hepatitis viruses B, C and D; the role of drug-induced liver damage; further specification of chronic cholestatic conditions, including primary biliary cirrhosis and primary sclerosing cholangitis; identification of numerous metabolic defects (like in glycogen storage diseases, hereditary fructose intolerance, tyrosinemia, Wolman's disease, cholesterol ester storage disease, protoporphyria, a_1-antitrypsin deficiency, peroxisomal disorders ...).

In spite of tremendous progress, any aetiological classification of cirrhosis today still ends with the category of "cryptogenic cirrhosis", awaiting the new discoveries still to be made.

Clinical and therapeutic aspects of cirrhosis

Until the early 19th century, the treatment of cirrhosis and ascites was based on the old concept of humoral pathology, and consisted of bleeding and application of leeches, believed to have a detoxifying effect, purgation and enemas based on Hippocrates' assumption that ascites could be removed via the intestinal veins, paracentesis and diuretics, often with harmful effects (Schaffner & Sieratzki, 1987).

The 20th century has seen an explosion of knowledge on the pathophysiology of portal hypertension and treatment of its complications, on liver function tests and search for means of monitoring of fibrosis; on techniques for imaging of the liver; on the pathophysiology and treatment of ascites and hepatic encephalopathy (Boyer & Bianchi, 1987) and on the relationship between cirrhosis and hepatocellular carcinoma. Most of what we know today has been discovered in the last few decades.

However, aside from prevention by hygiene and vaccination, no therapeutic approach to the underlying disease short of liver transplantation is available, and as the 20th century draws to a close, the answers seem to be still distant (Schaffner & Sieratzki, 1987).

FROM NOW TO THE FUTURE

Progress in basic and applied hepatology during the last two decades has brought an intense realization of the complexity of liver biology.

The transition of a normal liver into cirrhosis appears to involve an incredibly complex network of interactions between the diverse cell types constituting the normal liver, their surrounding biomatrix or ectoskeleton (Bissell, 1990), and cells of "inflammatory" type recruited into the changing organ (Popper & Martin, 1982; Popper & Acs, 1985).

The three old themes of cirrhotic morphogenesis (parenchymal damage, fibroplasia and parenchymal regeneration) (Rössle, 1930) are studied nowadays at higher levels of sophistication.

The mechanisms of parenchymal cell damage and necrosis are analysed at the level of organelles, intracellular signal systems and molecules (Popper, 1988; Popper & Keppler, 1986).

Inflammation is seen as an intricated network of mediators, effector cells and target cells, in which the epithelial parenchymal cells no longer remain the passive victims, but appear actively involved in strategies of immunomodulation (Volpes et al., 1990; Volpes et al., 1991).

Fibrosis is analyzed in terms of detailed biomatrix components, with due attention to new molecules like undulin (Schuppan et al., 1991), tenascin (Van Eyken et al., 1990) and elastin (Porto et al., 1990); in terms of cells involved in synthesis and breakdown of connective tissue constituents, with perisinusoidal cells (or Ito cells) as prime performers (Clement et al., 1986; Friedman, 1990; Gressner & Bachem, 1990), and in terms of signal molecules which modulate the complex cellular interactions in fibrosis, with transforming growth factor b emerging as a key director (Nakatsukasa et al., 1990).

Regeneration of parenchymal cells is analyzed in studies of hormones, growth factors (EGF, IGF) and protooncogenes (Fausto & Mead, 1989; Michalopoulos, 1990), with recent findings of new stimulators (Noji et al., 1990; Nagasaki & Lieberman, 1991) and inhibitors (TGFb) (Carr et al., 1986) of hepatocellular growth.

Because of the complexity of the interactions and their role in regulating liver cell function and structure, a new approach to the study of chronic liver disease is needed as proposed by Rojkind (Rojkind, 1987; Rojkind & Greenwel, 1988).

The liver should be considered as a small ecosystem within a greater universe composed of many ecosystems. Each ecosystem has its own homeostatic mechanisms; however, it is under the surveillance and control of the other ecosystems.

Accordingly, when one ecosystem fails, the others suffer functional modifications (Rojkind, 1987; Rojkind & Greenwel, 1988).

The hepatic ecosystem is a balanced, homeostatic, dynamic equilibrium of interactions between hepatocytes, bile duct cells, the diverse sinusoidal lining cells and the surrounding biomatrix.

A disturbance at one point in the network, especially if the trigger is chronic or repetitive, may lead to consequences with amplifying effect.

The cell-cell and cell-matrix interactions are governed by humoral and nervous factors, but also by local (autocrine and paracrine) effects, realized through cytokines and their specific receptors.

This symposium will review the latest advances in such mechanisms : the mediators of liver cell injury and the network of interacting key events (NIKE) involved in cell death (Popper & Keppler, 1986); the basic mechanisms of inflammation; the triggers, mechanisms and kinetics of fibrogenesis and fibrolysis, with the monokines (Tumor Necrosis Factor alpha; Interleukin-1) and cytokines (especially Transforming Growth Factor beta) involved; and the regulatory signals in regeneration of liver cells and growth of neoplastic cells.

The future will bring a bewildering wealth of information on the detailed steps of cellular actions, interactions and reactions : identification of signal molecules and their receptors, cloning of their genes and identification of their normal and altered activation, resulting in synthesis of lymphokines, monokines and cytokines, receptors and adhaesion molecules; and study of the role of oncogenes and growth factors in normal and neoplastic growth of cells.

The new approach to biology and pathobiology may necessitate a new philosophy of science : the introduction of deterministic chaos and chaotic attractors, since phenomena become so complex that there is no a priori rational way to determine their laws (Zajicek, 1991).

REFERENCES

Anthony, P.P., Ishak, K.G., Nayak, N.C., Poulsen, H., Scheuer, P.J. & Sobin, L.H. (1977): The morphology of cirrhosis: definition, nomenclature and classification. *Bull. WHO* 55, 521-540.

Bianchi, L., De Groote, J., Desmet, V.J., Gedigk, P., Korb, G., Popper, H., Poulsen, H., Scheuer, P.J., Schmid, M., Thaler, H. & Wepler, W. (1971): Morphological criteria in viral hepatitis. *Lancet* i, 333-337.

Bissell, D.M. (1990): Foreword. Connective tissue metabolism and hepatic fibrosis: an overview. *Semin. Liver Dis.* 10, iii-iv.

Boyer, J.L. & Bianchi, L. Editors (1987): Liver Cirrhosis. Lancaster: MTP Press Limited.

Carr, B.I., Hayashi, I., Branum, E.L. & Moses, H.L. (1986): Inhibition of DNA synthesis in rat hepatocytes by platelet-derived b transforming growth factor. *Cancer Res.* 46, 2330-2334.

Charcot, J.M. & Gombault, A. (1876): Contributions à l'étude des différentes formes de la cirrhose du foie. *Arch. Physiol. Norm. Pathol.* 2, Serie 3, 453-489.

Clement, B., Grimaud, J.-A., Campion, J.-P., Deugnier, Y. & Guillouzo, A. (1986): Cell types involved in collagen and fibronectin production in normal and fibrotic human liver. *Hepatology* 6, 225-234.

Desmet, V.J. (1985): New aspects of piecemeal necrosis. In *Trends in hepatology*, ed. L. Bianchi, W. Gerok & H. Popper, pp. 183-200. Lancaster: MTP Press Limited.

Desmet, V.J. (1990): Liver reaction patterns in infections. In *Infectious diseases of the liver*, ed. L. Bianchi, W. Gerok, K.-P. Maier & F. Deinhardt, pp. 31-47. Dordrecht: Kluwer Academic Publishers.

Desmet, V.J. (1991): Immunopathology of chronic viral hepatitis. *Hepatogastroenterology* 38, 14-21.

Desmet, V.J., Sciot, R. & Van Eyken, P. (1990): Differential diagnosis and prognosis of cirrhosis: role of liver biopsy. *Acta Gastroenterol. Belg.* 53, 198, 208.

Desoil, P. (1897): La cirrhose alcoolique graisseuse du foie. *Bull. Méd. du Nord*, Lille, sér. 2, tI, pg. 34.

Fausto, N. & Mead, J.E. (1989): Biology of disease. Regulation of liver growth: proto-oncogenes and transforming growth factor. *Lab. Invest.* 60, 4-13.

Friedman, S.L. (1990): Cellular sources of collagen and regulation of collagen production in liver. *Semin. Liver Dis.* 10, 20-29.

Gressner, A.M. & Bachem, M.G. (1990): Cellular sources of noncollagenous matrix proteins: role of fat-storing cells in fibrogenesis. *Semin. Liver Dis.* 10,30-46.

Hanot, V. (1876): Etude sur une forme de cirrhose hypertrophique du foie. Paris: Baillière.

Laënnec, R.T.H. (1837): Traité de l'Auscultation Mediate, et des Maladies des Poumons et du Coeur. 4th Edition, Vol. 2, Sect. 5, Observation 37, pg. 501. Paris: Chaude.

Michalopoulos, G.K. (1990): Liver regeneration: molecular mechanisms of growth control. *FASEB J.* 4, 176-187.

Moon, V.H. (1932): Histogenesis of atrophic cirrhosis. *Arch. Pathol.* 13, 691-706.

Morgagni, G.B. (1761): De sedibus et causis morborum per anatomen indagatis. *Venetus* epist. XXXVI, XXXVII, XXXVIII.

Nagasaki, T. & Lieberman, M.A. (1991): Liver contains heparin-binding growth factors as the major growth factor for cultured fibroblasts. *Hepatology* 13, 6-14.

Nakatsukasa, H., Nagy, P., Evarts, R.P., Hsia, C.-C., Marsden, E. & Thorgeirsson, S.S. (1990): Cellular distribution of transforming growth factor-b_1 and procollagen types I, III, and IV transcripts in carbon tetrachloride-induced rat liver fibrosis. *J. Clin. Invest.*, 85, 1833-1843.

Noji, S., Tashiro, K., Koyama, E., Nohno, T., Ohyama, K., Taniguchi, S. & Nakamura, T. (1990): Expression of hepatocyte growth factor gene in endothelial and Kupffer cells of damaged rat livers, as revealed by in situ hybridization. *Biochem. Biophys. Res. Commun.* 173, 42-47.

Popper, H. (1982): Summary of the conference. In *Connective tissue of the normal and fibrotic human liver*, ed. U. Gerlach, G. Pott, J. Rauterberg & B. Voss, pp. 246-258. Stuttgart: Georg Thieme Verlag.

Popper, H. (1988): Hepatocellular degeneration and death. In *The Liver; Biology and Pathobiology*, 2nd Ed, ed. I.M. Arias, W.B. Jakoby, H. Popper, D. Schachter & D.A. Shafritz, pp. 1087-1103. New York: Raven Press.

Popper, H. & Acs, G. (1985): Regulatory factors in pathologic processes of the liver. Modulators and interacting metabolic networks. *Semin. Liver Dis.* 5, 191-207.

Popper, H. & Keppler, D. (1986): Networks of interacting mechanisms of hepatocellular degeneration and death. In *Progress in Liver Diseases*, Vol. VIII, ed. H. Popper & F. Schaffner, pp. 209-235. Orlando: Grune & Stratton.

Popper, H. & Martin, G.R. (1982): Fibrosis of the liver: the role of the ectoskeleton. In *Progress in Liver Diseases*, Vol. VII, ed. H. Popper & F. Schaffner, pp. 133-156. New York: Grune & Stratton.

Popper, H. & Schaffner, F. (1957): Liver: Structure and function. New York: McGraw-Hill Book Company.

Popper, H., Elias, H. & Petty, D.E. (1952): Vascular patterns of the cirrhotic liver. *Am. J. Clin. Pathol.* 22, 717-729.

Porto, L.C., Chevallier, M., Guerret, S., Hartmann, D.J. & Grimaud, J.-A. (1990): Elastin in alcoholic liver disease. An immunohistochemical and immunoelectron microscopic study. *Pathol. Res. Pract.* 186, 668-679.

Rappaport, A.M., McPhee, P.J., Fisher, M.M. & Phillips, M.J. (1983): The scarring of the liver acini (cirrhosis). Tridimensional and microcirculatory considerations. *Virchows Arch. [A]* 402, 107-137.

Report of the Board of Classification and Nomenclature of Cirrhosis of the Liver (1956): 5th Pan-American Congress of Gastroenterology. *Gastroenterology* 31, 213-216.

Rojkind, M. (1987): Homeostasis of cells and connective tissue matrix in normal and cirrhotic liver. In *Liver cirrhosis*, ed. J.L. Boyer& L.Bianchi, pp. 39-45. Lancaster: MTP Press Limited.

Rojkind, M. & Greenwel, P. (1988): The liver as a bioecological system. In *The Liver; Biology and Pathobiology*, 2nd Ed., ed. I.M. Arias, W.B. Jakoby, H. Popper, D. Schachter & D.A. Shafritz, pp. 1269-1285. New York: Raven Press.

Rössle, R. (1930): Entzündungen der Leber. In: *Handbuch der speziellen pathologischen Anatomie und Histologie*, Vol. V, Part 1, ed. F. Henke & O. Lubarsch, pp. 243-505. Berlin: Julius Springer.

Savolainen, E.R., Leo, M.-A., Timpl, R. & Lieber, C.S. (1984): Acetaldehyde and lactate stimulate collagen synthesis of cultured baboon liver myofibroblasts. *Gastroenterology* 87, 777-787.

Schaffner, F. & Sieratzki, J.S. (1987): The early history of cirrhosis. In *Liver Cirrhosis*, ed. J.L. Boyer & L. Bianchi, pp. 57-72. Lancaster: MTP Press Limited.

Schuppan, D., Just, M. & Riecken, E.O. (1991): Der Verlust Undulins und sein Ersatz durch Tenaszin im interstitiellen Bindegewebe demarkiert Zonen des (irreversiblen) Umbaus bei der progredienten Leberfibrose. *Z. Gastroenterol.* 28, 722.

Sciot, R., Staessen, D., Van Damme, B., Van Steenbergen, W., Fevery, J., De Groote, J. & Desmet, V.J. (1988): Incomplete septal cirrhosis: histopathological aspects. *Histopathology* 13, 593-603.

Smetana, H. (1956): Histogenesis of coarse nodular cirrhosis. *Lab. Invest.* 5, 175-193.

Takahashi, T. (1978): Three-dimensional morphology of the liver in cirrhosis and related disorders. *Virchows Arch. [A]* 377, 97-110.

Tsukamoto, H., Matsuoka, M. & French, S.W. (1990): Experimental models of hepatic fibrosis: a review. *Semin. Liver Dis.* 10, 56-65.

Van Eyken, P., Sciot, R. & Desmet, V.J. (1990): Expression of the novel extracellular matrix component tenascin in normal and diseased human liver. An immunohistochemical study. *J. Hepatol.* 11, 43-52.

Virchow, R. (1858): Cellular Pathologie in ihrer Begründung auf Physiologie und pathologische Gewebslehre. Berlin: Hirschwald.

Volpes, R., Van den Oord, J.J. & Desmet, V.J. (1990): Immunohistochemical study of adhesion molecules in liver inflammation. *Hepatology* 12, 59-65.

Volpes, R., Van den Oord, J.J., De Vos, R., De Pla, E., De Ley, M. & Desmet, V.J. (1991): Expression of interferon-y receptor in normal and pathological human liver tissue. *J. Hepatol.* 12, 195-202.

Wanless, I.R. (1990): Micronodular transformation (nodular regenerative hyperplasia) of the liver: a report of 64 cases among 2.500 autopsies and a new classification of benign hepatocellular nodules. *Hepatology* 11, 787-797.

Yamamoto, T., Kobayashi, T. & Phillips, M.J. (1984): Perinodular arteriolar plexus in liver cirrhosis. Scanning electron microscopy of microvascular casts. *Liver* 4, 50-54.

Zajicek, G. (1991): Chaos and biology. *Methods Inf. Med.* 30, 1-3.

Résumé

Cette introduction passe en revue quelques points saillants dans l'évolution des aspects de la cirrhose hépatique depuis l'antiquité. Durant des siècles, la lenteur du progrès et la rareté de faits prouvés restaient le problème principal.
Connue depuis Hippocrate, la cirrhose hépatique n'a été mieux définie qu'après l'introduction de l'anatomie (Vésale, 16ème siècle) et de la pathologie (Morgagni, 18ème siècle), et a abouti à une diversité troublante de classifications au début de ce siècle.
La plus grande partie de ce que nous savons de la cirrhose provient de l'éclosion de "la science la plus jeune" (L. Thomas) de ce siècle : la reconnaissance de la souffrance hépatocellulaire, la fibrose et la régénération en tant que mécanismes majeurs de la morphogénèse ; la distinction entre la cirrhose et les maladies qui lui ressemblent ; l'identification de plusieurs étiologies ; des progrès dans le diagnostic et le traitement des complications ; et les études des mécanismes de la mort cellulaire, de l'inflammation, de la fibrose et de la régénération.
Les techniques récentes de la biologie moléculaire ont orienté des recherches nouvelles vers les mécanismes de base au niveau cellulaire et moléculaire : l'interaction fascinante entre les différents types de cellules hépatiques qui constituent un écosystème harmonieux à l'intérieur du système plus complexe de l'organisme vivant, et son dysfonctionnement par les maladies.
Aujourd'hui nous sommes confrontés à l'accélération du progrès, la divergence des techniques et l'abondance des informations nouvelles.

Cell damage and inflammation

Altérations cellulaires et inflammation

Cellular and Molecular Aspects of Cirrhosis. Eds B. Clément, A. Guillouzo. Colloque INSERM/John Libbey Eurotext Ltd. © 1992, Vol. 216, pp. 13-23

Chronic metal overload and hepatic damage

Pierre Brissot, Olivier Loréal, Noëlla Hubert, Isabelle Morel, Hervé Jouanolle, Romain Moirand, Dominique Guyader, Gérard Lescoat and Yves Deugnier

Clinique des Maladies du Foie and INSERM U 49, Hôpital Pontchaillou, 35033 Rennes, France

SUMMARY. Chronic excess in iron or copper is a classical etiology of human liver damage, resulting in fibrosis and cirrhosis. Genetic haemochromatosis (GH) and Wilson's disease are, respectively for iron and copper, the most representative disorders . *Hepatic iron toxicity* has been experimentally studied on animals submitted to parenteral (baboon, gerbil) or oral (rat) administration of iron and on iron overloaded hepatocyte cultures. Hepatocyte damage has been demonstrated morphologically by the lesion of sideronecrosis and biochemically by iron-induced lipid peroxidation towards the plasma membrane as well as the membranes of the various intracellular organelles, especially the mitochondria. Non-transferrin-bound iron is increasingly considered as a highly damaging iron species. Particularly prone to produce free radicals, this iron form has been shown , in case of iron overload, not only to remain avidly taken-up by the liver but also to be no longer excreted via the biliary route. Iron-related fibrosis is likely to occur through the role of aldehyde-protein adducts produced by hepatocyte damage. The role of non parenchymal cells, including lipocytes and endothelial cells, especially through cytokine release from kupffer cells, needs to be explored. *Hepatic copper toxicity* has been well documented in animal models developing inherited copper toxicosis such as the Bedlington terrier and the toxic milk mouse. The major cellular target is the hepatocyte with steatosis and mitochondrial damage. An oxidant injury to hepatocyte mitochondria may be one of the initiating factors in hepatocellular damage. Iron and copper overload realize quite separate clinical entities but are close in terms of their cellular targets and biochemical mechanisms of cytotoxicity.

Beside numerous other factors (among which alcohol, infectious - especially viral or parasitic-agents, autoantigens, drugs), chronic metal overload can generate hepatic damage, the main culprits being iron and copper. The present review will essentially focus on iron overload since it represents the most frequent encountered clinical situation.

1. CHRONIC IRON OVERLOAD AND HEPATIC TOXICITY

1.1. Clinical Background (Brissot & Deugnier, 1990).*Genetic Haemochromatosis* (GH) is the most typical situation . Characterized by iron excess, especially of the hepatocytes , it is genetically transmitted as an autosomal recessive trait and principally determined by a gene situated on the short arm of the sixth chromosome very close to the A locus of HLA system. Iron overload is certainly related to intestinal hyperabsorption of iron , but an associated increase of hepatic avidity for iron remains a possibility. The primary location for the expression of the genetic defect is not yet established in terms of organs (i.e intestine and/or the liver) as well of cellular type (parenchymal versus macrophagic cells). Likewise, the nature of the basic metabolic defect (i.e. the protein abnormality) making the link between the abnormal gene and the development of iron overload remains to be determined. A number of protein candidates (transferrin, transferrin receptor, L-ferritin, IRE-binding protein) appear to-day unlikely since their respective genes are not located on chromosome 6. No molecular biology data have provided arguments for the involvement of H-ferritin, despite the fact that some of its genes are situated on chromosome 6. The main candidates might be the ferritin receptor or mostly a protein abnormality resulting in excessive concentration and/or role of non-transferrin-bound iron Stremmel & al., 1991). Whatever the pathogenesis of iron overload, hepatic toxicity is a prominent feature of this disease. Clinically, the liver may be considerably enlarged. Biochemically, toxicity is only slightly expressed by an increase in serum aminotransferases which is usually less than two fold the upper normal limit. Pathologically, two types of lesions can develop (Deugnier & al. ,in press): sideronecrosis defined as eosinophilic or cytolytic necrosis of iron-loaded hepatocytes, and fibrosis (or cirrhosis). *Secondary iron overload* is mainly represented by iron-loading anaemias, either congenital such as thalassaemias major and at a lesser degree intermedia or acquired (acquired refractory sideroblastic anaemia, hypoplastic or myeloplastic disorders). Under these conditions, iron accumulation is related a) mainly to transfusions (e.g. aplastic anaemias), b) to increased iron absorption due to enhanced erythroid activity (thalassaemia intermedia) or c) to both mechanisms (thalassaemia major or sideroblastic anaemia). The excess absorbed iron is mainly deposited in the parenchymal sites in a similar fashion to GH. Transfused iron is initially deposited within macrophages in the mononuclear phagocytic system, but subsequently iron redistribution occurs, leading to parenchymal deposition and damage so that, eventually, the pattern of organ involvement resembles that encountered in GH (Schafer & al., 1981).

1.2. Experimental Models . Globally, experimental models reproducing the hepatic damage of iron overload proved difficult to be obtained. Interesting data have, however, been obtained both in vivo and in vitro. *In vivo,* three animal models can be mentioned: a) the baboon in which parenteral administration of iron produced a chronic elevation of serum aminotransferases and, in the most heavily loaded animal, a slight fibrosis in areas of massive sinusoidal siderosis (Brissot & al., 1983, 1987); b) the rat fed with carbonyl iron (Bacon & al., 1983). In this model, the distribution pattern of iron resembles that of GH (with predominant periportal and hepatocellular distribution) and, by 8 months of iron overloading, periportal fibrous tissue was present which became more pronounced at twelve months (Park & al., 1987); however, this fibrogenic effect seems inconstant (Iancu & al., 1987) and in no case cirrhosis was produced. c) the gerbil has been recently (Carthew & al., 1991) proposed as a promising model since, submitted to parenteral administration of iron-dextran complex, it developed fibrosis after 6 weeks and cirrhosis after 12. *In vitro* , primary cultures of iron overloaded liver cells represent also important experimental tools (Desvergne & al., 1989; Morel & al., 1990).

1.3. Cellular Targets for Iron Toxicity. *Iron-related hepatocyte damage* is illustrated , in the clinical situation of GH, by the recently characterized features of sideronecrosis. Deugnier & al.(in press), studying 135 patients with homozygous genetic haemochromatosis, reported that sideronecrosis was absent in moderate iron overload (liver iron concentration < 150 µmol/g dry liver weight ; N<36) and present in increasing proportion from important to massive haemochromatosis, being scarse and localized mainly in zone 1, often in the vicinity of iron-loaded macrophages. Sideronecrosis was found only in patients with a hepatocytic iron score superior to 17 (maximum theoretical score for this original grading: 36). It was associated with a slight but highly significant increase of AST and ALT. Extensive fibrosis or cirrhosis was present in 88 per cent of patients with sideronecrosis versus 31 per cent of patients without sideronecrosis (X2-p=10-3). Experimentally, using adult rat hepatocyte pure cultures supplemented with ferric nitrilotriacetate (Fe-NTA), Morel & al. (1990) observed a higher LDH, AST and ALT release into the culture medium than in the controls supplemented or not with NTA; moreover the extracellular leakage was well correlated with the intracellular enzyme decrease, especially for LDH and ALT. *The membrane* represents the major target of iron toxicity. This damaging effect affects the plasma membrane as well as the membranes of the various intrahepatocytic organelles. Iron-induced lipid peroxidation represents the main mechanism accounting for the membrane damage. This mechanism, already suggested by Golberg & al.(1962) in mice and rats injected with an iron-dextran complex, has been confirmed and precised by numerous investigators especially following the data obtained in the rats overloaded by Fe-NTA or carbonyl iron (Bacon & al., 1983). The following recent studies may serve to illustrate this iron-catalyzed lipid peroxidation: a) Using adult rat hepatocyte cultures supplemented with Fe-NTA, lipid peroxidation was evaluated by free malondialdehyde (MDA) using size exclusion chromatography (HPLC) as a specific and sensitive method (Morel & al., 1990). The ferric iron exhibited a prooxidant activity corresponding to an increase of free MDA recovery in the cells and in the culture medium . b) Levels of MDA in hepatocytes isolated from rats fed with carbonyl iron increased significantly after 21 days on the diet as compared with the controls (Fletcher & al., 1989). c) Using, in carbonyl iron fed rats, an antiserum specific for MDA-lysine protein adducts, Houglum & al.(1990) demonstrated by immunochemistry the presence of aldehyde-protein adducts in the cytosol of periportal hepatocytes, which colocalized with iron overload. These data provide strong evidence for the occurrence of iron-catalyzed lipid peroxidation in vivo. As to the intrahepatocytic organelles involved in this peroxidative process, mitochondria are a major target whereas microsomes are affected at a lesser degree (Bacon & al;1983). Impairment in mitochondrial oxidative metabolism as well as reduction in cytochrome P-450 could represent functional consequences of these organelle injuries (Bacon & Britton, 1990). Peroxidative injury might also be implicated in the increased lysosomal fragility reported in haemosiderin-laden lysosomes isolated from iron-loaded liver biopsies (Peters & al., 1986 ; Mak & Weglicki, 1985 ; Myers & al, 1991). This lysosomal fragility, which regresses with iron removal by phlebotomy, could result in hydrolytic enzyme leakage into the cytosol.

1.4. Nature of the Toxic Iron. *Transferrin iron* is ineffective in stimulating lipid peroxidation. The following forms could be candidates for toxicity: a) *Haemosiderin iron*: a correlation has been found between its concentration and enzymatic markers of lysosomal fragility (Peters & al; 1986). b) *Ferritin iron*: devoid of toxicity while stored within the protein core, iron- once released- may promote superoxide dependent lipid peroxidation (Thomas & al., 1985). c) *Cytosolic low-molecular-weight iron*: Ultrafiltrates from hepatic cytosol of carbonyl iron-loaded rats had greater prooxidant action, as reflected by MDA production, than did those from controls. These data support the view that iron overload results in an increase in a hepatic cytosolic pool of low-molecular-weight iron that is catalytically active in stimulating lipid peroxidation (Britton & al;, 1990). d) *Non-transferrin-bound iron (NTBI).* This iron species is increasingly considered as a major damaging form. NTBI, which is often found in the serum of haemochromatotic patients, may represent complexes of iron ions with low-molecular weight organic ligands (especially with citrate and acetate, Grootveld & al., 1989); other ligands such as carboxylated groups of albumin could also be involved (Singh & Hider, 1988). NTBI has been shown , in the isolated perfused rat liver, to be avidly taken-up by the liver (single-pass extraction 58-75 per cent versus <1 per cent for transferrin iron) (Brissot & al., 1985), without down-regulation of this hepatic uptake in case of iron-overloaded liver (Wright & al., 1986). Similar results were obtained using hypotransferrinemic mice (Craven & al., 1987). Moreover, recent results in the intact rat have shown that biliary excretion of plasma NTBI, which was a significant excretory pathway in normal animals, became negligible in chronically iron overloaded rats (Brissot & al., 1991). Collectively, these findings support the concept that , in chronic iron overload, non-transferrin-bound iron may present the liver with an obligatory iron load due not only to enhanced hepatic uptake, but also to absence of biliary excretion. Therefore, taking into account the high propensity of NTBI to stimulate the formation of hydroxyl radicals and lipid peroxidation (Gutteridge & al., 1985), this iron species may play an important harmful role towards the liver. Several possibilities exist concerning the ultimate oxidizing species responsible for initiation of lipid peroxidation in *in vivo* iron overload (Britton & al., 1990; Bacon & Britton, 1990; Tavill & Bacon, 1986): the classical mechanism involves the intermediate formation of oxygen free radical species such as the hydroxyl radical (.OH) produced either by the Fenton reaction, or by the Haber-Weiss reaction or both. Alternatively, a) Minotti & Aust (1986) have proposed that the initiation of lipid peroxidation is linked to hydrogen peroxide-mediated oxidation of iron and requires both reduced and oxidized forms of iron. b) Ferric iron could generate ferryl or perferryl radicals capable of attacking polyunsaturated fatty acids directly (Halliwell & Gutteridge, 1984). c) Iron can also react with preformed lipid hydroxyperoxides to yield lipid alkoxyl or peroxyl radicals, which in turn could initiate the peroxidation of neighbouring lipids, therefore propagating the reaction.

1.5. Mechanism of Fibrosis. The mechanism(s) whereby iron produces fibrosis remain(s) undefined. a) A direct and specific stimulating effect of iron (Fe-NTA) on *hepatocyte alpha-1-collagen 1 and bêta-1-laminin mRNAs* could not be found using primary cultures of adult rat hepatocytes (Loréal & Loyer, unpublished). However, in carbonyl iron fed rats (where hepatocytes are early and predominantly interested by iron deposition) Pietrangelo & al. (1990) reported a prompt activation of pro-alpha2(I)-collagen gene. b) The role of non specific *hepatocyte damage* itself is a likely possibility. On the basis that the highly reactive aldehydes that form as products of lipid peroxidation stimulate collagen gene expression in cultured fibroblasts (Brenner & Chojkier, 1987; Chojkier & al., 1989), Houglum & al. (1990) have proposed that lipid peroxidation could be a link between tissue injury and tissue fibrogenesis. c) Another attractive mechanism could involve *non parenchymal cells* and the role of lipocytes and endothelial cells, especially through the release of cytokines from other cells e.g. Kupffer cells, needs to be explored. Whatever the intimate mechanisms of iron-related fibrosis, iron per se is probably only slightly fibrogenic. This is particularly illustrated by: a) Experimentally, the major difficulties to find an adequate animal model for iron-related fibrosis; b) Clinically, the high "fibrogenic threshold" for liver iron concentration, estimated at 400 (Bassett & al., 1986) or even 500 (Loréal & al. submitted) µmol/g dry liver weight. It appears therefore possible that, in clinical situation, to become markedly fibrogenic, iron needs, besides high level and long duration of overload, cofactors such as alcoholism or viral infection.

2. CHRONIC COPPER OVERLOAD AND HEPATIC TOXICITY.

2.1. Clinical Background (Sternlieb, 1980; Sternlieb, 1990; Gollan, 1990). Wilson's Disease (Hepatolenticular Degeneration) is the most characteristic human copper overload syndrome. It is transmitted in an autosomal recessive fashion and is due to a gene located on chromosome 13 (Frydman & al., 1985; Bowcock & al., 1988). Copper overload is not caused by intestinal hyperabsorption of copper but by impairment of biliary excretion of the metal. It is likely that a hepatic lysosomal defect interfering with the excretion of copper from lysosomes to bile underlies the accumulation of hepatic copper. The primary defect does not appear to be directly related to ceruloplasmin (the gene for this protein is located on chromosome 13). The liver which is the site of the inherited metabolic defect is also the organ most frequently injured by the excessive tissue concentrations of copper. Hepatic manifestations can correspond to chronic active hepatitis, cirrhosis or fulminant hepatic failure. Other clinical conditions where copper can accumulate in the liver are represented by *chronic cholestatic syndromes* , either of intrahepatic (e.g. primary biliary cirrhosis) or extrahepatic origin. In cholestasis, copper excess is due to the fact that , normally, the biliary route is the major pathway for copper excretion.

2.2. Experimental Models. *In vivo*, two animal models are of special interest since they develop recessively inherited hepatic copper toxicosis : the Bedlington terrier (Twedt & al., 1979; Su & al., 1982), particularly interesting because a defect in biliary copper excretion accounts, like in Wilson's disease , for copper overload; the toxic milk mouse (Biempica & al., 1988) exhibits less hepatic morphologic similarities to Wilson's disease than the canine model and the defect leading to copper excess is unknown. Chronic dietary copper overload in the rat is of more questionable interest since excessive intake, and not defective biliary excretion , is responsible for copper accumulation. Chronic intraperitoneal administration of cupric nitrilotriacetate produced, in all rats surviving over 16 weeks extensive liver fibrosis or micronodular cirrhosis (Toyokuni & al, 1989). *In vitro*, isolated rat hepatocytes exposed to cupric chloride have been used (Sokol & al;, 1989).

2.3. Cellular Targets. Copper damages the *hepatocyte*. Evidence for this deleterious effect is provided by the conspicuous morphologic abnormalities of hepatocytes observed in Wilson's disease (Sternlieb, 1980). Early abnormalities consist of steatosis and ballooned glycogen nuclei. Mitochondria become markedly pleomorphic with large vacuoles containing granular material. Peroxisomes may be enlarged with flocculent matrices. Mallory's cytoplasmic hyalin may be found. The mechanisms by which excess copper results in hepatocyte toxicity have not been fully established. There is , however, growing evidence that *membrane lipid peroxidation* may be involved (Sokol & al.,1990). In copper fed rats, Dillard & Tappel (1984) have shown increased production of pentane and hepatic MDA. Generation of thiobarbituric acid-reactive substances have been reported by Sokol & al. (1989) in isolated rat hepatocytes exposed to cupric chloride. Recently, using a dietary model of chronic hepatic copper overload in the rat, Sokol & al. (1990) demonstrated significant peroxidation of mitochondrial lipids in the absence of microsomal lipid peroxidation, suggesting that the mitochondria may be a specific target organelle of copper hepatotoxicity. This copper-induced lipid peroxidation may in fact require iron as an intermediary factor. Beckman & al (1988) have provided data suggesting that the primary role of copper in the potentiation of iron-induced peroxidation is to provide enough reduced iron (and an optimal Fe^{2+}/ Fe^{3+} ratio) for initiation reactions to proceed. The mechanisms whereby copper is fibrogenic await more studies. It is, however, likely that, like for iron, a link exists between lipid peroxidation and fibrogenesis.

In conclusion, human genetic chronic overloads in iron and copper correspond to quite separate clinical entities. Marked similarities, however, exist between these metals concerning their hepatocellular targets as well as the biochemical mechanisms involved in their cytotoxicity.

REFERENCES

Bacon, B.R. & Britton, R.S. (1990): The pathology of hepatic iron overload : a free radical-mediated process? *Hepatology* 11, 127-137.

Bacon, B.R., Tavill, A.S., Brittenham, G.M., Park, C.H & Recknagel, R.O. (1983) : Hepatic lipid peroxidation in vivo in rats with chronic iron overload. *J. Clin. Invest.* 71, 429-439.

Bassett, M.L., Halliday, J.W. & Powell L.W. (1986) : Value of hepatic iron measurements in early hemochromatosis and determination of the critical iron level associated with fibrosis.Hepatology 6, 24-29.

Beckman, J.K., Borowitz, S.M., Greene, H.L. & Burr, I.M. (1988): Promotion of iron-induced rat liver microsomal lipid peroxidation by copper. *Lipids* 23, 559-563.

Biempica, L., Rauch, H., Quintana, N. & Sternlieb,I. (1988) : Morphologic and hepatic copper toxicosis. *Lab.Invest.* 59, 500-508.

Bowcock, A.M., Farrer, L.A., Hebert, J.M., Agger, M., Sternlieb, I., Scheinberg, H., Buys, C.H.C.M., Scheffer, H., Frydman, M., Chajek-Saul, T., Bonne- Tamir, B. & Cavalli-Sforza, L.L. (1988) : Eight closely linked loci place the Wilson disease locus within I3qI4-q21. *Am. J.Hum..Genet.* 43, 664-674.

Brenner, D.A. & Chojkier, M. (1987): Acetaldehyde increases collagen gene transcription in cultured human fibroblasts. *J. Biol. Chem.* 262, 17690-17695.

Brissot, P., Campion, J.P., Guillouzo, A., Allain, H., Messner, M., Simon, M., Ferrand, B. & Bourel, M. (1983) : Experimental hepatic iron overload in the baboon: results of a two- year study. Evolution of biological and morphologic hepatic parameters of iron overload. *Dig. Dis. Sci* 28, 616- 624.

Brissot, P. & Deugnier Y.(in press): Genetic Haemochromatosis. In *Oxford Textbook of Clinical Hepatology*, ed. N. McIntyre, J. Bircher, M. Rizzetto & J. Rodes Oxford: Oxford University Press.

Brissot, P., Farjanel, J., Bourel D., Campion, J.P., Guillouzo, A., Rattner, A., Deugnier, Y., Desvergne, B., Ferrand, B., Simon, M. & Bourel, M. (1987) : Chronic liver iron overload in the baboon by ferric nitrilotriacetate. Morphologic and functional changes with special reference to collagen synthesis enzymes. *Dig. Dis. Sci.*, 32, 620-627.

Brissot, P., Wright, T.L., Ma, W.L. & Weisiger, R.A. (1985): Efficient clearance of non-transferrin-bound iron by rat liver. Implications for hepatic iron loading in iron overload states. *J. Clin. Invest.* 76, 1463-1470.

Brissot, P., Zanninelli, G., Zeind, J. & Gollan, J. (1990): Biliary excretion of plasma-non-transferrin bound iron : a significant excretory pathway in normal but not in chronically iron overloaded rats. *Gastroenterology* 100, 724 A.

Britton, R.S., Ferrali, M., Magiera, C.J., Recknagel, R.O. & Bacon, B.R. (1990) : Increased prooxidant action of hepatic cytosolic low-molecular- weight iron in experimental iron overload. *Hepatology* 11, 1038- 1043.

Carthew, P., Edwards, R.E., Smith, A.G., Dorman, B.,& Francis, J.E. (1991) : Rapid induction of hepatic fibrosis in the gerbil after the parenteral administration of iron-dextran complex. *Hepatology* 13, 534-539.

Chojkier, M., Houglum, K., Solis-Herruzo, J. & Brenner, D.A. (1989) : Stimulation of collagen gene expression by ascorbic acid in cultured human fibroblasts. *J. Biol. Chem.* 264, 16957-16962.

Craven, C.M., Alexander, J., Eldridge, M., Kushner, J.P., Bernstein, S. & Kaplan, J. (1987) : Tissue distribution and clearance kinetics of non- transferrin-bound iron in the hypotransferrinemic mouse: a rodent model for hemochromatosis. *Proc. Natl. Acad. Sci. USA* 84, 3457-3461.

Desvergne, B., Baffet, G., Loyer, P., Rissel, M., Lescoat, G., Guguen-Guillouzo, C. & Brissot, P. (1989) : Chronic iron overload inhibits protein secretion by adult rat hepatocytes maintained in long-term primary culture. *Eur. J. Cell. Biol.* 49, 162-170.

Deugnier, Y., Loréal, Y., Turlin, B., Guyader, D., Jouanolle, H., Moirand, R., Jacquelinet, C. & Brissot, P. (in press): Liver pathology in genetic hemochromatosis : a review of 135 homozygous cases and their bio-clinical correlations. *Gastroenterology.*

Dillard, C.J. & Tappel, A.L. (1984): Lipid peroxidation and copper toxicity in rats. *Drug Chem. Toxicol.* 7, 477-487.

Fletcher, L.M., Roberts, F.D., Irving, M.G., Powell, L.W. & Halliday, J.W. (1989) : Effects of iron loading on free radical scavenging enzymes and lipid peroxidation in rat liver. *Gastroenterology* 97, 1011-1018.

Frydman, M., Bonné-Tamir, B., Farrer, L.A., Conneally, P.M., Magazanik, A., Ashbel, S. & Goldwitch, Z. (1985) : Assignment of the gene for Wilson disease to chromosome 13: linkage to the esterase D locus. *Proc. Natl. Acad. Sci. USA* 82, 1819-1821.

Golberg, L., Martin, L.E. & Batchelor, A. (1962): Biochemical changes in the tissues of animals injected with iron. *Biochem. J.* 83, 291-298.

Gollan, J.L. (1990): Copper metabolism, Wilson's disease, and hepatic copper toxicosis. In *Hepatology. A textbook of liver disease*, ed. D. Zakim & T.Boyer, vol.1, pp. 1249-1272.Philadelphia: W.B. Saunders Company.

Grootveld, M., Bell, J.D., Halliwell, B., Aruoma, O.I., Bomford, A. & Sadler, P.J.(1989) : Non-transferrin-bound iron in plasma or serum from patients with idiopathic hemochromatosis. Characterization by high performance liquid chromatography and nuclear magnetic resonance spectroscopy. *J. Biol. Chem.* 264, 4417-4422.

Gutteridge, J.M.C., Rowley, D.A., Griffiths, E. & Halliwell, B. (1985) : Low-molecular-weight complexes and oxygen radical reactions in idiopathic haemochromatosis. *Clin. Sci.* 68, 463-467.

Halliwell, B. & Gutteridge, J.M.C. (1984): Oxygen toxicity, oxygen radicals, transition metals and disease. *Biochem. J.* 219, 1-14.

Houglum, K., Filip, M., Witztum, J.L. & Chojkier, M. (1990) : Malondialdehyde and 4-hydroxynonenal protein adducts in plasma and liver of rats with iron overload. *J. Clin. Invest.* 86, 1991-1998.

Iancu, T., Ward, R.J. & Peters, T.J. (1987): Ultrastructural observations in the carbonyl iron-fed rat, an animal model for hemochromatosis. *Virchows Arch B(Cell Pathol.)* 53, 208-217.

Mak, I.T. & Weglicki, W.B. (1985): Characterization of iron-mediated peroxidative injury in isolated hepatic lysosomes. J. Clin. Invest. 75, 58-63.

Minotti, G. & Aust, S.D. (1987) : The requirement for iron III in the initiation of lipid peroxidation by iron II and hydrogen peroxide. *J. Biol. Chem.* 262, 1098-1104.

Morel, I., Lescoat, G., Cillard, J., Pasdeloup, N., Brissot, P. & Cillard, P. (1990) : Kinetic evaluation of free malondialdehyde and enzyme leakage as indices of iron damage in rat hepatocyte cultures. Involvement of free radicals. *Biochem.Pharmacol.* 39, 1647-1645.

Myers, B.M., Prendergast, F.G., Holman, R., Kuntz, S.M. & La Russo, N. (1991) : Alterations in the structure, physicochemical properties and pH of hepatocyte lysosomes in experimental iron overload. *J. Clin. Invest.* 88, 1207-1215.

Park, C.H., Bacon, B.R., Brittenham, G.M. & Tavill, A.S. (1987) : Pathology of dietary carbonyl iron overload in rats. *Lab. Invest.* 57, 555-563.

Peters, T.J., O'Connell, M.J. & Ward, R.J. (1986): Role of free-radical mediated lipid peroxidation in the pathogenesis of hepatic damage by lysosomal disruption. In *Free radicals in liver injury*, ed. G. Poli, K.H. Cheeseman, M.U. Dianzani & T.F. Slater, pp. 107-115. Oxford : ITP Press.

Pietrangelo, A., Rocchi, E., Schiaffonati, L., Ventura, E. & Cairo, G. (1990): Liver gene expression during chronic dietary iron overload in rats. *Hepatology* 11, 798-804.

Schafer, A.I., Cheron, R.G., Dluhy, R., Cooper, B., Gleason, R.E., Soeldner, J.S. & Bunnh, F. (1981) : Clinical consequences of acquired transfusional iron overload in adults. *N Engl. J. Med.* 304, 319-324.

Singh, S. & Hider, R.C. (1988): Colorimetric detection of the hydroxyl radical: comparison of the hydroxyl-radical-generating ability of various iron complexes. *Anal. Biochem.* 171, 47-54.

Sokol, R.J., Devereaux, M., Mierau, G.W., Hambidge, K.M. & Shikes, R.H. (1990): Oxidant injury to hepatic mitochondrial lipids in rats with dietary copper overload. Modification by vitamin E. *Gastroenterology.* 99, 1061-1071.

Sokol, R.J., Devereaux, M.W., Traber, M.G. & Shikes, R.H. (1989) : Copper toxicity and lipid peroxidation in isolated rat hepatocytes: effect of vitamin E. *Pediatr. Res.* 25, 55-62.

Sternlieb, I. (1980) : Copper and the liver. *Gastroenterology* 78, 1615-1628.
Sternlieb, I. (1990) : Perspectives on Wilson's disease. *Hepatology* 12, 1234-1239.
Stremmel, W., Teichmann, D., Arweiler, D., Vierbuchen, H.D., Diede, H.D., Niederau, C & Strohmeyer, G. (1991) Iron uptake by enterocytes represents a carrier mediated uptake mechanism: significance of the microvillous membrane iron protein in primary hemochromatosis. Third International Conference on Haemochromatosis. Düsseldorf (July 25-26). Abstract p17.
Su, L.-C., Owen, C.A., Zollman, P.E. & Hardy, R.M. (1982): A defect in biliary excretion of copper in copper-laden Bedlington terriers. *Am. J. Physiol.* 243, G 231-236.
Tavill, A.S & Bacon, R.B. (1986): Hemochromatosis: how much iron is too much? *Hepatology* 6, 142-145.
Thomas, C.E., Morehouse, L.A. & Aust, S.D. (1985): Ferritin and superoxide-dependent lipid peroxidation. *J. Biol. Chem.* 260, 3275-3280.
Toyokuni, S., Okada, S., Hamazaki, S., Fujioka, M., Li, J.L. & Midorikawa, O. (1989) : Cirrhosis of the liver induced by cupric nitrilotriacetate in wistar rats. An experimental model of copper toxicosis. *Am. J. Pathol.* 134, 1263-1274.
Twedt, D.C., Sternlieb, I & Gilbertson, S.R. (1979) : Clinical, morphologic, and chemical studies on copper toxicosis of Bedlington terriers. *J. Am. Vet. Med. Assoc.* 175, 269-275.
Wright, T.L., Brissot, P., Ma, W.L. & Weisiger, R.A. (1986) : Characterization of non-transferrin-bound iron clearance by rat liver. *J. Biol. Chem.* 261, 10909-10914.

Acknowledgements. The authors wish to thank the Association de la Recherche pour le Cancer, the Fondation Langlois, Bull Computers, the Caisse Régionale d'Assurance Maladie de Bretagne and the Conseil Régional de Bretagne for their generous support.

Résumé . La surcharge chronique en fer ou en cuivre constitue une étiologie classique d' hépatopathie fibrotique voire cirrhotique. L'hémochromatose génétique et la maladie de Wilson en sont respectivement les expressions cliniques les plus caractéristiques. *La toxicité hépatique du fer* a été étudiée sur des animaux soumis à une surcharge en fer parentérale (babouin, gerbil) ou orale (rat) ainsi que sur des cultures hépatocytaires surchargées en fer. L'atteinte hépatocytaire a été démontrée morphologiquement par la lésion de sidéronécrose et biochimiquement par une peroxydation lipidique ferro-induite qui s'exerce tant au niveau de la membrane plasmique hépatocytaire qu'à celui des membranes des divers organites intrahépatocytaires, au premier rang desquels les mitochondries. La toxicité du fer non lié à la transferrine est de plus en plus mise en avant. En effet, en cas de surcharge hépatique en fer, cette forme de fer, qui est particulièrement productrice de radicaux libres, voit non seulement se maintenir son haut niveau de captation hépatique mais aussi disparaître son excrétion biliaire. La fibrose hépatique pourrait, au moins en partie, être due à l'effet des dérivés protéiques aldéhydiques produits par la lésion hépatocytaire. Le rôle des cellules non parenchymateuses, notamment lipocytes et cellules endothéliales, sous l'effet des cytokines d'origine kupfférienne mérite d'être étudiée. *La toxicité hépatique du cuivre* a été bien démontrée sur des animaux présentant une surcharge génétique en cuivre tels que le terrier Bedlington ou la "toxic milk mouse". La cible cellulaire privilégiée est l'hépatocyte qui devient stéatosique et développe d'importantes altérations mitochondriales. La peroxidation lipidique des mitochondries pourrait constituer l'un des mécanismes déclenchants de la lésion hépatocytaire.

Il s'avère ainsi qu'en dépit d'expressions cliniques bien différentes, les surcharges en fer et en cuivre sont proches tant par leur cible hépatocytaire que par les mécanismes biochimiques impliqués dans leur cytotoxicité.

Cellular and Molecular Aspects of Cirrhosis. Eds B. Clément, A. Guillouzo. Colloque INSERM/John Libbey Eurotext Ltd. © 1992, Vol. 216, pp. 25-37

Metabolism of hepatic glutathione and its relevance in alcohol induced liver damage

Y. Israël, H. Speisky, A.J. Lança, S. Iwamura, M. Hirai and G. Varghese

Departments of Pharmacology and Medicine, University of Toronto and Addiction Research Foundation, Toronto, Ontario, M5S 1A8 Canada

Summary

The availability of glutathione in the liver determines the susceptibility of this organ to the toxic effects of many reactive electrophiles and peroxides. Glutathione also protects the liver against the oxygen radical damage that results from ischemia-reperfusion.

Acute alcohol administration markedly lowers hepatic glutathione levels. Rodents given alcohol chronically can compensate for the glutathione-depleting effects of ethanol such that after its continuous ingestion hepatic glutathione levels are either normal or even elevated. Humans presenting alcoholic liver disease do not compensate adequately for the effects of ethanol and thus, they present low levels of hepatic glutathione. Chronic alcohol consumption increases hepatic gamma-glutamyl transferase activity, both in humans and in rodents. We have demonstrated that this enzyme occurs on the sinusoidal surface of the liver cells and that it catalyzes the degradation of circulating glutathione into precursors for the re-synthesis of the tripeptide. We suggest that gamma-glutamyl transferase, localized preferentially in upstream (periportal) cells, serves as a mechanism to provide glutathione precursors to downstream (centrilobular) liver cells, and that its elevation by chronic alcohol consumption represents a compensatory mechanism to replenish intrahepatic glutathione.

In rodents, which are more resistant than humans to develop alcohol-induced liver injury, an additional protective mechanism involves increases in S-adenosyl-methionine synthetase, an enzyme of the transulfuration pathway which converts methionine into the glutathione-precursor cysteine. Humans presenting alcoholic liver disease show very low hepatic S-adenosyl-methionine synthetase activity and a severe impairment in this pathway. Administration of S-adenosyl-methionine reverses the glutathione depletion and normalizes indicators of liver injury.

We suggest that a reduction in the steady state levels of hepatocellular glutathione, in individuals who cannot support an adequate rate of synthesis or uptake of cysteine for glutathione synthesis, may act in synergy with other conditions (hypoxia for example) which lead to hepatocellular necrosis and liver injury.

Metabolism of Hepatic Glutathione

Glutathione, gamma-glutamyl-cysteinyl-glycine (Figure 1), a tripeptide present in liver cells at concentrations 500 times higher than in plasma, is known to play a major role in hepatocyte protection against toxic arylating and alkylating electrophiles produced in the liver during the metabolism of xenobiotics. Glutathione also participates in the detoxification of naturally occurring free radicals and soluble peroxides (Reed and Farris, 1984; Kaplowitz et al., 1985; Deneke and Farburg, 1990). A number of conditions which decrease the intrahepatic availability of glutathione (GSH) are associated with an increased susceptibility of the liver to the cytotoxic effects of compounds which require GSH for detoxification (Sakamoto et al., 1989; Reed, 1990). Glutathione also plays an important role in the protection against liver injury caused by ischemia and reperfusion where active oxygen radicals are generated (Werns and Lucchesi, 1990). Under such conditions, the ability of the liver to meet an enhanced demand for GSH depends largely on its capacity to replenish intracellular glutathione via de novo synthesis. Understanding the mechanisms by which the liver replenishes GSH is, therefore, of special relevance in hepatotoxicity induced by a number of mechanisms.

GSH is formed intracellularly in two consecutive ATP-requiring reactions. The first reaction leading to the synthesis of gamma-glutamyl-cysteine from glutamate and cysteine, constitutes the rate limiting step since cysteine levels in the hepatocytes are below the Km for gamma-glutamyl-cysteine synthetase (Meister, 1984; Beutler, 1989). In a second reaction, glutathione synthetase catalyzes the incorporation of glycine into gamma-glutamyl-cysteine to yield GSH.

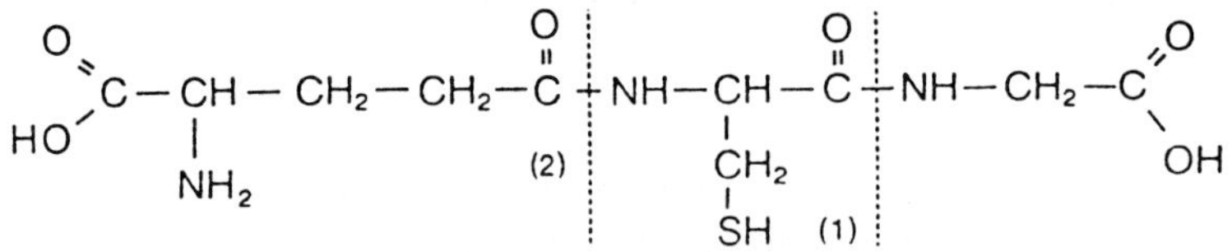

Figure 1. The structure of glutathione: γ-glutamyl-cysteinyl-glycine. (1) Cysteinyl thiol; (2) γ-glutamyl peptide linkage.

Despite the major need for glutathione in liver cell protection, hepatocytes export into the circulation most of the GSH they synthesize. In fact, over 80% of glutathione produced by the hepatocytes is exported into the blood (Adams et al., 1983; Lauterburg et al., 1984). The high turnover of hepatic glutathione, which results from a high efflux into the circulation and the maintenance of high intracellular levels, requires effective mechanisms to provide cysteine for GSH synthesis. Intracellular cysteine can be derived from two main mechanisms: (a) the transformation of methionine into cysteine through the transulfuration pathway and (b) uptake of cysteine by hepatocytes. Although the quantitative relationship between these two mechanisms in providing free cysteine for GSH synthesis has not been established, diverse conditions that reduce the transulfuration pathway markedly reduce the levels of intrahepatic glutathione (Henning et al., 1989; Friedel et al., 1989).

In the transulfuration pathway (Figure 2), methionine is converted into S-adenosyl-methionine by a reaction catalyzed by S-adenosyl-methionine synthetase (E-1). In mammals up to 50% of methionine utilized in the liver is converted into S-adenosyl-methionine (Zeisel and Poole, 1979). S-adenosyl-methionine donates its methyl group via a number of methylation reactions catalyzed by methyl-transferases (E-2). Amongst the methylation reactions is the transformation of phosphatidylethanolamine into phosphatidylcholine, a phospholipid essential in the regulation of cell membrane function and structure (Stramentinolini, 1987; Friedel et al., 1989). The product of S-adenosyl-methionine demethylation, S-adenosyl-homocysteine, is subsequently converted into homocysteine, a pivotal intermediate in the transulfuration pathway. Homocysteine can follow two routes: re-methylation into methionine, which leads to the preservation of this essential amino acid, or transformation into cystathionine, and further into cysteine, for the synthesis of glutathione. Two different substrates, N-methyl tetrahydrofolate and betaine serve as methyl-donor substrates to convert homocysteine back into methionine (E-4 and E-5, Fig. 1). In rodents, conditions of protein deprivation favour the re-methylation pathway at the expense of the transulfuration pathway (Finkelstein et al., 1974; Finkelstein and Martin, 1986). Chronic administration of diets marginally low in methionine (and choline) to rats has been shown to reduce by 50-60% both hepatic S-adenosyl-methionine and GSH levels, when compared with the administration of the same diet but supplemented with methionine (Henning et al., 1989). Depending on the stringency

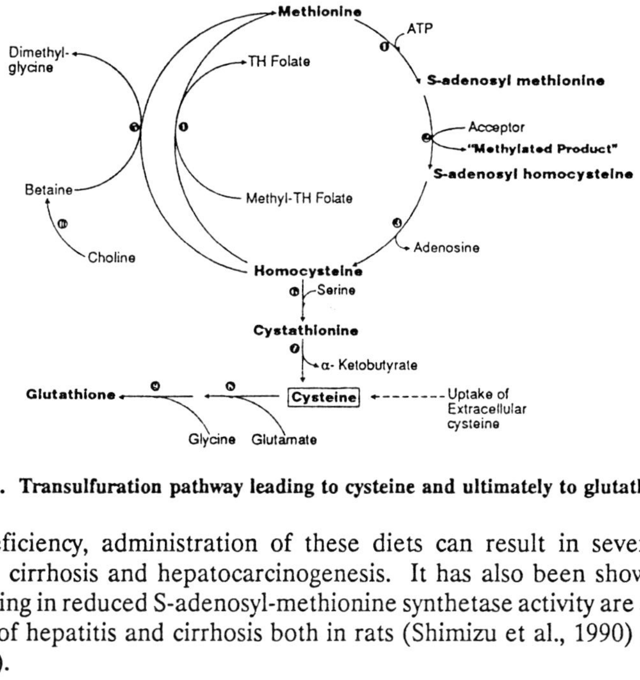

Figure 2. Transulfuration pathway leading to cysteine and ultimately to glutathione

of the dietary deficiency, administration of these diets can result in severe liver injury, including fibrosis, cirrhosis and hepatocarcinogenesis. It has also been shown that genetic deficiencies resulting in reduced S-adenosyl-methionine synthetase activity are associated with the development of hepatitis and cirrhosis both in rats (Shimizu et al., 1990) and in humans (Liau et al., 1979).

As indicated above, another important source of cysteine in hepatocytes is its uptake from the circulation. Recent studies in rat perfused livers have shown that at physiological concentrations ^{35}S-cysteine is rapidly taken up by the liver (Saiki et al., 1990). Zone 3 hepatocytes were shown to be 30-40% more effective in removing cysteine than zone 1 hepatocytes. Supporting the latter results, studies in isolated hepatocytes have shown that zone 3 hepatocytes are about 20% more efficient in taking up cysteine from the extracellular fluid than zone 1 hepatocytes (Penttilä, 1990). On the other hand, zone 1 hepatocytes are more active than zone 3 hepatocytes in the uptake (30%) and in the transformation (80%) of methionine into glutathione (Kera et al., 1988; Penttilä, 1990).

Studies in perfused rat livers (Iwamura and Israel, in preparation) have shown that, in the absence of externally added precursors, the concentration of cysteine in zone 3 hepatocytes is only one third that in zone 1 hepatocytes (80 ± 10 μM versus 220 ± 40 μM respectively, $p<0.005$). Since in vivo, zone 3 hepatocytes show only 10-15% less GSH than zone 1 hepatocytes (Schön et al., 1988; Penttilä, 1990; Iwamura and Israel, in preparation), effective mechanisms must exist in vivo to allow an efficient flow of cysteine to zone 3 hepatocytes, to retain high GSH levels. The maintenance of high GSH levels in hepatocytes in this acinar zone is essential since the endogenous production of free radicals and the activation of xenobiotics via the cytochrome - P-450 reaction is substantially higher in zone 3 than in zone 1 (see Gumucio and Chianale, 1988).

We have shown (Speisky and Israel, 1990, Speisky et al., 1990) that an important part of glutathione exported from the hepatocytes in the circulation is broken down by sinusoidal GGT ectoactivity in the liver itself. Gamma-glutamyl transferase is the only enzyme capable of hydrolyzing the gamma-glutamyl-amide group of GSH (Meister and Tate, 1976). The resulting dipeptide (cysteinyl-glycine) is quickly hydrolyzed into cysteine and glycine by ubiquitous dipeptidases. Rat liver, which presents only one-tenth of the GGT activity in human liver, degrades 20-25% of GSH released by the hepatocytes in the sinusoid while guinea pig liver, with a GGT activity comparable to that in humans, degrades up to 90% of GSH exported into the sinusoids. The liver is also able to degrade GSH made available through the systemic circulation (Table 1). Serine borate an inhibitor of GGT fully prevents the production of sinusoidal cysteine derived from circulating GSH (Figure 3).

Table 1. Removal of circulating glutathione by the perfused guinea pig liver. (From Speisky et al., 1990)

Portal glutathione (μmol/L)	Rate of hydrolysis (nmol/min/gm liver)	% Extraction ([glutathione]) portacaval × 100)
10	31.3 ± 2	90.0 ± 2.3
20	57.0 ± 3	86.1 ± 2.7
30	82.6 ± 2	78.0 ± 5.2
40	98.7 ± 5	71.9 ± 5.3
50	113.0 ± 4	71.8 ± 2.7

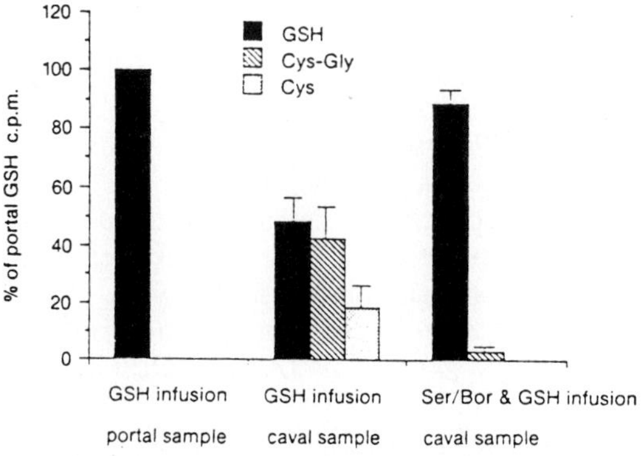

Figure 3. Products of γ-glutamyltransferase-mediated degradation of circulating glutathione in the perfused guinea pig liver. Livers depleted of glutathione (GSH) were portally perfused with 50 μmol/L ^{35}S-(cysteine)-labeled glutathione and the products of degradation cysteinyl-glycine (Cys-Gly) and cysteine (Cys) were assayed in the caval effluents (From Speisky et al., 1990).

Studies indicating that the liver is able to metabolize sinusoidal GSH, countered the view, derived from earlier histochemical observations in rat liver (Ronchi and Desnet, 1973; Mochizuki and Furukawa, 1983), that there would be no basolateral or sinusoidal GGT activity in the liver and that the enzyme would only be present in the canalicular membrane of the hepatocyte, thus not exposed to the sinusoidal circulation. We have demonstrated that such a conclusion actually results from a relative artifact of tissue fixation. By means of a novel GGT substrate-protection fixation approach (which equally protects the enzyme in the two poles) we have histochemically demonstrated the occurrence of GGT in the sinusoidal pole of rat hepatocytes (Lanca and Israel, 1991). Such sinusoidal activity could be observed in guinea pig liver even in the absence of substrate protection fixation. These studies also confirmed the preferential acinar localization of GGT in zone 1 of hepatic acinus.

On the basis of the above findings, we have proposed (Speisky et al., 1990) that glutathione released from zone 1 hepatocytes is converted by the action of sinusoidal GGT ectoactivity into GSH precursors (most importantly cysteine) which are available to zone 3 hepatocytes (Figure 4).

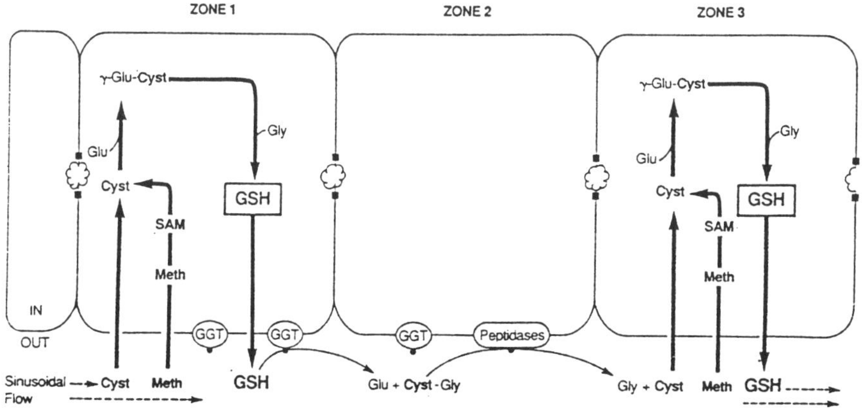

Figure 4. Proposed glutathione degradation by sinusoidal gammaglutamyl transferase activity and re-utilization of cysteine

Unpublished experiments from our laboratory (Hirai, Speisky and Israel) show that GSH-depleted guinea pig livers can recover intracellular GSH when perfused with exogenous GSH. This replenishment is also seen in vivo and it is blocked by the GGT inhibitor. It is of interest to note that recent reports show that lung tissue can also utilize circulating GSH by a mechanism in which extracellular GSH is broken down by GGT and its products are used for the synthesis of intracellular GSH (see Tsan et al., 1989).

Effects of Ethanol on Liver Glutathione

A number of studies have reported that the acute administration of ethanol to rodents leads to a 30-50% decrease in hepatic glutathione content (MacDonald et al., 1977; Guerri and Grisolia, 1980; Fernandez and Videla, 1981; Shaw et al., 1981; Kera et al., 1985). Lauterburg et al. (1984) and Speisky et al. (1985) showed that two major mechanisms mediate the GSH-depleting effects of ethanol: (a) an increased rate of GSH utilization, which is by a greater release of GSH from the liver into the circulation, and (b) a decreased rate of glutathione synthesis. During the early phase of glutathione depletion hepatic cysteine levels are minimally altered. However, as the depletion of GSH progresses a significant depletion of hepatic cysteine is also observed. In the naive rat liver, the acute administration of ethanol markedly increases the efflux of GSH, leading to a 50% higher concentration of GSH in plasma leaving the liver (Speisky et al., 1985). An increased hepatic efflux of GSH can account for the increased plasma GSH levels observed in human volunteers administered ethanol acutely (Vendemiale et al., 1989).

No studies have addressed the possible differential localization of the GSH-depleting effects of alcohol in zones 1 and 3 of the hepatic acinus. Knowledge of the latter is of importance since in alcoholic liver disease hepatocellular necrosis, inflammation and fibrosis are almost exclusively of zone 3 origin (see Orrego et al., 1981). Rats fed alcohol chronically, in conditions in which high blood levels of ethanol are maintained, also develop zone 3 necrosis (Tsukamoto et al., 1990, French et al., 1986). Glutathione depletion potentiates the hepatotoxic effects of ethanol given acutely; animals pretreated with the GSH depletor phorone show marked increases in serum enzymes characteristic zone 3 hepatocytes, following the administration of small doses of ethanol (Strubelt et al., 1987).

Rats fed alcohol chronically exhibit increased rates of hepatic GSH efflux, an effect that can be observed in perfused livers (Pierson & Mitchell, 1986; Fernandez-Checa et al., 1987) and in hepatocytes isolated (Fernandez-Checa, 1987; 1989) from these animals. Chronically alcohol fed rats also present increases (30-40%) in glutathione turnover which correlate highly with increases in the activity of hepatic gamma-glutamyl transferase (Morton & Mitchell, 1985; Callans et al., 1987). Elevations in plasma GSH and in plasma cysteine of 25-65% have been documented in chronically alcohol fed animals (Callans et al., 1987). Despite a continuously elevated efflux of hepatic GSH into the circulation, the levels of liver GSH in chronically alcohol fed animals have been shown to be either normal (Kaplan et al., 1980; Aykac et al., 1985; Pierson & Mitchell, 1986) or slightly elevated (Nichimura et al., 1981; Hetu et al., 1982; Muñoz et al., 1987; Speisky, 1986; Kawase et al., 1989), although some authors report the existence of somewhat lower GSH levels (Fernandez-Checa et al., 1987; 1989), possibly depending on blood alcohol on sacrifice. Hepatic GSH levels significantly increase above normal values following alcohol withdrawal (Callans et al., 1987).

Studies in our laboratory have shown that GGT ectoactivity is markedly elevated in the liver of alcohol-fed rats (Speisky & Israel, 1990). In perfused livers of these animals, the ability to degrade physiological concentrations of circulating GSH is increased by about 100% (Figure 5). Since most of the hepatic GGT activity is concentrated in zone 1 hepatocytes, the sinusoidal degradation of GSH is expected to start taking place in this area while the products of GSH degradation (precursors of GSH) are expected to be transported along the sinusoid towards zone 3 of the acinus (Fig. 4). According to this latter view, the increased efflux of GSH that occurs following chronic alcohol administration, combined with the increased GGT ectoactivity in the liver, would potentiate each other resulting in a greater availability of precursors for the resynthesis of GSH in zone 3.

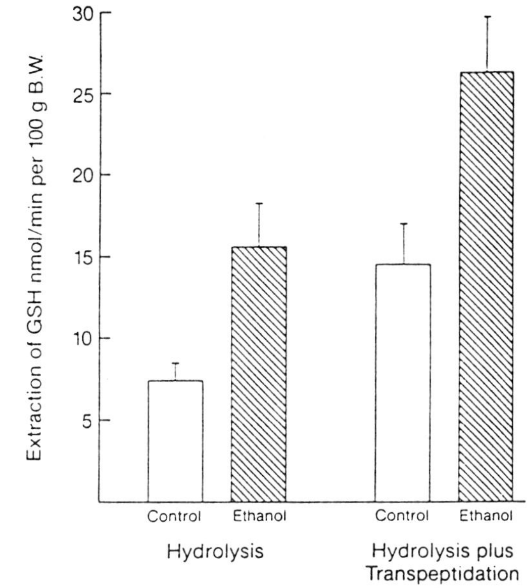

Figure 5. Effect of chronic ethanol administration on the rate of removal (Hydrolysis, and Hydrolysis plus Transpeptidation) of circulating GSH (10 μM) by the perfused rat liver. The results represent data obtained from 9 livers for each experiment condition. (From Speisky and Israel, 1990)

Rodents fed alcohol chronically also compensate for the GSH-depleting effects of ethanol by increasing the activity of enzymes of the transulfuration pathway, primarily, S-adenosyl-methionine synthetase (Fig. 2, E-1) (Finkelstein & Kyle, 1968) and cystathionine synthetase (E-6) (Finkelstein et al., 1984), thus leading to a greater ability to synthesize cysteine from methionine. The levels of gamma-glutamyl-cysteine synthetase remain unaltered (Morton & Mitchell, 1985; Speisky, 1986), although changes in this enzyme might be zone specific. It has also been reported that the incorporation of radioactivity from ^{35}S-methionine into GSH is increased in the liver of alcohol-fed rats (Vendemiale et al., 1984). However, since the specific activities of the precursors were not measured, it is difficult to conclude whether the effect reported indeed represents an increased transulfuration capacity or changes in precursor pool.

In humans presenting alcoholic liver disease and in baboons fed alcohol chronically, the compensatory mechanisms to maintain hepatic GSH appear not to function adequately, as the levels of hepatic GSH greatly reduced (Shaw et al., 1981; Woodhouse et al., 1983; Videla et al., 1984; Jewell et al., 1986). In alcoholics without liver disease hepatic glutathione levels may also be reduced, as seen by their low ability to differentially form acetaminophen-GSH metabolites. In these patients hepatic glutathione deficiency, in addition to microsomal induction, has been proposed to lead to the greater susceptibility to acetaminophen hepatotoxicity (Lauterburg and Velez, 1988). Individuals with alcoholic cirrhosis also present greatly reduced levels of hepatic S-adenosyl-methionine synthetase (Cabrero et al.,1988; Duce et al., 1988) and are unable to utilize methionine in the transulfuration reaction (Horowitz et al., 1981; Chawla et al., 1984), resulting in increased levels of circulating methionine. It is not clear, however, if these effects are pathogenic or result from the underlying disease. It has been reported that low hepatic S-adenosyl-methionine synthetase levels can also occur in hepatic cirrhosis of non-alcoholic etiology (Duce et al., 1988). Nevertheless, it is conceivable that the patients in whom these deficiencies occur, might be more susceptible to develop liver disease independently of the etiologic factor. Perhaps more important, is the demonstration that administration of S-adenosyl-methionine both to patients presenting alcoholic liver disease (Vendemiale et al., 1989) and to baboons fed alcohol chronically

(Lieber et al., 1990) results in increased hepatic GSH levels and in the normalization of a number of biological indicators of liver damage including serum transaminases, bile acids and serum albumin.

A normalization of hepatic GSH levels following S-adenosyl-methionine administration may occur not only because S-adenosyl-methionine is a precursor of homocysteine, but also since S-adenosyl-methionine is a potent activator (up to 300%) of cystathionine synthetase (Finkelstein et al., 1975) (Fig.2, E-6), a pivotal enzyme. Activation of cystathionine synthetase can divert homocysteine into cysteine synthesis rather than back into methionine. Conditions that favour homocysteine re-methylation would, in turn, be expected to be deleterious. In fact supplementation with dietary choline, a precursor of betaine, to baboons fed alcohol chronically increases the severity of alcohol induced liver injury (Lieber et al., 1985).

As expected from a normalization in hepatic GSH levels following S-adenosyl-methionine, GGT levels were reduced in these patients (Salerno et al., 1986; Frezza et al., 1987). An unexpected effect of S-adenosyl-methionine treatment was a reduction in circulating methionine levels. Such an effect might be explained on the basis of the recent findings that the active tetrameric form of hepatic S-adenosyl-methionine synthetase can be dissociated by sulfhydryl blocking agents into the 15-times less active dimeric form. Thus, sulfhydryl group protection of the enzyme, by an increase in GSH following S-adenosyl-methionine administration, might reactivate S-adenosyl-methionine synthetase, leading to a greater utilization of circulating methionine (Corrales et al., 1990). In cirrhosis, unlike in normal liver, hepatic S-adenosyl-methionine synthetase is found primarily in the dimeric form (Cabrero et al., 1988). Recent studies by Corrales et al., (1991) indicate that a small reduction (30%) in hepatic glutathione levels induced by inhibition of glutathione synthesis, results in marked reductions in S-adenosyl-methionine synthetase activity and S-adenosyl-methionine levels (60 and 40% reductions respectively). These studies might explain the protective effect of dietary lecithin (phosphatidyl choline), which spares S-adenosyl-methionine, on alcoholic cirrhosis in experimental animals (Lieber et al., 1990b).

In conclusion, we have shown that gamma-glutamyl transferase is present in the basolateral aspect of the hepatocyte, which endows it with the ability to degrade circulating glutathione. Acute administration of ethanol increases glutathione efflux from the liver while chronic administration of alcohol increases both the efflux of hepatic glutathione and the activity of basolateral gamma-glutamyl transferase. These, acting in concert, increase the sinusoidal availability of cysteine to centrilobular (zone 3) hepatocytes. These hepatocytes are most susceptible to hypoxic conditions, and toxic xenobiotics. Thus, increases in hepatic gamma-glutamyl transferase may constitute a protective mechanism to replenish intracellular glutathione.

REFERENCES

Adams, J.D., Lauterburg, B.H. & Mitchell, J.R. (1983): Plasma glutathione and gluthatione disulfide in the rat: regulation and response to oxidative stress. *J. Pharmacol. Exp. Ther.* 227, 749-754.

Anderson M.E., Powrie, F., Puri, R.N. & Meister, A. (1985): Gluthatione monoethyl ester: preparation, uptake by tissues and conversion to glutahione *Arch. Biochem. Biophys.* 239, 538-548

Aykac, G. (1985): The effect of chronic ethanol ingestion of hepatic lipid peroxide, glutathione, glutathione peroxidase and glutathione transferase in rats. *Toxicology* 36,

71-76.
Beutler, E. (1989): Nutritional and metabolic aspects of glutathione. *Ann. Rev. Nutr.* 9, 287-302.
Cabrero, C. Duce, A.M., Ortiz, P., Alemany, S. & Mato, J.M. (1988): Specific loss of the high-molecular-weight form of S-adenosyl-L-methionine synthetase in human liver cirrhosis. *Hepatology* 8, 1530-1534.
Callans, D.J., Wacker, L.S. & Mitchell, M.C. (1987): Effects of ethanol feeding and withdrawal on plasma glutathione elimination in the rat. *Hepatology* 7, 496-501.
Chawla, R.K., Lewis F.W., Kutner, M.H., Bate, D.M., Roy, R.G.B & Rudman, D. (1984): Plasma cysteine, cystine, and glutathione in cirrhosis. *Gastroenterology* 87, 770-776.
Corrales, F., Cabrero, C., Pajares, M.A., Ortiz, P., Duce, A.M. & Mato, J.M. (1990): Inactivation and dissociation of S-adenosylmethionine synthetase by modification of sulfhydryl groups and its possible occurrence in cirrhosis. *Hepatology* 11, 216-222.
Corrales, F., Ochoa, P., Rivas, C., Martin-Lomas, M., Mato, J.M. & Pajares, M.A. (1991): Inhibition of glutathione synthesis in the liver leads to s-adenosylmethionine synthetase reduction. *Hepatology* 14, 528-533.
Deneke, S.M. & Fanburg, B.L. (1989): Regulation of cellular glutathione. *Am. J. Physiol.* 257, L163-L173.
Duce, A.M., Ortiz, P., Cabrero, C. & Mato, J. (1988): S-adenosyl-L-methionine synthetase and phospholipid methyltransferase are inhibited in human cirrhosis. *Hepatology* 8, 65-68.
Fernandez, V. & Videla, L.A. (1981): Effect of acute and chronic ethanol ingestion on the content of reduced glutathione of various tissues of the rat. *Experientia* 37, 392-394.
Fernandez-Checa, J.C., Ookhtens, M. & Kaplowitz, N. (1987): Effect of chronic ethanol feeding on rat hepatocytic glutathione: compartmentation, efflux and response to incubation with ethanol. *J. Clin. Invest.* 80, 57-62.
Fernandez-Checa, J.C., Ookhtens, M. & Kaplowitz, N. (1989): Effects of chronic ethanol feeding on rat hepatocytic glutathione: relationship of cytosolic glutathione to efflux and mitochondrial sequestration. *J. Clin. Invest.* 83, 1247-1252.
Finkelstein, J.D. & Kyle, W.E. (1968): Ethanol effects on methionine metabolism in rat liver. *Proc. Soc. Exper. Biol. Med.* 129, 497-501.
Finkelstein, J.D., Cello, J.P. & Kyle, W.E. (1974): Ethanol-induced changes in methionine metabolism in rat liver. *Biochem. Biophys. Res. Comm.* 61, 525-531.
Finkelstein, J.D., Kyle, W.E., Martin, J.J., Pick A.M. (1975): Activation of cystathionine synthase by adenosylmethionine and adenosylthionine. *Biochem. Biophys. Res. Comm.* 66, 81-87.
Finkelstein, J.D. & Martin ,J.J. (1986): Methionine metabolism in mammals. *J. Biol. Chem.* 261, 1582-1587.
French, S.W., Miyamoto, K. & Tsukamoto, H. (1986): Ethanol-induced hepatic fibrosis in the rat: role of the amount of dietary fat. *Alcohol Clin. Exp. Res.* 10, 13S
Frezza, M., & DiPadova, C. (1987): Multicenter placebo controlled clinical trial of intravenous and oral s-adenosylmethionine (SAMe) in cholestatic patients with liver disease. *Hepatology* 7, 1105.
Friedel, H.A., Goa, K.L. & Benfield, P. (1989): S-adenosylmethionine. A review of its pharmacological properties and therapeutic potential in liver dysfunction and affective disorders in relation to its physiological role in cell metabolism. *Drugs* 38, 389-416.
Guerri, C. & Grisolia, S. (1980): Changes in glutathione in acute and chronic alcohol intoxication. *Pharmacol. Biochem. Behav.* 13, 53-61.
Gumucio, J.J. & Chianale, J. (1988): Liver cell heterogeneity and liver function. In *The Liver, Biology and Pathology* 2nd edn, eds. Arias, Jakoby, Popper, Schachter & Shafritz, pp 931-947, New York: Raven Press.

Henning, S.M., McKee, R.W., & Swendseid, M.E. (1989): Hepatic content of S-adenosylmethionine, S-adenosylhomocysteine and glutathione in rats receiving treatments modulating methyl donor availability. *J. Nutr.* 119, 1478-1482.
Hetu, C., Yalle, L. & Joly, J.C. (1982): Influence of ethanol on hepatic glutathione content and on the activity of glutathione S-transferases and epoxide hydrase in the rat. *Drug Metab. Disp.* 40, 246-250.
Horikawa, S., Ishikawa, M., Ozasa, H. & Tsukada, K. (1989): Isolation of a cDNA encoding the rat liver S-adenosylmethionine synthetase. *Eur. J. Biochem.* 184, 497-501.
Horowitz, J.H., Rypins, E.B., Henderson, J.M. et al., (1981): Evidence for impairment of transulfuration pathway in cirrhosis. *Gastroenterology* 81, 668-675.
Jewell, S.A., Di Monte, D., Gentile, A., Guglielmi, A., Altomare E. & Albano, O. (1986): Decreased hepatic glutathione in chronic alcoholic patients. *J. Hepatol.* 3, 1-6.
Kaplan, E., DeNaster, E.G. & Jagasawa, H.T. (1980): Effect of pargyline on hepatic glutathione levels in rats treated acutely and chronically with ethanol. *Res. Comm. Pathol. Pharmacol.* 30, 577-580.
Kaplowitz, N., Yee, A.W.T. & Ookhtens, M. (1985): The regulation of hepatic glutathione. *Ann. Rev. Pharmacol. Toxicol.* 25, 715-744.
Kawase, T., Kato, S. & Lieber C. (1989): Lipid Perodixidation and antioxidant defense systems in rat liver after chronic ethanol feeding. *Hepatology* 10, 815-821.
Kera, Y., Komara, S., Olibora, Y., Kiriyama, T. & Inoue, K. (1985): Ethanol induced changes in lipid peroxidation and nonprotein sulfhydryl content. *Res. Comm. Chem. Path.* Pharmcol. 47, 203-209.
Kera, Y., Penttilä, K. & Lindros, K.O. (1988): Glutathione replenishment capacity is lower in isolated perivenous than in periportal hepatocytes. *Biochem. J.* 254, 411-417.
Lanca, A.J. & Israel, Y. (1991): Histochemical demonstration of sinusoidal gamma-glutamyl transferase activity by substrate protection fixation: comparative studies in rat and guinea pig liver. *Hepatology* 14, 857-
Lauterburg, B.H. & Velez, M. (1988): Glutathione deficiency in alcoholics: risk factor for paracetamol hepatotoxicity. *Gut* 29, 1153-1157.
Lauterburg, B.H., Admas, J.D. & Mitchell, J.R. (1984): Hepatic glutathione homeostasis in the rat: efflux accounts for glutathione turnover. *Hepatology* 4, 586-590.
Lauterburg, B.H., Davies, S. & Mitchell, J.R. (1984): Ethanol suppresses hepatic glutathione synthesis in rats in vivo. *J. Pharmacol. Exp. Ther.* 230, 7-11.
Liau, M.C., Chang, C.F., Belangers, L & Grenier, A. (1979): Correlation of isozyme patterns of s-adenosylmethionine synthetase with fetal stages and pathological stages of the liver. *Cancer Res.* 39, 162-169.
Lieber, C.S., Leo, M.A., Mak, K.M., DeCarli, L.M. & Sato, S. (1985): Choline fails to prevent liver fibrosis in ethanol-fed baboons but causes toxicity. *Hepatology* 5, 561-572.
Lieber, C.S., Casini, A., De Carli, L.M., Kim, C., Lowe, N., Sasaki, R. & Leo, M.A. (1990): S-adenosyl-L-methionine attenuates alcohol-induced liver injury in the baboon. *Hepatology* 11, 165-172.
Lieber, C.S., De Carli, L.M., Mak, K.M., Kim, C. & Leo, M.A. (1990): Attenuation of alcohol-induced hepatic fibrosis by polyunsaturated lecithin. *Hepatology* 12, 1390-1398.
MacDonald, C.M., Dow, J. & Moore, M.R. (1977): A possible protective role for sulphydryl compounds in acute alcoholic liver injury. *Biochem. Pharmacol.* 26, 1529-1531.
Meister, A. & Tate, S.S. (176): Glutathione and related γ-glutamyl compounds: biosynthesis and utilization. *Ann. Rev. Biochem.* 45, 559-604.
Meister, A. (1984): New aspects of glutahtione biochemistry and transport: selective alteration of glutathione metabolism. *Fed. Proc.* 43, 3031-3042.
Mochizuki, Y. & Furukawa, K. (1983): Histochemical investigation of hepatic gamma-

glutamyl-transpeptidase of rats treated with high dose of phenobarbital. *Acta Histochem. Cytochem.* 16, 155-162.
Morton, S.B. & Mitchell, M.C. (1985): Effects of chronic ethanol feeding on glutathione turnover in the rat. *Biochem. Pharmacol.* 34, 1559-1563.
Muñoz, M.E., Martin, M.I., Fermoso, J., Gonzalez, J. & Esteller, A. (1987): Effect of chronic ethanol feeding on glutathione and glutathione-related enzyme activities. *Drug and Alcohol Depend.* 20, 221-226.
Nishimura, M., Stein, H., Berges, W. & Teschke, R. (1981): Gamma-glutamyltransferase activity of liver plasma membrane: induction following chronic alcohol consumption. *Biochem. Biophys. Res. Comm.* 99, 142-148.
Orrego, H., Israel, Y. & Blendis, L.M. (1981): Alcoholic liver disease: information in search of knowledge? *Hepatology* 1, 267-283.
Orrego, H., Israel, Y., Blake, J.E. & Medline, A. (1983): Assessment of prognostic factors in alcoholic liver disease: toward a global quantitative expression of severity. *Hepatology* 3, 896-905.
Pentillä, K. (1990): Role of cysteine and taurine in regulating glutathione synthesis by periportal and perivenous hepatocytes. *Biochem. J.* 269, 659-664.
Pierson, J.L. & Mitchell, M.C. (1986): Increased hepatic efflux of glutathione after chronic ethanol feeding. *Biochem. Pharmacol.* 35, 1533-1537.
Reed, D.J. (1990): Glutathione: toxicological implications. *Ann. Rev. Pharmacol. Toxicol.* 30, 603-631.
Reed, D.J. & Farris, M.W. (1984): Glutathione depletion and susceptibility. *Pharmacol. Rev.* 36, 25S-33S.
Ronchi, G. & Desnet, V.J. (1973): Histochemical study of gammaglutamyl transpeptidase (GGT) in experimental intrahepatic and extrahepatic cholestasis. *Beitr. Pathol.* 150, 316-321.
Saiki, H., Chan, E.T., Wong, E., Yamauro, W., Ookhtens, M. & Kaplowitz, N. (1990): Unique transport of cysteine in acinar zone III. *Hepatology* 12(4), 893.
Sakamoto, Y., Higashi, N. & Meister, A. (1989): in *Glutathione Centennial: Molecular Perspectives and Clinical Implications*, New York: Academic Press.
Salerno, M.T., Vendemiale, G., Amendola, A., Trione, T. et al., (1986): Effect of orally administered s-adenosyl-L-methionine (SAMe) in patients with alcoholic liver disease. *Digest. Dis. Sci.* 31, 192S
Schön, M.R., Kaufman, F.C. & Thurman, R.G. (1988): Selective depletion and measurement of glutathione in periportal and pericentral regions in the perfused rat liver. *Toxicol. Lett.* 42, 265-272.
Shaw, S., et al., (1981): Ethanol-induced lipid peroxidation: potentiation by long-term alcohol feeding and attenuation by methionine. *J. Lab. Clin. Med.* 98, 417-424.
Shaw, S., Rubin, K.P. & Lieber C.S. (1983): Depressed hepatic glutathione and increased diene conjugates in alcoholic liver disease. Evidence of lipid peroxidation. *Digest. Dis. Sci.* 28, 585-589.
Shimizu, K., Abe, M., Yokoyama, S., Sawada, N., Mori, M. & Tsukada, K. (1990): Decreased activities of S-adenosylmethionine synthetase isozymes in hereditary hepatitis in long-evans rats. *Life Sci.* 46, 1837-1842.
Speisky, H., Macdonald, A., Giles, H.G., Orrego, H. & Israel, Y. (1985): Increased loss and decreased synthesis of hepatic glutathione after acute ethanol administration turnover studies. *Biochem. J.* 25, 565-572.
Speisky, H. & Israel, Y. (1990): Gamma-glutamyl transferase ectoactivity in the intact rat liver: effect of chronic alcohol consumption. *Alcohol* 7, 339-347.
Speisky, H., Shackel, N., Varghese, G., Wade, D. & Israel, Y. (1990): Role of hepatic gamma-

glutamyl transferase in the degradation of circulating glutathione: studies in the intact guinea pig perfused liver. *Hepatology* 11, 843-849.
Stramentinoli, G. (1987): Pharmacological aspects of s-adenosylmethionine. Pharmokinetics and pharmacodynamics. *Am. J. Med.* 83, 35-42.
Strubelt, O., Younes, M. & Pentz, R. (1987): Enhancement by glutathione depletion of ethanol-induced acute hepatotoxicity in vitro and in vivo. *Toxicology* 45, 213-223.
Tietze, F. (1969): Enzymic method for quanititative determination of nanogram amounts of total and oxidized glutathione: applications to mammalian blood and other tissues. *Anal. Biochem.* 27, 502-522.
Tsan, M.F., White, J.E. & Rosano, C.L. (1989): Modulation of endothelial GSH concentrations: effect of exogenous GSH and GSH monoethyl ester. *J. Appl. Physiol.* 66, 1029-1034.
Tsukamoto, H., Gaal, K. & French, S.W. (1990): Insights into the pathogenesis of alcoholic liver necrosis and fibrosis: status report. *Hepatology* 12, 599-608.
Vendemiale, G., Jayatielleke, E., Shaw, S. & Lieber, C-S. (1984): Depression of biliary glutathione excretion by chronic ethanol feeding in the rat. *Life Sci.* 34, 1065-1073.
Vendemiale, G., Altomare, E., Grattagliano, I. & Albano, O. (1989): Increased plasma levels of glutathione and malondialdehyde after acute ethanol ingestion in humans. *J. Hepatology* 9, 359-365.
Vendemiale, G., Altomare, E., Trizio, T., Grazie, L.E., De Padova, C., Salarno, M.T., Carrieri, V. & Albano, O. (1989): Effects of oral s-adenosyl-L-methionine on hepatic glutathione in patients with liver disease. *Scand. J. Gastroenterol.* 24, 407-415.
Videla, L., Iturriaga, H., Pino, M.E., Bunout, D., Valenzuela, A. & Ugarte, G. (1984): Content of hepatic reduced glutathione in chronic alcoholic patients: influence of the length of abstinence and liver necrosis. *Clin. Sci.* 66, 283-290.
Werns, S.W., & Lucchesi, B.R. (1990): Free radicals and ischemic tissue injury. *Trends in Pharmacol. Sci.* 11, 161-166.
Woodhouse, K.E., Faith, M.W., Mutch, E., Wright, P., James, O.F.W. & Rawlins, M.D. (1983): The effect of alcoholic cirrhosis on the activities of microsomal aldrin epoxidase, 7-ethoxycoumarin 0-de-ethylase and epoxide hydrolase, and on the concentrations of reduced glutathione in human liver. *Br. J. Clin. Pharmacol.* 15, 667-672.
Zeisel, S.H. & Poole, J.R. (1979): in *Transmethylation*, eds. E. Usdin, R.T. Borchardt, C.R. Crevelin, The Netherlands:Elsevier/North Holland 59.

Résumé

La disponibilité en glutathion dans le foie détermine sa prédisposition aux effets toxiques de nombreux électrophiles et peroxydes réactifs. Le glutathion protège également le foie contre les dommages des radicaux oxygénés qui résultent des perfusions après ischémie.
L'administration aiguë d'alcool diminue fortement les taux de glutathion hépatique. Les rongeurs traités de manière chronique à l'alcool peuvent compenser les effets d'épuisement du glutathion par l'éthanol de telle façon qu'après ingestion continue les niveaux de glutathion hépatique sont normaux, voire plus élevés. Les hommes ayant une maladie hépatique alcoolique ne compensent pas efficacement les effets de l'éthanol et donc ont un niveau réduit de glutathion hépatique. La consommation chronique d'alcool augmente l'activité de la gamma-glutamyl transférase hépatique chez l'homme et les rongeurs. Nous avons démontré que cet enzyme est présent sur la surface du pôle sinusoïdal des cellules hépatiques et qu'il catalyse la dégradation du glutathion circulant en précurseurs pour la re-synthèse de ce tripeptide. Nous suggérons que la gamma-glutamyl transférase qui est localisée préférentiellement en amont, dans les cellules périportales, agit comme un fournisseur de précurseurs de glutathion en aval, pour les cellules centrolobulaires, et que son augmentation par une consommation chronique d'alcool représente un mécanisme de compensation pour le réapprovisionnement en glutathion intrahépatique.
Chez les rongeurs qui sont plus résistants que l'homme au développement de lésions hépatiques liées à l'alcool, un mécanisme de protection supplémentaire met en jeu une augmentation de synthétase S-adénosyl-méthionine, un enzyme de la voie de transulfuration qui transforme la méthionine en cystéine, précurseur du glutathion. Les hommes qui ont une maladie hépatique alcoolique ont une activité très basse de synthétase S-adénosyl-méthionine et une forte altération de cette voie de transulfuration. L'administration de S-adénosyl-méthionine inverse la perte en glutathion et normalise les signes des lésions hépatiques.
Nous suggérons qu'une réduction dans les niveaux stables du glutathion hépatocellulaire chez ceux qui n'ont pas un taux normal de synthèse ou de captation de cystéine pour la synthèse de glutathion, peut agir en synergie avec d'autres facteurs (par exemple l'hypoxie) qui conduisent à la nécrose hépatocellulaire et aux lésions hépatiques.

Cellular and Molecular Aspects of Cirrhosis. Eds B. Clément, A. Guillouzo. Colloque INSERM/John Libbey Eurotext Ltd. © 1992, Vol. 216, pp. 39-48

Molecular basis of granuloma formation in schistosomiasis : interaction of T cells, their α-idiotypic regulatory and subsequent T suppressor factor activity

S. Michael Phillips [(1)], Peter J. Perrin [(2)], Ligang Shi [(1)] and Taghrid Gaafar [(3)]

[(1)] Allergy and Immunology Section, University of Pennsylvania School of Medicine, Philadelphia, PA 19104, USA; [(2)] Navy Medical Research Institute, Immune Cell Biology Program, Bethesda, MD 20889, USA; [(3)] Dr. Osman Hospital, Maadi, 16 Road 107, Maadi, Cairo, Egypt

Morbidity in schistosomiasis, a helminthic disease effecting an estimated 200 individuals (World Health Organization, Technical Report No. 728, Geneva, Switzerland (1985), and Kenneth (1989), is principally due to hepatic granulomatous inflammation and fibrosis (Warren (1961), Phillips and Lammie (1986), and Perrin and Phillips (1989). This host response, directed against the parasite eggs and egg products, which have embolized to small capillaries in the liver, is a delicately orchestrated reaction. We have been studying the cellular and soluble components which play precise and interreactive roles in granulomatous hypersensitivity (Perrin and Phillips (1989), Doughty and Phillips (1982), Bentley, **et al.** (1982), Bentley, **et al.** (1985), Perrin and Phillips (1988), Perrin, **et al.** (1989), Perrin and Phillips (1989), and Perrin, **et al.** (1989).

I. THE CELLULAR CONSTITUENTS OF GRANULOMATOUS HYPERSENSITIVITY: Although many aspects of the complex relationships between infection and morbidity remain poorly understood, it is clear that the pathophysiologic scenario is dependent upon multiple subpopulations of distinct subsets of T lymphocytes (Perrin and Phillips (1989), Boros (1989), Ragheb and Boros (1989), and Phillips and Lammie (1986). Initial granulomas increase to a maximum size as disease progresses; subsequent granulomas are smaller. Granulomas are produced by TH1 (T-Helper cells) cells, $L3T4^+$, bearing IL-2 high affinity receptors and producing IL-2 and interferon-γ as a consequence of antigenic stimulation. These cells recruit and activate eosinophils, macrophages, and fibroblasts thru cytokine production. The reaction is subsequently regulated by $Lyt\text{-}2^+$ TS (T-Suppressor cells) cells, which express little IL-2 or IL-5. We have been studying these subpopulations, utilizing a variety of in vitro depletion and adoptive transfer studies and in vitro analyses of immune mediated granuloma formation. Figure 1 summarizes the maximum size of granulomas in mice which had been depleted of various subpopulations of T lymphocytes 10 weeks after their exposure to *S. mansoni* cercariae. These results demonstrate the importance of various subpopulations of T cells in creating and regulating granulomatous hypersensitivity. As can also be noted the sizes of the animals spleens, the hydroxyproline content of liver and splenic portal pressure are consonant with the notion that clinical disease is similarly effected by the same populations.

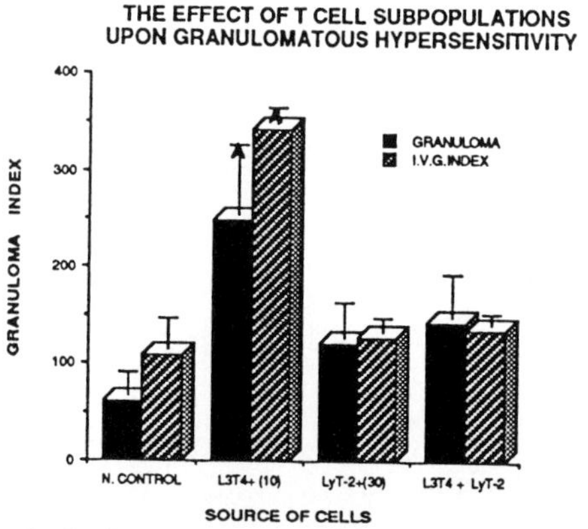

Figure 1: Animals were depleted of lymphocyte subpopulations by in vivo administration of monoclonal antibodies during the period of maximum granulomatous hypersensitivity (12 wks after exposure). Results are expressed as a percent of the given parameter shown by similarly exposed, untreated animals.

Utilizing the in vitro model of granuloma formation similar results were obtained. Figure 2 demonstrates a well-developed in vitro granuloma surrounding an antigen-coated nidus. These reactions faithfully recapitulate in vivo events in terms of cell content, kinetics of development, lymphokine elaboration, and susceptibility to regulation.

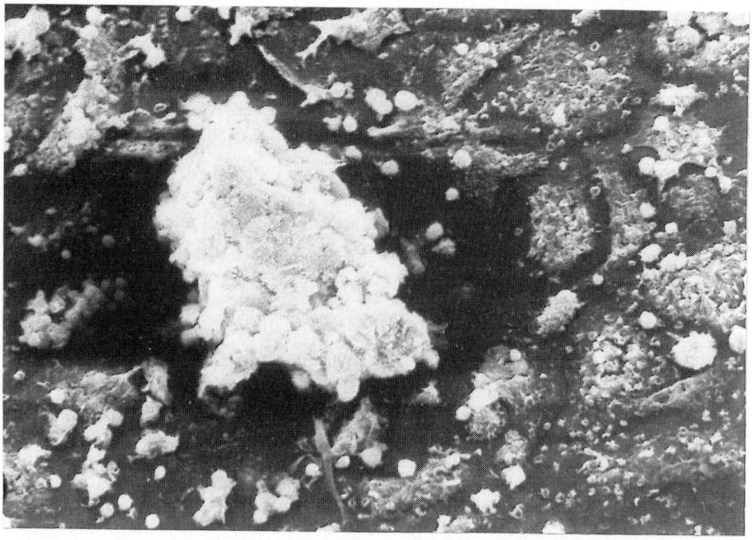

Figure 2: Mature well-formed in vitro granuloma, 3 days after initiation of culture. A schistosome egg antigen-coated bead was incubated in the presence of spleen cells from an exposed animal. Note the multitude of cell populations including mononuclear cells, lymphocytes, and fibroblasts migrating to these surface of the egg and encapsulating it in a multilayered granuloma.

Histologically this lesion is identical to a delayed type hypersensitivity granuloma, with antigen reactive T helper cells most closely juxtaposed to the central covalently-bound antigen, closely associated with activated macrophages, many of which are undergoing fusion into multinuclear giant cells, small numbers of recruited eosinophils of macrophages, and an external ring of lymphocytes dominated by T suppressor cells. One can also note a variety of other populations including fibroblasts migrating toward the center of the lesion.

The ability of various subpopulations of cells to create and regulate the granuloma are summarized in Figure 3. The data is expressed as a granuloma size and as an index which is a quantitative enumeration of carefully defined morphometric parameters of reactivity. Note that $L3T4^+$ cells adoptively transfer larger granulomas and form them <u>in vitro</u>. $Lyt\text{-}2^+$ cells transfer no reactivity but can suppress the granuloma formation capability of the $L3T4^+$ cells when admixed <u>in vitro</u> or coadoptively transferred <u>in vivo</u>.

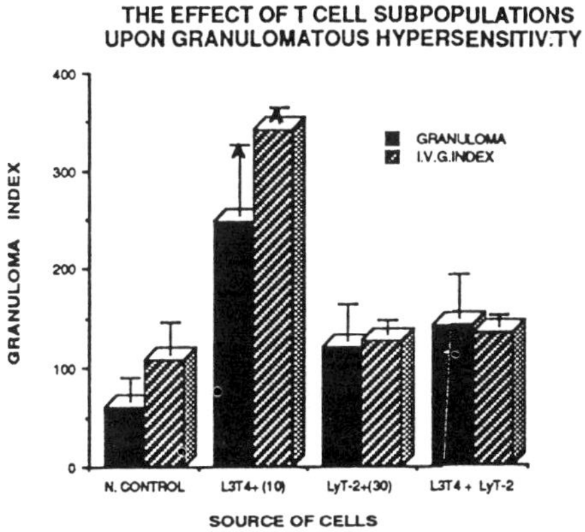

<u>Figure 3</u>: T helper cells ($L3T4^+$) obtained from acutely infected animals (10 wks) and T suppressor cells ($Lyt\text{-}2^+$) obtained from chronically infected animals (30 wks) were assessed for their ability to adoptively transfer granulomatous hypersensitivity <u>in vivo</u> or to produce granulomas <u>in vitro</u>. L3T4 cells formed large granulomas and that granuloma formation was actively suppressed by the T suppressor cells when cocultured <u>in vitro</u> or coadoptively transferred <u>in vivo</u>.

II. IMMUNOLOGIC REGULATION OF GRANULOMATOUS HYPERSENSITIVITY: The regulation of these reactions is based primarily on specific receptor ligand interactions. Infection or immunization with egg antigens generates populations of antigenically reactive cells and a regulatory anti-idiotypic response. This response is characterized by the development of anti-clonotypic T cells and anti-idiotypic antibodies. These anti-idiotypic reactants specifically interact with the receptors of the SEA reactive TH cells, inactivate these latter cells and prevent the formation of granulomas. Anti-idiotypic immunization with T cell receptors directed against egg antigens induces a regulatory anti-idiotypic response and decreases a variety of immune responses to the egg. These decreased exposure include DTH to egg antigens, <u>in vivo</u> granuloma formation, type 3 and type 1 hepatic collagen accumulation, IL-2 and interferon-γ production in response to antigen and <u>in vitro</u> granuloma formation and incorporation of hydroxyproline into collagenase sensitive protein. There is no effect on IL-4 or IL-5 production (Figure 4).

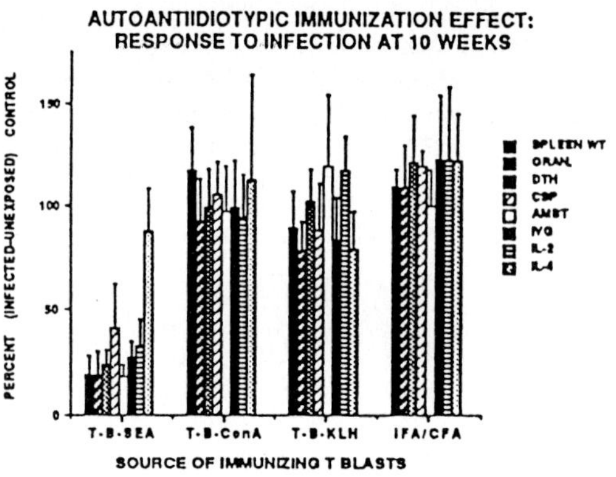

Figure 4: Animals were actively immunized with a variety of T blasts bearing specific receptors. Specifically these receptors were directed against SEA (Soluble Schistosome Egg Antigen), Conconavalin A blasts, keyhole limpet hemocyanin. Following the induction of the anti-auto-idiotypic response, they were challenged with S. mansoni and assessed 10 weeks later for a variety of parameters including: spleen weight, granuloma size, delayed type hypersensitivity to egg antigens, coagenase sensitive protein, antigen mediated blast transformation, in vitro granuloma formation, IL-2 and IL-4 production.

Additional studies have indicated that anti-idiotypic immunization with specific T cell receptors can also lead to the autoregulation of T suppressor activity. In this instance granulomatous hypersensitivity, hepatic fibrosis, morbidity, and the other parameters demonstrated above demonstrate changes opposite to those in Figure 4. Thus the induction of anti-idiotypic regulation at various points in the evolution of granuloma formation, have differing effects. These findings suggest that the granuloma formation and its subsequent regulation are contingent on waves of sequentially developing subpopulations of cells. Initially reactions are dominant by T-Helper populations and subsequent reactions are dominated by suppressor elements (Figure 5).

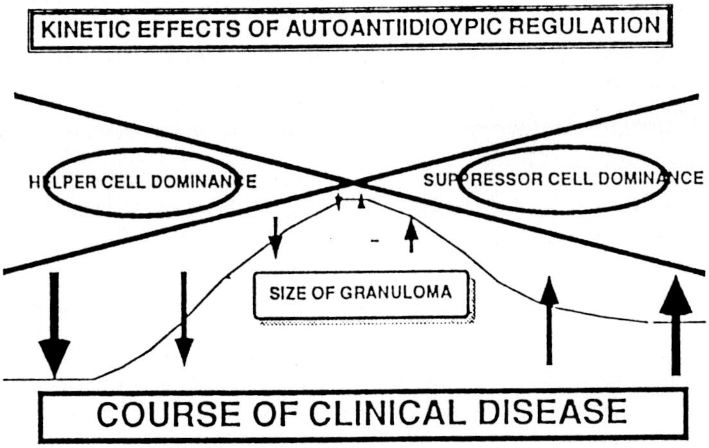

Figure 5: The clinical course of schistosomiasis is characterized initially by dominance of helper cell influences and the gradual production of granulomas of increased size. Later in the course the granulomas modulated become smaller under the influence of suppressor cell dominance. Auto-anti-idiotypic regulation during, periods of helper cell dominance, result in strong suppression of granuloma size, hepatic inflammation, and clinical disease. Regulatory phenomenon are relatively balanced in the mid course of disease. During chronic disease auto-anti-idiotypic regulation suppresses the negative regulatory aspects of the disease and result in increasing immunologic reactivity and morbidity.

III. THE MOLECULAR REGULATION OF GRANULOMATOUS REACTIVITY: TS cells regulate granuloma modulation via an antigenically and genetically restricted cascade of suppressor-inducer and suppressor-effector factors. There has been considerable interest in these factors (Perrin and Phillips (1989), Chensue, **et al.** (1983), Abe and Colley (1984), Mathew and Boros (1986). Perrin and Phillips (1988), Perrin, **et al.** (1989), Perrin and Phillips (1989), Perrin, **et al.** (1989), and Fidel and Boros (1991) as they regulate immune reactivity in schistosomiasis. The suppressor-effector factor (TseF) directly suppresses granuloma formation both in vitro and in vivo. Using a variety of techniques of heterodimeric chain reduction, immunoadsorptive chromatography, and in vitro functional complementation, the dimeric molecules have been analyzed. By analyzing genetic restriction, antigenic specificity, and phenotypic markers, the contributions of the component chains to the 72KD TseF reactivity have been determined. One chain bears antigenic receptors and imparts antigenic specificity. The other chain bears IJ determinants, a TCR β chain allotypic determinant, and impart genetic restriction and function. Exogenous IL-2 prevents the formation of TseF but not its action. Anti-idiotypic antibody directed against either the T cell receptor or the T3ϵ chain could abrogate functional activity. Since TseF bears no T3 phenotypic marker, the results suggest that the factor works through transmembrane signal induction. It is also of interest that TseF can be recovered from T suppressor cells obtained from chronically infected animals, which show small granulomas. Little TseF is made during the acute phase of infection when granulomas are large and dominated by T helper cells.

Additional studies have indicated that TseF is the result of the action of a second, inducting lymphokine, TsiF (T suppressor-inducer factor) which acts upon an L3T4$^+$, 14-30$^+$ T cell. TsiF does not directly suppress but induces the formation of the TseF. TsiF is also a non-immunoglobulin heterodimer composed of an α and a β chain. TsiF shows many of the same characteristics of TseF. The molecule can induce the production of TseF only if L3T4$^+$ cells which produce the TseF are genetically compatible with the cells which produced the TsiF. The TseF which is produced demonstrates the same antigenic specificity as the TsiF. Several characteristics of TseF and TsiF are summarized in the accompanying Table I. When α and β chains from TseF and TsiF are recombined, the β chain determines the functional activity of the molecule.

Additional studies have demonstrated that the addition of TseF to antigen reactive cells results in a decreased expression of the IL-2 high affinity receptor by heterogenous and cloned L3T4$^+$ target cells. These changes are associated with subsequent decreased amounts of IL-2 and interferon-γ production. TseF does not effect IL-4 or IL-5 production. These changes are associated with a decreased accumulation of activated IL-2R$^+$, L3T4$^+$ antigen reactive T lymphocytes at the site of initial granuloma formation and by subsequent diminution of the recruitment of the other cell populations and OH-proline incorporation into collagenase sensitive protein (Figure 6).

Table I: Comparison of TsiF and TseF

	TsiF	TseF
General Structure	Disulfide Bonded Heterodimer M.W. 68-72 KD	Disulfide Bonded Heterodimer 68-72 KD
Source	L3T4^{+}, IL-2R^{+}	L3T4^{-}, Lyt-2$^{\pm}$, IL-2R^{+}
Alpha Chain	Bears Antigenic Receptor and 14-12 Determinant Imparts Antigenic Specificity	Bears Antigenic Receptor Imparts Antigenic Specificity
Beta Chain	Bears IJ, TCR Determinants Determines Suppressor Inducer Mode	Bears IJ, TCR, 14-30 Determinants Determines Suppressor Effector Mode
IL-2 Interaction	Prevents Production not Effect	Synergystic Action
Mode of Action	Direct Transmembrane Signaling Induction of TseF	No effect on Antigen Direct Transmembrane Signaling Recognition Induction of Differentiation Protein Kinase C Induction

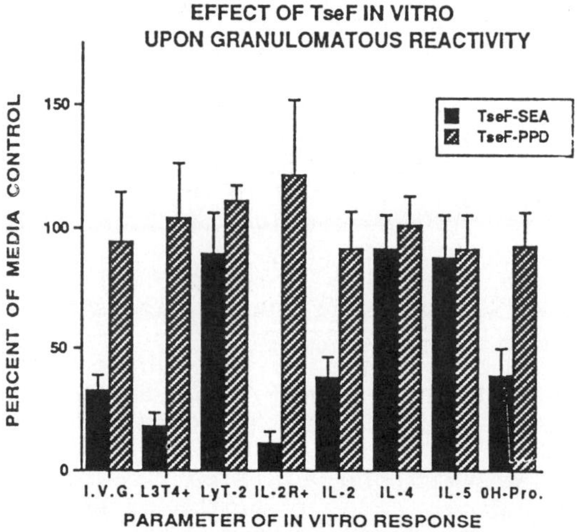

Figure 6: TseF was added to *in vitro* granuloma cultures and assessed for the effects on a variety of immune parameters. In comparison to control media, TseF decreased numbers of activated T helper cells at the site of lesion as well as other measurements of cell recruitment and activation.

Our more recent studies have addressed the mechanisms whereby TseF and TsiF suppress functional immune responses, i.e. the consequence of altered membrane signal transduction. Although antigen mediated blast transformation by lymphoid cells derived from actively infected animals is high, both glutathione (GSH) and ornithine decarboxylase (ODC) levels are only marginally elevated. Conversely, the proliferative response to antigen by cells derived from chronically infected animals is less than that of cells derived from acutely infected animals but associated with higher levels of ODC and glutathione. These results suggested that cells derived from chronically infected animals are in a non-reactive state of increased differentiation (Table II).

Table II

GSH and ODC Levels in Lymphocytes
Derived from Acutely and Chronically Infected Animals

Cells[a]	Stimulation[b]	Parameter[c] GSH	ODC	AMBT	IVGF
N	KLH	1.24±0.04	5±4	0.52±0.06	1.23±0.07
A	KLH	1.36±0.06	11±3	2.01±0.09	1.34±0.12
C	KLH	1.49±0.03	15±4	1.74±0.84	1.26±0.05
N	SEA	1.64±0.14	7±2	0.64±0.09	1.25±0.10
A	SEA	3.57±0.28	32±6	25.43±0.07	3.68±0.23
C	SEA	4.31±0.25	52±16	18.38±0.14	2.31±0.14

[a]Source of cells: N: Normal, unexposed animals. A: Acutely infected mice, 10 weeks post infection with 30 *Schistosoma mansoni* cercariae. C: Chronically infected mice, 25 weeks post infection with 30 *Schistosoma mansoni* cercariae.
[b]Studies were performed in the presence or absence of schistosome antigen (SEA) or a control Ag (KLH).
[c]Parameters assessed were intracellular glutathione (nm/10^7 cells), ornithine decarboxylase (pm/10^7 cells), antigen mediated blast transformation (CPM incorporated ^{3}H-TdRx10^{-3}), and IVG formation. In the IVG assay, antigen is covalently linked to polyacrylamide beads, serving as the nidus of the reaction.

Incubation of lymphocytes derived from acutely infected animals or defined T cell clones with TseF results in a marked increase in GSH and ODC levels. Since these molecules are elevated in chronic disease, they may be responsible for the differentiation and decreased morbidity associated with chronic disease states. The increase in ODC and GSH do not require antigen presenting cells indicating that TseF interacts directly with this target cell. Furthermore, TseF synergized with IL-2 to increase further ODC and GSH. These effects are independent of antigen mediated blast transformation, suggesting that increases in ODC and GSH induce cellular differentiation without effecting antigenic recognition (Table III).

Table III: Elevation of GSH and ODC Levels By TseF

Cells[a]	Stimulation	GSH	ODC	AMBT	IVGF
N	KLH	1.18±0.03	6±3	0.26±0.09	1.05±0.03
A	KLH	1.42±0.03	8±2	4.26±0.26	1.27±0.10
A	SEA	2.41±0.10	36±5	29.11±3.10	3.81±0.22
A	SEA+TseF	3.57±0.08	149±23	27.64±2.66	2.28±0.12
A	KLH+TseF	3.01±0.20	66±16	1.67±0.04	1.21±0.03

[a]Source of cells: N: Normal, unexposed animals. A: Acutely infected mice, 10 weeks post infection with 30 *Schistosoma mansoni* cercariae.

[b]Studies were performed in the presence or absence of schistosome antigen (SEA) or a control antigen (KLH) in the presence or absence of SEA specific TseF.

[c]Parameters assessed were intracellular glutathione (nm/10^7 cells), ornithine decarboxylase (pm/10^7 cells), antigen mediated blast transformation (CPM incorporated ^{3}H-TdRx10^{-3}), and IVG formation. In the IVG assay, antigen is covalently linked to polyacrylamide beads, serving as the nidus of the reaction.

These events ultimately are associated with increased protein kinase C dependent phosphorylation. Our recent ability to produce TsiF by a recombinant suppressor-inducer clone has opened the doors to the analysis of the true molecular basis of idiotypic regulation. This cloned factor demonstrates similar physical chemical characteristics to those of the naturally produced material, similar genetic and antigenic restriction, and *in vivo* activity.

In summary, granuloma formation and fibrosis is a highly regulated immune event, contingent on precise receptor ligand (anti-idiotypic) responses. Inflammation is produced by specific subsets of activated T lymphocytes and mediated by specific subsets of T suppressor cells and the soluble T cell analogs which they secrete. These T cell analogs augment differentiation but decrease function. Our current studies are directed toward the clonal expression of the suppressor substances and a definition of the preferential TCR genes utilized to regulate granulomatous hypersensitivity. A greater understanding of mechanisms of granuloma formation and fibrosis in schistosomiasis will provide important insights into a more general understanding of hepatic immunopathology.

Acknowledgement: The authors would like to thank Ms. Anne Barr for her terrific secretarial assistance and patience in preparing this manuscript.

REFERENCES

Abe, T., and Colley, D.G. (1984): Modulation of Schistosoma mansoni egg-induced granuloma formation. III. Evidence for an anti-idiotypic, I-J positive, I-J restricted soluble T suppressor factor. J. Immunol. 132:2084.

Bentley, A.G., Doughty, B.L., and Phillips, S.M. (1982): Ultrastructural analysis of the cellular response to Schistosomiasis mansoni. III. The in vitro granuloma. Am. J. Trop. Med. Hyg. 31:1168.

Bentley, A.G., Phillips, S.M., Kaner, R.J., Theodorides, V.J., Linette, G.P., and Doughty, B.L. (1985): In vitro delayed hypersensitivity granuloma formation: development of an antigen-conjugated bead model. J. Immunol. 134:4163.

Boros, D.L. (1989): Immunoregulatory mechanisms active in the suppression of the schistosome egg granuloma, in Basic mechanisms of granulomatous inflammation, T. Yoshida and M. Torisu, eds., Elsevier Science Publishers, B.V. (Biomedical Division), p. 143.

Chensue, S.W., Boros, D.L., and David, C.S. (1983): Regulation of granulomatous inflammation in murine schistosomiasis. II. T suppressor cell derived, I-C subregion-encoded soluble suppressor factor mediates regulation of lymphokine production. J. Exp. Med. 157:219.

Doughty, B.L., and Phillips, S.M. (1982): Delayed hypersensitivity granuloma formation around Schistosoma mansoni egg in vitro. I. Definition of the model. J. Immunol. 128:30.

Fidel, P.L., and Boros, D.L. (1991): Regulation of granulomatous inflammation in murine schistosomiasis. V. Antigen-induced T cell derived suppressor factors down regulate proliferation and IL-2, but not IL-4 production by CD4+ cells. J. Immunol. 146:1941.

Kenneth, E. (1989): Contrasts in the control of schistosomiasis. Mem. Inst. Oswaloo Cruz 84(Suppl. 1):3.

Mathew, R.C., and Boros, D.L. (1986): Regulation of granulomatous inflammation in murine schistosomiasis. III. Recruitment of antigen-specific IJ+ suppressor cells of the granulomatous response by an IJ+ granulomatous response by an IJ+ soluble suppressor factor. J. Immunol. 136:1093.

Perrin, P.J., and Phillips, S.M. (1988): The molecular basis of granuloma formation in schistosomiasis. I. T cell derived regulatory factors. J. Immunol. 141:1717.

Perrin, P.J., and Phillips, S.M. (1989): The molecular basis of granuloma formation in schistosomiasis. III. In vivo effects of a T cell-derived suppressor effector factor and IL-2 on granuloma formation. J. Immunol. 143:649.

Perrin, P.J., Phillips, R.J., and Phillips, S.M. (1989): The molecular basis of granuloma formation in schistosomiasis. IV. T cell derived suppressor-inducer and suppressor-effector factor reactivities are regulated by a TCR β chain analog. Cell. Immunol. 124:345.

Perrin, P.J., Prystowsky, M.B., and Phillips, S.M. (1989): The molecular basis of granuloma formation in schistosomiasis. II. Analogies of a T suppressor effector factor to the T cell receptor. J. Immunol. 142:985.

Phillips, S.M., and Lammie, P.J. (1986): Immunopathology of granuloma formation and fibrosis in schistosomiasis. Parasitol. Today 2:296.
Phillips, S.M., Lin, J., Galal, N., Linette, G.P., Walker, D.J., and Perrin, P.J. (1990): The regulation of resistance to Schistosoma mansoni by auto-anti-idiotypic immunity. III. An analysis of effects on epitopic recognition, idiotypic expression, and anti-idiotypic reactivity at the clonal level. J. Immunol. 145:2272.
Ragheb, S., and Boros, D.L. (1989): Characterization of granuloma T lymphocyte function from Schistosoma mansoni-infected mice. J. Immunol. 142:3239.
Warren, K.S. (1961): The etiology of hepatosplenic schistosomiasis in mice. Am. J. Trop. Med. Hyg. 10:870.
World Health Organization (1985): The Control of Schistosomiasis, Technical Report Series No. 728, Geneva, Switzerland.

Résumé

La formation du granulome de la Schistosomiase ainsi que la fibrose sont le résultat d'un processus immunitaire complexe qui dépend des réponses de type récepteur/ligand (anti-idiotypique). L'inflammation est induite par l'intermédiaire des lymphocytes T activés et médiés par des cellules suppressives T et des analogues solubles T qu'elles sécrètent. Ces analogues cellulaires T ont une action positive sur la différenciation et négative sur les fonctions. Nos études actuelles s'intéressent à l'expression des substances suppressives et aux gènes préférentiels TCR servant à réguler l'hypersensitivité granulomateuse. Une meilleure compréhension de la formation du granulome et de la fibrogénèse dans la Schistosomiase permettra de mieux connaître l'immunopathologie du foie.

Cellular and Molecular Aspects of Cirrhosis. Eds B. Clément, A. Guillouzo. Colloque INSERM/John Libbey Eurotext Ltd. © 1992, Vol. 216, pp. 49-59

Regulation of liver acute phase genes by interleukin 6 and leukemia inhibitory factor

Gertrud Hocke, Mei-Zhen Cui, Georges Baffet, Raymond Fletcher, David Barry and Georg H. Fey

Department of Immunology, The Scripps Research Institute, La Jolla, California 92037, USA

SUMMARY

The acute phase proteins are a group of plasma proteins with greatly altered concentrations during acute and chronic inflammations in response to tissue injury and infections. They are produced by liver hepatocytes and provide protective functions for containment and elimination of the cause of damage. The acute phase genes are induced in the liver by the cytokines interleukin 1 (IL1), interleukin 6 (IL6), leukemia inhibitory factor (LIF), glucocorticoids and possibly other mediators of inflammation. They fall into two groups. Group 1 genes are mainly regulated by IL1 and combinations of IL1 and IL6, group 2 genes mainly by IL6, LIF and combinations of these agents. Induction of group 1 genes involves the nuclear transcription factor NF-IL6/IL6-DBP/LAP. The mechanism of induction of group 2 genes is different and the responsible nuclear factors are still unknown. The IL6-response element (IL6-RE) of the prototype group 2 gene, the rat α2-macroglobulin (α2M) gene, had previously been mapped. Here we mapped the LIF-response element (LIF-RE) of the rat α2M gene and showed it to be contained in or identical with the 18 base pair IL6-RE sequence. The same characteristic nuclear protein-DNA complex was observed between the IL6-RE/LIF-RE sequence and nuclear factors from IL6 or LIF-treated cells. The IL6 and LIF receptors are different, and therefore we concluded that the IL6 and LIF signal cascades converged at a common endpoint in hepatocytes. The rat LIF gene was cloned, sequenced and characterized, and LIF mRNA was detected in regenerating rat livers after partial hepatectomy, but not in control rat livers.

INTRODUCTION

The acute phase proteins and their induction by interleukin 6 in liver cells have recently been reviewed (Baumann & Gauldie, 1990; Heinrich *et al.*, 1990; Fey & Gauldie, 1990). The acute phase genes fall into two groups: group 1 genes are mainly regulated by IL1 and combinations of IL1 plus IL6; group 2 genes mainly by IL6 or LIF and by combinations of IL1 plus IL6 or IL1 plus IL6 plus glucocorticoids, or combinations including LIF (Baumann & Gauldie; 1990). The nuclear factor involved in mediating the cytokine response of group 1 genes, NF-IL6/IL6-DBP/LAP, has recently been cloned and characterized (Akira *et al.*, 1990; Descombes *et al.*, 1990; Poli *et al.*, 1990). The IL6-response element (IL6-RE) of the prototype rat liver acute phase gene, the α2-macroglobulin (α2M) gene, has also been mapped and characterized (Kunz ***et al.***, 1989; Ito ***et al.***, 1989; Hattori ***et al.***, 1990). It differs in sequence from the IL6-RE of group 1 genes, and the factors binding at the group 2 IL6-RE are distinct from NF-IL6/IL6-DBP/LAP (Brechner ***et al.***, 1991). LIF-response elements (LIF-RE's) of liver acute phase genes had so far not been identified and mapped. Here we demonstrate that the LIF-RE of the rat α2M gene is contained in and possibly identical with the 18 base pair (bp) sequence of its IL6-RE.

RESULTS

The IL6-response element of the rat α2M gene is located between -150 to -200 bp upstream of the transcription start site (Figure 1). The element consists of two regions, called the core- and core-homology regions, which are each approximately 18 bp long and constitute binding sites for nuclear factors, probably transcription factors. Mutagenesis and transfection studies revealed that the central hexanucleotides of these two regions are essential for protein binding and the transcriptional activation of the gene by IL6. These sequences, CTGGAAA and CTGGGAA are identical in 6/7 nucleotides and are referred to as the core-homology and core-sites, respectively. Multiple copies of the core region were sufficient to confer IL6-responsiveness to heterologous promoters that were not normally responsive to IL6 (Figures 3,4 below). Sequences closely related to the core-site have also been detected in other rat liver acute phase genes and have been shown to mediate the IL6-response of those genes (Won & Baumann, 1990; Wilson ***et al.***, 1990).

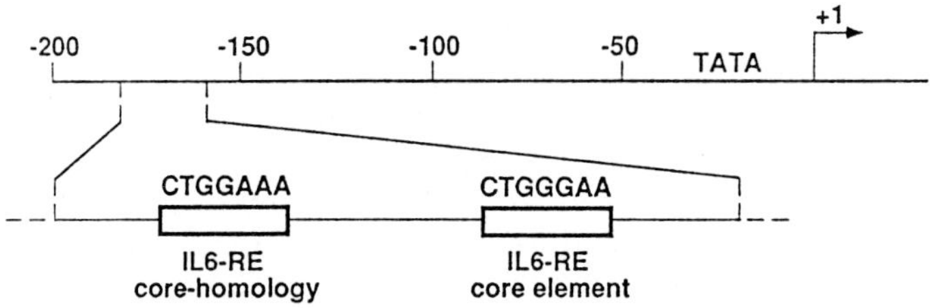

Figure 1. The IL6-RE of the rat α2M gene consists of two subelements. TATA, TATA-box, +1, transcription start site.

Nuclear protein extracts from normal and acute phase rat livers (Figure 2, tracks 1 and 2) were allowed to react with a radiolabeled, double-stranded synthetic oligonucleotide probe that represented two tandem copies of the 18 bp core region. This probe called TB2 was designed to maintain the same 20 bp distance between the two sites as in the native α2M gene between the core and core-homology sites. A characteristic protein DNA complex induced under acute phase conditions was obtained in gel mobility shift experiments (Figure 2, complex II). A complex of identical mobility was also observed with nuclear protein extracts from IL6-treated Hep3B human hepatoma cells, but not from control cultures (Figure 2, tracks 3 and 4). The kinetics of induction of this complex was compatible with the hypothesis that this complex may also occur *in vivo* and play a functional role in the induction of this gene by IL6, both in rat and human liver cells. This complex was specific for the core sequence as shown by competition gel mobility shift experiments using appropriate wildtype and mutated oligonucleotides as competitors. The other complexes of lower mobility did not show the same competition behavior, and thus probably represented non-specific protein DNA complexes. Complex II was also induced by IL6 treatment of FAO rat hepatoma cells and the IL6-responsive human lymphoid cell lines CESS and U266, but not of the IL6-non-responsive lymphoid cell lines Raji and Namalwa. Complex II was the only complex that was consistently observed with nuclear protein extracts from different IL6-responsive cell lines of the same species (humans) and IL6-responsive liver-derived cultures from different species (rats, humans) as well as primary rat livers. All the properties known so far for this com-

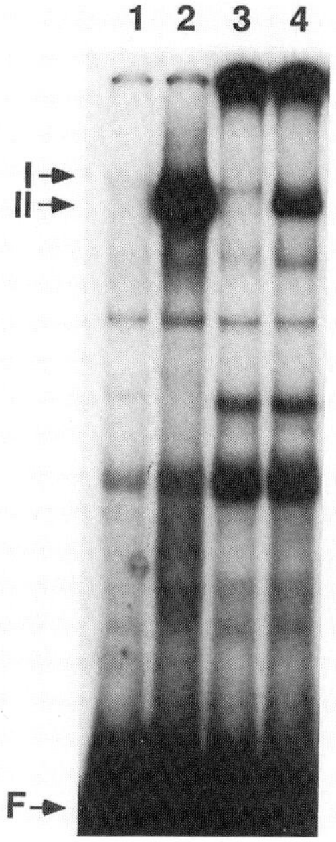

Figure 2. Acute phase conditions and IL6 induce a characteristic protein-DNA complex. The double stranded, end-labeled oligonucleotide probe TB2 (Brechner *et al.*, 1991) represented two tandem copies of the 18 bp core-region. F=free probe, II=specifically induced protein DNA-complex; complex II. Rat liver nuclear extracts from untreated and acute phase rats (tracks 1 and 2) and untreated and IL6-treated human Hep3B hepatoma cells (tracks 3,4) were reacted with this probe.

plex suggest very strongly that it plays a role in gene activation by IL6. However, the proteins that assemble complex II, have not yet been purified and cloned, and therefore it is not yet possible to make definitive statements about their functions as transcriptional regulators. Additional studies (Brechner *et al.*, 1991) have shown that most likely the same or very similar proteins bind at the two sites, and that both sites were occupied in complex II. Binding was cooperative, and the core site was the stronger binding site than the core homology site. Complex II was also obtained with DNA fragments containing the native configuration of one core-site and one core-homology site, but complexes of the same mobility and greater intensity were obtained with synthetic oligonucleotides such as TB2 that contained two tandem copies of the stronger core-site. Additional studies demonstrated that the proteins contained in complex II were distinct from the known transcription factors NF-κB and NF-IL6/IL6-DBP/LAP as well as DBP1, another member of the C/EBP-family of factors. Thus, while group 1 acute phase genes apparently are mainly regulated by IL6 through the factor NF-IL6, group 2 genes are regulated through an element differing in sequence from the consensus binding site for

NF-IL6 and a different factor. Therefore, the same cytokine, IL6, can activate different subsets of genes in liver cells by utilizing different target sequences and different nuclear proteins binding at these target sequences. Further studies demonstrated that the factor preexisted in liver cells, and probably required a cytokine-induced secondary modification to form complex II and to activate transcription. Appearance of complex II was prevented by blocking protein synthesis with cycloheximide. It is not clear whether complex formation was prevented because *de novo* synthesis of the factor itself or of a modifying activity or both were required.

Mapping the LIF-RE of the rat α2M gene. IL6 and LIF induce a similar spectrum of liver acute phase genes (Baumann & Gauldie, 1990) and have common effects on hemopoietic cells (Metcalf, 1989; Lord ***et al.***, 1991). Therefore, we suspected that they may act via a common response element and signalling mechanism, and attempted to map the LIF-RE of the rat α2M gene. For this purpose a series of constructs were already available from a previous study mapping the IL6-RE of this gene (Hattori ***et al.***, 1990). All constructs used the firefly luciferase coding sequence as the reporter gene. In a first series of transfection experiments constructs containing 5' flanking sequences from +17 to -1151 bp and +17 to -209 bp of the rat α2M gene, respectively, were transfected into FAO rat hepatoma and human HepG2 hepatoma cells. After treatment with IL6 or LIF, a strong induction was obtained with both constructs and both cytokines. The result suggested that a LIF-RE was contained in the 209 bp region upstream of the transcription start site. Additional constructs were prepared that contained one of three different minimal promoters driving the expression of the luciferase reporter gene: the promoters of thymidine kinase gene (TK), the simian virus 40 early gene (SV40e) and the rat α2M gene. In front

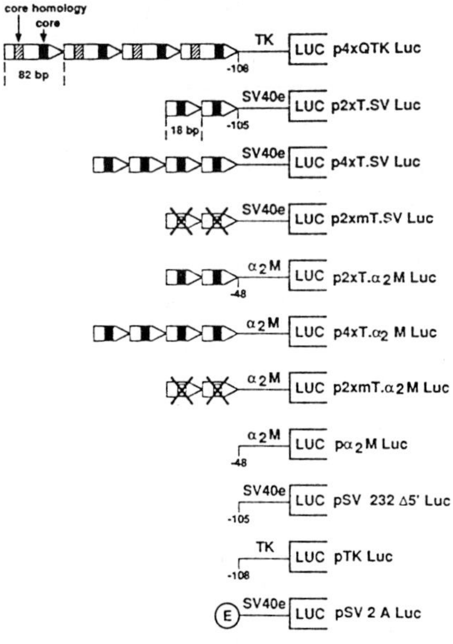

Figure 3. Constructs used to map the LIF-response element. Luc=coding sequence for the firefly luciferase gene. TK, α2M, SV40e=minimal promoters without upstream control elements; E=enhancer of the SV40 early gene.

of these minimal promoters were placed either 4 copies of an 82 bp gene fragment containing both the core- and core-homology regions in their native configuration (Figure 3, construct p4xQTKLuc); two or four tandem copies of the 18 bp core region (p2xT.SVLuc; p4xT.SVLuc; p2xT.α2MLuc; p4xT.α2MLuc); or two tandem copies of a mutated 18 bp core region (p2xmT.SVLuc; p2xmT.α2MLuc). This 6 bp substitution mutation of the core site had previously been shown to abolish the IL6-response of the IL6-RE (mutant m205; Hattori ***et al.***, 1990). As negative controls, constructs were prepared that carried only the minimal promoters without any added control-elements. The construct pSV2ALuc carrying the complete SV40 early promoter and enhancer was used as a positive, cytokine independent control. These constructs were transfected into HepG2 human hepatoma cells, and transient expression was allowed to develop overnight. One group of cultures was then treated with either IL6 or LIF, and a control group were mock-treated with buffer. At variable times after addition of the cytokines (0 to 36 hours), cell extracts were prepared and assayed for luciferase activity as a measure of cytokine-induced promoter activity. The following results were obtained (Table 1):

a) The 18 bp IL6-RE element comprised a LIF-response element. Two copies of this element driving the α2M gene's own minimal promoter in the construct p2xT.α2MLuc gave a 44.6 fold induction with IL6 and a 7.7 fold induction with LIF. Four tandem copies of the same element in the construct p4xT.α2MLuc resulted in a 187.3 fold induction by IL6 and a 37.9 fold induction by LIF. b) This 18 bp element functioned in combination with three different promoters: It conferred inducibility by both IL6 and LIF to the α2M gene's own minimal promoter, as well as to the SV40 early and herpes virus TK gene's minimal promoters. c) The hexanucleotide core of the element was essential for both the IL6 and LIF-responsiveness. When it was replaced by an unrelated hexanucleotide sequence that had previously been demonstrated to abolish its IL6-responsiveness, then LIF-responsiveness was also abolished (constructs p2xmT.α2MLuc and p2xmT.SVLuc, Table 1).

Table 1. The 18 bp IL6-RE contains the LIF-RE and confers IL6- and LIF-responsiveness to three different minimal promoters. a) Treatment with recombinant human LIF and IL6 was for 3 to 4 hours. Luciferase activities were measured with 200 mg protein extract in a standard luciferase assay. b) Relative inductions: activities obtained after treatment with the cytokine divided by the activity obtained after transfection of the same constructs in control cultures.

Construct transfected	Luciferase activity after treatment with			Relative Induction[b]	
	Medium alone	LIF[a]	IL6	LIF	IL6
p4xQ.TKLuc	519,232	1,536,514	2,858,572	3.0	5.5
p2xT.SVLuc	79,100	218,564	523,602	2.8	6.6
p2xmT.SVLuc	92,477	90,064	114,684	1.0	1.2
p4xT.SVLuc	261,866	1,083,518	2,434,943	4.1	9.3
p2xT.α2MLuc	7,234	55,477	322,938	7.7	44.6
p2xmT.α2MLuc	5,064	5,285	7,616	1.0	1.5
p4xT.α2MLuc	7,743	293,685	1,450,274	37.9	187.3
pα2MLuc	9,207	9,796	14,499	1.1	1.6
pSV232Δ5'Luc	103,247	111,534	122,361	1.1	1.2
pTKLuc	238,884	259,950	293,822	1.1	1.2
pSV2ALuc	19,777,802	18,964,833	23,483,519	1.0	1.2

From these data we concluded that a LIF-RE was contained within the 18 bp IL6-RE, and that this element was sufficient to confer LIF-responsiveness to heterologous promoters. These data do not yet allow us to claim that the LIF-RE sequence is identical with the IL6-RE, since saturation mutagenesis at all positions has not yet been performed. However, since the same hexanucleotide core was essential for the responses to both hormones, and since this hexanucleotide was also essential for sequence-specific protein binding, we believe that the IL6- and LIF-RE's of the α2M gene may in fact be identical. We do not yet know, whether the same or different proteins (nuclear transcription factors) bind at this element to mediate the IL6 and LIF-responses. However, the currently available data indicate that the same or very similar nuclear factors binding at this sequence may be responsible for its IL6- and LIF-controlled transcriptional inducer function.

Indistinguishable complex II - formation was induced by treatment of HepG2 cells with both IL6 and LIF. HepG2 cells were separately treated with either IL6 or LIF and nuclear protein extracts were prepared. These were then used to perform gel mobility shift experiments with a variety of probes, including the TB2 probe. Complexes II of indistinguishable mobilities were obtained from acute phase rat livers, from FAO rat hepatoma cells treated with either IL6 or LIF and from HepG2 human hepatoma cells treated with either IL6 or LIF. In addition, a complex II of indistinguishable mobility was also formed with nuclear protein extracts from a LIF-treated murine embryonal stem cell. These data suggested that either the same nuclear proteins or nuclear proteins of very similar molecular weights must bind at the 18 bp IL6-RE = LIF-RE after the cellular IL6 or LIF-signalling cascades have been triggered. Moreover, this factor is likely to be present in a wide range of LIF-responsive tissues, including liver cells, embryonal stem cells and others, and a wide range of species (humans, rats, mice). Therefore, this is probably a factor or a family of factors of widespread importance in the response to cytokines. It appears to be different from the so-far known general or cytokine-specific transcription factors.

Structure and expression of the rat LIF gene. The human and murine LIF cDNAs and genes had previously been cloned by others, and the expression of the LIF gene in various producer cell types has been studied (Gearing **et al.**, 1987; Gough **et al.**, 1988; Yamamori **et al.**, 1989; Gearing **et al.**, 1988; Moreau **et al.**, 1988; Lowe **et al.**, 1989; Stahl **et al.**, 1990). During the course of those studies it had become obvious that LIF and IL6 expression were induced in certain producer cell types by a similar set of signals, including lipopolysaccharides (LPS), IL1, and others. We had previously cloned the rat IL6 gene and discovered that rat IL6 was inducible in certain rat hepatoma cell lines by IL1 and LPS, and that this induction was prevented by glucocorticoids (Northemann **et al.**, 1989; Northemann **et al.**, 1991; Baffet **et al.**, 1991). Therefore, we decided to clone the rat LIF gene, to study its expression in hepatoma cells and macrophages, and to compare it with the expression of the IL6 gene in these cells. The long-range objective was to determine whether both genes contained in their control regions similar response elements for IL1, glucocorticoid and LPS-control, and whether rat hepatoma cells could provide a suitable model to unravel the elusive LPS signaling mechanism. The rat LIF gene was cloned and sequenced including a stretch of approximately 2.5 kilo base pairs of 5' flanking sequences that is expected to contain relevant control elements. We discovered that accumulation of LIF mRNA was stimulated by treatment with LPS in the rat hepatoma cell lines H5 and HTC, in primary cultures of peritoneal rat macrophages, in the rat macrophage derived cell line RM-SV1, and in the murine macrophage-derived cell line RAW 254.7. The stimulatory effect of LPS in the rat hepatoma cell lines was blocked to a significant extent by treatment with the synthetic glucocorticoid dexamethasone. Secretion of LIF protein by LPS-stimulated rat hepatoma cell lines was demonstrated by metabolic labeling with ^{35}S-methionine and immunoprecipitation with anti-rat LIF antibodies. These antibodies were raised in rabbits against a peptide deduced from the rat LIF coding sequence (Baffet *et al.*,1992). Thus, LIF mRNA and LIF-protein were expressed in hepa-toma cells after appropriate stimulation (IL1, LPS), but they were not expressed at detectable levels in normal adult rat livers. It is known that LIF as well as IL6 are expressed in many tumor-derived cell lines (Kishimoto, 1989; Gascan *et al.*, 1990), but it is not clear whether this expression in tumor-derived cell lines is part of the course or the consequence of their altered growth and differentiation properties. Although our findings showed that the LIF gene was inducible by LPS in hepatoma cells, we do not yet know whether it is also inducible by LPS in primary hepatocytes and what the physiological significance of such an induction might be, if any. However, the mechanism of induction of the LIF gene by LPS and its inhibition by glucocorticoids can now be studied in rat hepatoma cells, and this is a convenient system for such studies.

Finally, we have discovered the presence of LIF mRNA by Northern blot analysis in regenerating rat livers four hours after partial hepatectomy. No LIF mRNA was detected in control rat livers. Using the anti-rat LIF peptide antibody, preliminary evidence was also obtained for the presence of LIF antigen in regenerating rat liver, but not in control rat livers.

DISCUSSION

LIF is an interesting multifunctional cytokine with recognized effects on a wide variety of cell types. It derives its name from its characteristic ability to induce terminal differentiation of M1 murine myeloid leukemia cells and thereby to suppress their clonogenicity and self-renewal (for review see: Metcalf, 1989). LIF is also a differentiation inducing agent for cholinergic neurons (Yamamori *et al.*, 1989) and participates in the regulation of the normal development of hemopoietic cells (Metcalf, 1989b; Metcalf *et al.*, 1990) and mouse embryos (Conquet & Brulet, 1990; Murray *et al.*, 1990). In contrast to its differentiation-promoting effects on leukemia cells, hemopoietic cells and neurons and its induction of the acute phase genes in liver, LIF has the striking property of a growth-promoting and differentiation-inhibiting factor for embryonal stem cells (ES-cells) and ES-cell lines (Metcalf, 1989a; Moreau *et al.*, 1988; Williams *et al.*, 1988; Smith *et al.*, 1988; Pease *et al.*, 1990). In addition, LIF has other effects on bone resorption and lipid metabolism, and has therefore an unusually broad range of activities. It functions at the earliest stages of mammalian development and therefore is an exciting agent to study in fundamental biological research. At the other end of the spectrum of reasons generating interest in this molecule is its potentially useful property of preventing the proliferation of certain types of leukemia cells. Therefore, it is very important to study the intracellular signal cascade for LIF. Until now, not much was known about this cascade. The LIF receptor has recently been cloned and sequenced, and shown to be distinct from the IL6-receptor (Gearing *et al.*, 1991). It belongs into the same cytokine receptor super-family as the IL6 receptor, but the detailed cascade of intracellular events that follow the binding of ligand to the receptor is still completely unknown. Therefore, our discovery that the LIF-RE of the α2M gene is contained in its IL6-RE is significant because it shows that both cascades have one common endpoint. Apart from this mechanism, both IL6 and LIF may utilize additional other signalling mechanisms, but they share at least one common effect, the activation of the IL6-RE of the rat α2M gene. This provides us with a model system to study the LIF signalling cascade in biochemical detail because rat liver cells are available in sufficient supply for detailed biochemical studies. Our current efforts are directed at the purification and cloning of the IL6-response factor of the rat α2M gene, the protein that binds at the IL6-RE and participates in the formation of complex II. We will then attempt to answer the question, whether the same protein, or a similar but distinct protein constitutes the endpoint of the LIF cascade and mediates the LIF response through this 18 bp element.

Our discovery that LIF mRNA is expressed in regenerating rat liver but not in normal rat liver will be further explored. We will attempt to determine which cells produce LIF in regenerating rat livers, and whether LIF is the consequence or participates in the cause of liver regeneration.

ACKNOWLEDGEMENTS
This work was supported by research grants AI22166 and AI23351 from the National Institutes of Health to G.H.F. G.B. was supported by INSERM, the French National Institute for Science, Education and Medical Research, by the American Liver Foundation and the Philippe Foundation. G.H. was the recipient of postdoctoral research fellowships from the DAAD (German Academic Exchange Service) and the DFG (Deutsche Forschungsgemeinschaft). We thank the veterinary staff of the Scripps Division of Animal Resources and Gene Jensen for help with the VAX computer. The VAX facility was supported by our General Clinical Research Center's NIH grant MO1 RR00833. We thank Keith Dunn for expert help with the preparation of the manuscript. This is publication number 7105-IMM from the Department of Immunology, The Scripps Research Institute.

REFERENCES

Akira, S., Isshiki, H., Sugita, T., Tanabe, O., Kinoshita, S., Nishio, Y., Nakajima, T., Hirano, T. & Kishimoto, T. (1990): A nuclear factor for IL6 expression (NF-IL6) is a member of the C/EBP family. EMBO J. 9, 1897-1906.

Baffet, G., Braciak, T.A., Fletcher, R.G., Gauldie, J., Fey, G.H. & Northemann, W. (1991): Autocrine activity of interleukin 6 secreted by hepatocarcinoma cell lines. Mol. Biol. Med. 8, 141-156.

Baffet, G., Fletcher, R., Cui, M.-Z., Northemann, W. & Fey, G.H. (1992): Structure of the gene coding for rat leukemia inhibitory factor and its expression in hepatoma cells and macrophages. J. Biol. Chem., submitted.

Baumann, H. & Gauldie, J. (1990): Regulation of hepatic acute phase plasma protein genes by hepatocyte stimulating factors and other mediators of inflammation. Mol. Biol. Med. 7, 147-160.

Brechner, T., Hocke, G., Goel, A. & Fey, G.H. (1991): Interleukin 6 response factor binds cooperatively at two adjacent sites in the promoter upstream region of the rat α2-macroglobulin gene. Mol. Biol. Med. 8, in press.

Conquet, F. & Brulet, P. (1990): Developmental Expression of Myeloid Leukemia Inhibitory Factor Gene in Preimplantation Blastocysts and in Extraem-bryonic Tissue of Mouse Embryos. Mol. Cell. Biol. 10, 3801-3805.

Descombes, P. Chojkier, M., Lichtsteiner, S., Falvey, E. & Schibler, U. (1990): LAP, a novel member of the C/EBP gene family, encodes a liver-enriched transcriptional activator protein. Genes & Development 4, 1541-1551.

Fey, G.H. & Gauldie, J. (1990): The acute phase response of the liver in in-flammation. In *Progress in Liver Disease,* ed. H. Popper & F. Schaffner, pp. 89-116. Philadelphia: W.B. Saunders.

Gascan, H., Anegon, I., Praloran, V., Naulet, J., Godard, A., Souillou, J.-P. & Jacques, Y. (1990): Constitutive Production of Human Interleukin for DA Cells/Leukemia Inhibitory Factor by Human Tumor Cell Lines Derived from Various Tissues. J. Immunol. 144, 2592-2598.

Gearing, D.P., Gough, N.M., King, J.A., Hilton, D.J., Nicola, N.A., Simpson, R.J., Nice, E.C., Kelso, A. & Metcalf, D. (1987): Molecular Cloning and Expression of cDNA Encoding a Murine Myeloid Leukemia Inhibitory Factor (LIF). EMBO J. 6, 3995-4002.

Gearing, D.P., King, J.A. & Gough, N.N. (1988): Complete Sequence of Murine Myeloid Leukemia Inhibitory Factor. Nucl. Acids Res. 16, 9857.

Gearing, D.P., Thut, C.J., VandenBos, T., Gimpel, S.D., Delaney, P.B., King, J., Price, V., Cosman, D. & Beckmann, M.P. (1991): Leukemia Inhibitory Factor Receptor is Structurally Related to the IL6 Signal Transducer, gp130. EMBO J. 10, 2839-2848.

Gough, N.M., Gearing, D.P., King, J.A., Willson, T.A., Hilton, D.J., Nicola, N.A. & Metcalf, D. (1988): Molecular Cloning and Expression of the Human Homo-logue of the Murine Gene Encoding Myeloid Leukemia Inhibitory Factor. Proc. Natl. Acad. Sci. U.S.A. 85, 2623-2627.

Hattori, M., Abraham, L.J., Northemann, W. & Fey, G.H. (1990): Acute phase reaction induces a specific complex between hepatic nuclear proteins and the interleukin 6 response element of the rat α2-macroglobulin gene. Proc. Natl. Acad. Sci. U.S.A. 87, 2364-2368.

Heinrich, P.C., Castell, J.V. & Andus, T. (1990): Interleukin 6 and the acute phase response. Biochem. J. 265, 621-636.

Ito, T., Tanahashi, H., Misumi, Y. & Sakaki, Y. (1989): Nuclear factors interac-ting with an interleukin 6 response element of the rat α2-macroglobulin gene. Nucl. Acids Res. 17, 9425-9435.

Kishimoto, T. (1989): The biology of interleukin 6. Blood 74, 1-10.

Kunz, D.R., Zimmermann, R., Heisig, M. & Heinrich, P.C. (1989): Identification of the promoter sequences involved in the intreleukin 6 dependent expression of the rat α2-macroglobulin gene. Nucl. Acids Res. 17, 1121-1138.

Lord, K.A., Abdollahi, A., Thomas, S.M., DeMarco, M., Brugge, J.S., Hoffman-Liebermann, B. & Liebermann, D. (1991): Leukemia inhibitory factor and interleukin 6 trigger the same immediate early response, including tyrosine phosphorylation, upon induction of myeloid leukemia differentiation. Mol. Cell. Biol. 11, 4371-4379.

Lowe, D.G., Nunes, W., Bombara, M., McCabe, S., Rauges, G.E., Henzel, W., Tomida, M., Yamaoto-Yamaguchi, Y., Hozumi, M. & Goeddel, D.V. (1989): Genomic Cloning and Heterologous Expression of Human Differentiation Stimulating Factor. DNA 8, 351-359.

Metcalf, D. (1989a): The Molecular Control of Cell Division, Differentiation Commitment and Maturation in Hemopoietic Cells. Nature 339, 27-30.

Metcalf, D., Nicola, N.A. & Gearing, D.P. (1990): Effects of Injected Leukemia Inhibitory Factor on Hemopoietic and Other Tissue in Mice. Blood 76, 50-56.

Metcalf, D. (1989b): Actions and Interactions of G-CSF, LIF and IL6 on Normal and Leukemic Murine Cells. Leukemia 3, 349-355.

Moreau, J.F., Donaldson, D.D., Bennett, F., Wittek-Giannotti, J., Clark, S.C., & Wong, G.G. (1988): Leukemia Inhibitory Factor is Identical to the Myeloid Growth Factor Human Interleukin for DA Cells. Nature 336, 690-692.

Murray, R., Lee, F. & Chiu, C.-P. (1990): The Genes for Leukemia Inhibitory Factor and Interleukin6 are Expressed in Mouse Blastocysts Prior to the Onset of Hemopoiesis. Mol. Cell. Biol. 10, 4953-4956.

Northemann, W., Braciak, T.A., Hattori, M., Lee, F. & Fey, G.H. (1989): Structure of the rat interleukin 6 gene and its expression in macrophage-derived cells. J. Biol. Chem. 264, 16072-16082.

Northemann, W., Hattori, M., Baffet, G., Braciak, T.A., Fletcher, R.G., Abraham, L.J., Gauldie, J., Baumann, M. & Fey, G.H. (1990): Production of interleukin 6 by hepatoma cells, Mol. Biol. Med. 7, 273-286.

Pease, S., Braghetta, P., Gearing, D., Grail, D. & Williams, R.L. (1990): Isolation of Embryonic Stem (ES) Cells in Media Supplemented with Recombinant Leukemia Inhibitory Factor (LIF). Developmental Biol. 141, 344-352.

Poli, V., Mancini, F.P. & Cortese, R. (1990): IL6-DBP, a nuclear protein involved in interleukin 6 signal transduction, defines a new family of leucine zipper proteins related to C/EBP. Cell 63, 643-653.

Smith, A.G., Health, J.K., Donaldson, D.D., Wong, G.G., Moreau, J., Stahl, M. & Rogers, D. (1988): Inhibition of Pluripotential Embryonic Stem Cell Differentiation by Purified Polypeptides. Nature 336, 688-690.

Stahl, J., Gearing, D.P., Willson, T.A., Brown, M.A., King, J.A. & Gough, N.M. (1990): Structural Organization of the Genes for Murine and Human Leukemia Inhibitory Factor. J.Biol. Chem. 265, 8833-8841.

Williams, R.L., Hilton, D.J., Pease, S., Willson, T.A., Stewart, C.L., Gearing, D.P., Wagner, E.F., Metcalf, D., Nicola, N.A. & Gough, N.M. (1988): Myeloid leukemia inhibitory factor maintains the developmental potential of embryonic stem cells. Nature 336, 684-687.

Wilson, D.R., Juan, T.S.C., Wilde, M.D., Fey, G.H. & Darlington, G.J. (1990): A 58 basepair region of the human C3 gene confers synergistic inducibility by interleukin 1 and interleukin 6. Mol. Cell. Biol. 10, 6181-6191.

Won, K.A. & Baumann, H. (1990): The cytokine response element of the rat α1 acid glycoprotein gene is a complex of several interacting regulatory sequences. Mol. Cell. Biol. 10, 3965-3978.

Yamamori, T., Fukada, K., Aebersold, R., Korsching, S., Fann, M.-J. & Patterson, P. (1989): The cholinergic neuronal differentiation factor from heart cells is identical to leukemia inhibitory factor. Science 246, 1412-1416.

Résumé

Les protéines de la phase aigüe sont un ensemble de protéines plasmatiques dont les concentrations sont fortement modifiées durant l'inflammation aigüe et chronique en réponse à une lésion tissulaire ou à une infection. Elles sont produites par les hépatocytes et ont une fonction de protection afin de contenir et d'éliminer les agents responsables des dommages.

Les protéines de la phase aigüe sont induites dans le foie par les cytokines, telles l' Interleukine 1 (IL 1), l' Interleukine 6 (IL 6), le Leukemia Inhibitory Factor (LIF), les glucocorticoïdes et aussi probablement par d'autres médiateurs de l'inflammation. Elles se répartissent en deux groupes. Les gènes du groupe 1 sont principalement régulés par l'IL 1 seul et par l'association IL 1/IL 6. Les gènes du groupe 2 sont principalement régulés par l'IL 6, le LIF ou l'association de ces deux agents. L'induction des gènes du groupe 1 met en jeu le facteur de transcription NF-IL 6/IL 6-DBP/LAP. Le mécanisme d'induction des gènes du groupe 2 est différent et les facteurs nucléaires responsables toujours inconnus. L'élément de réponse à l'IL 6 (IL 6-RE) d'un gène "prototype" du groupe 2, l'alpha 2-macroglobuline de rat, a été identifié. Dans ce travail nous avons caractérisé l'élément de réponse au LIF (LIF-RE) et montré qu'il est contenu dans, ou identique à la séquence de 18 paires de bases de l'IL 6-RE. Le même complexe proteine nucléaire-ADN est observé entre IL 6-RE/LIF-RE et les facteurs nucléaires après induction par l'IL 6 ou le LIF. Les récepteurs IL 6 et LIF étant différents, nous pouvons donc conclure que dans l'hépatocyte, les cascades de signaux induits par l'IL 6 et le LIF convergent à un point commun final. Le gène LIF de rat a été cloné, séquencé, caractérisé et l'ARN messager du LIF a pu être détecté dans les foies de rat en régénération après hépatectomie partielle.

Cellular and Molecular Aspects of Cirrhosis. Eds B. Clément, A. Guillouzo. Colloque INSERM/John Libbey Eurotext Ltd. © 1992, Vol. 216, pp. 61-68

Expression of acute-phase proteins in cultured liver cells

André Guillouzo, Pascal Loyer, Ziad Abdel-Razak, François Delers *, Alain Fautrel and Christiane Guguen-Guillouzo

*INSERM U 49, Unité de Recherches Hépatologiques, Hôpital Pontchaillou, 35033 Rennes Cedex, and *Laboratoire des Protéines de la Réaction Inflammatoire, UER Biomédicale, 45, rue des Saints-Pères, 75006 Paris, France*

ABSTRACT

The development of *in vitro* methods that reproduce regulatory properties of the acute-phase liver has received major attention over the last years. Several hepatoma cell lines of both rat and human origin have been reported to regulate a spectrum of acute-phase plasma proteins ; they offer the avantages of continuous growth *in vitro* and of being phenotypically relatively stable. However, these cells invariably differ from the normal hepatocytes. The expression of certain genes has been silenced or their regulation has been modified. Moreover, the spectrum of expressed and regulated acute-phase proteins never coincides in independent cell lines.

Therefore many investigators have selected primary cultures of adult hepatocytes since these cells have nontransformed phenotype and can be obtained in large yields. A number of experiments have demonstrated that stimulation of a variety of acute-phase proteins can be accomplished in short-term conventional cultures using rodent hepatocytes. Similar conclusion has also recently raised from studies on human hepatocytes. Interleukin-6 stimulates a large spectrum of proteins while interleukin 1 and tumor necrosis factor α have a moderate effect on several acute-phase proteins. The two last cytokines inhibit fibrinogen synthesis in addition to the negative acute-phase proteins albumin and transferrin. Transforming growth factor β has also an inhibitory effect on albumin, fibrinogen, haptoglobin and increases fibronectin production.

Since the results obtained in short-term conventional cultures do not exactly reproduce the *in vivo* response, the use of more sophisticated culture conditions that preserve longer the normal phenotype can be more appropriate. When cocultured with another rat liver cell type, rat hepatocytes remain capable of secreting various proteins, including albumin, haptoglobin, hemopexin and transferrin at relatively constant rates for at least 3 weeks. Addition of a conditioned medium (CM) from lipopolysaccharide-activated human monocytes results in increased secretion of α_2-macroglobulin and α_1-acid glycoprotein and in decreased secretion of albumin and transferrin. CM treatment also alters the glycosylation pattern of α_1-glycoprotein. Such alterations are comparable with the inflammatory response *in vivo*.

INTRODUCTION

The acute-phase response is the answer of the organism to disturbances of its homeostasis. These disturbances can be due to infection, tissue injury, neoplastic growth or immunological disorders. The acute-phase response consists of a local reaction at the site of injury. This reaction results in activation of mononuclear cells and granulocytes which in turn release cytokines. In addition to leukocytes, activated fibroblasts and endothelial cells are able to produce cytokines. These mediators act on specific receptors on different target cells, leading to a systemic reaction (Heinrich et al., 1990). Among the target cells are hepatocytes which exhibit dramatic changes in the production of some plasma proteins designed as acute-phase proteins.

Species	Increase	No change	Decrease
Human	C-reactive protein (*) Serum amyloid A (*) α_1-acid glycoprotein α_1-antichymotrypsin Fibrinogen Haptoglobin	α_2-macroglobulin Hemopexin	Albumin Transferrin α_1-lipoprotein
Rat	α_2-macroglobulin (*) α_1-acid glycoprotein (*) Fibrinogen Haptoglobin Hemopexin	Serum amyloid P	Albumin Transferrin

(*) 10-100 fold increase

TABLE I : Response of some acute-phase plasma proteins in human and rat

Acute-phase protein patterns vary from one species to another (Table I). Thus C-reactive protein (CRP) and serum amyloid A show the highest increase in man whereas in the rat α_2-macroglobulin and α_1-acid glycoprotein exhibit the most spectacular changes. In many species plasma levels of fibrinogen, haptoglobin α_1-antitrypsin and α_1-antichymotrypsin increase during the acute-phase response. Simultaneously albumin and transferrin concentrations decrease. The major cytokines which stimulate synthesis of acute-phase proteins are interleukin-6 (IL-6), interleukin-1 (IL-1) and tumor necrosis factor α (TNF-α). Interleukin 6 induces the broadest range of proteins ; in man these include CRP, serum amyloid A, haptoglobin, fibrinogen, α_1-antitrypsin and α_1-antichymotrypsin. More recently leukemia inhibitory factor (LIF) and transforming growth factor β (TGF-β) have also been reported to affect the production of acute-phase proteins. It appears that although less potent on a molecular weight basis, LIF induces the same set of proteins as found with IL-6.

Over the last few years major progress has been made toward i) identification of the potential mediators of the liver regulation ; ii) - reproduction of the liver cell reaction *in vitro* and iii) - delineation of the cellular and molecular mechanisms by which the acute-phase protein genes are regulated (Baumann, 1989).

In vitro studies of the hepatic acute-phase response have been performed on both primary hepatocyte cultures and hepatoma cell lines. The focus of this review is to discuss their advantages and limitations as model systems to reproduce the *in vivo* acute-phase reaction.

I - THE CAPACITY OF NORMAL HEPATOCYTES AND HEPATOMA CELLS TO SECRETE PLASMA PROTEINS.

Hepatoma cell lines from both rodent and human origin have been widely used. Some of them express a broad range of proteins. However these cells invariably differ from normal hepatocytes (Table II). Moreover, the set of expressed proteins may vary between the subclones of a given hepatoma cell line. These limitations of tumoral cells explain why many investigators have preferred to use primary hepatocyte cultures. Indeed these cells have a nontransformed phenotype and can be obtained in large yields. When put in culture adult hepatocytes retain the ability to regulate most of the plasma protein genes. However, compared to the *in vivo* situation, both quantitative and qualitative variations are observed as soon as the first hours following cell seeding. They can be attributed to the trauma of initial culture adaptation resulting from cell dissociation and changes in structural and soluble external environment of the hepatocytes. Thus, CRP production is elevated during the first days then dramatically drops (Moshage et al., 1988, 1991 ; Loyer et al., unpublished observations). Alterations also affect the glycosylation pattern of glycoproteins which shows an inflammatory pattern (Le Breton et al., 1985).
Hepatocytes do not remain functionnally stable *in vitro* ; within a few days they exhibit marked phenotypic changes leading to a decrease or a loss of most liver-specific functions (Guguen-Guillouzo and Guillouzo, 1983). Early changes include production of both positive and negative acute-phase proteins. As an example we have reported that secretion rates of albumin, haptoglobin and α_2-macroglobulin are dramatically affected in rat hepatocytes after 3-4 days of culture (Figure 1) (Guillouzo et al., 1984). By contrast human hepatocytes are more stable. No marked variation was observed in haptoglobin and α_1-acid glycoprotein secretion levels over a 2 weeks period (Guillouzo et al., 1986).

Species	Hepatoma cell line	Major modifications of the phenotype
Rat	Reuber H_{35} cells - some subclones - FaO cells HTC cells	 No synthesis of albumin No synthesis of hemopexin Express only α_1-acid glycoprotein (sensitive to glucocorticoids)
Human	HepG2 cells PLC/PRF/5 cells	No synthesis of CRP Restricted set of plasma proteins but synthesis of CRP

TABLE II : **Some major modified properties of widely used rat and human hepatoma cell lines.**
These modifications are reviewed in Baumann (1989).

More sophisticated culture conditions have been devised that allow better preservation of liver specific functions over a prolonged period ; they include supplementation of the nutrient medium, with soluble factors such as hormones, growth factors and ligands, the use of organic substrates, e.g. matrigel and addition of other cell types in order to recreate specific cell-cell interactions (Guillouzo et al., 1990). Thus, when co-cultured with another liver cell type, rat hepatocytes remain capable of secreting various proteins, including albumin, haptoglobin, hemopexin, complement component C3 for at least three weeks (Guillouzo et al., 1984 ; Le Breton et al., 1985) (Figure 1). Alterations related to cell dissociation are observed as found in pure cultures but the glycosylation

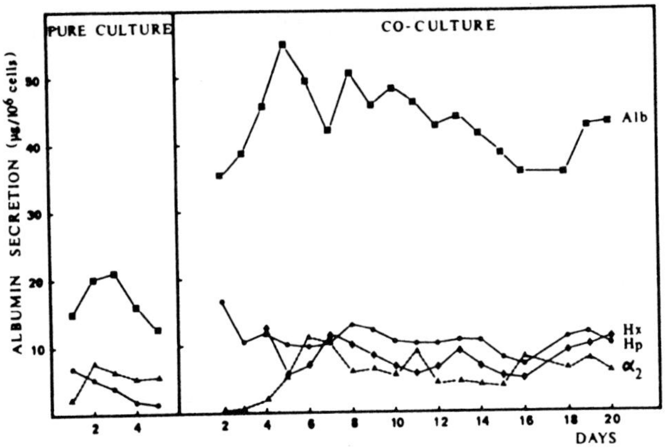

Figure 1 : **Secretion of plasma proteins in the medium of pure cultures and cocultures of adult rat hepatocytes.**
Amounts of albumin, haptoglobin, α_2-macroglobulin and hemopexin were determined by an electroimmunoassay. The values are expressed in µg/day/10^6 hepatocytes and are means of two independent experiments performed in duplicate. The number of attached hepatocytes was evaluated by measuring intracellular lactate dehydrogenase content before addition of rat liver epithelial cells. Cultures were maintained in serum-free medium (Taken from Guillouzo et al., 1984).

pattern of glycoproteins return to a normal one and reexpression of α_2-macroglobulin, although consistently observed, is lower than in standard culture conditions and remains constant over the coculture time. Its production could be due to the presence of high corticosteroid concentration in the medium (Guillouzo et al., 1984).

II - EFFECTS OF CYTOKINES ON THE ACUTE-PHASE RESPONSE IN VITRO.

Both hepatoma cells and normal hepatocytes have been shown to respond to cytokines. However, as for the basal expression of plasma proteins variations in the response to cytokines were found in different clones of a given hepatoma cell line (Baumann, 1989 ; Ganapathi et al., 1988 ; Sehgal, 1990). Wide variations have, for example, been reported among stocks of HepG3 cells (Ganapathi et al., 1988). Stimulation of acute-phase protein genes can be observed even when there are silenced in untreated cells (Baumann, 1989).
The maximum regulation of acute-phase proteins by cytokines being usually elicited within 24 h primary hepatocyte cultures are a suitable *in vitro* model. A number of studies have reported stimulation of acute-phase proteins in rodent hepatocyte cultures by IL-6, IL-1 and TNF-α when added either individually or as a mixture in a conditioned medium from human monocytes stimulated with bacterial lipopolysaccharides (Conner et al., 1990 ; Koj et al., 1987 ; Lin et al., 1990 ; Ramadori et al., 1985 ; Mortensen et al., 1988).
Thus in our laboratory we have studied the response of rat hepatocytes cocultured with rat liver epithelial cells to conditionned medium (CM) from liposaccharide-activated human peripheral blood monocytes by measuring the concentration of α_2-macroglobulin, α_1-acid glycoprotein, albumin and transferrin, as well as the changes in glycosylation of α_1-acid glycoprotein. In co-cultures treated with CM concentrations of α_2-macroglobulin, and α_1-acid glycoprotein were increased while those of albumin and

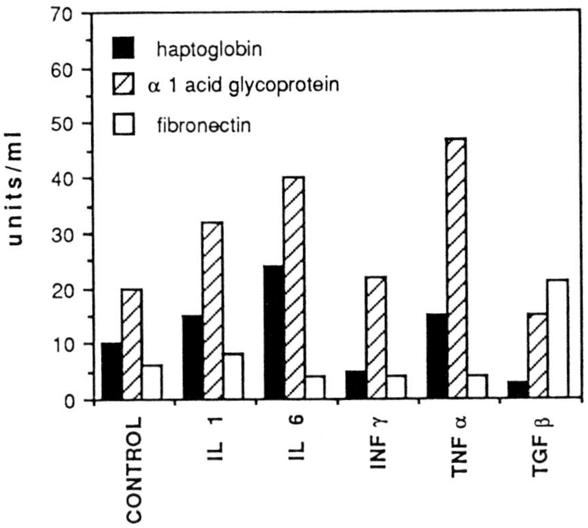

Figure 2 : **Effects of various cytokines on accumulation of haptoglobin, α_1-acid glycoprotein and fibronectin in the medium of adult human hepatocyte cultures.**
Hepatocyte monolayers were treated after 24 h with the indicated factors. After a 24 h stimulation the medium added with the cytokines was renewed and was collected after an additional 24 h. Cultures were treated with 100 U/ml IL-1, 500 U/ml IL-6, 100 ng/ml TNF-α, 50 U/ml or 2 ng/ml TGF-β. The proteins were measured by electroimmunoassay. The values are expressed as arbitrary units/ml of medim and are mean of two cultures.

transferrin were decreased. The glycosylation pattern of α_1-acid glycoprotein as shown by crossed immunoaffinity chromatograpy indicated an important relative increase of the concanavalin A-strongly-reactive variant upon treatment, as found during the acute-phase response. When CM addition was stopped the concentrations of the four proteins and the glycosylation pattern of α_1-acid glycoprotein reverted to those of control cultures. Resumption of CM treatment increased the secretion of α_2-macroglobulin and decreased that of albumin and transferrin (Conner et al., 1990).
By contrast only a few studies have dealt with adult human hepatocytes (Busso et al., 1990 ; Castell et al., 1988, 1989, 1990 ; Moshage et al., 1988) and are based either on only one cell population (Castell et al., 1989) or on typical experiment without information on interindividual variations (Moshage et al., 1988 ; Castell et al., 1990). Moshage et al (1988) have reported a stimulation of CRP and SAA production after exposure of human hepatocytes to IL-1 or IL-6 for 24 h. Castell et al. (1988, 1989, 1990) found that IL-6 but not IL-1 and TNF-α, exerted an induction of both CRP mRNA and CRP-protein levels in cultured human hepatocytes. Corticosteroids were not a prerequisite but when present modulated IL-6 effect in a dose-dependent manner. Concommitantly fibrinogen and α_1-antitrypsin levels were increased while those of albumin were markedly decreased. The direct effect of IL-6 was verified by adding a conditioned medium of Kupffer cells. No difference was observed suggesting that IL-6 did not act on hepatocytes via induction of other mediators in contaminant Kupffer cells. Similarly we have shown that rat liver epithelial cells did not alter the response of rat hepatocytes to cytokines in a coculture system (Conner et al., 1990). We have confirmed the stimulating effect on IL-6, IL-1 and TNF-α on other acute- phase proteins, namely hepatoglobin and α_1-acid-glycoprotein

(Figure 2) as well as that of IL-6 on fibrinogen (unpublished observations) in adult human hepatocyte cultures.

More recently another multifunctional molecule, TGF-β, secreted by mononuclear phagocytes and though to play a central role in inflammatory events was also proved to affect production of acute-phase proteins in cultured human liver cells. This molecule decreased both albumin mRNA content and albumin protein levels in human hepatocyte cultures (Busso et al., 1990). In addition TGF-β was found to decrease haptoglobin and α_1-acid glycoprotein production and to augment fibronectin (Figure 2). The inhibitory effect of TGF-β was confirmed in human hepatoma cells (Busso et al., 1990 ; Morrone et al., 1989 ; Mackiewitz et al., 1990) and in fetal human hepatocyte cultures (Bauer et al., 1991). Mackiewitz et al. (1990) also reported the absence of stimulation by TGF-β of haptoglobulin and α_1-acid-glycoprotein in HepG2 cells which did not express these two proteins in control conditions.

ACKNOWLEDGMENTS

We are indebted to Mrs A. Vannier for typing the manuscript. Personal work was supported by Institut National de la Santé et de la Recherche Médicale, Ministère de la Recherche et de la Technologie and Fondation de la Recherche Médicale Française

REFERENCES

Bauer, J., Lengyel, G., Thung, S., Jonas, U., Gerok, W. & Acs, G. (1991): Human fetal hepatocytes respond to inflammatory mediators and excrete bile. *Hepatology* 13, 1131-1141.

Baumann, H. (1989): Hepatic acute-phase reaction in vivo and in vitro. *In Vitro Cell Development. Biol.* 25, 115-126.

Busso, N., Chesné, C., Delers, F., Morel, F. & Guillouzo, A. (1990): Transforming growth-factor-β (TGF-β) inhibits albumin synthesis in normal human hepatocytes and in hepatoma HepG2 cells. *Biochem. Biophys. Res. Commun.*, 171, 647-654.

Castell, J.V., Gomez-Lechon, M., David, M., Hirano, T., Kishimoto, T. & Heinrich, P.C. (1988): Recombinant human interleukin-6 (IL-6/BSF-2/HSF) regulated the synthesis of acute-phase proteins in human hepatocytes. *FEBS Lett.* 232, 347-350.

Castell, J.V., Gomez-Lechon, M., David, M., Andus, T., Geiger, T., Trullenque, R., Fabra, R. & Heinrich, P.C. (1989): Interleukin-6 is the major regulator of acute-phase protein synthesis in adult human hepatocytes. *FEBS Lett.* 242, 237-239.

Castell, J.V., Gomez-Lechon, M.J., David, M., Fabra, R., Trullenque, R. & Heinrich, P.C. (1990): Acute-phase response of human hepatocytes : regulation of acute-phase protein synthesis by interleukin-6. *Hepatology* 12, 1179-1186.

Conner, J., Vallet-Collom, I., Daveau, M., Delers, F., Hiron, M., Lebreton, J.P. & Guillouzo, A. (1990): Acute-phase response induction in rat hepatocytes co-cultured with rat liver epithelial cells. *Biochem. J.* 266, 683-688.

Ganapathi, M.K., May, L.T., Schultz, D., Brabenec, A., Weinstein, J., Seghal P.B. & Kushner, I. (1988): Role of interleukin-6 in regulating synthesis of C-reactive protein and serum amyloid A in human hepatoma cell lines. *Biochem. Biophys. Res. Commun.* 157, 271-277.

Guguen-Guillouzo, C. & Guillouzo, A. (1983): Modulation of functional activities in cultured rat hepatocytes. *Mol. Cell Biochem.*53/54, 35-56.

Guillouzo, A., Delers, F., Baffet, G., Engler, R. & Guguen-Guillouzo, C. (1986): Production of acute-phase proteins by hepatocytes. In *Marker Proteins in Inflammation*, eds. J. Bienvenu, J.A. Grimaud, P. Laurent, vol. 3, pp. 253-259. New-York: Walter de Gruyter.

Guillouzo, A., Delers, F., Clément, B., Bernard, N. & Engler, R. (1984): Long-term production of acute-phase proteins by adult rat hepatocytes co-cultured with another liver cell type in serum-free medium. *Biochem. Biophys. Res. Commun.*, 120, 311-317.

Guillouzo, A., Morel, F., Ratanasavanh, D., Chesné, C. & Guillouzo, C. (1990): Long-term culture of functional hepatocytes. *Toxicol. In Vitro 4*, 415-427.

Heinrich, P.C., Castell, J.V. & Andus, T. (1990): Interleukin-6 and the acute-phase response. *Biochem. J.* 265, 621-636.

Koj, A., Kurdowska, A., Magielska-Zero, D., Rokita, H., Sipe, J.D., Dayer, J.M., Demezuk, S. & Gauldie, J. (1987): Limited effects of recombinant human and murine interleukin 1 and tumor necrosis factor on production of acute-phase proteins by cultured rat hepatocytes. *Biochem. Internat.* 14, 553-560.

Le Breton, J.P., Daveau, M., Hiron, M., Fontaine, M., Biou, M., Gilbert, D. & Guguen-Guillouzo, C. (1985): Long-term biosynthesis of complement component C3 and α_1-glycoprotein by adult rat hepatocytes in a co-culture system with an epithelial liver cell-type. *Biochem. J.*, 235, 421-427.

Lin, B.F., Ku N.O., Zahedi K., Whitehead A.S. & Mortensen R.F. (1990): IL-1 and IL-6 mediate increased production and synthesis by hepatocytes of aute-phase reactant mouse serum amyloid-P component (SAP). *Inflammation* 14, 297-313.

Mackiewitz, A., Ganapathi, M.K., Schultz, D., Brabenec, A., Weinstein, J., Kelley, M.F. & Kushner, I. (1990): Transforming growth factor β1 regulates production of acute-phase proteins. *Proc. Natl. Acad. Sci.* 87, 1491-1495.

Morrone, G., Cortese, R. & Sorrentino, V. (1989): Post-transcriptional control of negative acute-phase genes by transforming growth factor beta. *EMBO J.* 8, 3767-3771.

Mortensen, R.F., Shapiro, J., Lin, B.F., Douches, S. & Neta, R. (1988): Interaction of recombinant IL-1 and recombinant tumor necrosis factor in the induction of mouse acute-phase proteins. *J. Immunol.* 140, 2260-2666.

Moshage, H.J., Roelofs, H.M.J., Van Pelt, J.F., Hazenberg, B.P.C., Van Leeuwen, M.A., Limburg, P.C., Aarden, L.A. & Yap, S.H. (1988): The effect of interleukin-1, interleukin-6 and its relationship on the synthesis of serum amyloid A and C-reactive protein in primary cultures of adult human hepatocytes. *Biochem. Biophys. Res. Commun.* 155, 112-117.

Ramadori, G., Sipe, J.D., Dinarello, C.A., Mizel, S.B. & Colten, M.R. (1985): Pretranslational modulation of acute-phase hepatic protein synthesis by murine recombinant interleukin 1 (IL-1) and purified human IL-1. *J. Exp. Med.* 162, 930-942.

Sehgal, P.B. (1990): Interleukin-6 : A regulator of plasma protein gene expression in hepatic and non-hepatic tissues. *Mol. Biol. Med.* 7, 117-130.

Résumé

Les modèles *in vitro* capables de reproduire la stimulation des protéines de la phase aiguë au cours de la réaction inflammatoire ont, ces dernières années, suscité beaucoup d'intérêt. Certaines lignées d'hépatome d'homme ou de rat ont conservé la capacité d'exprimer et de réguler de nombreuses protéines de la phase aiguë ; elles offrent l'avantage d'avoir une croissance continue et de posséder un phénotype relativement stable. Néanmoins, elles diffèrent toujours des hépatocytes normaux. Certains gènes ne sont pas exprimés ou ne sont pas normalement régulés. De plus, les protéines exprimées sont différentes d'une lignée à l'autre.

Aussi, pour contourner ces difficultés, de nombreux auteurs ont choisi d'utiliser des cultures primaires d'hépatocytes. Ceux-ci peuvent être obtenus en grand nombre et ont un phénotype non transformé. Les protéines de la phase aiguë peuvent être stimulées dans des cultures à court terme d'hépatocytes de rongeurs ou d'homme. L'IL-6 agit sur un nombre élevé de protéines tandis que l'IL-1 et le TNF-α n'affectent qu'un nombre restreint. Ces deux dernières cytokines inhibent la production des protéines négatives de l'inflammation telles que l'albumine et la transferrine mais aussi celle du fibrinogène. Le TGF-β a également un effet inhibiteur sur l'albumine et le fibrinogène et augmente la production de fibronectine.

L'utilisation de conditions de culture plus sophistiquées permet un maintien prolongé d'un phénotype plus différencié. Lorsqu'ils sont cultivés avec des cellules épithéliales de foie de rat, les hépatocytes restent capables de sécréter des protéines plasmatiques à des taux élevés et relativement constants pendant 3 semaines ou plus. L'addition d'un milieu conditionné (CM) de monocytes humains activés par des liposaccharides bactériens provoque une augmentation de la sécrétion d'α_2-macroglobuline et d'α_1-glycoprotéine acide et une réduction de celle de l'albumine et de la transferrine. Les traitements par un milieu conditionné altèrent en outre le profil de glycosylation de l'α_1-glycoprotéine acide. De telles altérations sont comparables à celles observées *in vivo* au cours de la réaction inflammatoire.

Cellular and Molecular Aspects of Cirrhosis. Eds B. Clément, A. Guillouzo. Colloque INSERM/John Libbey Eurotext Ltd. © 1992, Vol. 216, pp. 69-75

Heterogeneity of the hepatic lobule : a valuable concept for the synthesis of plasma proteins

D. Bernuau, I. Tournier, L. Legrès, Y. Lamri and G. Feldmann

Laboratoire de Biologie Cellulaire, INSERM U 327, Faculté de Médecine Xavier Bichat, Paris, France

SUMMARY

The liver lobule represents the smallest structural unit of the liver. Functional heterogeneity among hepatocytes of the lobule has long been recognized for metabolic and enzymatic functions, leading to the concept of "metabolic zonation" within the lobule. Lobular functional heterogeneity with regard to plasma protein synthesis, an important function of hepatocytes, has been debated. Using the in situ hybridization and immunoperoxidase techniques, we have detected in situ the products of several plasma protein genes on rat liver sections. In the adult, although all hepatocytes are engaged in plasma protein synthesis, a zonal heterogeneity exists for the expression of albumin and 3 acute phase proteins, α_2-macroglobulin, α_1-inhibitor 3 and α_1-antitrypsin. Such heterogeneity is visible at the mRNA and/or protein level, with patterns specific to each gene. Modulation of the expression of the acute phase genes after a turpentine-induced acute inflammatory reaction takes place almost exclusively in the zones of the liver lobule expressing preferentially these genes in basal conditions. During liver development, the zonal heterogeneity for albumin gene is not visible before the first post-natal week, in parallel with maturation of the fetal liver. Moreover, transcriptional inactivation of the AFP gene during the first post-natal weeks seems to occur more rapidly in periportal hepatocytes than in the other lobular areas. These data suggest that functional lobular heterogeneity is a concept valuable not only for enzymatic or metabolic functions, but also to plasma protein synthesis.

The hepatic lobule represents the smallest functional unit of the liver. The lobule receives a dual blood supply, from the hepatic artery and the portal vein, both located into the portal space. The incoming blood drains into the central vein, at the center of the lobule. This unidirectional flow of blood through the lobule is thought to create gradients of oxygen and hormones along the porto-central distance. The hepatic lobule has thus been divided into 3 functional zones : a periportal zone, made of the hepatocytes around the portal vein, a pericentral zone including hepatocytes around the central vein, and an intermediate zone, in-between, the mediolobular zone .

It has long been recognized that hepatic metabolism differs in these 3 zones of the liver lobule, leading to the concept of metabolic zonation of the liver. Thus, periportal hepatocytes are involved in glucose release, urea synthesis, and hepatic oxidative energy metabolism, whereas the metabolic pathways involved in glucose uptake, glutamine synthesis and biotransformation have been localized to the pericentral zone(Jungermann & Katz, 1989). By contrast the existence of a lobular heterogeneity for plasma protein synthesis, one major function of hepatocytes, has remained unknown for many years.

It is well known that the liver is the main source of the majority of plasma proteins in the body. However, not all liver cells participate to the synthesis of plasma proteins. Hepatocytes, which represent about 78 % of the hepatic volume, are the main cells involved in this function. They synthesize virtually all plasma proteins, except immunoglobulins. Sinusoidal cells, which include endothelial cells and Kupffer cells, also produce small amounts of plasma proteins, such as α_1-antitrypsin, the retinol-binding protein, and factor VIII. Biliary cells do not synthesize any plasma proteins.

This review is focused on hepatocyte lobular heterogeneity for plasma protein synthesis, although it is quite possible that a lobular heterogeneity also exists for sinusoidal cells.

The first data supporting a lobular heterogeneity for plasma protein synthesis was the demonstration of an heterogeneous distribution of albumin mRNA in the normal rat liver, by in situ hybridization (Poliard *et al.*, 1986). Although all hepatocytes express albumin mRNA, the transcripts are more abundant in the periportal zone than in the pericentral zone. Similarly, immunostaining of albumin demonstrates the same zonal distribution of the protein. Since then, several studies have confirmed and extended these observations to several plasma proteins. With the exception of serum amyloid A, for which no lobular heterogeneity has been recorded (Meek *et al.*, 1989), the majority of plasma proteins studied so far display a lobular heterogeneity. The expression of plasma proteins within the lobule is not confined to a single compartment, as is often the case for enzyme activities. Rather, a gradient of expression over the entire porto-central distance is present. Albumin, α_2-macroglobulin and α_1-inhibitor 3 are predominantly expressed in the periportal zone, both at the mRNA and protein levels (Bernuau *et al.*, 1989). Fibrinogen and α_1-acid glycoprotein display also a predominant periportal pattern, at least at the protein level (Courtoy *et al.*, 1981). Alpha-fetoprotein (Poliard *et al.*,1986) and α_{2u}-macroglobulin (Mancini *et al.* 1991) mRNA and protein are found predominantly in the pericentral zones. The pattern of expression of α_1-antitrypsin is more complex. While the mRNA are homogeneously distributed within the lobule (Bernuau, *et al.* 1989)., the protein is more intensely stained in the pericentral zones (Lamri *et al.* , 1986, Bernuau *et al.*, 1989)

In order to get an insight into the mechanisms of lobular heterogeneity for plasma protein synthesis, we have looked at the expression of alpha-fetoprotein and albumin during the perinatal period, at a time when maturation of the fetal liver towards an adult architecture is taking place. Moreover during this period transcriptional inactivation of alpha-fetoprotein gene occurs, while transcription of albumin gene is at its maximum by the end of gestation. The fetal liver consists of irregularly arranged hepatocyte plates, which are several cells thick. At the end of gestation, both AFP mRNA and protein are homogeneously distributed within the liver. The same homogeneous distribution is observed for albumin (Poliard *et al.*, 1986). During the first post-natal week, hepatocyte plates become thinner and more regularly arranged from the portal space to the centrilobular vein. This is the period when lobular heterogeneity for AFP and ALB expression becomes first visible. As inhibition of AFP gene transcription proceeds, a gradual decrease of AFP mRNA is observed, but the lobular pericentral heterogeneity persists. By 3 weeks of post-natal life, a few cells expressing appreciable amounts of AFP mRNA are still visible around the pericentral vein, while all the remaining hepatocytes express a very small number of AFP transcripts. In the adult liver, there is a weak residual signal for AFP, but the pericentral heterogeneity is no longer visible. These results demonstrate that the development of the lobular heterogeneity for AFP and albumin is parallel with the maturation of the neonatal liver. During this period, changes in blood circulation, wich lead to the establishment of hormonal gradients , and changes in cellular contacts are known to occur.

Therefore, one can postulate that modulatory factors specific to each gene become preferentially expressed in some parts of the lobule. With respect to AFP gene localization, repression of the gene transcription is thought to be mediated by negative regulatory factors, and particularly steroid hormones. Among other mechanisms, it could be postulated that there is a higher amount of, or a higher sensitivity to these factors in the periportal zone, leading to a more rapid extinction of the gene in these areas.

In order to analyze the dynamics of plasma protein lobular heterogeneity in another situation, we have also investigated whether modulation of the expression of acute phase genes induced by an acute inflammatory reaction could modify the pattern of lobular expression of these genes. Two positive acute phase genes, α_2-macroglobulin and α_1-antitrypsin, and one negative acute phase gene, α_1-inhibitor 3 were studied. During acute inflammatory reaction in rat, α_2-macroglobulin and α_1-antitrypsin hepatic mRNA increase, while α_1-inhibitor 3 transcripts decrease. We observed in situ that at 24 h, the peak of the inflammatory reaction, α_2-macroglobulin mRNA increase significantly in the periportal and mediolobular zones, while no quantitative changes are observed in the pericentral zones, as compared with unstimulated liver ; the protein follows the same zonal pattern (Bernuau *et al.*, 1989). For α_1-inhibitor 3, an opposite modulation is observed in the periportal and mediolobular zones, while again the pericentral zone remains unchanged during inflammation. Stimulation of α_1-antitrypsin synthesis is reflected in situ by an increase in the number of mRNA in the 3 lobular zones, and by a disappearance of the preferential pericentral expression of the protein (Bernuau *et al.*, 1989). In summary, these results suggest that the environment of the periportal zone is more favorable to the basal expression of α_2-macroglobulin and α_1-inhibitor 3 than the pericentral area. They also demonstrate that modulation of the expression of the 2 genes induced by an acute inflammatory reaction takes place in the lobular areas where they are preferentially expressed in basal conditions. Signals for modulation of both genes during the acute inflammatory reaction appears to spread from the portal space to the pericentral zones. Thus, predominant expression of several acute phase genes in the periportal and mediolobular zones could be explained by the arrival of cytokines in the liver through the portal triads. One of these cytokines, interleukin 6, is now considered as the main inflammatory mediator controlling the expression of many acute phase genes (Fey & Gauldie, 1989,

Heinrich *et al.*, 1990) The distribution and activity of interleukin 6 receptors in the liver lobule remain unknown. Finally, α_1-antitrypsin expression within the lobule appears to be mediated by different molecular mechanisms. The factors involved in the regulation of lobular heterogeneity for plasma protein synthesis remain almost completely unknown. It is admitted that the regulation of plasma protein expression by hepatocytes *in vivo* is modulated by several factors. Circulating factors, such as hormones, cytokines or growth factors, are important modulators. Other factors include cellular communication between hepatocytes and the other liver cells, such as Kupffer cells, endothelial cells, or Ito cells, and interaction between hepatocytes and the extracellular matrix components. In this context, lobular heterogeneity for plasma protein synthesis could be explained by differences between the periportal and the pericentral environment of the liver lobule for the intrinsic capacity of hepatocytes to respond to circulating factors, or the composition of the extracellular matrix, or the phenotype and/or functional capacity of sinusoidal cells. There is no information available, up to now, on the distribution of cytokine, hormone or growth factor receptors in different areas of the liver lobule. The only available data concerns EGF receptor. It has been reported that the density of this receptor is higher on hepatocytes of the periportal area than in the other lobular zones. Whether differences exist between the periportal and the pericentral zone as concerns the composition of the extra-cellular matrix or the phenotype and/or functional activity of Kupffer cells and endothelial cells remains to be defined.

It is clear that many questions remain opened concerning the mechanisms of lobular heterogeneity. Clarification of these mechanisms will allow a better understanding of the pathobiology and consequences of zonal damage to the liver, such as for example, those occuring during the alcoholic liver disease, or during some toxic injuries.

REFERENCES

Bernuau, D.,*et al* (1989) : Heterogeneous lobular distribution of hepatocyte expressing acute-phase genes during the acute inflammatory reaction. *J. Exp. Med.* 170, 349-354.

Courtoy, P.J., *et al.* (1981) : Synchronous increase of four acute phase proteins synthesized by the same hepatocytes during the inflammatory reaction. A combined biochemical and morphologic kinetics study in the rat. *Lab. Invest.* 44, 105-115.

Fey, G. & Gauldie, J. (1989) : The acute phase of the liver in inflammation. In *Progress in liver diseases,* ed. H. Popper & F. Schaffner, vol IX, pp.89-116. Philadelphia : Saunders.

Heinrich, P.C., *et al.* (1990) : Interleukin-6 and the acute phase response. *Biochem. J.* 265, 621-636.

Jungermann, K., & Katz, N. (1989) : Functional specialization of different hepatocyte populations. *Physiol. Rev.* 69, 708-764.

Lamri, Y., *et al.* (1986) : Cellular and subcellular distribution of alpha-antitrypsin in the normal rat liver and during the acute inflammatory reaction. A light and electron microscopic study with peroxidase labelled antibodies. *Cell. Mol. Biol.* 32, 691-699.

Mancini, M.A., *et al.* (1991) : Age-dependent reversal of the lobular distribution of androgen-inducible α_2u-macroglobulin and androgen-repressible SMP-2 in rat liver. *J. Histochem. Cytochem.* 39, 401-405.

Meek, R.L., *et al* (1989) : Serum amyloid A in the mouse. Sites of uptake and mRNA expression. *Am. J. Pathol.* 135, 411-419.

Poliard, A. *et al.* (1986) : Cellular analysis by in situ hybridization and immunoperoxidase of alpha-fetoprotein and albumin gene expression in rat liver during the perinatal period. *J. Cell Biol.* 103, 777-786.

Résumé

Le lobule hépatique représente la plus petite unité structurale du foie. L'existence d'une hétérogénéité fonctionnelle des hépatocytes des différentes zones du lobule hépatique en ce qui concerne de nombreuses activités enzymatiques ou métaboliques a conduit au concept de "zonation métabolique" du foie. La question d'une possible hétérogénéité fonctionnelle lobulaire en ce qui concerne la synthèse de protéines plasmatiques a été longtemps débattue. A l'aide des techniques d'hybridation *in situ* et d'immunoperoxydase, nous avons détecté *in situ* les produits de plusieurs protéines plasmatiques dans des coupes de foie de rat. Chez l'adulte, bien que tous les hépatocytes soient engagés dans la synthèse des protéines plasmatiques, il existe une zonation d'expression de l'albumine et de 3 protéines de la phase aiguë, l'α_2-macroglobuline, l'α1-inhibiteur 3 et l'α_1-antitrypsine. Cette hétérogénéité est visible au niveau à la fois des ARNm et de la protéine, avec une topographie spécifique pour chaque gène. La modulation d'expression des gènes de la phase aiguë au cours d'une réaction inflammatoire aiguë se fait presque exclusivement dans les zones du lobule hépatique exprimant préférentiellement ces gènes à l'état basal. Au cours du développement du foie, l'hétérogénéité lobulaire d'expression du gène albumine n'apparait qu'au cours de la première semaine post-natale, parallèlement à la maturation du foie foetal. De plus, l'inhibition de transcription du gène alpha-foetoprotéine semble se faire plus rapidement dans les zones périportales. Ces observations suggèrent que le concept d'hétérogénéité fonctionnelle lobulaire s'applique non seulement aux fonctions métaboliques et enzymatiques, mais aussi à la synthèse des protéines plasmatiques.

Cellular and Molecular Aspects of Cirrhosis. Eds B. Clément, A. Guillouzo. Colloque INSERM/John Libbey Eurotext Ltd. © 1992, Vol. 216, pp. 77-80

Selenium induced liver damage : cirrhosis or nodular regenerative hyperplasia ?

P. Bioulac-Sage, L. Dubuisson, C. Bedin, P. Gonzalez and C. Balabaud

Laboratoire des Interactions Cellulaires, Université de Bordeaux II, 33076 Bordeaux Cedex, France

INTRODUCTION

Liver pathology of animals chronically exposed to selenium (Se) varies according to the species ; it can lead eventually to fibrosis, cirrhosis and tumor formation (Smith et al 1937, Nelson et al 1943). Examination of the livers of rats fed 4 ppm of Se for 2 months for the prevention of lipid peroxidation revealed the formation of nodules highly suggestive of nodular regenerative hyperplasia (NRH). NRH is a clinical condition characterized by diffuse micronodular transformation of the hepatic parenchyma without fibrosis septa between the nodules but with atrophic hepatocytes (Wanless 1990). The exact pathogenesis of NRH has not yet been established. It is however accepted that the common factor is an apparent heterogeneity of the blood supply with atrophy in the poorly supplied and hypertrophy in the well vascularized zone (Wanless et al 1980, Wanless 1990).Of the different mechanisms involved in these variations in blood supply, the obliteration of small portal veins has been the most documented (Wanless et al 1980). Other vessels damage has been suspected such as in veno-occlusive disease (Wanless et al 1980), in Budd-Chiari syndrome (De Sousa et al 1991), in peliosis (Cadranel et al 1990) and in arterial lesions (Solis-Herruzo et al 1986).To the best of our knowledge there is no animal model of NRH. The aim of this study was therefore to investigate whether Se intoxication could represent such a model.

MATERIAL AND METHODS

We used weaned male Sprague Dawley rats weighing 50 g . These rats were divided into 2 groups with a specific diet for each group. Group 1 was fed a control diet containing 0.4 ppm of Se, group 2 a 4 ppm Se enriched diet . Rats were sacrificed at 2 weeks, 1, 2 and 6 months . Liver function tests (total bilirubin, ASAT, ALAT, alkaline phosphatase, GGT) and liver histology were performed. The liver was routinely fixed for light microscopy (HES, reticulin and picro Sirius red), and part of a lobe was perfusion-fixed with 1.5 % glutaraldehyde : a) for light microscopy (on 1µm sections stained with toluidine blue) and b) for electron microscopy . Portal pressure was measured at 1, 2 and 6 months.

RESULTS

Growth. Rats from group 2 grew more slowly for the first 2 weeks but their growth then paralleled that of the control group. None died.

Liver function tests. These were in the control range except at 2 weeks when bilirubin was slightly elevated.

Portal pressure. There was a significant increase at 1 (9.28 ± 1.3 versus 6.2 ± 0.17cm H_2O), 2 (11.3 ± 0.74 versus 6.2± 0.36 cm H_2O), and 6 months (17.23 ± 1.73 versus 5.5 ± 0.38 cm H_2O)

Liver weight/body weight. This was mildly but significantly increased at 2 weeks (6.82 ± 1.28 versus 6.14 ± 0.41) and 2 months (3.65 ± 0.26 versus 3.31 ± 0.1)

Macroscopy. At 2 weeks and 1 month, one could observe reddish patches on the surface of the liver. At 2 and 6 months, the liver appeared macroscopically abnormal. In the most severe cases, atrophic micronodular reddish lobes coexisted with others which were hypertrophic with a slightly irregular surface. In the least severe cases, the surface was only slightly irregular.

Light microscopy. By light microscopy, lesions were heterogeneous from animal to animal, from lobe to lobe and from parts of a same lobe.

2 weeks. Sinusoids were congestive; lesions were, however, difficult to visualize on paraffin sections. On 1µm sections, the Disse space was often enlarged, and contained a few cells. In some cases the endothelial wall appeared to be detached from it (Fig. 1a).

1 month. In addition to the above lesions, there were areas of peliosis (more or less severe) (Fig. 1b).

2 and 6 months. *Atrophic lobes*. These could be divided into 2 areas: a peripheral nodular zone, with micronodules less than 3 mm in diameter, limited at their periphery by atrophic hepatocyte plates separated by a condensed reticulin network , corresponding to NRH, and a central atrophic zone, with an increased perisinusoidal network in between atrophic hepatocytes, containing numerous large portal tracts and hepatic veins (Fig.1 c, d). Portal veins, hepatic veins and arteries were normal.

In the nodules, hepatocytes appeared nearly normal, sometimes arranged in more than one cell-thick plates. The perisinusoidal network was very faint. At 6 months, damage was more pronounced than at 2 months.

Hypertrophic lobes and lobes with some macroscopic abnormalities. Liver histology was either relatively normal, or with some peliotic areas; however on reticulin staining one could see some zones of complete or incomplete NRH, often located at the periphery of the lobe. In non-nodular areas the reticulin network was slightly increased.

Electron microscopy

2 weeks , 1 month. The Disse space limited by a flattened sinusoidal membrane of hepatocytes was very much enlarged, particularly at 1 month, and contained extravasated cells such as red blood cells and a few macrophages (Fig. 1e). Sinusoids were often entirely or partially capillarized: endothelial cell processes had few or no fenestrae, and these could even be occluded by diaphragms. These cells with large overlapping processes sent out short digitations into the lumen. Some of these extensions formed a complicated network of channels and pouches; endothelial cells were surrounded by a continuous or almost continuous basement membrane, occasionally in several layers. Perisinusoidal cells had a well developed RER and cytoskeleton in their cell body and thin processes.

2 and 6 months. *Nodular areas*. In nodules the majority of sinusoids were normal without signs of capillarization. Quite often endothelial cells sent out processes in between hepatocytes.

In atrophic zones at the rim of nodules, numerous small capillarized sinusoids and portal vein sections could be seen in between atrophic hepatocytic plates.

Non-nodular areas. Sinusoidal damage was less marked than at 2 weeks or 1month but was of the same nature

DISCUSSION

Se administered to weaned rats at a dose 10 times higher than the recommended dose induces micronodular transformation of the liver without fibrotic septa between the nodules but with atrophic hepatocytes; it is associated with portal hypertension, normal liver function tests and normal liver weight/body weight. These lesions described by Smith et al in 1937 and by Nelson et al in 1943 have always been interpreted as cirrhosis. In fact they have the morphological characteristics of NRH and represent, to our knowledge, the first experimental model of this syndrome.

NRH is thought to be a secondary and non specific tissue adaptation to heterogeneous distribution of blood flow (Wanless et al 1980). In 80 % of cases, NRH is associated with histological evidence of portal vein thrombosis (Wanless et al 1980). Other vascular lesions have been reported in association with NRH such as arterial lesions, Budd Chiari syndrome, veno-occlusive disease and peliosis. It would thus seem that there are probably several mechanisms which can cause heterogeneity of blood flow.

In the Se model, no lesions were found on the portal vein, hepatic artery or hepatic vein. It is very possible that there is damage at the sinusoidal level. Electron microscopy at 2 weeks and 1 month, showed severe sinusoidal lesions such as capillarization and the presence of red blood cells in the Disse space. Drug-induced and hepatotoxins-induced NRH has also been reported for several drugs such as azathioprine (Haboubi et al 1988), and hepatotoxins including inorganic arsenic, copper sulfate, toxic oil (Solis-Herruzo et al. 1990).

Because a dose 10 times higher is obviously toxic for the liver and, perhaps, for other organs such as the nervous system, the safety margin is relatively narrow (Koller & Exon 1986). Until now Se toxicity has not been thought to play a role in human liver disease. It is however a major ecological problem in areas where the water has a high Se content, inducing severe liver damage, for example, in aquatic birds (Ohlendorf et al 1988) and fish (Sorensen et al 1983). Regenerative nodules have occasionally been reported in these birds (Ohlendorf et al 1988). Liver toxicity, from elevated liver enzymes (Baker et al 1989) to focal necrosis and congestion of sinusoids (Dafalla & Adam 1986) has also been reported in various species fed a high Se diet.

REFERENCES

Baker, D.C.J. et al. (1989): Toxicosis in pigs fed selenium-accumulating astragalus plant species or sodium selenate. Am J. V. Res. 50, 1396-1399.

Cadranel, L. J. F., et al. (1990): Nodular regenerative hyperplasia of the liver, peliosis hepatis and perisinusoidal fibrosis. Gastroenterology 99, 268-273.

Dafalla, R. & Adam, S.E.I. (1986): Effects of various levels of dietary selenium on hybro-type chicks.Vet. Hum. Toxicol. 28, 105-108.

De Sousa, J.M., et al. (1991): Nodular regenerative hyperplasia of the liver and the Budd-Chiari syndrome. J. Hepatol. 12, 28-35.

Haboubi, N. Y. et al. (1988): Role of endothelial cell injury in the spectrum of azathioprine-induced liver disease after renal transplant : light microscopy and ultrastructural observations. Am J Gastroenterol. 83, 256-261.

Koller, L.D. & Exon, J.H. (1986): The two faces of selenium - deficiency and toxicity - are similar in animal and man. Cancer J. Vet. 50 , 297-306.

Nelson, A.A., et al. (1943): Liver tumors following cirrhosis caused by selenium in rats. Cancer Res. 1943, 230-236.

Ohlendorf H.M., et al. : Selenium toxicosis in wild aquatic birds. J. Toxicol. Environ. Health 24, 67-92.

Smith, M. I., et al. (1937): The toxicity and pathology of selenium ; J. Pharm. Exper. Ther. 60, 449-471.

Solis-Herruzo, J. A., et al. (1986): Nodular regenerative hyperplasia of the liver associated with the toxic oil syndrome : report of five cases. Hepatology 6, 687-693.

Sorensen, E.M.B, et al. (1983): Histopathological changes in selenium-exposed fish. Amer. J. Forensic Medicine Pathology 4, 111-123.

Wanless, I.R., et al. (1980) Nodular regenerative hyperplasia of the liver in hematologic disorders : a possible response to obliterative portal venopathy. A morphometric study of nine cases with an hypothesis on the pathogenesis. Medicine 59, 367-379.

Wanless, I.R. (1990) Micronodular transformation (nodular regenerative hyperplasia) of the liver: a report of 64 cases among 2, 500 autopsies and a new classification of benign hepatocellular nodules. Hepatology 11, 787-797

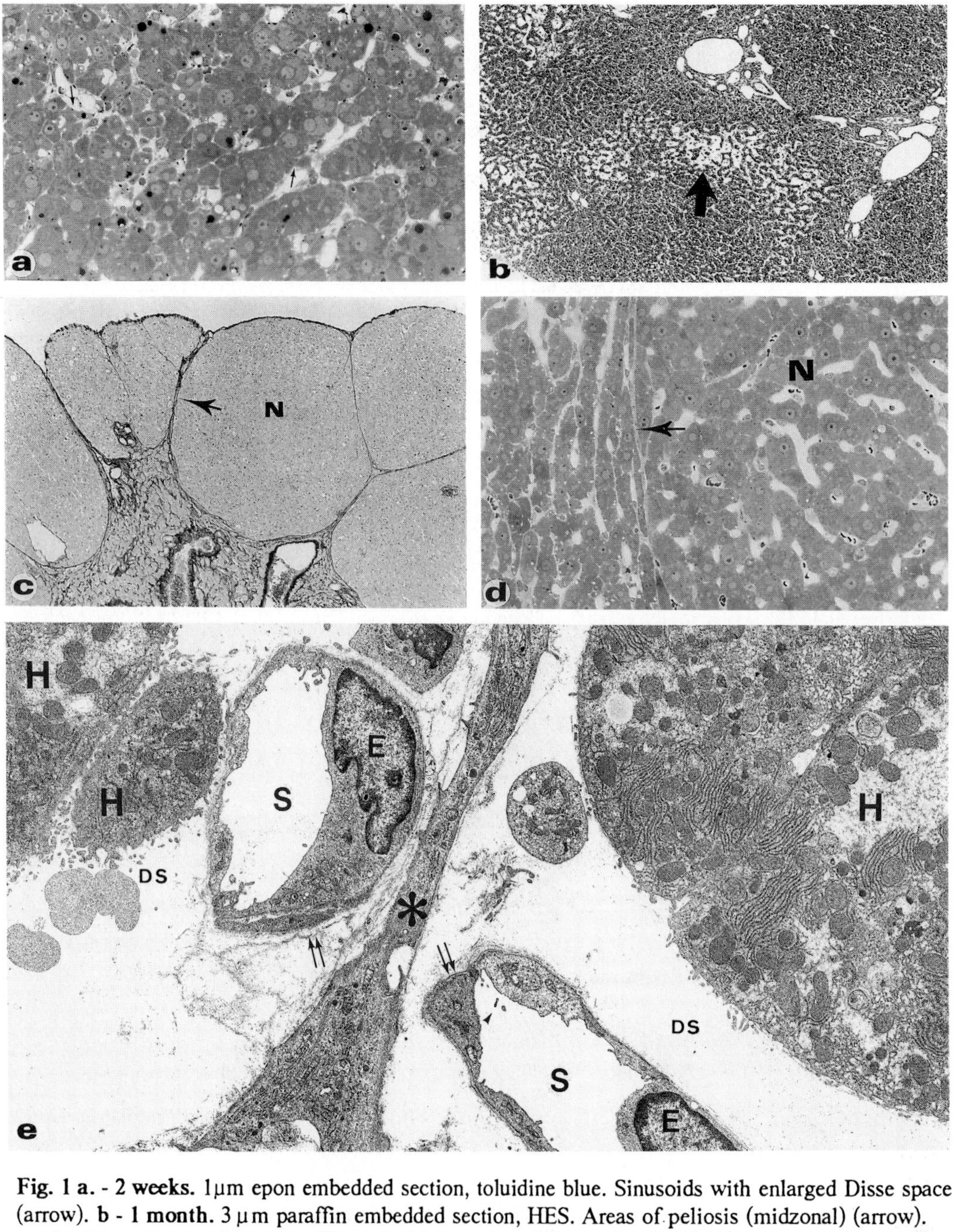

Fig. 1 a. - 2 weeks. $1 \mu m$ epon embedded section, toluidine blue. Sinusoids with enlarged Disse space (arrow). **b - 1 month.** $3 \mu m$ paraffin embedded section, HES. Areas of peliosis (midzonal) (arrow).
c , d - 6 months. c - $3 \mu m$ paraffin embedded section, Sirius red stain and **d** - $1 \mu m$ epon embedded section, toluidine blue. Nodules (N) are separated by bands of atrophic hepatocytes, very thin in **c** , clearly visible in **d** (arrow). The atrophic center of the lobe (**c**) contains large portal tracts.
e - 1 month. Electron microscopy. Parts of two capillarized sinusoids (S), separated by a perisinusoidal process (asterisk) seem to float in an enlarged Disse space (DS). H: hepatocyte; E: endothelial cell ; double arrow: basement membrane. **a:** x 200 ; **b:** x 35 ; **c:** x 35 ; **d:** x 160 ; **e:** x 4,600

Cellular and Molecular Aspects of Cirrhosis. Eds B. Clément, A. Guillouzo. Colloque INSERM/John Libbey Eurotext Ltd. © 1992, Vol. 216, pp. 81-84

Antioxidant activity of iron chelating agents on iron loaded hepatocyte cultures. Study of their free radical scavenging properties

Isabelle Morel (1), Josiane Cillard (1), Gérard Lescoat (2), Aydin Z. Ocaktan (3), Nicole Pasdeloup (2), Mohamed A. Abdallah (3), Pierre Brissot (2) and Pierre Cillard (1)

(1) Laboratoire de Biologie Cellulaire et de Botanique, UFR des Sciences Pharmaceutiques, 2, avenue du Pr. L. Bernard, 35043 Rennes Cedex; (2) Unité de Recherches Hépatologiques, INSERM U 49, Hôpital Pontchaillou, 35033 Rennes Cedex; (3) Laboratoire de Chimie Microbiologique, URA 31 CNRS, Institut de Chimie, Université Pasteur, 67008 Strasbourg Cedex, France

Ferric iron supplementation of rat hepatocyte cultures is known to induced lipid peroxidation, which has already been evaluated by free malondialdehyde (MDA) measurement, as an indice of cellular damage (Morel et al., 1990). The mechanism whereby iron stimulates lipid peroxidation seems to involve the intermediate formation of reactive oxygen species such as O_2^-, OH° and H_2O_2.

In the present study, the investigation of the protective effect of four iron chelators (deferoxamine: Desferal®: DFO; hydroxypyrid-4-ones: CP20 & CP22; pyoverdin A: Pyo A) was estimated according 3 points:

1- the reduction of lipid peroxidation

2- the chelating efficiency

3- the free radical scavenging activity

MATERIAL AND METHODS

-Hepatocyte supplementation :

Rat hepatocyte cultures were obtained as previously described (Guguen et al., 1975). Ferric iron was used under its complexed form with nitrilotriacetic acid (NTA). The hepatocytes were supplemented by 100 µM of Fe-NTA during 24 hours, with and without an iron chelator (DFO: 50 µM; CP 20, CP 22, Pyo A: 200 µM).

- Lipid peroxidation evaluation :

Free MDA measurement was performed at the end of the incubation using a size exclusion chromatography (HPLC) of ultrafiltrated samples (500 daltons) from culture media and cell lysates (Morel et al., 1990).

- Iron chelating activity :

The iron chelating activity was evaluated at various incubation times by following the level in culture media of low affinity iron complexes, representing iron non-specifically bound to transferrin, ferritin, or an iron chelator.The determination of these low affinity iron complexes was based on an HPLC procedure where an on-column derivatization took place (Singh et al., 1990).

- Free radical scavenging ability :

This property was tested on two models:

- *a cell free system* ,where the hydroxyl radical scavenging activity was investigated; OH° was generated by photolysis of H_2O_2 (0.3%, 88 µM) and spin-trapped by DMPO (36 mM) in the presence and in the absence of an iron chelator (DFO or Pyo A : 150 mM; CP22: 50 mM) as a potentially free radical scavenger, in comparison to ethanol (150 mM), a well established OH° scavenger. Spin adduct DMPO-OH° was evaluated using an HPLC procedure including an electrochemical detection (+400 mV)(Husain et al., 1987).

- *an hepatocyte model*: the MDA production was evaluated in the culture after 24 hours of supplementation with Fe-NTA (100 µM) in the presence of an iron chelator associated to a free radical scavenger (SOD : 500 IU/ml or Mannitol : 50 mM). This assay was performed in order to exhibit a possible addition or potentialization of the antilipoperoxidant activity of both agents.

RESULTS AND DISCUSSION

1- the reduction of lipid peroxidation

In comparison to the control cultures only supplemented with iron and representing 100% of MDA production, the presence of an iron chelator considerably reduced MDA level (table 1); the efficiency could be classified as follow: DFO>> CP 20 > CP 22 > Pyo A.

	Fe-NTA (100µM)				
	-	DFO	CP 20	CP 22	Pyo A
Free MDA (%)	100 ± 0	7.9 ± 0.7	14.1 ± 3.7	39.3 ± 8	53.9 ± 7.1

Table 1. Total free MDA production in cultures supplemented with Fe-NTA in the presence and in the absence of an iron chelator (DFO : 50 µM; CP 20, CP 22 or Pyo A : 200 µM). Results were expressed as mean ± SEM of 3 experiments.

2- the chelating efficiency

The study of the chelating activity showed that among the four agents tested, DFO appeared to be the farthermost efficient chelator (fig. 1). As early as the first 30 minutes of incubation, 100% of iron has desappeared under a complexed form in the presence of DFO, 58% with Pyo A and 0% with CP 20 & CP 22. It should be noted that at this same time in the cultures without any chelator, only 62.7 µM of low affinity iron complexes remained in the medium, suggesting that the other 37.3 µM already were inside the cells or bound to culture medium components.

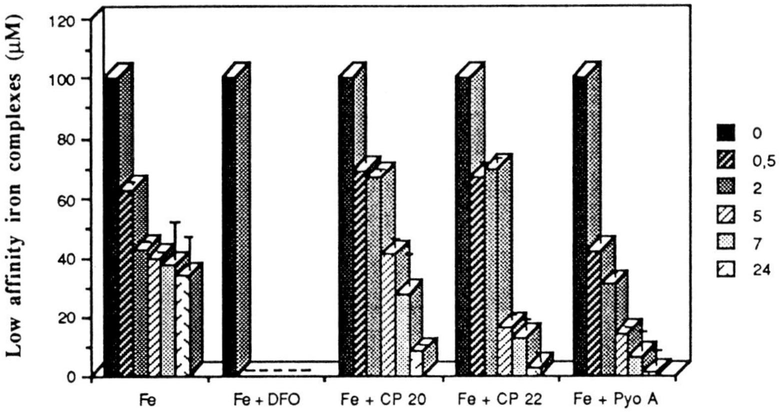

Fig. 1. Evolution with time of low affinity iron complexes in culture media supplemented with DFO (50 µM), CP 20, CP 22 or Pyo A (200 µM).

3- the free radical scavenging activity

- *on the cell-free system,* the three iron chelators tested (DFO, CP 22, Pyo A) revealed a good capacity to scavenge OH° as compared to the same concentration of ethanol, a well known OH° scavenger (fig.2). Moreover, CP 22 and Pyo A appeared to be more efficient than DFO.

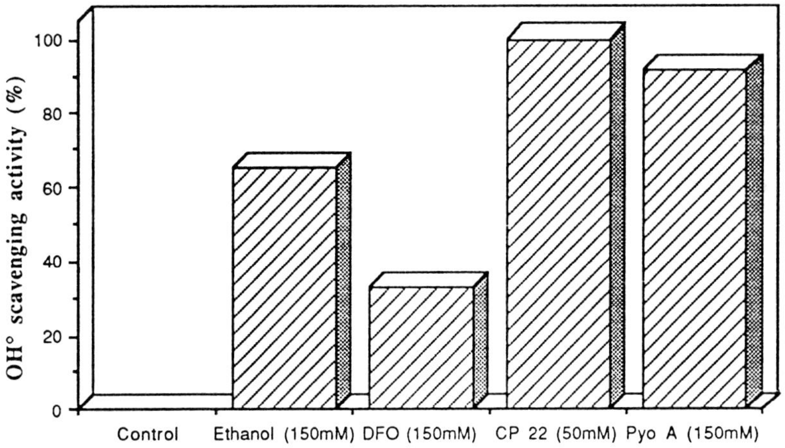

Fig. 2. Percentage of hydroxyl radical (OH°) scavenged by ethanol, DFO, CP 22 or Pyo A.

- *on an hepatocyte model;* the addition of a free radical scavenger (SOD or Mannitol) to the hepatocyte culture supplemented with iron and DFO or CP 22 had no significant influence on the free MDA level (fig. 3). This could be explained by a dual behavior of DFO and CP 22, acting simultaneously as iron chelators and as free radical scavengers. However, when the chelator was Pyo A , the combination with a free radical scavenger increased the reduction of MDA level, suggesting that the inhibitory mechanism on lipid peroxidation by Pyo A was represented more by its iron chelating property than by its free radical scavenging activity.

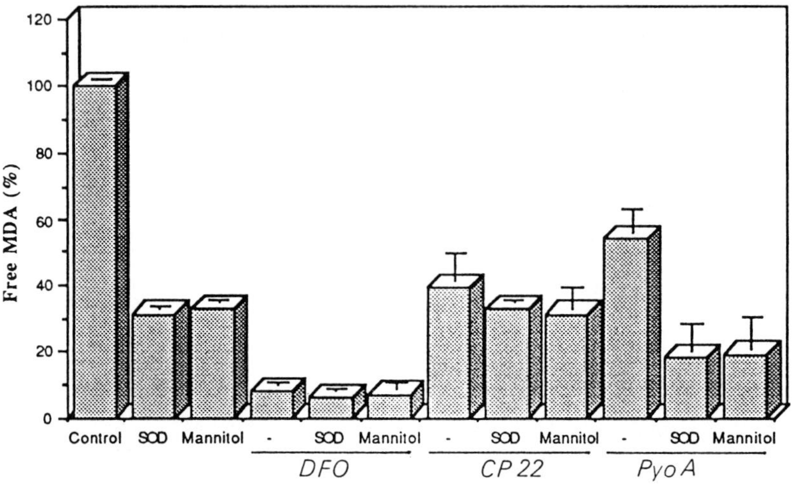

Fig. 3. Effect of the association of an iron chelator (DFO:50 μM; CP 22 or Pyo A: 200 μM) and a free radical scavenger (SOD : 500 IU/ml, Mannitol : 50 mM) on free MDA level in Fe-NTA (100 μM) supplemented hepatocyte cultures.

CONCLUSION

Each iron chelator tested was able to *reduce lipid peroxidation* in iron supplemented hepatocyte cultures with an efficiency classified as follow : DFO>> CP 20 > CP 22 > Pyo A. The high effectiveness of DFO could be assumed to its high *chelating activity* , whereas its *OH° scavenging efficiency* was lower than for the hydroxypyrid-4-ones (CP 20 - CP 22). This implied that both the chelating activity and the free radical scavenging capacity were involved in the reduction of lipid peroxidation ; however, each property seemed to be more or less influent according to the iron chelator considered : for CP 22, on the opposite to DFO and Pyo A, the antilipoperoxidant activity could mainly be represented by its free radical scavenging capability and poorly by its iron chelating effectiveness.

REFERENCES

Guguen C., Guillouzo A., Boisnard M., Le Cam A. and Bourel M. (1975): Etude ultrastructurale de monocouches d'hépatocytes de rat adulte cultivés en présence d'hémisuccinate d'hydrocortisone. Biol. Gastroenterol.8: 223-231.

Husain S.R., Cillard J. and Cillard P. (1987): Hydroxyl radical scavenging activity of flavonoids. Phytochem.26 : 2489-2491.

Morel I. , Lescoat G., Cillard J., Pasdeloup N., Brissot P. and Cillard P. (1990): Kinetic evaluation of free malondialdehyde and enzyme leakage as indices of iron damage in rat hepatocyte cultures. Biochem. Pharmacol.39: 1647-1655.

Singh S., Hider R.C. and Porter J.B. (1990): A direct method for quantification of non-transferrin bound iron (NTBI). Anal. Biochem.186, 320-323.

Cellular and Molecular Aspects of Cirrhosis. Eds B. Clément, A. Guillouzo. Colloque INSERM/John Libbey Eurotext Ltd. © 1992, Vol. 216, pp. 85-88

Inhibition of iron overload toxicity in rat hepatocyte cultures by desferrioxamine B and pyoverdin Pf, the siderophore of *Pseudomonas fluorescens*

Patrick Jego [1], Noëlla Hubert [1], Isabelle Morel [3], Nicole Pasdeloup [1], Aydin Z. Okactan [4], Mohamed Abdallah [4], Pierre Brissot [1,2] and Gérard Lescoat [1]

[1] Unité de Recherches Hépatologiques, INSERM U 49; [2] Clinique des Maladies du Foie, Hôpital Pontchaillou, 35033 Rennes Cedex; [3] Laboratoire de Biologie Cellulaire et de Botanique, Département de Pharmacologie, 2, avenue du Pr. L. Bernard, 35043 Rennes Cedex; [4] Laboratoire de Chimie Microbiologique, CNRS URA 31, Institut de Chimie, Université Louis Pasteur, 67008 Strasbourg Cedex, France

In genetic as well as secondary hemochromatosis, iron overload leads to hepatotoxicity. Desferrioxamine B (DFO), a siderophore isolated from *Streptomyces pilosus*, is currently used in case of secondary hemochromatosis because of its high specificity for Fe^{3+} and to its ability to achieve negative iron balance by removing iron under a non toxic form. However, DFO half-life is very short and this iron chelator is ineffective when administered orally. Thus, there is a need for a better iron chelator. The present work was undertaken to study the effect on iron overloaded rat hepatocyte cultures of one pyoverdin, a bacterial iron chelating agent isolated from *Pseudomonas fluorescens* (pyoverdin Pf). The pyoverdin Pf is a chromopeptide possessing three bidentate groups which bind iron (III) giving very stable octahedral complexes (K Assoc. = 10^{32}) (Demange et al., 1990 a,b).

Since the liver is the major target of iron overload toxicity, hepatocyte cultures have been used for assessing desferrioxamine B and pyoverdin Pf effects.

MATERIAL AND METHODS

Ferric nitrilotriacetate solution

The final concentration of ferric iron was 10 mM and the molar ratio nitrilotriacetic acid/ferric iron was 2/1.

Hepatocyte cultures

Rat hepatocytes were isolated from 2 month-old Sprague-Dawley male rats. For experimental purpose, the cultures were maintained in Multiwell plates for 24 hours in the control conditions, in the presence of iron alone or iron plus chelators at indicated concentrations. Iron or chelators were added on day 1 of culture ; the culture medium and the hepatocytes were collected on day 2.

Iron chelators

Desferrioxamine B (DFO) was purchased from Ciba-Geigy. Pyoverdin Pf was isolated from *Pseudomonas fluorescens*.

Enzyme assay

Lactate dehydrogenase (LDH) activity was measured in the culture medium and inside the hepatocytes as an index of toxicity, employing LDH kits (Roche) adapted to the Cobas - bio analyzer.

Protein assay

The total protein content per well was determined by the bio-rad protein assay using bovine serum albumin as standard.

Albumin assay

Albumin was quantified by immunonephelemetry.

Lipid peroxydation evaluation

Total free malondialdehyde (MDA) production was performed using a size exclusion chromatography (HPLC) of ultrafiltrated samples (500 Da) from culture media and cell lysates (Morel et al., 1990).

Statistics

Experimental values are means $\pm$ SEM. Significance was assessed using Student t-test at the level of 0.05.

RESULTS

Evaluation of iron toxicity in hepatocyte cultures

In the cultures maintained in the presence of iron concentrations ranging from 0 to 80 µM, a significant increase ($p < 0.001$) in LDH release was observed (Table 1). This release was accountable to a significant cellular decline ($p < 0.001$) in LDH activity (Table 1). Under similar conditions, albumin secretion was decreased ($p < 0.001$) as compared to the control (Table 1).

It appeared clearly that iron overload, particularly at the concentration of 80 µM was highly toxic for rat hepatocyte cultures. This toxic effect was also confirmed by the increase observed in total free MDA production of the cultures treated with 80 µM of iron ($p < 0.001$; Table 2).

Iron centration (μM)	Extracellular LDH (mIU/ml medium)	Intracellular LDH (mIU/mg protein)	Albumin secretion (μg/ml medium)
0	60 ± 15	3.8 ± 0.1	18 ± 2
5	122 ± 20	2.5 ± 0.2	14 ± 1.5
10	240 ± 21	2.6 ± 0.2	11 ± 2
20	418 ± 20	2.5 ± 0.2	10 ± 1.5
40	550 ± 35	2.3 ± 0.2	9 ± 1
80	715 ± 45	1.6. ± 0.2	9 ± 0.5

TABLE 1 : Extra- or intracellular level of LDH and albumin secretion in rat hepatocyte cultures maintained for 24 hours in the control conditions or in the presence of increasing concentrations of iron. Each experimental point is the mean ± SEM of quadruplicate cultures.

Experimental conditions	Total free MDA (ng/dish ; % of control)
C	100 ± 0
Fe	1379 ± 2
Fe + DFO	186 ± 11
Fe + Pf	91 ± 16

TABLE 2 : Total free MDA production in rat hepatocyte cultures maintained for 24 hours in the control conditions (C), in the presence of 80 μM of iron (Fe) or 80 μM of iron plus 100 μM of desferrioxamine B or pyoverdin Pf (Fe + DFO or Pf). Each experimental point is the mean ± SEM of triplicate cultures and is expressed in per cent of total free MDA measured in the control cultures.

Protective effect of desferrioxamine B and pyoverdin Pf

In the cultures treated with 80 μM of iron, a highly significant release ($p < 0.001$) of LDH was observed (Table 3).

This release due to iron overload was inhibited by 100 μM of DFO or pyoverdin Pf ($p < 0.001$; Table 3). This protective effect of DFO and pyoverdin Pf was concomitantly seen on the decrease in the albumin secretion ($p < 0.001$; Table 3) as well as on the total free MDA production ($p < 0.001$; Table 2).

Experimental conditions	Extracellular LDH (mIU/ml medium)	Albumin secretion (μg/ml medium)
C	33 ± 8	19 ± 3
Fe	538 ± 109	8 ± 1
Fe + DFO	34 ± 2	18 ± 4
Fe + Pf	47 ± 8	20 ± 3

TABLE 3 : Extracellular LDH and albumin secretion in rat hepatocyte cultures maintained for 24 hours in the control conditions (C), in the presence of 80 μM of iron (Fe) or 80 μM of iron plus 100 μM of desferrioxamine B or pyoverdin Pf (Fe + DFO or Pf). Each experimental point is the mean ± SEM of quadruplicate cultures.

DISCUSSION

The present study provides evidence that iron overload was toxic for adult rat hepatocyte cultures since the release of LDH in the culture medium was increased while its intracellular level was decreased. This toxicity was also confirmed by a decrease in albumin secretion and an increase in total free MDA production.

We have demonstrated that the toxic effect of iron overload in rat hepatocyte cultures was inhibited by desferrioxamine B. The present data shows also that pyoverdin Pf was as effective as desferrioxamine B in the protection of hepatocyte cultures against this toxic effect.

The mechanisms by which desferrioxamine B and pyoverdin Pf may act are very certainly related to their powerful ability to chelate iron. However, iron toxicity is known to be mediated by the induction of lipid peroxydation which involves formation of oxygene free radicals species such as hydroxyl radical or superoxyde anion (Dianzani, 1987). Desferrioxamine B can also inhibit iron toxicity by blocking the generation of these free radicals involved in tissue injury observed in human diseases (Halliwell, 1989).

In conclusion, the present data indicates that pyoverdin Pf is a valuable substance preventing iron toxicity in hepatocyte cultures.

REFERENCES

Demange, P., Bateman, A., Mertz, C., Dell, A., Piemont, Y., and Abdallah, M.A. (1990a) : Bacterial siderophores : the structure of pyoverdins Pt siderophores of *Pseudomonas tolaasii* NCPPB 2192 and pyoverdins Pf, siderophores of *Pseudomonas fluorescens* CCM 2798. Identification of an unusual natural amino acid. Biochemistry 46: 11057-11067.

Demange, P., Bateman, A., Macleod, J.K., Dell, A., and Abdallah, M.A. (1990b) : Bacterial siderophores : Unusual 3,4,5,6-tetrahydropyrimidine-based amino acids in pyoverdins from *Pseudomas fluorescens*. Tetrahedron Lett. 31: 7611-7614.

Dianzani, M.U. (1987): The role of free radicals in liver damage. Proc. Nutr. Soc. 46: 43-52.

Halliwell, B. (1989): Protection against tissue damage *in vivo* by desferrioxamine : What is its mechanism of action ? Free Radical Biol. Med. 7: 645-651.

Morel, I., Lescoat, G., Cillard, J., Pasdeloup, N., Brissot, P., and Cillard, P. (1990): Kinetic evaluation of free malondialdehyde and enzyme leakage as indices of iron damage in rat hepatocyte cultures. Biochem. Pharmacol. 39: 1647-1655.

Fibrogenesis

Fibrogenèse

Cellular and Molecular Aspects of Cirrhosis. Eds B. Clément, A. Guillouzo. Colloque INSERM/John Libbey Eurotext Ltd. © 1992, Vol. 216, pp. 91-101

Ultrastructure of sinusoids in human cirrhotic nodules

P. Bioulac-Sage, B. Le Bail, J. Carles, P. Bernard, G. Janvier, C. Brechenmacher, J. Saric, C. Balabaud and the PATH group

Laboratoire d'Anatomie Pathologique et Unité de Transplantation hépatique, Hôpital Pellegrin CHRU Bordeaux et Laboratoire des Interactions Cellulaires, Université de Bordeaux II, 33076 Bordeaux Cedex, France

SUMMARY

Livers from 21 patients transplanted for cirrhosis were studied. 1,5 % glutaraldehyde was perfused inside a single nodule, part of it was cut into small blocks and processed for electron microscopy. Although the morphology of sinusoids was rather heterogeneous, both within a single nodule and amongst different nodules, it appeared that some patterns could be identified: - **1** - normal sinusoids - **2** - capillarized sinusoids - **3** - sinusoids in inflammatory zones - **4** - sinusoids in regenerative areas; here, sinusoids could be normal or showed varying degrees of abnormality or presented signs of regeneration. Quite apart from this categorization, sinusoidal cells can present ultrastructural changes such as signs of endothelial cell damage, capillarization and regeneration. In view of this heterogeneity - true capillarization being a rare event, often limited to the periphery of the nodule - functional results should be interpreted with caution, particularly when morphology is taken as a strong argument to support a hypothesis (intact-hepatocyte theory, intrahepatic shunts, capillarization)

INTRODUCTION

The morphology of sinusoids in cirrhotic nodules has not been extensively studied (Bioulac-Sage et al 1988) for at least 3 reasons - **a** - the concept of capillarized sinusoids formed by Schaffner & Popper (1963) has been so widely accepted that it seems hazardous to take the risk of destroying a dogma - **b** - perfusion-fixation of sinusoids, essential for electron microscopic studies, is even more difficult in this than in any other pathological condition - **c** - there are so many different types of nodules (Millward-Sadler 1987) (variations in size, the degree of inflammation, necrosis, cholestasis, regeneration etc...) that it seems impossible to cover all the morphological aspects.

It is now widely accepted that sinusoidal cells and the matrix play a vital role in maintaining the normal homeostasis of the liver (Clement et al 1988, Rojkind & Greenwell 1988). It would thus seem appropriate to reevaluate the morphology of sinusoids and sinusoidal cells in a disease characterized by the breakdown of normal architecture and blood supply (Rappaport et al 1983, Hirooka et al 1986), an acceleration in the process of death and regeneration, the extension of fibrosis and vascular proliferation (Yamamoto et al 1984, Sherman et a1 990), the remodelling of hepatocytes into biliary hepatocytes (Phillips et al 1987), the proliferation of ductular hepatocytes possibly from progenitor cells (Vandersteenhoven et al 1990) and perhaps also important, a clear association with hepatocellular carcinoma (Millward-Sadler 1987) by both hepatocyte "de-differentation" and the abnormal differenciation of progenitor cells (Fausto 1990).

This review is a brief summary of our own experience.

MATERIAL AND METHODS

Livers from 21 patients transplanted for end-stage liver cirrhosis constituted the material for this study. All patients but one were adult. Cirrhosis was of viral origin in 8 cases (6 HBV, 2 HCV), alcoholic in 4, autoimmune in 1, biliary in 2 (1 primary biliary cirrhosis, 1 congenital hepatic fibrosis), hemochromatotic in 2 and unknown in 4. Sixty % of cases were macro or mixed nodular.

A wedge biopsy was taken during hepatectomy and a 5 mm section then examined under a binocular lens. A chosen nodule was perfused using several needles inserted superficially through the capsule just inside the nodule. 1.5 % glutaraldehyde was perfused for 15 to 30 min until the entire cut section of the nodule appeared hardened - The upper part of the nodule was cut into small blocks of 1 mm^3 which were routinely processed for electron microscopy. 1 um sections stained with toluidine blue were used to select areas (rim of the nodule, areas of regeneration, etc...) for ultrastructural examination. The unfixed part of the biopsy was used for light microscopic examination to appreciate the size of the nodules, the degree of inflammation, necrosis, cholestasis, etc...

RESULTS

This technique enabled satisfactory fixation of a sufficient number of sinusoids. Although the morphology of sinusoids was rather heterogeneous (Fig. 1 - 6) both within a single nodule and amongst different nodules from different patients, albeit in the same etiological class, it appeared that some patterns could be identified.

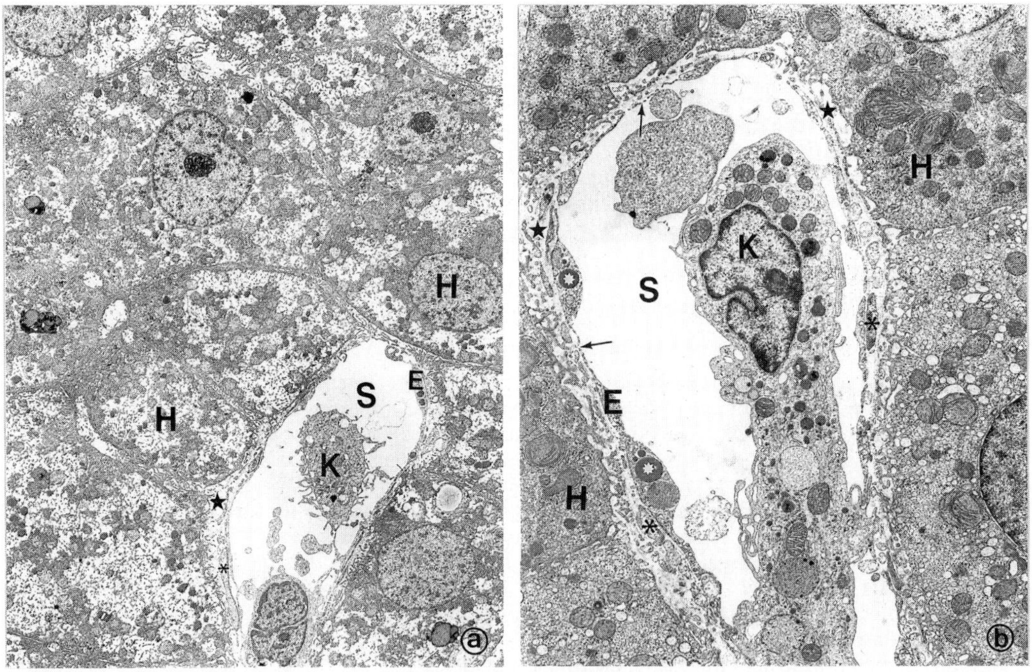

Fig.1 a, b: normal sinusoids. Two nearly normal sinusoids (S) inside cirrhotic nodules. Endothelial cells (E) are thin, fenestrated (arrow) and contain some dense bodies (white star). Kupffer cells (K) are floating into the lumen. The narrow Disse space (star) contains thin perisinusoidal processes (asterisk) and is limited by the sinusoidal pole of hepatocytes (H) covered by numerous microvilli.
a: x 2, 300; **b**: x 4, 500

1 - **Normal sinusoids.**

Normal sinusoids which could not be morphologically distinguished from sinusoids of control livers (Balabaud et al 1988) were visible in all cases . Particularly striking was the presence of normal hepatocyte microvilli, a narrow Disse space and fenestrated endothelial cells (Fig. 1 a, b).

2 - **Capillarized sinusoids.**

True capillaries could be observed at or close to the edge of the nodule. These were defined by a non-fenestrated endothelial wall, an absence of Kupffer cells anchored to the sinusoidal wall, the presence of a continuous basement membrane, transformation of perisinusoidal cells into pericytes, widening of the Disse space containing abundant extracellular matrix (ECM), and a decrease in or absence of hepatocytic microvilli (Fig. 2 a, b). Hepatocytes around these capillaries could be in a rosette formation or even transformed into biliary hepatocytes. Not all sinusoids of the margin were capillarized. Some were normal, others presented varying degrees of capillarization affecting one or several sinusoidal cells particularly endothelial and perisinusoidal cells (progressive loss of fenestrae, irregular thickness of processes which often overlapped for the former, transition from a normal perisinusoidal cell to a fibro/myofibroblast for the latter) and transformation of the extracellular matrix (extension of the fragments of basement membrane like material , deposit of fibrillar and collagenous material...).

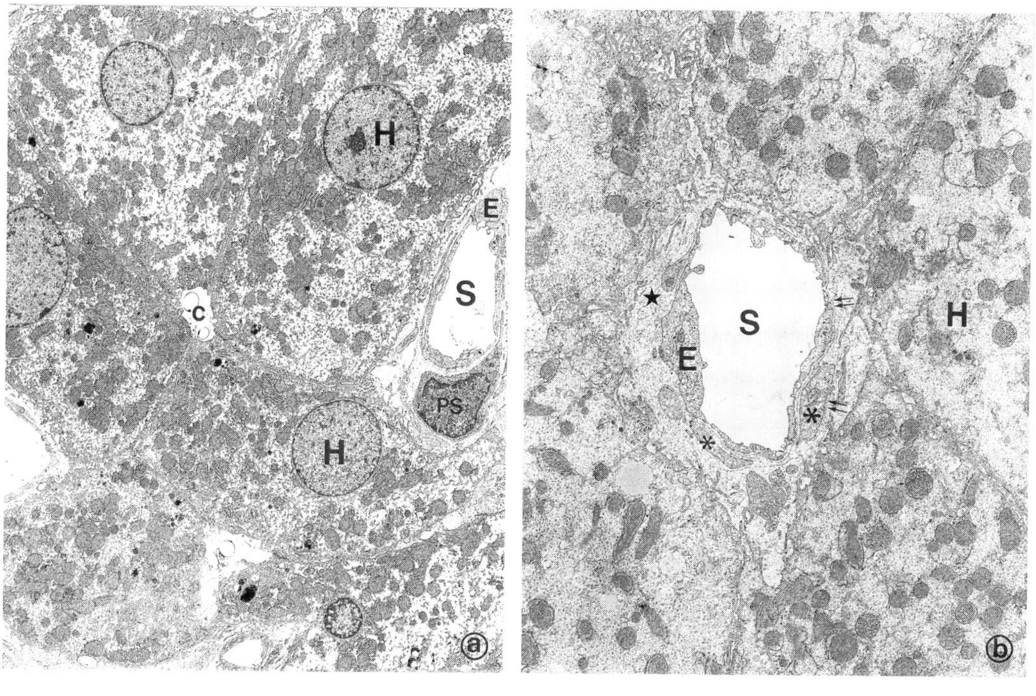

Fig. 2 a, b: capillarized sinusoids. These 2 capillarized sinusoids (S) are located near the margin of a nodule. Non-fenestrated endothelial cells (E) are underlain by a continuous basement membrane (double arrow) duplicated around myofibroblastic processes (asterisk) of perisinusoidal cells (PS). An enlarged Disse space (star) contains a loose, granular, filamentous extracellular matrix and fragments of basement membrane. In **a**, hepatocytes (H) are arranged in a rosette formation around a canalicular lumen (c). **a**: x 2, 300; **b**: x 4, 500

3 - **Sinusoids in inflammatory zones.**
In active cirrhosis, the Disse space was enlarged and contained an abundant ECM, numerous fibro/myofibroblastic cells with several layers of processes, cellular debris, macrophages often loaded with large phagolysosomes and occasional red blood cells (Fig. 3 a, b).The variety of sinusoids was impressive: some were capillarized; others, often large, contained active Kupffer cells or other inflammatory cells and cellular debris; others were normal or presented varying degrees of damage, in some cases so severe that only remnants were visible.

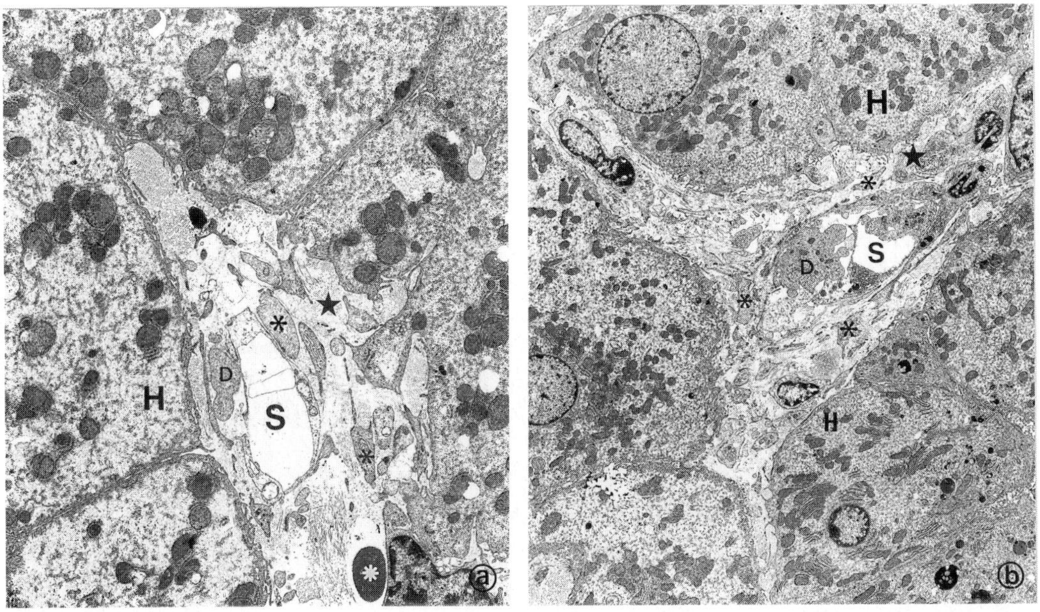

Fig. 3 a, b : sinusoids in active cirrhosis. These 2 small sinusoids (S) are located in an enlarged Disse space (star) containing abundant extracellular matrix with collagen fascicles, fibrils and granular material, numerous perisinusoidal processes (asterisk), cellular debris (D), inflammatory cells, and red blood cells (white star). The sinusoidal membrane of hepatocytes (H) is flattened.
a: x 4, 100; **b**: x 2, 300

4 - **Sinusoids in regenerative areas** .
In areas in which hepatocytes are arranged in plates more than one cell-thick, in contrast with the surrounding parenchyma, sinusoids could be normal (Fig. 5 a) or showed varying degrees of abnormality (Fig. 5 b) or presented signs of regeneration (Fig. 6), which on some occasions, were difficult to evaluate. Criteria used to define regeneration were the following :

a- well formed sinusoids: endothelial cells with digitations formed neo cavities with or without fenetrae (Fig. 6 a).

b- sinusoids with ill defined or with no sinusoidal lumen were recognized by their location. One could observe, in between sinusoidal poles of hepatocytes covered by microvilli containing an ECM with no or few collagen bundles, fragments of basement membrane material and perisinusoidal cell processes of transitional types, fairly active cell fragments (active RER) that could reasonably be attributed to endothelial cells (size of the mitochondria, the presence of a lumen with or without fenestrae, these sometimes showing a diaphragm) (Fig. 6 b, c, d). These cells were or were not associated with other cell types such as Kupffer cells or lymphocytes. These sinusoids had initially been interpreted as sinusoidal remnants, as it was not rare to observe on the same section part of a dying endothelial cell close to a regenerative one.
Quite apart from this categorization, sinusoidal cells can present ultrastructural changes which are presented in table 1 and Fig. 4.

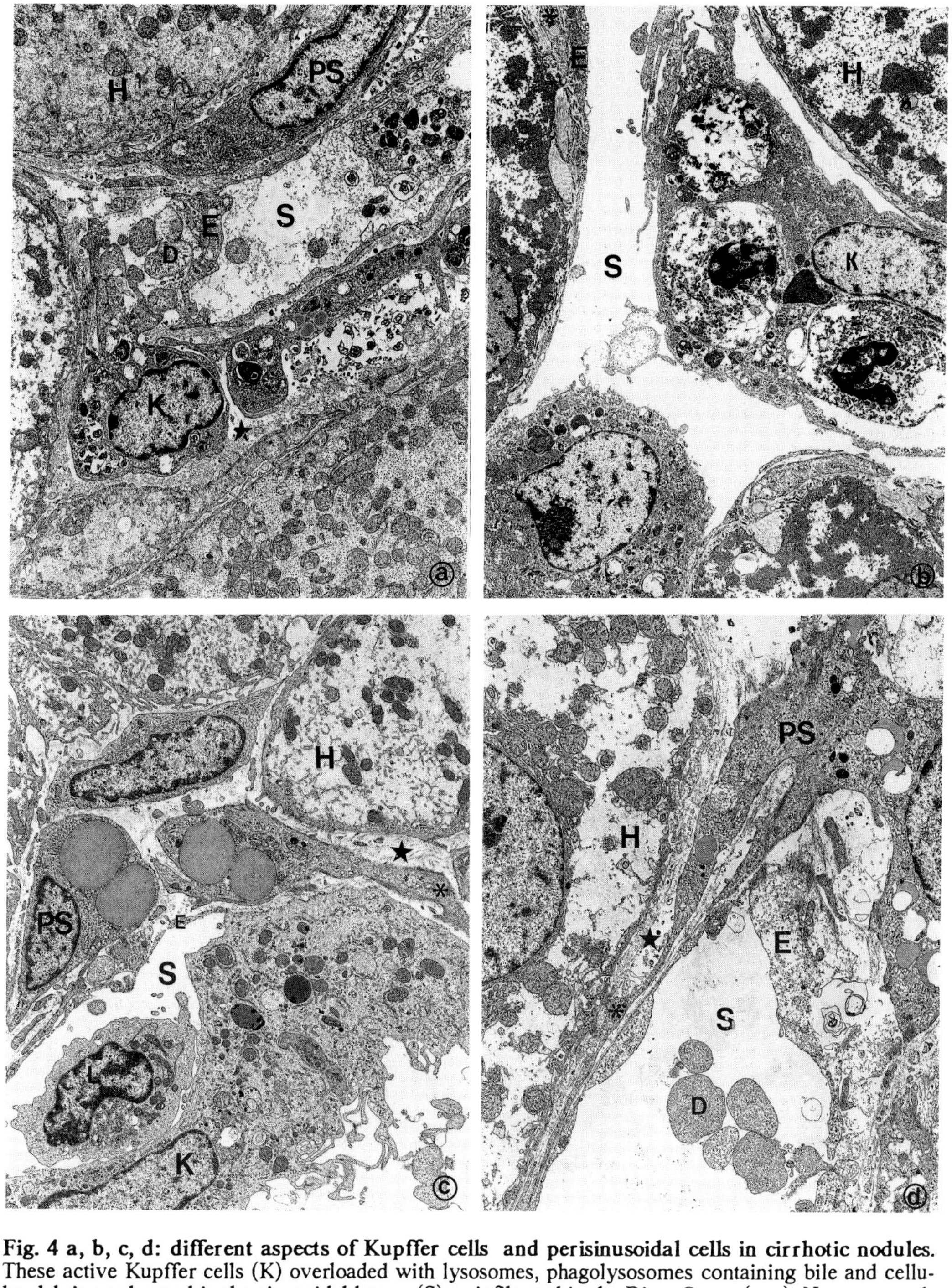

Fig. 4 a, b, c, d: different aspects of Kupffer cells and perisinusoidal cells in cirrhotic nodules. These active Kupffer cells (K) overloaded with lysosomes, phagolysosomes containing bile and cellular debris are located in the sinusoidal lumen (S) or infiltrated in the Disse Space (star). Numerous cellular debris (D) can be seen in the Disse space and the lumen. Perisinusoidal cells (PS) are of transitional (**c**) or of myofibroblastic (**d**) aspect. H: hepatocyte; E: endothelial cell; L: lymphocyte; asterisk: perisinusoidal process . **a**: x 4, 100; **b**: x 3, 300; **c**: x 4, 400; **d**: x 5, 500

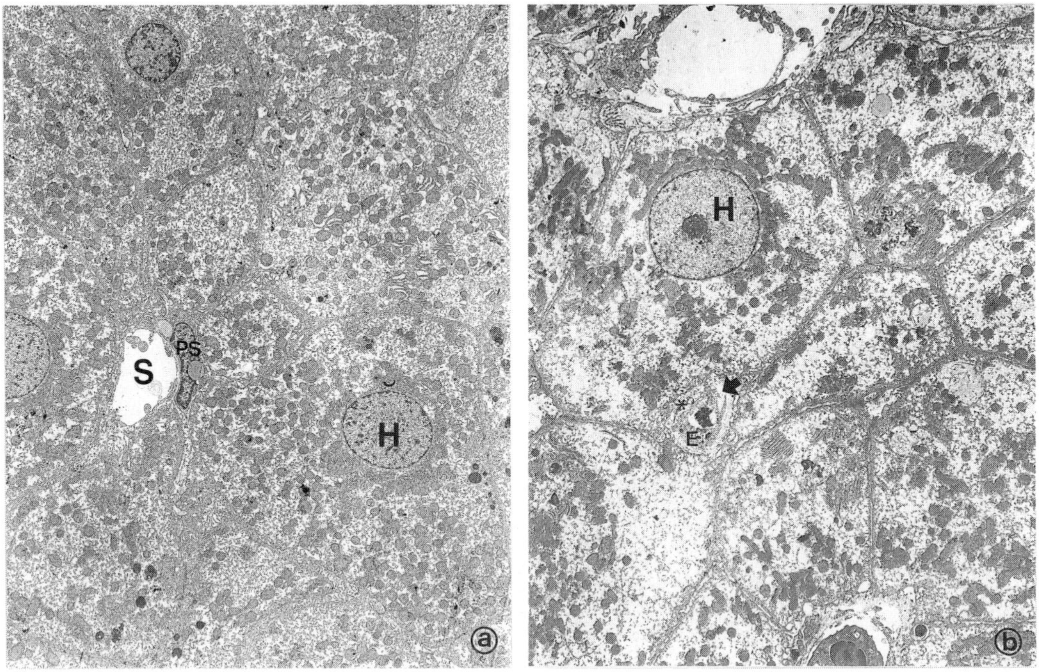

Fig. 5 a, b : sinusoids in regenerative areas. Hepatocytes (H) are arranged in more than one cell - thick plates. **a** - This small, compressed sinusoid (S) is nearly normal with a perisinusoidal cell (PS) containing lipids; **b** - In this small lumen (arrow), fragments of perisinusoidal processes (asterisk) and endothelial cell (E) can be recognized.
a:x 1, 800; **b**:x 2, 200

DISCUSSION

The fine ultrastructure of sinusoids in cirrhotic nodules can be studied by the transnodular perfusion - fixation technique. The morphology of sinusoids is extremely heterogeneous, but some patterns can by identified: in active cirrhosis, in regenerative areas, at the rim or close to the rim of the nodule. Elsewhere in the nodule, sinusoids can be normal or show some of the sinusoidal cell alterations we have described. In addition and this was true of all types of sinusoids, even in regenerative areas, endothelial cells could present evidence of damage. There are several interesting elements in this study :
1 -Even in end-stage cirrhosis, there are sinusoids which are, morphologically speaking, normal
2 -True capillarization is a rare event, often limited to the periphery of the nodule. This corroborates the recent data obtained by light microscopy using Ulex (UEA 1) (Petrovic et al 1989) and factor VIII RAg (Petrovic et al 1989, Babbs et al 1990) staining. Capillarization is often accompanied by phenotypic damage to hepatocytes (rosette formation, biliary hepatocytes) (Phillips at al 1987)
3 -Whilst comporting certain accepted views [loss of Kupffer cells (Lough et al 1987), transformation of perisinusoidal cells into fibro/myofibroblasts (Bioulac- sage et al 1988), loss of hepatocyte microvilli (Phillips et al 1987), enlargement of the Disse space (Bioulac-Sage et al 1988), increase in the number of collagen bundles (Schaffner and Popper 1963)], this study has also revealed the extraordinary morphological diversity of sinusoidal cells (number, activity, phenotype), the scarcity of collagen bundles inside the nodule compared to the periphery and an increase in the deposit of non-collagenous material. Immunocytological studies on the localization of Kupffer cells (Mills & Scheuer 1985, Triger et al 1989), the phenotypic transformation of perisinusoidal cells (Schmitt-Gräff et al 1991) and modification of the ECM (Peyrol & Grimaud 1988) have confirmed our results. In view of

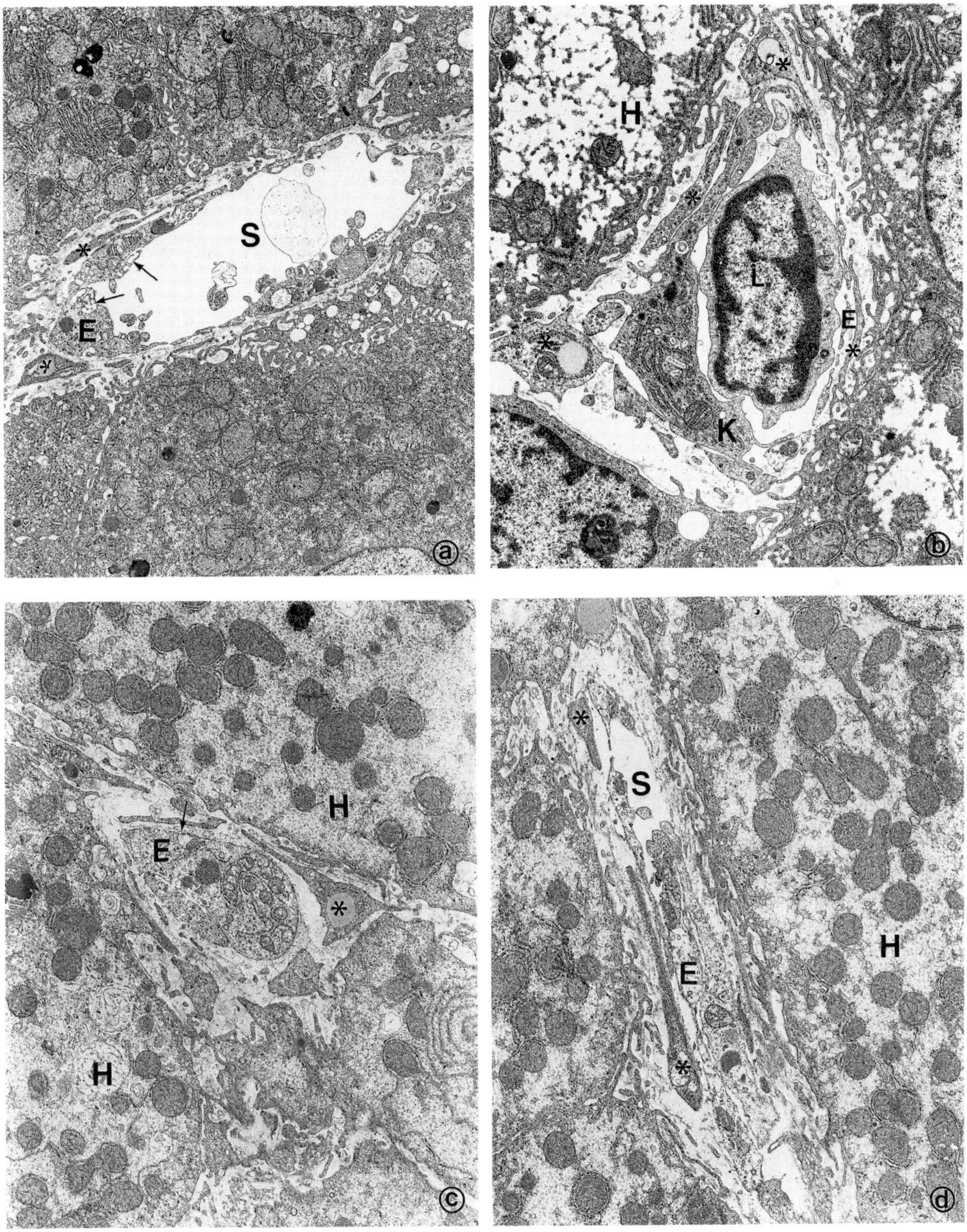

Fig. 6 a, b, c, d: sinusoidal cells in regenerative areas. a : this endothelial cell is active with fenestrated neocavities (arrow) and digitations reaching into the sinusoidal lumen (S) - **b** : this lumen containing a lymphocyte (L) is principally formed by a Kupffer cell (K) in continuity with a fenestrated endothelial (E) process underlain by transitional perisinusoidal cell processes (asterisk). Hepatocyte (H) microvilli are numerous - **c** : this fragment of E can be recognized by its fenestrae (arrow) - **d** : this E is of irregular thickness and seems to form one or several lumens. **a:** x 5, 500; **b:** x 7,300; **c:** x 6, 800; **d:** x 6, 800

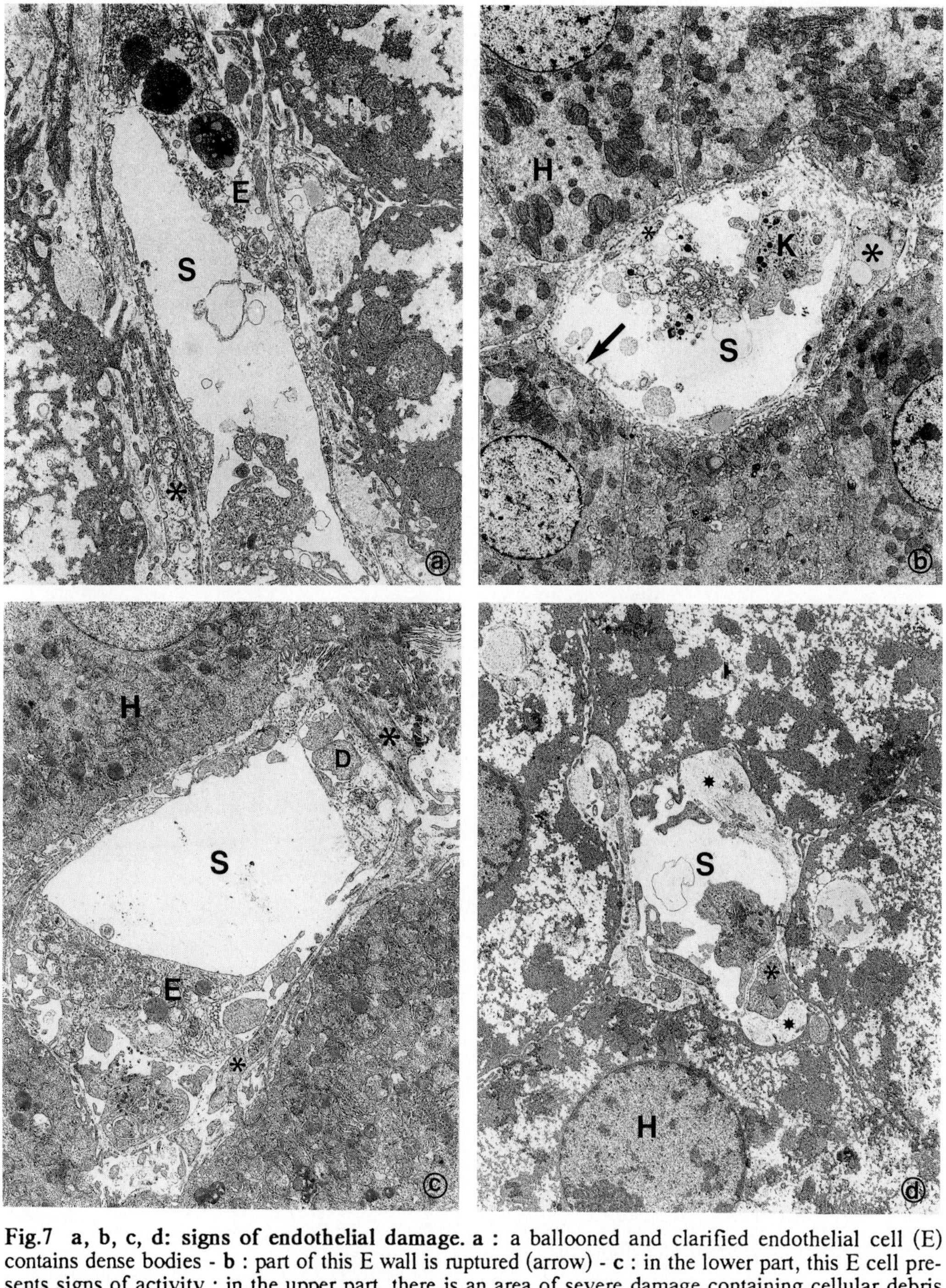

Fig.7 a, b, c, d: signs of endothelial damage. a : a ballooned and clarified endothelial cell (E) contains dense bodies - **b** : part of this E wall is ruptured (arrow) - **c** : in the lower part, this E cell presents signs of activity ; in the upper part, there is an area of severe damage containing cellular debris (D) - **d** : this sinusoid is still recognizable by the presence of perisinusoidal cell processes (asterisk) and extracellular matrix (star) in spite of the fact that the endothelial wall can no longer be identified.
K: Kupffer cell. **a**: x 7, 800; **b**: x 3, 000; **c**: x 4, 400; **d**: x 5, 500

this heterogeneity, functional results obtained by the multiple indicator dilution technique (Villeneuve et al 1990), hepatic clearances, quantitation of intrinsic drug-metabolizing capacity (Meyer et al 1991) etc..., should be interpreted with caution, particularly when morphology is taken as a strong argument to support a hypothesis (intact-hepatocyte theory, intrahepatic shunts, capillarization...).

4 - In spite of the interesting data provided by electron microscopic studies of sinusoids and especially the newer elements: evidence of sinusoidal regeneration, endothelial cell damage..., the study of ultrastructure alone will not explain certain crucial features of cirrhosis - namely, extension of fibrosis (Friedman 1990, Gressner &Bachem 1990), regeneration, malignant transformation (Fausto &Mead 1990). The combination of *in vivo* microscopy (McCuskey 1988), electron microscopy (scanning, transmission), immunocytochemistry (Sakakibara et al 1986, Al-Adnani 1989, Martinez-Hernandez et al 1991), in situ hybridization (Milani et al 1989) to cellular (Shiratori et al 1986, Matsuoka & Tsukamoto 1990) and molecular biology (Maher & McGuire 1990) and to *in vivo* experiments (Huet et al 1982, Reichen & Lee 1986, Marteau et al 1989), should help to resolve these important issues.

Table 1. Different types of sinusoidal cell damage observed in cirrhotic nodules

<u>Endothelial cells</u>
- signs of damage : dense bodies, ballooning, blebs, gaps of varying size, rupture, cell remnants, necrotic areas, disappearance.
- signs of capillarization : decrease in or even loss of fenestrae, diaphragmated fenestrae, increased thickness, overlap.
- signs of regeneration : formation of neocavities (with or without fenestrae, with or without diaphragm), active RER.

<u>Kupffer cells</u>
- progressive to complete disappearance.
- signs of overload: large and numerous lysosomes, phagolysosomes containing bile or cellular debris.
- signs of hyperactivity : large and numerous pseudopodes sometimes infiltrated in the Disse space.

<u>Perisinusoidal cells</u>
- from a normal perisinusoidal cell to a transitional cell (lipids and active RER) and to a fibro / myofibroblast.

REFERENCES

Al Adnani , M.S. (1989): Differential immunohistochemical localization of cytokeratins and collagen types I and III in experimentally-induced cirrhosis. J. Pathol. 159, 151-158.

Babbs, C. et al. (1990): Endothelial cell transformation in primary biliary cirrhosis : a morphological and biochemical study. Hepatology 11, 723-729.

Balabaud, C. et al. (1988): Light and transmission electron microscopy of sinusoids in human liver. In Sinusoids in human liver : health and disease, eds. P. Bioulac-Sage, C. Balabaud, pp. 87-110. Rijswijk: The Kupffer cell foundation.

Bioulac-Sage, P. et al. (1988): Ultrastructure of sinusoids in liver disease. In Sinusoids in human liver:health and disease, eds. P. Bioulac-Sage, C.Balabaud, 223-279. Rijswijk : The Kupffer cell foundation.

Clement, B. et a!. (1988): Interaction of cells and extracellular matrix in the liver. In Sinusoids in human liver : health and disease, ed. P. Bioulac-Sage, C. Balabaud, pp. 111-137. Rijswijk : The Kupffer cell foundation.

Fausto, N. (1990): Hepatocyte differentiation and liver progenitor cells. Current opinion in cell biology 2, 1036-1043.

Fausto, N. & Mead, J. E. (1990): Role of protooncogenes and transforming growth factors in normal and neoplastic liver growth. In Liver diseases, eds. H. Popper, F. Schaffner, pp. 57-71. New-york : W.B. Saunders company.

Friedman, S. L. (1990): Cellular sources of collagen and regulation of collagen production in liver. Seminars liver disease 10, 20-29.

Gressner, A. M. & Bachem M. D. (1990): Cellular sources of noncollagenous matrix proteins : role of fat storing cells in fribrogenesis. Seminars liver disease 10, 30-46.

Hirooka, N. et al. (1986): Hepatic microcirculation of liver cirrhosis studied by corrosion cast scanning electron microscope examination. Acta Pathol. Jpn 36, 375-387.
Huet, P.M. et al. (1982): Assessment of liver microcirculation in human cirrhosis. J. Clin. Invest. 70, 1234-1244.
Lough, J. et al. (1987): Kupffer cell depletion associated with capillarization of liver sinusoids in carbon tetrachloride-induced rat liver cirrhosis; J. Hepatol. 5, 190-198.
Maher, J.J., McGuire, R.F. (1990): Extracellular matrix gene expression increases preferentially in rat lipocytes and sinusoidal endothelial cells during hepatic fibrosis in vivo. J. Clin. Invest. 86, 1641-1648.
Martinez-Hernandez, A. et al (1991): The extracellular matrix in hepatic regeneration. Localization of collagen types I, III, IV, laminin and fibronectin. Lab. Invest. 64, 157-166.
Marteau, P. et al. (1989): Effect of vasodilators on hepatic microcirculation on cirrhosis : a study in the isolated perfused rat liver. Hepatology 9, 820-823.
Matsuoka, M. & Tsukamoto, H. (1990): Stimulation of hepatic lipocyte collagen production by Kupffer cell-derived transforming growth factor beta : implication for a pathogenetic role in alcoholic liver fibrogenesis. Hepatology 11, 599-605.
Mc Cuskey, R. S. (1988): Hepatic microcirculation in disease. In Sinusoids in human liver : health and disease, eds. P. Bioulac-Sage, C. Balabaud, pp. 315-321. Rijswijk : The Kupffer cell foundation.
Meyer, B. et al. (1991): Quantitation of instrinsic drug-metabolizing capacity in human liver biopsy specimens : support for the intact-hepatocyte theory. Hepatology. 13, 475-481.
Milani, S. et al. (1989): In situ hybridization for procollagen types I, III and IV mRNA in normal and fRbrotic rat liver : evidence for predominant expression in non parenchymal liver cells. Hepatology 10, 84-92.
Mills, L.R. & Scheuer, P.J. (1985): Hepatic sinusoidal macrophages in alcoholic liver disease. J. Pathol. 147, 127-132.
Millward-Sadler, G. H. (1987): Cirrhosis. In Pathology of the liver, eds. R.N.M. MacSween, P.P. Anthony, P.J. Scheuer pp. 821-860. London :Churchill Livingstone.
Petrovic, L.M. et al. (1989): Hepatic sinusoidal endothelium : ulex lectin binding. Histopathology 14, 233-243.
Peyrol, S. &Grimaud, J. A. (1988): Perisinusoidal connective matrix. In Sinusoids in human liver : health and disease, eds. P. Bioulac-Sage, C. Balabaud, pp. 323-340. Rijswijk : The Kupffer cell foundation.
Phillips, M. J. et al (1987): The liver. An atlas and text of ultrastructural pathology, eds. M. J. Phillips, S. Poucell, J. Paterson, P. Valencia. New York : Raven Press.
Rappaport, A.M. et al. (1983): The scarring of the liver acini (cirrhosis). Tridimentional and microcirculatory considerations. Virchows Arch. A. 402, 107-137.
Reichen, J. & Le, M. (1986): Verapamil favorably influences hepatic microvascular exchange and function in rats with cirrhosis of the liver; J. Clin. Invest. 78, 448-455.
Rojkind, MK & Greenwell, P. (1988) : The liver as a bioecological system . In The liver biology and pathobiology , eds. I. M. Arias, W. B. Jakoby, H. Popper, D. Schachter, D. A. Shafritz, pp. 1269-1285. New York : Raven Press.
Sakakibara, K. et al. (1986): Immunolocalization of type III collagen and procollagen in cirrhotic human liver using monoclonal antibodies. Virchows Arch. A. 409, 37-46.
Schaffner, F. & Popper, H. (1963): Capillarization of hepatic sinusoids in man. Gastroenterology 44, 239-242.
Schmitt-Gräff, A. et al. (1991): Modulation of alpha smooth muscle actin and desmin expression in perisinusoidal cells of normal and diseased human livers. Am. J. Pathol. 138, 1233-1242.
Sherman, I.A. et al. (1990): Hepatic microvascular changes associated with development of liver fibrosis and cirrhosis. Am. J. Physiol. 258, 460-465.
Shiratori, Y. et al. (1986): Kupffer cells from CC14-induced fibrotic livers stimulate proliferation of fat storing cells. J. Hepatol. 3, 294-303.
Triger, D.R. et al.. (1989): Hepatic reticulo-endothelial function : a correlation of radioscopic and immunohistochemical assessment. Liver 9, 86-92.
Vandersteenhoven, A. M. et al. (1990): Characterization of ductular hepatocytes in end-stage cirrhosis. Arch. Pathol. Lab. Med.: 138, 1233-1242.
Villeneuve, J. P. et al. (1990): Isolated perfused cirrhotic human liver obtained from liver transplant patients : a feasibility study. Hepatology 12 : 257-263.
Yamamoto, T. et al (1984): Perinodular arteriolar plexus in liver cirrhosis. Scanning electron microscopy of microvascular casts. Liver 4, 50-54.

Résumé

Les foies de 21 patients transplantés pour cirrhose ont été examinés. Un nodule bien individualisé a été fixé par perfusion d'une solution à 1,5 % de glutaraldéhyde puis pour partie découpé en petits fragments et préparé pour un examen en microscopie électronique. La morphologie des sinusoïdes est apparue plutôt hétérogène ; néanmoins au sein d'un seul nodule et d'un nodule à l'autre, différentes zones pouvaient être identifiées : 1 - des sinusoïdes normaux ; 2 - des sinusoïdes capillarisés ; 3 - des sinusoïdes avec des zones inflammatoires ; 4 - des sinusoïdes avec des zones de régénération. En dehors de cette classification, les cellules sinusoïdales pouvaient présenter des modifications ultrastructurales telles que des signes de lésions des cellules endothéliales, de capillarisation et de régénération. Au regard de cette hétérogénéïté, une vraie capillarisation était un évènement rare, souvent limité à la périphérie du nodule ; aussi, les données fonctionnelles doivent être interprétées avec précaution, notamment lorsque la morphologie est utilisée comme un solide argument pour étayer une hypothèse (théorie de l'hépatocyte intact, shunt intrahépatique, capillarisation).

Cellular and Molecular Aspects of Cirrhosis. Eds B. Clément, A. Guillouzo. Colloque INSERM/John Libbey Eurotext Ltd. © 1992, Vol. 216, pp. 103-113

Microcirculation in perfused liver

P. Michel Huet, Jean-Pierre Villeneuve and Bernard Willems

André-Viallet Clinical Research Center, Hôpital Saint-Luc, 264 René-Lévesque Boulevard, East, Montréal, Quebec, H2X 1P1 Canada

WHAT DO WE KNOW ABOUT PARENCHYMAL BLOOD FLOW IN CIRRHOSIS?

1) ABSTRACT

To be honest, the answer to this question is: not much. However there are some new insights which can help to understand a little more about the complex mechanisms leading to alterations of parenchymal blood flow in cirrhosis. When we refer to parenchymal blood flow, we refer to blood perfusing the parenchymal cells (the hepatocytes) through normal sinusoids, ie. through specific hepatic capillaries which are perforated by a multitude of small fenestrae, without basement membrane. In such a case, red blood cells remain within the sinusoidal lumen; plasma and plasma-dissolved substances diffuse freely in the extravascular space (the space of Disse) and reach directly the underlying hepatocytes where uptake processes can take place. Using the multiple indicator dilution technique (MIDT), vascular, extravascular and cellular water spaces can be measured following injection of indicators in the inflow vessels as well as extraction of various substances during a single passage through the liver. Under normal conditions parenchymal blood flow is equivalent to sinusoidal blood flow; also, all blood flowing through the portal vein and hepatic artery must flow through the sinusoidal bed and consequently parenchymal or sinusoidal blood flow and hepatic blood flow are equal. In chronic liver disease blood flowing through the liver will not necessarily flow through sinusoids, because of intrahepatic shunts and blood that will flow through sinusoids may flow through abnormal sinusoids. Large intrahepatic shunts can demonstrated in vivo by a modification of the MIDT using labelled microspheres larger than the sinusoidal diameter. In presence of shunts, part of the microspheres will flow through these large channels along with red blood cells. On the other hand, abnormal sinusoids can be found with disappearance of endothelial fenestrae and formation of a basement membrane underlying endothelial cells (capillarization), also new collagen fibers can fill up the space of Disse (collagenization). In such conditions, plasma and plasma-dissolved substances may not have a direct access to hepatocytes and the space of distribution of albumin will be markedly restricted as demonstrated by the MIDT. Thus, because of intrahepatic shunts and capillarization with collagenization of sinusoids, hepatic blood flow and sinusoidal blood flow are not any more equal. Moreover, sinusoidal and parenchymal blood flows may also be different: plasma-dissolved substances may diffuse differently through the new barrier between endothelial lumen and hepatocytes. Capillarization and collagenization may well restrict diffusion of albumin in the extravascular space without restriction for small molecules such as sucrose and water. Moreover selective restriction to diffusion can be found for protein-bound substances. In addition, blood entering the liver through hepatic artery and portal vein may not flow through the same vascular bed before reaching the efferent hepatic veins: in humans as well as in experimental cirrhosis, intrahepatic shunts were never found from hepatic artery to the hepatic veins, even in presence of large shunts from portal veins to hepatic veins. Also, terminal hepatic arteries end at different length along sinusoids where capillarization and collagenization may differ from periphery to center of regenerating nodules. Thus if we take into account variable degrees of shunts, collagenization and capillarization, and different routes of flow through the liver, an objective analysis becomes rather difficult if not impossible for a given patient.

2) ANATOMIC CHANGES IN CIRRHOSIS

Cirrhosis is characterized by the destruction of the normal architecture of the hepatic parenchyma, the development of large fibrous septa, and abnormal hepatocyte regeneration in nodules. Liver cell plates are no longer one cell thick, but appear to be formed of two or more rows of hepatocytes. The ultrastructural appearance of hepatocyte in the cirrhotic nodules is considered by most investigators to be virtually normal, except for non-specific mitochondrial alterations (such as increased size, varied shapes, and paracrystalline inclusions). Thus, it is generally thought that cirrhosis is primarily characterized by a disturbed hepatic circulation and architecture, rather than cellular alterations.

In the cirrhotic liver, both afferent (portal veins and hepatic arteries) and efferent (hepatic veins) are found within the fibrous septa. Although it is thought that blood supplied to the regenerating nodules is derived mainly from the portal vein (Mitra, 1966), the manner in which it leaves the nodules and drains into the hepatic veins is still not fully understood. In fibrous septa, vascular casts have demonstrated a dense network of vessels with some anastomoses between branches of the portal and hepatic veins and between those of the hepatic artery and portal veins (Popper et al, 1952). Anastomoses between branches of the hepatic artery and hepatic veins have only been found in cirrhotic rats. A noticeably enlarged arterial bed and peribiliary capillary plexus has been reported around proliferating bile ductules (Baldus & Hoffbauer, 1963; Mitra, 1966).

Large anastomoses (20-100μm in diameter) between afferent and efferent vessels were primarily demonstrated using vascular corrosion casts of human cirrhotic livers obtained on autopsy. However, cast preparations with gelatin, latex or plastic substances require high pressure injection to obtain satisfactory penetration of all vascular systems. Extrapolation of such findings to the in vivo situation should therefore be viewed with caution.

Other structural changes have been reported in cirrhotic nodules, in addition to intrahepatic shunts, particularly in the space of Disse. Schaffner and Popper (1963) first described the development of a continuous membrane at the margin of the microvascular channels in long-standing cirrhosis. The endothelial cells form a non-fenestrated lining separating the capillary lumen from the space of Disse and the liver cells. The space of Disse shows varying degrees of dilatation with increased deposits of collagen, mainly as bundles of fibrils. At the vascular pole of the hepatocyte, microvilli are smaller in number and irregular in shape (Schaffner & Popper, 1963). The vascular changes within the cirrhotic nodules tend to be regional: capillarization is mainly found at the periphery of the nodules and more normal sinusoidal sieve plates are found in their centre (Huet et al, 1982; Philips & Steiner, 1965). Capillarization probably progresses from the periphery of the nodule to its centre, as the cirrhotic process develops.

Scanning electron microscopy should be an ideal tool in assessing capillarization of the microvascular bed and the disappearance of fenestrae from the endothelial lining. However, using the freeze fracture technique is difficult because of the increase in fibrous tissue, and the literature reveals only a few scanning electron microscopic investigations of human hepatic sinusoidal lining cells. Eguchi et al. (1975) and Henriksen et al. (1984) have shown a decreased number of fenestrae in cirrhotic human liver. Recently, Horn et al. (1987) have demonstrated a significant reduction of fenestrae in the hepatic sinusoidal lining wall in the acinar zone 3 area of biopsies taken from non-cirrhotic alcoholic livers as compared with non-alcoholics. There was also a significant decrease in the porosity of the sinusoidal wall (Horn et al, 1987). A reduction in the area of fenestration per nm^2 of endothelial surface has likewise been reported in baboons chronically fed alcohol (Mak & Lieber, 1984).

Therefore, all anatomical changes occurring in cirrhosis contribute to the impairment of the exchange between sinusoidal blood and the hepatocytes. Following acute injury (from either alcohol, virus or toxic substances) and the disappearance of inflammation, cirrhosis is primarily characterized by a disturbed hepatic circulation (Popper & Orr, 1970).

3) APPLICATION OF THE MULTIPLE INDICATOR DILUTION TECHNIQUE IN CIRRHOSIS

The liver's ability to remove substances from the blood is impaired in cirrhotic patients and the hepatic uptake of most substrates during a single passage through the liver is generally decreased. Capillarization (and collagenization) of sinusoids and intrahepatic shunts may both contribute to this reduced uptake. However their relative roles in impaired blood-liver exchange in cirrhosis has not been evaluated.

a) Capillarization. The multiple indicator dilution technique (Mastaï and Huet, 1988) can be used to evaluate the progressive transformation of sinusoids into capillary-like channels in vivo by studying the distribution of plasma-dissolved substances into the extravascular and intracellular spaces. In cirrhosis, anatomic alterations will limit the diffusion of substances into the space of Disse by transforming the microvascular bed into a two-barrier system, as in other organs with a capillary system. Then, the space of distribution and/or distribution into the accessible space should be limited by each substance's diffusion properties in relation to the new barrier, contrasting with the flow-limited distribution observed in normal liver.

Albumin is a large molecule and it can be assumed that capillarization will limit its diffusion into the space of Disse. In such cases, the labeled albumin curve will be slightly delayed when compared with the corresponding labeled RBCs (fig. 1), as occurs in organs with a capillary circulation where no significant albumin exchange takes place during a single passage.

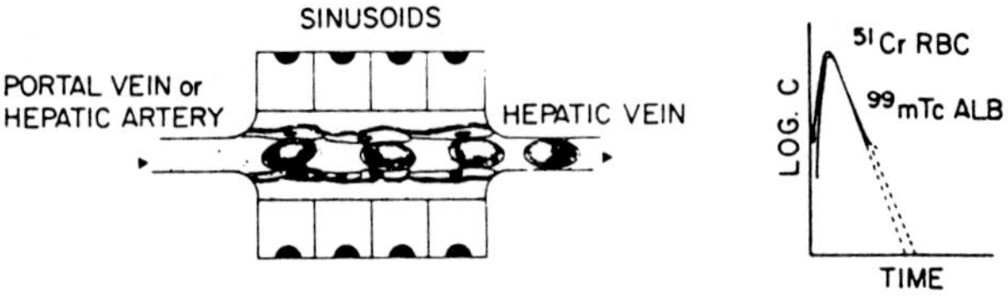

Figure 1: Schematic representation of the liver microcirculation in a cirrhotic liver. The development of a "new barrier" between the vascular space and hepatocyte will limit the diffusion of ^{99m}Tc albumin (^{99m}Tc ALB) into the space of Disse. The albumin curve is slightly delayed in relation to ^{51}Cr red blood cells (^{51}Cr RBC). Reproduced with permission from Mastaï and Huet (1988).

The diffusion of small molecules such as sucrose and water into their distribution space is much more difficult to predict in cirrhosis. If their distribution becomes diffusion-limited, time/concentration symmetry with respect to the distortion of the diffusible labeled curves will be lost when compared with that of the vascular reference substances (RBC curve), as occurs in organs with a capillary system such as the coronary circulation. Estimation of the extravascular sucrose volumes using the Goresky's flow-limited model can be incorrect in such circumstances and will differ systematically from those calculated in a more direct manner from the transit time (model-independent analysis). Sucrose dilution curves will not superimpose on RBC curves when transformed.

At the same time, it is difficult to appraise the potential contribution of intrahepatic shunts; this has to be evaluated, since a similar pattern could also have resulted from the transit through shunts.

b) Intrahepatic shunts. The modification to Goresky's technique that we proposed recently, provides a new approach to studying intrahepatic shunts in vivo (Huet et al, 1986; Varin & Huet, 1985). The modification involved the use of labeled microspheres (15 to 20μm in diameter) larger than normal sinusoids and labeled lidocaine, in addition to vascular and extravascular reference substances. Lidocaine was used to focus on the blood-to-hepatocyte diffusion transfer since, as we have already pointed out, it penetrates the liver cell membrane freely under normal conditions, only trace amounts being recovered in the hepatic outflow (Varin & Huet, 1985).

In the presence of intrahepatic shunts in a cirrhotic liver, the hepatic outflow pattern can be expected to result from the transit of blood via two different pathways: one related to the blood flowing through the intrahepatic shunts, considered to be poorly permeable, short-circuit type channels; and two, a later component, related to the blood coming through the sinusoids (fig. 2). When considering blood passing through intrahepatic shunts, there should be no significant exchange for the vascular reference substances and extravascular diffusible substances during a single passage; these substances can be expected to flow together, with no separation. Whether labeled microspheres should accompany the other test substances or not depends on their diameter relative to that of the intrahepatic shunts. When considering blood flowing through the sinusoidal bed, labeled RBCs should emerge first, followed by labeled albumin, sucrose and water, and substantially later, by a small amount of lidocaine released from the liver.

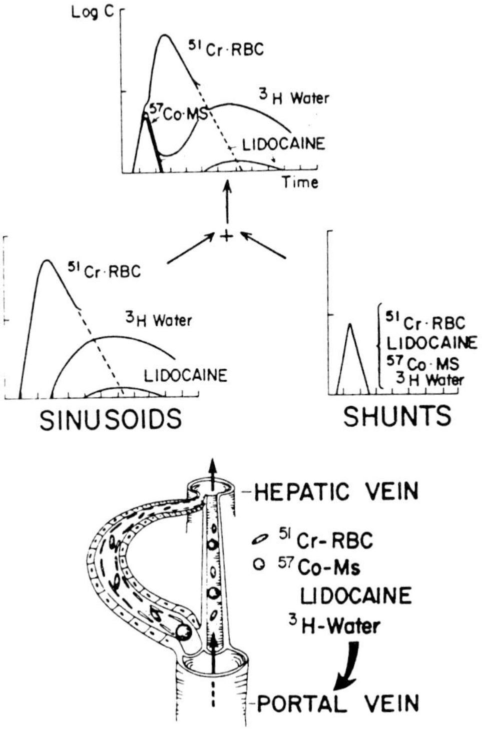

Figure 2: Schematic representation of the intrahepatic microcirculation in a cirrhotic liver. The outflow pattern obtained in the hepatic vein can be resolved in two parts: An early throughput component that has come through intrahepatic shunts (right) and a later compoment that has come through a more normal sinusoidal bed (left). Log C: logarithm to the base 10 of the concentrations of the various markers; MS: microsphere. Reproduced with permission from Huet et al (1986).

c) Animal studies using IPRL. Using IPRL in cirrhotic rats (following phenobarbital and CCl_4 exposure), the vascular space and extravascular spaces accessible to albumin were decreased significantly compared with non-cirrhotic rats (Varin & Huet, 1985). Albumin curve profiles, however, were compatible with flow-limited diffusion, indicating that the diffusion of albumin into its accessible interstitial space was not altered, despite its marked reduction in size. In some rats, the albumin curve was only slightly delayed in relation to RBC curve as shown on fig. 3, suggesting capillarization of most sinusoids.

The diffusion of labeled sucrose and water into their distribution spaces was much more difficult to analyze in these cirrhotic rats. In some rats, diffusion of sucrose and water was still compatible with flow-limited distribution; in other cirrhotic rats, sucrose and water curve profiles were not compatible with a flow-limited diffusion, the time/concentration symmetry for distortion of their dilution curves being lost when compared with RBC curves. However, the total space accessible to sucrose and water did not differ from that measured in non-cirrhotic rats (Varin & Huet, 1985). It therefore appears that sucrose and water are still able to diffuse into a near normal extravascular space, unlike albumin.

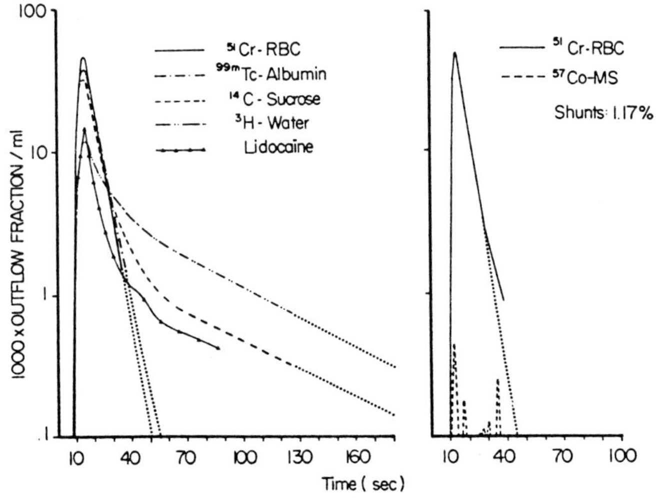

Figure 3: Multiple indicator dilution pattern (left panel) and outflow recovery of microspheres (MS) (right panel) obtained in an in situ perfused cirrhotic rat liver. The outflow recovery of lidocaine was 41.4% and of microspheres was 1.17%. Reproduced from Varin and Huet (1985).

The potential contribution of intrahepatic shunts was also directly appraised by the simultaneous use of labeled microspheres (15μm in diameter). The recovery from the outflow of injected labeled microspheres into the portal vein was never >1.2%. Moreover, outflows did not attain dilution curve profiles in any of the rats, whether cirrhotic or not, and the late activity might represent breakdown products smaller than sinusoidal diameter (fig. 3). The possible development of small shunts (less than 15μm in diameter) with poorly permeable walls was then evaluated, using lidocaine. In all cirrhotic rats, lidocaine was no longer able to penetrate the liver cell membrane freely and completely, and a substantial proportion emerged in the outflow related in time to the peak RBC curve (fig. 3).

The early peak of unchanged lidocaine can be interpreted as part of the substance flowing through poorly permeable, hepatocyte-free channels, without leaving the vascular bed. The proportion of lidocaine recovered in the outflow varied greatly (2 to more than 50%) and appeared to increase with the progression of the liver disease (Varin & Huet,

1985). The lidocaine throughput might also have resulted from complete capillarization and collagenization of all sinusoids, changing the liver microcirculation into a well-capillarized system. However, such stereotyped alteration of hepatic sinusoids was not demonstrated by light and electron microscopic studies. In this model, most of the sinusoids remain structurally unaltered, the space of Disse being widened with extensive collagen deposits (Stenger, 1966; Varin & Huet 1985). Occasional capillarized channels were found in a number of thin fibrotic bands dissecting the parenchymal modules, as well as in the internodular fibrotic septa (7 to 10μm in diameter).

Thus, in rats with CCl_4-induced cirrhosis, indicator dilution data are compatible with two kinds of alterations: 1) a decreased vascular space, with collagenization of the extravascular space limiting the diffusion of large molecules such as albumin; and 2) the development of small channels with poorly permeable walls limiting the diffusion of small molecules such as lidocaine, sucrose and water. Large intrahepatic shunts (>15μm in diameter) are not a common feature in this animal model.

d) Human studies using isolated perfused liver. Isolated perfused rat liver is a valuable tool for exploring the physiology and pathophysiology of the liver microcirculation and clearance functions in the cirrhotic rat (Gores et al, 1986). These studies are based on the assumption that animal models provide an accurate reflection of human cirrhosis, but the comparability of animal models and human disease remains uncertain (Perez Tammayo, 1983).

The advent of orthotopic liver transplantation has made the procurement of cirrhotic human livers feasible for isolated perfused organ studies. We have recently reported our preliminary experience with such studies, in which we examined the hepatic microcirculation and drug elimination in the cirrhotic human liver (Villeneuve et al, 1990).

Cirrhotic livers obtained from eight patients who underwent liver transplantation were perfused through the portal system and hepatic artery in a closed recycling system for periods ranging from 2 to 7 hours.

The perfusate consisted of Krebs bicarbonate buffer containing 20% (vol/vol) prewashed human RBCs, 20 gm/L bovine serum albumin and 5.5 mmol/L glucose. The perfusate was oxygenated with a pediatric blood oxygenator fitted with a thermostat which also served as a reservoir for the perfusate. The temperature was kept constant at 37°C.

The liver was placed on a 75-μm nylon mesh tray and perfused through the hepatic artery and portal vein, using two independent roller pumps with siliconized tubing. For the portal vein, a flow integrator was used to eliminate pulsation caused by the pump. Portal vein and hepatic artery flows were set to obtain perfusion pressures similar to those measured or anticipated in vivo. Outflow was collected underneath the liver and returned to the oxygenator by gravity. Portal vein and hepatic artery pressures were monitored continuously with strain-gauge transducers.

After 20-min of stabilization, we evaluated the presence of intrahepatic shunts from the outflow recovery of microspheres (MSs) using the multiple-indicator dilution technique (Varin & Huet, 1985). The injection mixture consisted of ^{51}Cr-labeled RBCs and ^{141}Ce-labeled, 15-μm MSs rapidly flushed into the portal vein or hepatic artery. PE-90 polyethylene tubing was placed in a right hepatic vein and samples were collected in serial tubes at 1-sec intervals for 40 sec. The samples were counted as described previously (Varin & Huet, 1985).

The livers were perfused over an average of 5 hours and appeared to remain viable as assessed by gross appearance, stable portal pressure, oxygen consumption and bile production. However, the parameters varied considerably from liver to liver. Perfusion flow averaged 451 ml/min, with about 80% coming from the portal vein and 20% from the hepatic artery. The addition of sodium bicarbonate was required to maintain pH at 7.4 throughout the experiments. During perfusion, there was a uniform, progressive rise in transaminase and lactic acid concentrations in the reservoir, whereas hematocrit, electrolytes and glucose concentrations remained constant.

Indicator dilution curves with MSs demonstrated the presence of significant intrahepatic shunts (> 15μm in diameter) from the portal vein to the hepatic vein in six of eight livers, whereas shunts from the hepatic artery to the hepatic vein were uniformly absent. Shunts varied between 1.2 and 32.2% (mean 16.7%). A representative example is illustrated in figure 4. The mean transit time of MSs was markedly faster during a single passage through the liver than that of RBCs through the sinusoids. There was no apparent relationship between RBC transit time and perfusion flow or portal pressure. On three occasions, dilution curves were obtained from the right and left hepatic lobes, and differences in shunting were found in one case (right vs. left: 25.4% vs. 25.3%, 32.2% vs. 22.6% and 1.2% vs. 1.0%).

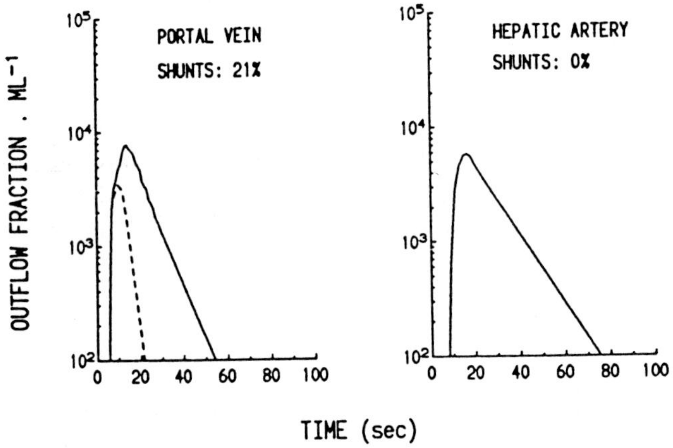

Figure 4: Red blood cell indicator dilution curve (—) and outflow recovery of microspheres (---) obtained in an isolated perfused cirrhotic human liver. After portal vein injection, large intrahepatic shunts were demonstrated, with 21% of microspheres appearing in the hepatic effluent. After hepatic artery injection, no shunt was present.

This is in contrast to the rat CCl_4 model of cirrhosis, in which large portohepatic shunts are rarely found (Varin & Huet, 1985). As one would expect, these shunts were fast-flowing channels. Shunts between the hepatic artery and hepatic veins were absent; this is in agreement with previous observations in humans in vivo, using invasive catheterization of portal vein, hepatic artery and hepatic veins (Huet et al, 1985; Huet et al, 1986).

The availability of cirrhotic livers obtained at liver transplantation offers a unique opportunity to gain insights into the pathophysiology of human disease. Isolated perfused liver studies are feasible, although some refinement of the procedure will be needed to prevent ischemic damage at harvest. Additional studies of normal and cirrhotic liver microcirculation will be of particular interest in examining possible differences in the pattern of anomalies, according to the origin of cirrhosis being compared.

ACKNOWLEDGMENTS

The authors thank L. Giroux, A. Brault and D. Piché for their technical assistance, and F. Trotier for preparing the manuscript.

REFERENCES

Baldus WP, Hoffbauer FW (1963): Vascular changes in the cirrhotic liver as studied by the injection technic. Am J Dig Dis 8: 689-700.

Eguchi T, Ikejiri N, Kawaguchi M, Miyahodo V, Abe H, Tanikawa K (1975): Scanning and transmission electron microscopic observation of human and rat liver sinusoid in liver cirrhosis. J Clin Elec Microsc 8: 5-6.

Gores GJ, Kost LJ, Larusso NF (1986): The isolated perfused rat liver: conceptual and practical consideration. Hepatology 6: 511-517.

Henriksen J, Horn T, Christoffersen P (1984): The blood-lymph barrier in the liver. A review based on morphological and functional concepts of normal and cirrhotic liver. Liver 4: 221-232.

Horn T, Christoffersen P, Henriksen J (1987): Alcoholic liver injury: defenestration in non cirrhotic livers - A scanning electron microscopy study. Hepatology 7: 77-82.

Huet PM, Goresky CA, Villeneuve JP, Marleau D., Lough JO (1982): Assessment of liver microcirculation in human cirrhosis. J Clin Invest 70: 1235-1244.

Huet PM, Villeneuve JP, Pomier Layrargues G, Marleau D (1985): Hepatic circulation in cirrhosis. Clin Gastroenterol 14: 155-168.

Huet PM, Pomier Layrargues G, Villeneuve JP, Varin F, Viallet A (1986): Intrahepatic circulation in liver disease. Semin Liver Dis 6: 277-286.

Mak KM, Lieber CJ (1984): Alterations in endothelial fenestrations in liver sinusoids of baboons fed alcohol: A scanning electron microscopy study. Hepatology 4: 386-391.

Mastaï R, Huet PM: a) Hepatic Circulation: Applicable Human Methodology. b) Hepatic Circulation in Disease (1988). In: P Bioulac-Sage, C Balabaud (Eds): Sinusoids in Human Liver: Health and Disease. The Kupffer Cell Foundation pp 139-150 and pp 299-314.

Mitra SK (1966): Hepatic vascular changes in human and experimental cirrhosis. J Pathol Bacteriol 92: 405-415.

Perez Tammayo R (1983): Is cirrhosis of the liver experimentally produced by CCl_4 an adequate model of human cirrhosis? Hepatology 3: 112-120.

Philips MJ, Steiner JW (1965): Electron microscopy of liver cells in cirrhotic nodules. Am J Pathol 46: 985-1005.

Popper H, Elias H, Petty DE (1952): Vascular pattern of the cirrhotic liver. Am J Clin Pathol 22: 717-729.

Popper H, Orr W (1970): Current concepts in cirrhosis. Scand J Gastroenterol Suppl. 6: 203-222.

Schaffner F, Popper H (1963): Capillarization of hepatic sinusoids. Gastroenterology 44: 239-242.

Stenger RJ (1966): Hepatic sinusoids in carbon tetra-chloride induced cirrhosis. Arch Pathol 81: 439-447.

Varin F, Huet PM (1985): Hepatic microcirculation in the perfused cirrhotic rat liver. J Clin Invest 76: 1904-1912.

Villeneuve JP, Huet PM, Gariépy L, Fenyves D, Willems B, Côté J, Lapointe R, Marleau D (1990): Isolated perfused cirrhotic human liver obtained from liver transplant patients: A feasibility study, Hepatology 12: 257-263.

Résumé

A la question sur l'étendue de nos connaissances sur le flux sanguin chez le cirrhotique, la réponse actuelle ne peut être que peu. Néanmoins, quelques données récentes permettent de comprendre un peu mieux les mécanismes complexes qui conduisent aux altérations du flux sanguin dans le parenchyme hépatique au cours de la cirrhose. Ce flux doit être défini par le sang qui perfuse les cellules parenchymateuses (hépatocytes) via les sinusoïdes normaux c'est-à-dire les capillaires hépatiques qui sont perforés d'une multitude de petites fenêtres et non entourés d'une lame basale. Dans ce cas, les globules rouges restent dans la lumière sinusoïdale ; le plasma et les composés dissous dans celui-ci diffusent librement dans l'espace extravasculaire (espace de Disse) et atteignent directement les hépatocytes sous-jacents où ils sont captés. Grâce à la technique de marquage de dilution multiple (MIDT) l'eau des compartiments vasculaire, extravasculaire et cellulaire et l'extraction de diverses substances au cours d'un seul passage intrahépatique peuvent être mesurés après injection de traceurs dans les vaisseaux afférents.

Dans des conditions normales, le flux sanguin dans le parenchyme hépatique est équivalent au flux sinusoïdal. En d'autres termes, tout le sang de la veine porte et de l'artère hépatique doit passer dans le sinusoïde, ce qui a pour conséquence un flux parenchymateux ou sinusoïdal égal au flux sanguin hépatique. Dans les maladies chroniques de foie le sang qui atteint le foie ne passe pas forcément dans les sinusoïdes, en raison de l'existence de shunts intrahépatiques ; aussi le sang qui passe dans les sinusoïdes peut passer par des sinusoïdes anormaux. Des shunts intrahépatiques de grande taille peuvent être révélés *in vivo* par une modification de la MIDT qui consiste en l'utilisation de microsphères marquées d'un diamètre supérieur à celui des sinusoïdes. Lorsque des shunts sont présents, une partie des microsphères est véhiculée dans ces larges vaisseaux avec les globules rouges. En outre, l'existence de sinusoïdes anormaux peut être associée à la disparition des fenêtres endothéliales et à la formation d'une lame basale sous les cellules endothéliales (capillarisation) et des fibres de collagène peuvent s'accumuler dans l'espace de Disse (collagénisation). Dans de telles conditions, le plasma et les substances dissoutes qu'il véhicule peuvent ne pas avoir un accès direct aux hépatocytes et l'espace de distribution de l'albumine est considérablement réduit comme le montre la MIDT.

Ainsi en raison de la présence de shunts intrahépatiques et de la capillarisation avec collagénisation des sinusoïdes, les flux sanguins hépatique et sinusoïdal ne peuvent être identiques. De plus, les flux sanguins sinusoïdal et parenchymateux peuvent également être différents : les substances dissoutes dans le plasma peuvent diffuser différemment à travers la nouvelle barrière qui s'est formée entre la lumière endothéliale et les hépatocytes. La capillarisation et la collagénisation peuvent très bien restreindre la diffusion de l'albumine dans l'espace extracellulaire sans réduire celles de petites molécules telles que le sucrose et l'eau. Une diffusion restreinte sélective peut aussi intéresser les substances fixées aux protéines. En outre, le sang selon qu'il pénètre dans le foie par l'artère hépatique et la veine porte peut utiliser des circuits vasculaires différents pour atteindre la veine hépatique efférente : chez l'homme et dans des cirrhoses expérimentales, il n'a jamais été observé de shunt intrahépatique entre l'artère et les veines hépatiques, même lorsque des shunts de grande taille existent entre les veines porte et hépatique. De plus, les artères hépatiques terminales peuvent s'interrompre à des distances différentes dans les sinusoïdes dans la mesure où la capillarisation et la collagénisation peuvent différer de la périphérie au centre des nodules de régénération. Ainsi, en prenant en compte l'étendue variable des shunts, de la capillarisation et de la collagénisation, ainsi que les différents circuits de flux dans le foie, une analyse objective est plutôt difficile sinon impossible pour un patient donné.

Cellular and Molecular Aspects of Cirrhosis. Eds B. Clément, A. Guillouzo. Colloque INSERM/John Libbey Eurotext Ltd. © 1992, Vol. 216, pp. 115-134

The extracellular matrix : a major signal transduction network

Detlef Schuppan, Rajan Somasundaram and Martin Just

Klinikum Steglitz, Medizinische Klinik, Abteilung für Gastroenterologie und Hepatologie, Hindenburgdamm 30, 1000 Berlin 45, Germany

Recent interest in cell biology centers on the interplay between cells and their extracellular matrix (ECM). It has been shown that defined epitopes on ECM molecules interact with specific cell surface receptors that transmit signals of position and differentiation to the interior of the cell. The components of the ECM can be classified as collagens, glycoproteins, proteoglycans and elastin. Of the 14 collagen types described so far the *collagens I, III, IV, V and VI* have been found in the liver. *Types I, III and V* form interstitial fibrils, which are interconnected and linked to cellular surfaces by microfibrils of collagen *type VI*, whereas collagen *type IV* serves as the scaffold for basement membranes. The mechanisms that disturb the finely tuned equilibrium of collagen biosynthesis and degradation and finally lead to hepatic cirrhosis are currently under intensive study. The large *ECM glycoproteins* bear several domains connected by flexible arms. These domains contain recognition sequences for cell surface receptors, collagens, proteoglycans/glycosaminoglycans and plasma proteins. *Fibronectins* play a pivotal role in early fibrogenesis and stabilization of the mesenchymal phenotype. *Laminins* anchor preferentially epi- and endothelial cells to basement membranes, directing their growth and maintaining the polarized and differentiated phenotype. *Tenascins* are expressed by undifferentiated mesenchyme and their synthesis is induced in fibrogenesis and in the vicinity of carcinomas, whereas *undulins are* associated with the highly differentiated mesenchyme. Several of the recently described proteoglycans such as *syndecan* and *decorin* have been found in the liver, part of them beeing implicated as cellular receptors or reservoirs for growth factors. Finally, the heterodimeric *integrins* serve as transmembrane signal transmitters by binding to peptide sequences of certain ECM proteins via their extracellular and to the cytoskeleton via their intracellular domains. Our knowledge about the molecular biology of the ECM opens promising new avenues for early detection and effective treatment of previously uncurable hepatic fibrosis and malignancy.

Introduction

The presence of extracellular matrix (ECM) is a basic requirement for multicellular organisms. The maintenance of tissue architecture, cellular polarization and processes such as embryogenesis, differentiation, inflammation and wound healing are dependent on a specialized ECM. Cells are endowed with sets of ECM receptors that transduce signals of position and differentiation generated by constituents of the ECM, thus initiating or modulating genetic programs. On

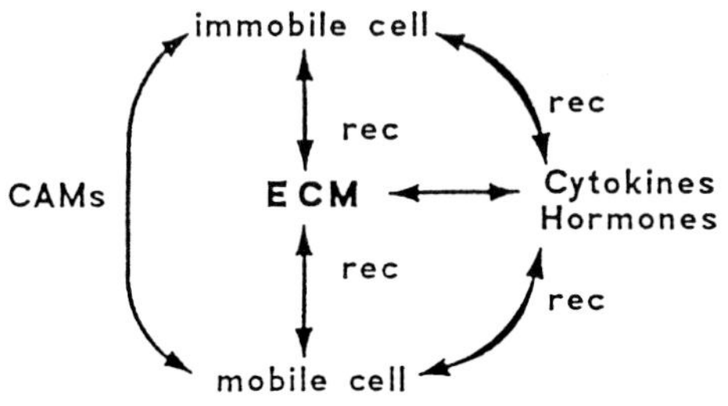

Fig.1 : The role of the ECM in intercellular communication. Cell2 receives signals from cell1 that are transduced by a particular ECM secreted by cell1, and vice versa. Furthermore, cells exchange information via soluble mediators (cytokines, hormones) or directly through cellular adhesion molecules (CAMs). The signals are transferred into the interior of the cell by special transmembrane receptors (rec), except for CAMs which themselves serve as cellular receptors. In addition, cytokine activity may be modulated by binding to ECM molecules.

the other hand these cells may influence the behaviour of their neighbours by secreting a characteristic subset of ECM molecules. Thus eukaryotic cells are interwoven in an interactive network of signal transduction involving the ECM, cellular adhesion molecules, cytokines, hormones and their cellular receptors (Fig.1). In recent years research on ECM has boomed and brought us exciting insight into the structure and function of ECM molecules, their receptors and subsequent cellular responses. It became clear that during evolution most ECM molecules have by exon shuffling aquired a specialized set of interactive domains which have been tailored to the requirements of the particular cellular environment. Such molecules may for example contain A domains of von Willebrand factor that bind collagenous sequences and fibronectin-like type III homologies that interact with heparansulfate proteoglycans or cellular integrin receptors, adding to the continuously growing number of ECM constituents. Molecular diversity is further enhanced by a tissue-specific pattern of differential splicing which may e.g. generate 20 different isoforms of the glycoprotein fibronectin from a single gene. This chapter is intended to provide a tiny overview of the major ECM components (collagens, glycoproteins, proteoglycans) and their cellular receptors that appear relevant for for the liver. Finally, some data on signal transduction and the modulation of growth factor activity by ECM will be mentioned.

Collagens

Collagens constitute the major ECM proteins in the normal adult liver, representing roughly 0.5% of wet liver weight and increasing up to 8% in advanced cirrhosis. Collagens are characterized by their rod-like core structures composed of a triple helix of three identical or homologous polypeptide chains. Formation of such triple helices requires a repetitive sequence with a glycine at every third position and frequent prolines and hydroxyprolines at the first and second positions, respectively. All of the 14 known collagen types bear covalently linked noncollagenous domains which may comprise more than 70% of the molecular weight in the case of collagens type VI, XII and XIV (Fig. 2). Thus far, only collagen types I, III, IV, V and VI have been described in the liver. Once exported from cells the so-called procollagens undergo homo- or heterotypic association to structures of higher order. The resulting kind of assembly is dictated by the collagenous as well as the noncollagenous domains, the latter of which may be proteolytically processed or completely removed. Thus the homo-

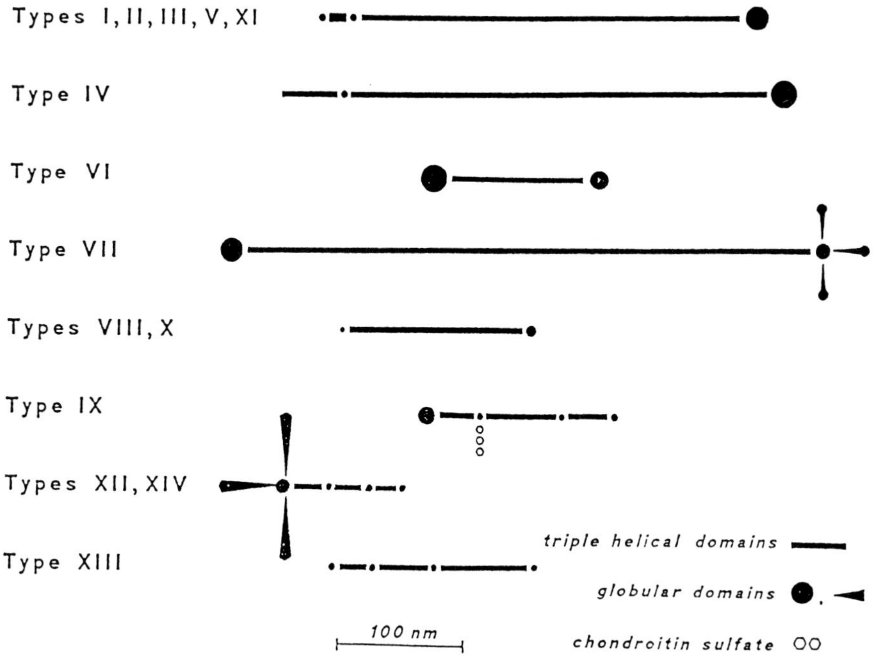

Fig. 2 : Structural models of collagen types I-XIV. The models are based on protein chemical data, sequence information derived from cDNA and the electron-microscopical visualization of single molecules. Only collagen types I, III, IV, V and VI have been found in the liver. Types II, IX, X and XI are limited to cartilage and vitreous body, type VII is a component of epidermal anchoring fibrils and type VIII occurs mainly in neuroectodermal tissues. Types XII and XIV appear to be associated with collagen fibrils in tendon and loose connective tissues and type XIII is expressed in growing and fetal tissues. Modified and actualized from Burgeson (1988).

logous fibril forming *collagen types I, III and V* loose their terminal propeptides by action of extracellular procollagen propeptidases allowing for fibril growth by lateral and end-to-end alignment. Recent data indicate that types I, III and V may form composite fibrils with type V as a core and types I and III as an outer shell. Furthermore, the aminoterminal propeptide of type III is only partly removed at the fibril surface, possibly limiting fibril growth by sterically hindering lateral association of newly synthesized collagen molecules. The fibril for-

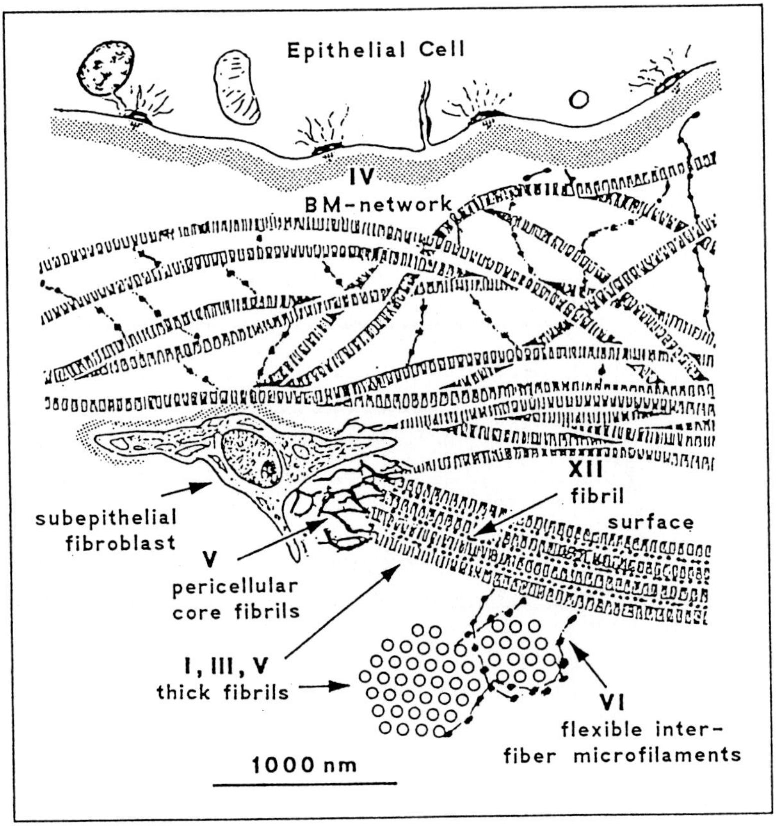

Fig. 3 : Ultrastructural correlate of the liver collagens. Partly processed (pro-) collagen type III is mainly localized at the surface of collagen fibers, whereas type V forms pericellular core fibrils around some mesenchymal cells, which appear to be the starting point for fibril growth by lateral association of collagens type I and III. It is most probable that traces of collagen type XII and/or XIV are also present on certain hepatic collagen fibers. Type VI collagen appears to link individual collagen fibrils to each other and to cellular integrin receptors. Modified from Schuppan (1990).

ming collagens represent more than 90% of total liver collagen with an approx. 40-45% each of types I and III and 5-10 % of type V in normal individuals, and with a shift in favor of type I in cirrhosis. Although *collagen types IV* and *VI* represent a minor fraction of the liver collagens, they fulfill important structural and functional roles as the major scaffold of basement membranes and as interconnecting interstitial microfilaments, respectively (Fig. 3). While procollagen type IV assembles to a flexible three-dimensional network by tetramerization of its aminoterminal and by dimerization of its carboxylterminal propeptides, collagen type VI associates to a chain-like macromolecule by lateral alignment to antiparallel tetramers and subsequent end-to end association. Presently, an ever increasing number of sequence domains is beeing uncovered that, apart from contributing to the particular structural feature of the respective collagen, mediate biologically important interactions such as with other ECM-constituents and cellular receptors. Examples are von Willebrand factor A domains of about 200 amino acids length that are known to interact with collagenous sequences. Repetitive A domains are found in the propeptides of the three constituent chains of collagen type VI, where they obviously mediate homotypic assembly via lateral alignment and heterotypic association with fibrillar collagens, whereas the frequent occurrence of the sequence Arg-Gly-Asp in the triple helical region, which is recognized by several integrins (see below), suggests a role of collagen type VI in cell attachment (Bonaldo et al. 1990). A domains that are separated by fibronectin-like type III homologies (see below) have been discovered in collagen types XII and XIV (Yamagata et al., 1991; Olsen BR, personal communication). Even smaller interactive peptides have been defined in collagen type IV, including a dodecapeptide in the carboxylterminal noncollagenous domain of the a1 chain that inhibits binding of procollagen type IV to heparin and to a yet undefined cellular receptor, and that prevents lateral assembly of the basement membrane collagen network (Tsilibary et al., 1990). A short peptide from the triple helix of the a1(IV) chain promotes melanoma cell attachment and motility (Chelberg et al., 1990), and the domain in collagen type IV interacting with the integrins a1ß1 and a2ß1 has been traced down to an aminoterminal triple helical segment (Vandenberg et al., 1991). Surprisingly, also the highly repetitive fibrillar collagens bear adhesive recognition sequences, such as the tetrapeptide Asp-Gly-Glu-Ala in the triple helical region of the a1 chain of collagen type I that binds to the integrin a2ß1 (Staatz et al., 1991).

ECM glycoproteins

Multifunctional glycoproteins play key roles in the organization of the ECM and in signal transduction processes. As multidomain structures they mediate interactions with other ECM constituents as well as with a variety of transmembrane receptors on sessile and inflammatory cells. Most of them exist in several molecular forms that have been generated by differential splicing of a common gene (as in the case of the fibronectins, tenascins and undulins) or are products of initially common, but subsequently divergent genes (as with the laminins). The major ECM glycoproteins found in the liver are illustrated in table 1.

Fibronectins

Among the ECM glycoproteins the fibronectins have been most extensively investigated (Ruoslahti, 1988). They bind via specific sequence domains to interstitial collagens, heparin, fibrinogen, to the transmembrane proteoglycan

	Structure	Mr (Da)	Localization
Fibronectin		540.000	Interstitium
Tenascin	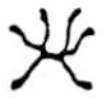	1.200.000	
Undulin	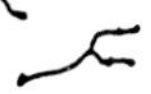	650.000	
Thrombospondin	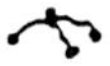	450.000	
Laminin	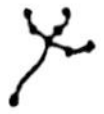	900.000	Basement Membrane
Entactin		150.000	

Table 1 : Electronmicroscopical visualization, molecular weight and localization of the major ECM glycoproteins of the liver. Fibronectin and thrombospondin, isoforms of which circulate as plasma proteins, are also found in most basement membranes, where part of them may have been trapped from the bloodstream.

syndecan and to seven different integrin receptors (see below). Apart from the cellular fibronectins, there exist isoforms that as a product mainly of hepatocytes circulate in plasma at levels between 200 and 400 mg/l. Besides their role in enhancing macrophage opsonic activity fibronectins are involved in blood coagulation and the formation of granulation tissue, where fibronectin-homopolymers and fibronectin-fibrinogen heteropolymers that are formed by a transglutaminase-catalyzed reaction constitute the predominant primary ECM. Anchoring to a fibronectin matrix appears to be important for the maintenance of a differentiated cellular phenotype, since the deficiency of pericellular fibronectin or its high affinity integrin receptor a5ß1 is associated with enhanced metastatic potential and invasiveness (Giancotti and Ruoslahti, 1990). Alternative splicing may produce up to 20 variant fibronectin-chains giving rise to a theoretical 400 species of the dimeric molecule (Fig. 4). This allows for a fine-tuning of the molecule's interactive potential that is tailored to the functional demands of the respective tissue. In addition to repetitive sequence domains, called type I and type II homologies, which bind to fibrin, heparin and collagens, the major portion of the fibronectin molecule is made up of 15 to 17 so-called type III homologies, stretches of about 90 amino acids length, that mediate the interaction with cellular integrin receptors and contain a second heparin-binding domain for the transmembrane proteoglycan syndecan (Saunders and Bernfield, 1988). The classical tripeptide recognition motive RGD (Arg-Gly-Asp) for several integrin receptors has originally been identified in the tenth (eleventh) type III homology of fibronectin (Pierschbacher and Ruoslahti, 1984). Although the presence of the RGD-motive is conditional for binding to the integrin a5ß1, in vitro expression of truncated and mutagenized fibronectin fragments demonstrated that the type III homologies located immediately aminoterminal are necessary for specificity and high avidity of this interaction (Kimizuka et al., 1991). Recently, other short peptide sequences have been defined such as LDV (Leu-Asp-Val) in the first fifth and REDV (Arg-Glu-Asp-Val) in the last fifth of the variable region of fibronectin (Mould et al., 1991; Komoriya et al., 1991). Both LDV and REDV bind to the same or to adjacent regions of the integrin a4ß1, a function of which is that of a lymphocyte homing receptor (Guan and Hynes, 1990). It has also been shown that the presence of the extradomain EIIIA which is found in most forms of tissue fibronectin strengthens cell binding (Mugnai et al., 1988), whereas the extradomain EIIIB, which is mainly expressed during embryogenesis and dedifferentiation, might allow for cell migration by downregulating the avidity for the fibronectin receptors (Carnemolla et al., 1989).

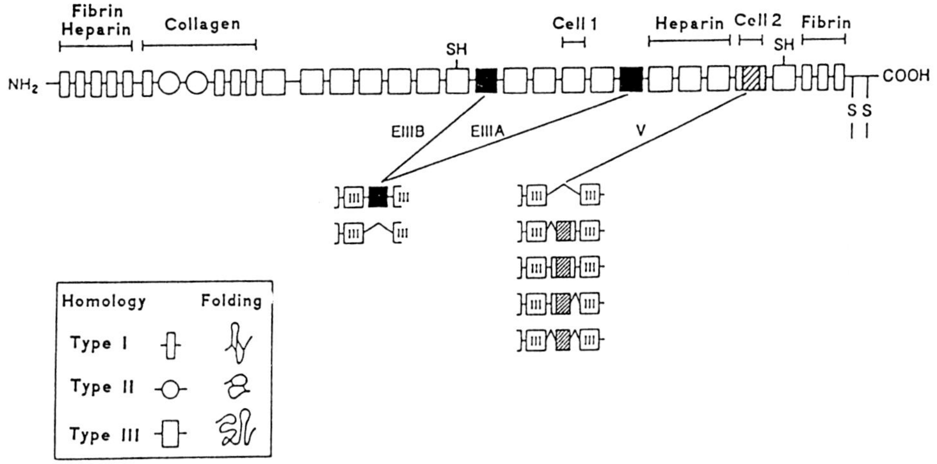

Fig. 4 : Multidomain structure of the fibronectins. The binding sites for fibrin, heparin, collagens and the type III homology with the classical tripeptide recognition motiv (Arg-Gly-Asp) for the cellular fibronectin receptor ('cell1') are indicated. Differential splicing of the extradomains EIIIA, EIIIB and of the variable region V that habours two more cell attachment sequences ('cell2') may give rise to 20 isoforms which are derived from a single gene. S, intermolecular disulfides; SH, free sulfhydryl group. Modified from Ruoslahti (1988).

Tenascins

Tenascins are macromolecules composed of six identical subunits, which are interconnected at their aminoterminal ends, hence the synonym hexabrachions. The various tenascins are generated from one gene by differential splicing of up to four of 15 fibronectin-like type III homologies. In addition, they harbour a carboxylterminal domain with similarity to fibrinogen, possibly mediating binding to the transmembrane proteoglycan syndecan, and 14½ repeats of 31 amino acids length with homology to epidermal growth factor (EGF) (Fig.5). These EGF-like repeats may transmit a growth stimulus to certain cells as has been shown for the respective domains in laminin (see below). The tissue distribution of the tenascins is much more restricted than that of the fibronectins. They are expressed in transitional mesenchyme that is in close contact with rapidly proliferating or migrating epi- and endothelium. Thus tenascins are found during morphogenesis and in the ECM of invasive tumours (Chiquet-Ehrismann, 1990). In the liver they are constitutively expressed in the perisinusoidal space and reexpressed around vascular proliferations during hepatic fibrogenesis (Ramadori et al., 1991). Interestingly, tenascins weaken the strong interaction of fibronectins with cells, thus setting the stage for cell migration and tissue remodeling (Chiquet-Ehrismann et al., 1988). This inhibition appears to be mediated by the EGF-like repeats (Spring et al., 1989). Together with thrombospondin (see below) and osteonectin, tenascins belong to a group of glycoproteins that by modulating cell-matrix interactions enhance cellular motility (Sage and Bornstein, 1991). Accordingly, cells do adhere to but not spread on a tenascin substrate (Bourdon and Ruoslahti, 1989).

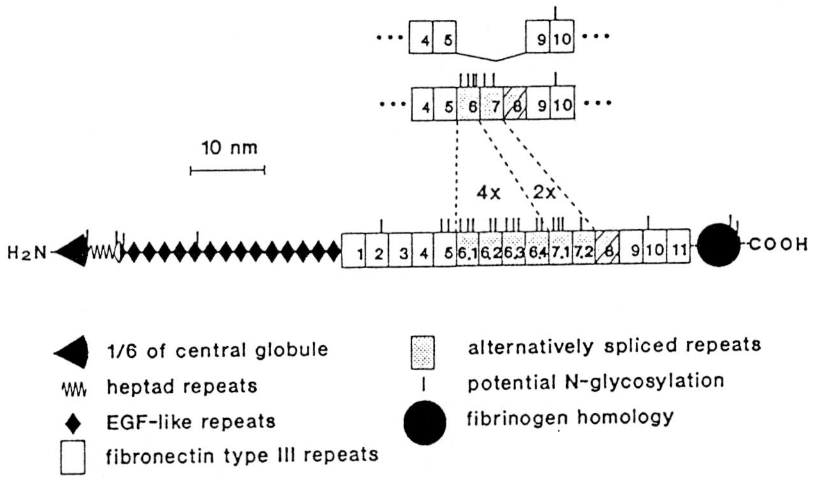

Fig. 5: Multidomain structure of human tenascins. Differential splicing has been observed for the highly glycosylated type III homologies, of which the seven numbered 6.1-6.4, 7.1-7.2 and 8 may be spliced out, leading to variants with Mr 200.000-280.000 Da. Hexamerization is mediated by the aminotermnal globular domains. From the data of Chiquet-Ehrismann (1990) and Nies et al. (1991).

Undulins

Contrary to tenascins, undulins are found almost exclusively in well differentiated connective tissues, and, consequently, their patterns of distribution are exclusive of each other (Schuppan et al., 1990). In the liver undulin decorates regular collagen fiber bundles in the portal field, with prominence in the adventitial sheath of vessels, and single fibers in the perisinusoidal space. Undulins form trimers, the chains of which arise from two or three of at least four known differentially spliced transcripts of a common gene. Sequence analysis of two carboxylterminal polypeptides that cover about 40% of the largest transcript revealed, among domains without similarity to other proteins, up to seven fibronectin-like type III homologies that are bordered at the aminoterminus by a von Willebrand factor A domain (Just et al., 1991). These A domains seem to be operative in mediating binding of undulin to short sequences in the interstitial collagens type I, III, V and VI. One of these sequences is the single cleavage site for the vertebral collagenase in the a2 chain of collagen type I, a finding which inaugurated the intruiging hypothesis that undulins may help to maintain the differentiated interstitial mesenchyme by preventing the degradation of regularly aligned collagen fibrils (Schuppan et al., 1991). In addition, undulins are adhesion proteins for mesenchymal cells, a function which appears to be mediated by one or more integrins, possibly a4ß1, since one of the two isoforms that have been partially sequenced so far, bears the sequence Leu-Asp-Val that has been identified as the recognition motive for the a4ß1 integrin in the CS1 region of fibronectin (Just et al., 1991).

Thrombospondin

Thrombospondin is synthesized by endothelial cells and activated thrombocytes. Accordingly, it is found on the surface of these cells as well as in basement membranes. Thrombospondin is a homotrimeric, three-armed structure with a large central domain and small terminal globules (table 1). Sequence analysis revealed the presence of EGF-like repeats (as in tenascin), minor homologies with fibronectin, von Willebrand factor and the aminoterminal propeptide of type I procollagen, and eight carboxylterminal Ca-binding domains with similarity to those in calmodulin (Lawler and Hynes, 1986). Once Ca is bound by these domains, thrombospondin enhances platelet aggregation, probably exposing an RGD-sequence that interacts with the platelet integrin aVß3 (see below). In addition, the large globule that is composed of the three disulfide-linked aminoterminal domains binds to heparin, collagen type V, laminin, fibronectin, plasminogen and fibrinogen (Lawler, 1986). Reminiscent of tenascin, thrombospondin has been shown to prevent cell spreading and to destabilize focal adhesions, integrin-mediated contacts of the ECM with the cytoskeleton. This effect appears to be facilitated by an interaction of the heparin-binding domain of thrombospondin with the transmembrane proteoglycan syndecan (Bacon-Baguley et al., 1990).

Laminins

Due to their potential to influence the cellular phenotype, laminins have attracted much interest in cell biology (Kleinman et al., 1985; Timpl, 1989). Together with collagen type IV they represent the majority of the basement membrane proteins. Laminin, as originally characterized from a murine tumour, is composed of three distinct polypeptide chains, namely A (M_r 440.000 Da), B1 (M_r 220.000 Da) and B2 (M_r 210.000 Da), that are intertwined to a structure resembling an asymmetric cross (Fig.6). Laminin stabilizes the differentiated phenotype of most epithelial cells, induces cellular polarization and is the most potent stimulator for neurite outgrowth. Thus, hepatocytes seeded on a laminin-rich 'biomatrix' maintain a high expression of albumin and cytochrome P450 for up to four weeks (Bissell et al., 1986). Elucidation of the complete primary structure and functional studies with proteolytic fragments allowed mapping of the laminin molecule for peptide regions with biological activity (Yamada, 1991).

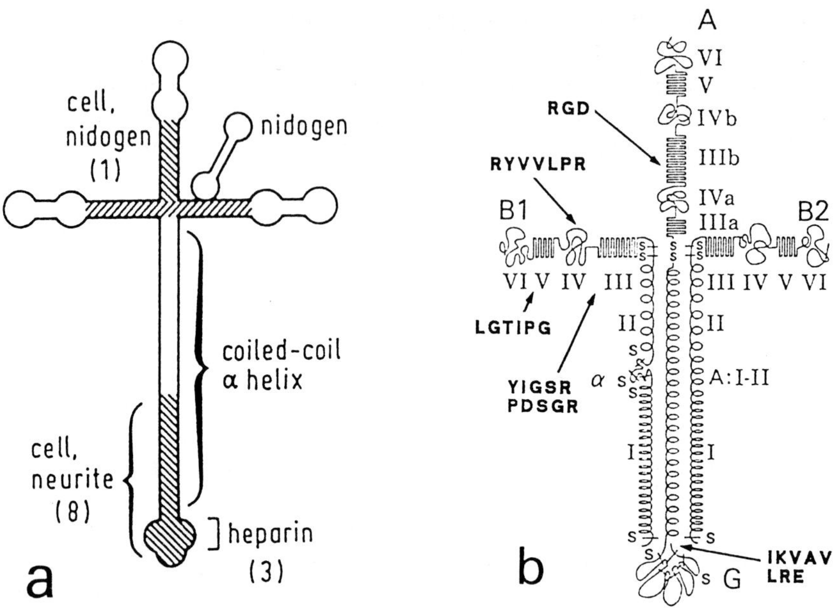

Fig. 6 : Structural model and interactive domains of mouse tumor laminin.

(a) Illustration of protease-resistant fragments 1, 3 and 8 (hatched) that mediate interactions with cellular receptors, heparin/heparansulfate proteoglycan and nidogen/entactin. Binding, and occasionally covalent cross-linking, of the basement membrane glycoprotein nidogen/entactin to domain 1 appears to modulate the interaction with cellular receptors.

(b) Structural organization of laminin that consists of the partially homologous chains A, B1 and B2 with globular domains (G, IV and VI), EGF-like repeats (III and V) and a long a-helical segment made up by the carboxyltermini of all three chains (I and II). The regions bearing biologically active peptides are indicated. Modified from Timpl (1989) considering references cited in the text.

At present, eight adhesive recognition sequences have been identified (Fig. 6b) that bind to cellular acceptor or receptor molecules that transmit functional and positional signals. In this context cellular adhesion to vascular basement membranes plays a crucial role in the multistep process of metastasis. It has been shown in a murine *in vivo* model of metastasis that the laminin peptides YIGSR (Tyr-Ile-Gly-Ser-Arg) and RYVVLPR (Arg-Tyr-Val-Val-Leu-Pro-Arg) that occur in domains III and IV of the B1 chain (Fig.6b) inhibit metastasis (Graf et al., 1987; Skubitz et al., 1990), whereas the peptide IKVAV (Ile-Lys-Val-Ala-Val) from the A chain stimulates release of collagenase IV, which via degradation of the basement membrane scaffold enhances tumor cell invasion and spread (Kanemoto et al., 1990). The finding that experimental metastasis can also be prevented by RGD-peptides points either to a function of this normally cryptic sequence in the A chain of native laminin or to the importance of early or late tumor cell interactions with other RGD-containing proteins such as fibronectin that are exposed in plasma or the interstitium (Humphries et al., 1988). Other biologically active structures are the EGF-like repeats in domains III and V of the laminin chains. Proteolytic fragments containing these repeats have been shown to act via the EGF-receptor and to be as potent as EGF proper in terms of mitogenic stimulation and effective molar concentrations (Panayotou et al., 1989).

Since most studies used the mouse tumor-derived laminin, with the chain composition AB1B2, the finding that the A chain was almost absent and that the B1 and B2 chains occurred in variable relative quantities in most normal adult tissues came as a surprise (Kleinman et al., 1987). Shortly thereafter homologous but genetically distinct members of the laminin family were discovered, such as merosin consisting of B1, B2 and a novel A chain of M_r 385.000 Da that is limited to basement membranes of nerve sheaths, placental trophoblast and cross-striated muscle (Leivo and Engvall, 1988), and S-laminin, an oligomer of only B3 chains that appears to be involved in the structural and functional organization of the synaptic cleft (Hunter et al., 1989).

Proteoglycans and regulation of growth factor activities

Proteoglycans (PG) are hybrid-molecules in which glycosaminoglycans, repetitive acidic carbohydrates, are covalently linked to a core protein. This linkage occurs via O-glycosidic bonds to serine or threonine, or via N-glycosidic bonds to asparagine. PG may be categorized according to their glycosaminoglycan moieties (heparan sulfate, dermatan sulfate, chondroitin sulfate and keratan sulfate) or according to the ever growing list of core proteins (Ruoslahti, 1989). The molecular weight of the various core proteins ranges from 19.000 Da for the intercellular *serglycin* (with dermatan and chondroitin sulfate side chains) to 500.000 Da for the basement membrane proteoglycan *perlecan* (with heparan sulfate side chains). The core proteins contain distinct functional domains. In the case of the large interstitial chondroitin/dermatan sulfate PG *versican* there are two EGF-like repeats and regions with homology to complement factor H, to lectin-binding proteins and to cartilage link protein. Complement factor H-like and lectin binding domains are also found in a class of lymphocyte homing receptors of postcapillary high endothelial venules (Bevilacqua et al., 1989), whereas the Hermes homing receptor functions as a receptor for hyaluronic acid, an interaction that is mediated by a domain with homology to cartilage link protein (Jalkanen et al., 1988). *Syndecan*, with single extracellular side chains of heparan and chondroitin sulfate, belongs to a family of transmembranous PG that similar to the integrins (see below) transmit signals to the cytoskeleton (Saunders and Bernfield, 1988). The binding of syndecan to fibronectin, which is mediated by the heparan sulfate chain, enhances integrin-induced cell adhesion. Certain PGs bear multiple side chains of the highly negatively charged heparan sulfate, and therefore interact with cytokines that bear certain arrays of basic amino acids. Such interactions are found between basement membrane heparan sulfate PG or heparin and basic fibroblast growth factor (b-FGF, Saksela et al., 1988) as well as interferon gamma (Lortat-Jacob et al., 1991). This binding protects b-FGF from rapid degradation by cell surface-bound plasmin and even promotes binding to the high affinity receptor for b-FGF. In addition, the release of growth factors from proteolytically modified heparan sulfate PG has been shown to initiate angiogenesis (Folkman et al., 1988). Interactions with growth factors can also be mediated by the core protein as demonstrated for the structurally related chondroitin/dermatan sulfate PGs decorin and biglycan that bind to and thus neutralize transforming growth factor beta 1 (TGFß1, Yamaguchi et al., 1990). Since TGFß1 that is considered the major mediator in hepatic fibrogenesis causes a severalfold stimulation of collagen and PG synthesis, decorin and biglycan appear to be members of a regulatory loop producing a feedback inhibition of an excessive fibrogenic reaction. Thus by imposing a tight spacial constraint PGs exert a crucial control on growth factor and cytokine activities (Ruoslahti and Yamaguchi, 1991). How this kind of autoregulation of ECM homeostasis is fine-tuned during pattern formation in embryogenesis, stabilized in differentiated tissues and invalidated during progressive fibrosis is currently of great interest.

Integrin receptors for extracellular matrix molecules

As mentioned before the ECM transmits to the cell signals that induce polarization and initiate or modulate migration, differentiation and proliferation. The cell selects ist proper biotope by an individual set of receptor molecules. Receptor-mediated adhesion does not merely imply attachment to the substrate, but also cell spreading, a process that is associated with a rearrangement of the cytoskeleton and an altered gene expression. The integrins and some transmembrane proteoglycans fulfil the criteria of true receptors, since extracellular ligand binding induces activation of their cytoplasmic domains. Other molecules such as the laminin and elastin binding proteins are peripheral membrane proteins. Although they appear to play a role in providing a first matrix anchor for malignant and metastasizing cells (see the overview of Mecham, 1991), they shall not be further discussed in this context.

The integrins are a family of non-covalently associated heterodimers of one a- and one ß-subunit with molecular weights of 90.000-220.000 Da. They mediate cell-matrix and cell-cell interactions. Originally, the integrins had been subdivided into three subfamilies according to their common ß-subunit (table 2). The classical ECM-receptors are found in the ß1-subfamily (synonymous with VLA, the 'very late activation antigens')(Albelda and Buck, 1990; Hemler, 1990), the leukocyte cell-cell adhesion integrins in the ß2-subfamily (Kishimoto et al., 1989) and the thrombocyte integrins (cytoadhesins) in the ß3-subfamily (Ginsberg et al., 1988). Recently at least three more integrin ß chains, which up to now have only been found associated with a single a-subunit, have been characterized. The known combinations of alfa and beta are illustrated in Fig.7a. The availability of cDNA sequences for all integrin chains as well as electronmicroscopical and innumerable functional studies have lead to a clearcut structural model of the integrin heterodimer (Fig.7b). The chains posess a large extracellular domain, a transmembranous segment and, except for ß4, a short cytoplasmic domain of maximally 45 amino acids. Chemical crosslinking showed that the ligand binding site is a pocket formed by the aminotermini of both chains (Smith

β-subfamily	α-subunit	ligand
β1 (CD 29)	α1 (CD 49a)	Lam, Col, FN
	α2 (CD 49b)	Col, Lam
	α3 (CD 49c)	FN, Lam, Col
	α4 (CD 49d)	FN, V-CAM
	α5 (CD 49e)	FN
	α6 (CD 49f)	Lam
	αV (CD 51)	FN
β2 (CD 18)	αL (CD 11a)	I-CAM
	αM (CD 11b)	C3bi, FB, Col
	αX (CD 11c)	C3bi, (Col?)
β3 (CD 61)	αIIb (CD 41)	VWF, FB, FN, VN
	αV (CD 51)	VN, FB, VWF, TSP
β4	α6 (CD 49f)	Lam
β5	αV (CD 51)	VN, FN
βP	α4 (CD 49d)	(ELAM?)

Tab. 2: Subfamily of integrins and their ligands.
Lam, laminin; Col, collagen; FN, fibronectin; C3bi, proteolytic fragment of complement C3; VWF, von Willebrand factor; FB, fibrinogen; VN, vitronectin; TSP, thrombospondin; V-CAM, venular endothelial adhesion molecule; I-CAM, intercellular adhesion molecule 1; ELAM, endothelial leukocyte adhesion molecule. Modified from Albelda and Buck (1990).

and Cheresh, 1988). This interaction is modulated by Ca, Mg or Mn that bind to an adjacent region of three or four sequence motives that are homologous to divalent cation-binding EF-hands (Kirchhofer et al., 1990). The adhesive recognition sequences such as RGD (Arg-Gly-Asp), LDV (Leu-Asp-Val) and LRE (Leu-Arg-Glu) that are contributed by the ligand always bear an aspartic or glutamic acid residue that appears to complement the tetravalent cation binding site, thus inducing a conformational change in the cytoplasmic domain of the integrin (Mould et al., 1991). The cytoplasmic domain of the ß1 chain contains a consensus sequence for tyrosin phosphorylation and is highly conserved among species, with 100% identity between man and mouse. It has been demonstrated that ras-induced tyrosine phosphorylation leads to decreased substrate adhesion in fibroblasts (Tapley et al., 1989), whereas serine- or threonine-phosphorylation of the cytoplasmic a-subunit by protein kinase C strenghtens this interaction (Chatila et al., 1989; Shaw et al., 1990). Both integrin subunits interact with talin and fibulin, cytoplasmic components of adhesion plaques that are coupled to the intermediate filament proteins a-actinin and vinculin. A subsequent structural change of the nuclear membrane induced by phosphorylation of the nuclear membrane protein lamin is possible but still has to be proven. Only recently has it been demonstrated that additional signal transduction pathways such as the induction of the AP-1 transcription factor may be operative upon integrin activation (Yamada et al., 1991).

At least 400 different proteins have been found that contain one or more of the

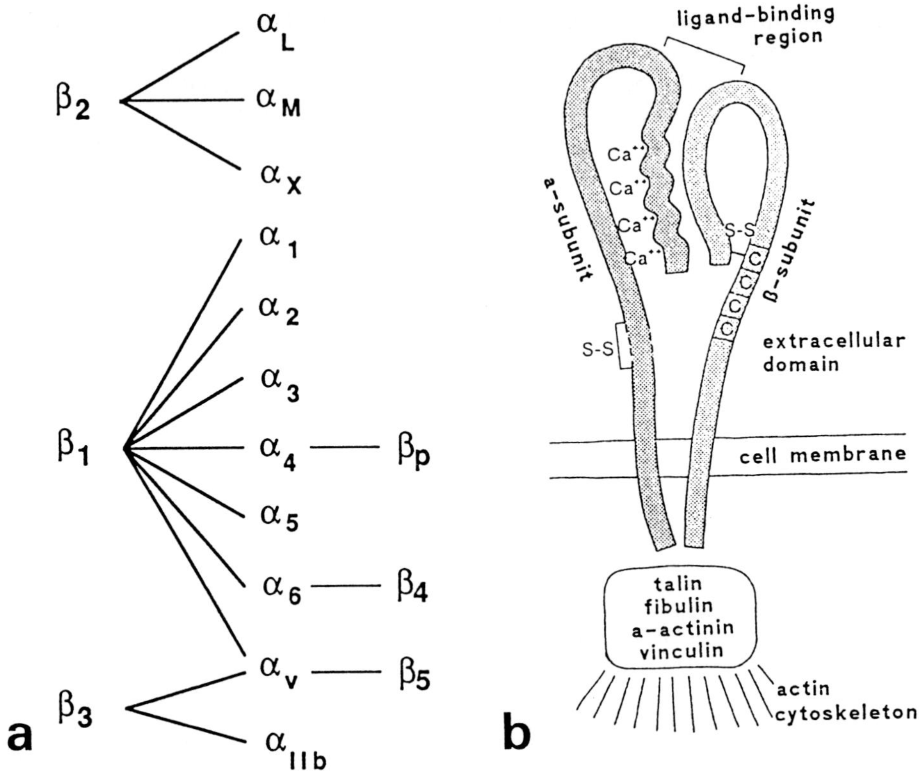

Fig. 7: (a) Known combinations of integrin subunits.
(b) Structural model of the integrins.
S-S, disulfide bridge; C, cystein-rich domain. For details refer to the text.
(a) and (b) have been modified from Albelda and Buck (1990).

copies of the classical adhesive recognition motive RGD, among them the majority of ECM molecules. In addition there are other recently defined (as LDV for a4ß1, see 'fibronectin') or still undefined (as in the ligands for a3ß1 and a6ß1) adhesive sequences. As can be seen from table 2 and Fig. 7 fibronectins can bind to seven different integrin receptors, and a single integrin may have several ligands with different adhesive sequences. Chemical crosslinking showed that the platelet integrin aIIbß3 binds the peptide Lys-GlN-Ala-Gly-Asp-Val of the a-chain of fibrinogen between positions 109-171 of the a-subunit, and the peptide Arg-Gly-Asp-Val of fibronectin between positions 294-314 of the ß-subunit (D'Souza et al., 1990). Furthermore, a1ß1, a2ß1 and the ß2-integrins bear inserted domains with homology to the A domains of von Willebrand factor (see 'collagens' and 'glycoproteins') that may be expected to interact with fibrillar collagens. Such an interaction has been shown between the leukocyte integrin aMß2 and collagens type II and VI (Ley and Schuppan, unpublished data). On the other hand, the classical matrix-receptors a1ß1 and a3ß1 may function as cell-cell adhesion molecules (Larjava et al., 1990).

Ligand binding to integrins can stimulate the secretion of collagenases and consequently allows a cell to invade or restructure the ECM. This has been demonstrated after binding of fibronectin fragments to the classical fibronectin receptor a5ß1 (Werb et al., 1989). That the equipment with integrins is linked to the state of cellular differentiation has been shown by several groups. As an example the polyspecific receptor a3ß1 is highly expressed on osteosarcoma cells, whereas the fibronectin specific a5ß1 is downregulated (Heino and Massague', 1989). This pattern of integrin expression can be reversed by addition of TGF-ß1. Certain types of integrins as the laminin specific a6ß4 (Hemler et al., 1989) and the fibrinogen/fibronectin specific aVß5 (Freed et al., 1989) appear to be associated with the transformed or undifferentiated cellular phenotype. Elegant experiments used transfection of the collagen receptor a2ß1 into rhabdomyosarcoma cells of low invasiveness and metastatic potential to produce a highly malignant phenotype (Chan et al., 1991), whereas transfection of the fibronectin receptor a5ß1 reduced the malignant potential of chinese hamster ovary cells (Giancotti and Ruoslahti, 1990).

Acknowledgement: We thank Fatuma Schuppan for excellent type work.

REFERENCES

Albelda, S.M., Buck, C.A. (1990): Integrins and other cell adhesion molecules. *FASEB J.* 4, 2868-2880.

Bacon-Baguley, E., Ogilvie, M.L., Gartner, T.K., Walz, D.A. (1990): Thrombospondin binding to specific sequences within the Aa- and Bß-chains of fibrinogen. *J. Biol. Chem.* 265, 2317-2323.

Bevilacqua, M.P., Stengelin, S., Gimbrone, M.A., Seed, B. (1989): Endothelial leukocyte adhesion molecule 1: an inducible receptor for neutrophils related to complement regulatory proteins and lectins. *Science* 243, 1160-1165.

Bissell, D.M., Stamatoglu, S., Nermut, M., Hughes, C. (1986): Interaction of rat hepatocytes with type IV collagen, fibronectin and laminin matrices. *Eur. J. Cell Biol.* 40, 72-78.

Bonaldo, P., Russo, V., Buciotti, F., Doliana, R., Colombatti, A. (1990): The carboxylterminus of the chicken a3 chain of collagen type VI is a unique mosaic structure with glycoprotein Ib-like, fibronectin type III, and Kunitz modules. *J. Biol. Chem.* 264, 20235-20239.

Bourdon, M.A., and Ruoslahti, E. (1989): Tenascin mediates cell attachment through an RGD-dependent receptor. *J. Cell Biol.* 108, 1149-1155.

Burgeson, R.E. (1988): New collagens, new concepts. *Annu. Rev. Cell Biol.* 4, 551-577.

Carnemolla, B., Balza, E., Siri, A., Zardi, L., Nicotra, M.R., Bigotti, A., Natali, P.G. (1989): A tumor-associated fibronectin isoform generated by alternative splicing of mRNA precursors. *J. Cell Biol.* 108, 1139-1148.

Chan, B.M.C., Matsuura, N., Takada, Y., Zetter, B.R., Hemler, M. (1991): In vitro and in vivo consequences of VLA-2 expression on rhabdomyosarcoma cells. *Science* 251, 1600-1602.

Chatila, T.A., Geha, R.S., Arnaout, M.A. (1989): Constitutive and stimulus-induced phosphorylation of CD11/CD18 leukocyte adhesion molecules. *J. Cell Biol.* 109, 3435-3443.

Chelberg, M.K., McCarthy, J.B., Skubitz, A.P.N., Furcht, L.T., Tsilibary, L.C. (1990): Characterization of a synthetic peptide from type IV collagen that promotes melanoma cell adhesion, spreading and motility. *J. Cell Biol.* 111, 262-270.

Chiquet-Ehrismann, R., Kalla, P., Pearson, C.A., Beck, K., Chiquet, M. (1988): Tenascin interferes with fibronectin action. *Cell* 53, 383-390.

Chiquet-Ehrismann, R. (1990): What distinguishes tenascin from fibronectin ? *FASEB J.* 4, 2598-2604.

D'Souza, , S.E., Ginsberg, M.H., Burke, T.A., Plow, E.F. (1990): The ligand binding site of the platelet integrin receptor GPIIb-IIIa is proximal to the second calcium binding domain of its a subunit. *J. Biol. Chem.* 265, 3440-3446.

Folkman, J., Klagsbrunn, M., Sasse, J., Wadzinski, M., Ingber, D., Vlodavsky, I. (1988): A heparin-binding angiogenic protein-basic fibroblast growth factor-is stored within basement membrane. *Am. J. Pathol.* 130, 393-400.

Freed, E., Gailit, J., van der Geer, P., Ruoslahti, E., Hunter, T. (1989): A novel integrin ß subunit is associated with the vitronectin receptor a subunit (aV) in a human osteosarcoma cell line and is a substrate for protein kinase C. *EMBO J.* 8, 2955-2965.

Giancotti, F.G., and Ruoslahti, E. (1990): Elevated levels of the a5ß1 fibronectin receptor suppress the transformed phenotype of Chinese hamster ovary cells. *Cell* 60, 849-859.

Ginsberg, M.H., Loftus, J.C., Plow, E,F. (1988): Cytoadhesins, integrins and platelets. *Thromb. Haemostasis* 59, 1-6.

Graf, J., Ogle, R.C., Robey, F.A., Sasaki, M., Martin, G.R., Yamada, Y, Kleinman, H.K. (1987). A pentapeptide from the laminin B1 chain mediates cell adhesion and binds the 67000 laminin receptor. *Biochemistry* 26, 6896-6900.

Guan, J.L., and Hynes, R.O. (1990): Lymphoid cells recognize an alternatively spliced segment of fibronectin via the integrin receptor a4ß1. *Cell* 60, 53-60.

Heino, J., Massague', J. (1989): Transforming growth factor-ß switches the pattern of integrins expressed in MG-63 human osteosarcoma cells and causes selective loss of cell adhesion to laminin. *J. Biol. Chem.* 264, 21806-21811.

Hemler, M.E. (1990): VLA proteins in the integrin family: structures, functions and their role on leukocytes. *Annu. Rev. Immunol.* 8, 365-400.

Hemler, M.E., Crouse, C., Sonnenberg, A. (1989): Association of the VLA a6 subunit with a novel protein. A novel alternative to the common VLA ß1 subunit on certain cell lines. *J. Biol. Chem.* 264, 6529-6535.

Humphries, M.J., Yamada, K.M., Olden, K. (1988): Investigation of the biological effects of anti-cell adhesive synthetic peptides that inhibit experimental metastasis of B16-F10 murine melanoma cells. *J. Clin. Invest.* 81, 782-790.

Hunter, D.D., Shah, V., Merlie, J.P., Sanes, J.R. (1989): A laminin-like adhesive protein concentrated in the synaptic cleft of the neuromuscular junction. *Nature* 338, 229-234.

Jalkanen, S., Jalkanen, M., Bargatze, R., Tammi, M., Butcher, E.C. (1988): Biochemical properties of glycoproteins involved in lymphocyte recognition of high endothelial venules in man. *J. Immunol.* 141, 1615-1623.

Just, M., Herbst, H., Hummel, M., Dürkop, H., Stein, H., Schuppan, D. (1991): Undulin is a novel member of the fibronectin-tenascin gene family of extracellular matrix glycoproteins. *J. Biol. Chem.* 266, 17326-17332.

Kanemoto, T., Reich, R., Greatorex, D., Adler, S.H., Shiraishi, N., Martin, G.R., Yamada, Y., Kleinman, H.K. (1990): Identification of an amino acid sequence from the laminin A chain that stimulates metastasis and collagenase IV production. *Proc. Natl. Acad. Sci. USA* 87, 2279-2283.

Kimizuka, F., Ohdate, Y., Kawase, Y., Shimojo, T., Taguchi, Y., Hashino, K., Goto, S., Hashi, H., Kato, I., Sekiguchi, K., Titani, K. (1991): Role of type III homology repeats in cell adhesive function within the cell-binding domain of fibronectin. *J. Biol. Chem.* 266, 3045- 3051.

Kirchhofer, D., Gailit, J., Ruoslahti, E., Pierschbacher, M.D. (1990): Cation-dependent changes in the binding specificity of the platelet receptor GPIIb/IIIa. *J. Biol. Chem* 265, 18525-18530.

Kishimoto, T.K., Larson, R.S., Corbi, A.L., Dustin, M.L., Staunton, D.E., Springer, T.A. (1989): The leukocyte integrins. *Adv. Immunol.* 46, 149-182.

Kleinman, H.K., Cannon, F.B., Laurie, G.R., Hassel, J.R., Aumailley, M., Terranova, V.P., Martin, G.R., Dubois-Dalc, M. (1985): Biological activities of laminin. *J. Cell. Biochem.* 27, 317-325.

Kleinman, H.K., Ebihara, I., Killen, P., Sasaki, M., Cannon, F.B., Yamada, Y., Martin, G.R. (1987): Genes for basement membrane proteins are coordinately expressed in differentiing F9 cells but not in normal adult murine tissues. *Dev. Biol.* 122, 373-378.

Larjava, H., Peltonen, J., Akiyama, S.K., Yamada, S.S., Gralnick, H.R., Uitto, J., Yamada, K.M. (1990): Novel functions for ß1-integrins in keratinocyte cell-cell interactions.*J. Cell Biol.* 110, 803-815.

Lawler, J. (1986): The structural and functional properties of thrombospondin. *Blood* 67, 1197-1209.

Lawler, J., and Hynes, R. (1986): The structure of human thrombospondin, an adhesive glycoprotein with multiple calcium-binding sites and homologies with several different proteins. *J. Cell Biol.* 103, 1635-1648.

Leivo, I., Engvall, E. (1988): Merosin, a protein specific for basement membranes of Schwann cells, striated muscle, and trophblast, is expressed late in nerve and muscle development. *Proc. Natl. Acad. Sci. USA* 85, 1544-1547.

Lortat-Jacob, H., Kleinman, H.K., Grimaud, J.A. (1991): High-affinity binding of interferon-gamma to a basement membrane complex (matrigel). *J. Clin. Invest.* 87, 878-883.

Mecham, R.P. (1991): Receptors for laminin on mammalian cells. *FASEB J.* 5, 2538-2543.

Mould, A.P., Komoriya, A., Yamada, K.M., Humphries, M.J. (1991): The CS5 peptide is a second site in the IIICS region of fibronectin recognized by the integrin a4ß1. *J. Biol. Chem.* 266, 3579-3585.

Mugnai, G., Lewandowska, K., Carnemolla, B., Zardi, L., Culp, L.A. (1988): Modulation of matrix adhesive responses of human neuroblastoma cells by neighbouring sequences in the fibronectins. *J. Cell Biol.* 106, 932-943.

Nies, D.E., Hemesath, T.J., Kim, J.H., Gulcher, J.R., Stefansson, K. (1991): The complete cDNA sequence of human hexabrachion (tenascin). A multidomain protein containing unique epidermal growth factor repeats. *J. Biol. Chem.* 266, 2818-2823.

Panayotou, P., End, G., Aumailley, M., Timpl, R., Engel, J. (1989): Domains of laminin with growth factor activity. *Cell* 56, 93-101.

Pierschbacher, M.D., and Ruoslahti, E. (1984): Cell attachment activity of fibronectin can be duplicated by small synthetic fragments of the molecule. *Nature* 309, 30-33.

Ramadori, G., Schwögler, S., Veit, T., Chiquet-Ehrismann, R., Mackie, E.J., Knittel, T., Rieder, H., Meyer zum Büschenfelde, K.H. (1991): Tenascin gene expression in rat liver cells. *Virchows Arch. B* 60, 145-153.

Ruoslahti, E. (1988): Fibronectin and its receptors. *Annu. Rev. Biochem.* 57, 375-413.

Ruoslahti, E. (1989): Proteoglycans in cell regulation. *J. Biol. Chem.* 264, 13369-13372.

Ruoslahti, E., Yamaguchi, Y. (1991): Proteoglycans as modulators of growth factor activities. *Cell* 64, 867-869.

Sage, H., and Bornstein, P. (1991): Extracellular proteins that modulate cell-matrix interactions. *J. Biol. Chem.* 266, 14831-14834.

Saksela, O., Moscatelli, D., Sommer, A., Rifkin, D.B. (1988): Endothelial cell-derived heparan sulfate binds basic fibroblast growth factor and protects it from degradation. *J. Cell Biol.* 107, 743-751.

Saunders, S., and Bernfield, M. (1988): Cell surface proteoglycan binds mouse mammary epithelial cells to fibronectin and behaves as a receptor for interstitial matrix. *J. Cell Biol.* 106, 423-430.

Schuppan, D. (1990): Structure of the extracellular matrix in normal and fibrotic liver: collagens and glycoproteins. *Sem. Liver Dis.* 10, 1-10.

Schuppan, D., Cantaluppi, M.C., Becker, J., Veit, A., Bunte, T., Troyer, D., Schuppan, F., Ackermann, R, Schmid, M., Hahn, E.G. (1990): Undulin, an extracellular matrix glycoprotein associated with collagen fibrils. *J. Biol. Chem.* 265, 8823-8832.

Schuppan, D., Schmid, M., Ackermann, R. : Binding of undulin to interstitial collagens type I, III, V and VI is mediated by specific sequence domains. Submitted.

Shaw, L.M., Messier, J.M., Mercurio, A.M. (1990): The activation dependent adhesion of macrophages to laminin involves cytoskeletal anchoring and phosphorylation of the a6ß1 integrin. *J. Cell Biol.* 110, 2167-2174.

Skubitz, A.P.N., McCarthy, J.B., Zhao, Q., Yi, X.Y., Furcht, L.T. (1990): Definition of a sequence, RYVVLPR, within laminin peptide F-9 that mediates metastatic fibrosarcoma cell adhesion an spreading. *Cancer Res.* 50, 7612-7622.

Smith, J.W., Cheresh, D.A. (1988): The Arg-Gly-Asp-binding domain of the vitronectin receptor. *J. Biol. Chem.* 263, 18726-18731.

Spring, J., Beck K., Chiquet-Ehrismann R. (1989): Two contrary functions of tenascin: dissection of the active sites by recombinant tenascin fragments. *Cell* 59, 325-334.

Staatz, W.D., Fok, K.F., Zutter, M.M., Adams, S.P., Rodriguez, B.A., Santoro, S. A. (1991): Identification of a tetrapeptide recognition sequence for the a2ß1 integrin in collagen. *J. Biol. Chem.* 266, 7363-7367.

Tapley, P., Horwitz, A., Buck, C., Duggan, K., Rohrschneider, L. (1989): Integrins isolated from Rous sarcoma virus-transformed chicken embryo fibroblasts. *Oncogene* 4, 325-333.

Timpl, R. (1989): Structure and biological activity of basement membrane proteins. *Eur. J. Biochem.* 180, 487-502.

Tsilibary, E.C., Reger, L.A., Vogel, A.M., Koliakos, G.G., Anderson, S.S., Charonis, A.S., Alegre, J.N., Furcht, L.T. (1990): Identification of a multifunctional, cell-binding peptide sequence from the a1(NC1) of type IV collagen. *J. Cell Biol.* 111, 1583-1591.

Vandenberg, P., Kern, A., Ries, A., Luckenbill-Edds, L., Mann, K., Kühn, K. (1991): Characterization of a type IV collagen major cell binding site with affinity to the a1ß1 and a2ß1 integrins. *J. Cell Biol.* 113, 1475-1483.

Werb Z., Tremble, P.M., Behrendtsen, O., Crowley, E., Damsky, C.H. (1989): Signal transduction through the fibronectin receptor induces collagenase and stromelysin gene expression. *J. Cell Biol.* 109, 887-889.

Yamada, K. (1991). Adhesive recognition sequences. *J. Biol. Chem.* 266, 12809-12812.

Yamada, A., Nikaido, T., Schlossmann, S.F., Morimoto, C. (1991): Activation of human CD4 T lymphocytes. Interaction of fibronectin with VLA-5 receptor on CD4 cells induces the AP-1 transcription factor. *J. Immunol.* 146, 53-56.

Yamagata, M., Yamada, K.M., Yamada, S.S., Shinomura, T., Tanaka, H., Nishida, Y., Obara, M., Kimata, K. (1991): The complete primary structure of type XII collagen shows a chimeric molecule with reiterated fibronectin type III motifs, von Willebrand factor A motifs, a domain homologous to a noncollagenous region of type IX collagen, and short collagenous domains with an Arg-Gly-Asp site. *J. Cell Biol.* 115, 209-221.

Yamaguchi, Y., Ruoslahti, E. (1990) : Negative regulation of transforming growth factor-ß by the proteoglycan decorin. *Nature* 346, 281-284.

Résumé

Les interactions cellules-matrice extracellulaire (ECM) constituent un centre d'intérêt récent en biologie cellulaire. Il a été montré que des épitopes bien définis des molécules matricielles interagissent avec des récepteurs cellulaires spécifiques qui transmettent des signaux de situation et de différenciation à l'intérieur de la cellule. Les constituants de l'ECM sont regroupés en différentes classes qui sont les collagènes, les glycoprotéines, les protéoglycanes et les élastines. Sur les 14 types de collagènes décrits jusqu'ici, les collagènes I, III, IV, V et VI ont été trouvés dans le foie. Les types I, III and V forment les fibres intersticielles qui sont interconnectées et liées aux surfaces cellulaires par des microfibrilles de collagène VI ; le collagène IV constitue la trame des lames basales. Les mécanismes qui perturbent l'équilibre très fin entre biosynthèse et dégradation et finalement conduisent à la cirrhose font actuellement l'objet d'études approfondies. Les glycoprotéines matricielles de grande taille possèdent plusieurs domaines reliés par des bras flexibles. Ces domaines contiennent les séquences de reconnaissance des récepteurs de la surface cellulaire, des collagènes, des protéoglycanes/glycosaminoglycanes et des protéines plasmatiques. Les fibronectines jouent un rôle primordial au cours des premiers stades de la fibrogénèse et dans la stabilisation du phénotype mésenchymateux. Les laminines attachent préférentiellement les cellules épithéliales et endothéliales aux lames basales, dirigent leur croissance et maintiennent le phénotype polarisé et différencié. Les ténascines sont exprimées par le mésenchyme indifférencié et leur synthèse est induite au cours de la fibrogénèse et à proximité des carcinomes tandis que les undulines sont associées au mésenchyme hautement différencié. Parmi les protéoglycanes récemment décrites plusieurs tels que le syndecan et la décorine ont été retrouvés dans le foie, une partie d'entre eux servant de récepteurs cellulaires et de réservoirs de facteurs de croissance. Enfin, les intégrines hétérodimériques agissent comme transmetteurs de signaux transmembranaires en se fixant à des séquences peptidiques de certaines protéines matricielles par leurs domaines extracellulaires et au cytosquelette par leurs domaines intracellulaires. La connaissance de la biologie moléculaire d'ECM ouvre des voies nouvelles très prometteuses pour la détection précoce et le traitement effectif de la fibrose hépatique jusqu'ici incurable et du cancer.

Cellular and Molecular Aspects of Cirrhosis. Eds B. Clément, A. Guillouzo. Colloque INSERM/John Libbey Eurotext Ltd. © 1992, Vol. 216, pp. 135-145

Basement membrane genes and transcription factors

Peter Burbelo [1], Gary Gabriel [1], J. Wujeck [2], Vishram V. Kedar, Benjamin S. Weeks [1], Hynda K. Kleinman [1] and Yoshihiko Yamada [1]

[1] *Laboratory of Developmental Biology, National Institute of Dental Research, National Institutes of Health;* [2] *Laboratory of Molecular Biology, National Institute of Neurological Disorders and Strokes, Bethesda, Maryland, USA*

SUMMARY

Basement membrane gene expression is of critical importance in cell differentiation, growth and development. The 5'-end of the laminin B1 and B2 gene and of the α1 and α2(IV) collagen genes have been isolated in order to understand the regulation of these genes. Using transfection analysis, DNA footprinting and gel shift assays, several DNA regulatory elements have been identified. Work in progress will ellucidate the transcription factors which bind to these regulatory elements.

Laminin induces differentiation, but the exact mechanisms are unclear. Using a differential screen, a transcription factor induced by laminin, Lilzip-1, has been identified in neural cells. A complete Lilzip-1 cDNA has been obtained and characterized as having a serine-rich domain, a highly basic DNA-binding domain and a leucine zipper dimerization domain. Anti-lilzip antibodies detected a 46 kDa protein in tissues rich in basement membrane such as brain, kidney, and lung. DNA binding experiments indicate Lilzip has a high affinity for AP-1 and CRE /ATF DNA sequences. Thus, laminin-induced differentiation may involve the induction of specific transcription factors.

INTRODUCTION

Basement membranes are thin layers a of extracellular matrix underlying endothelial, epithelial, muscular, and neural cells (Martin and Timpl, 1987). Basement membranes are the first extracellular matrices produced during embryonic development. These structures serve important structural and functional roles. For example, the glomerular basement membrane serves as an important filtration barrier. Basement membranes also effect a variety of processes including cellular differentiation, growth, and tissue development.

Elucidation of the mechanisms regulating basement membrane gene expression is critical in understanding the role of this structure in cellular differentiation, and tissue development. In this chapter, we will focus on the transcriptional regulation of the genes for basement components. The identification of regulatory elements for basement membrane genes and transcription factors which bind to these elements should help us understand the expression of these components during development and in disease. In addition, the role of the basement membrane in inducing differentiation via the induction of specific genes including transcription factors will also be discussed.

STRUCTURAL COMPONENTS OF THE BASEMENT MEMBRANE

The major constituents of basement membranes are entactin/nidogen, collagen IV, laminin, and perlecan (Table I). Entactin (nidogen) is a dumbbell-shaped protein (Mr= 150,000) which forms a stable complex with laminin. Collagen IV, the major structural component in basement membrane, belongs to a gene family comprising at least five distinct members. The most abundant form of collagen IV contains two α1(IV) and one α2(IV) chains. Laminin, a large glycoprotein, also appears to have several different forms. The most well characterized form is from the EHS tumor and consists of three distinct peptide chains, A(Mr= 400,000), B1(Mr= 210,000), and B2(Mr= 200,000), which form a cross-shaped structure that is held together by disulfide linkages. Additional laminin homologues have also been identified such as s-laminin, and merosin. S-laminin is present in high concentrations in the neuromuscular junction and appears to be a homologue of the B1 chain. Merosin, an apparent homologue of the A chain, may be more abundant in adult tissues than the A chain. Perlecan (basement membrane heparan sulfate proteoglycan) consists of a 400 kDa core protein, which shows two regions with similarity to the A chain. Perlecan has three or four heparan sulfate glycosaminoglycan chains attached to the core protein giving the molecule an average molecular weight of 600 kDa.

Table I Major Components of the Basement Membrane

Component	Molecular Size	Function
Entactin (Nidogen)	150,000	Binds to laminin
Collagen IV	540,000	Structural
Laminin	800,000	Cell Adhesion
Perlecan (HSPG)	800,000	Filtration

Gene Regulation of Basement Membrane Components

In order to explore the transcriptional regulation of basement membrane components, the 5'-end of the genes for the B1 and B2 laminin genes and α1(IV) and α2(IV) have been isolated. A schematic representation of the bidirectional promoter for the α1(IV) and α2(IV) collagen and laminin B1 and B2 promoters are shown in Figure 1.

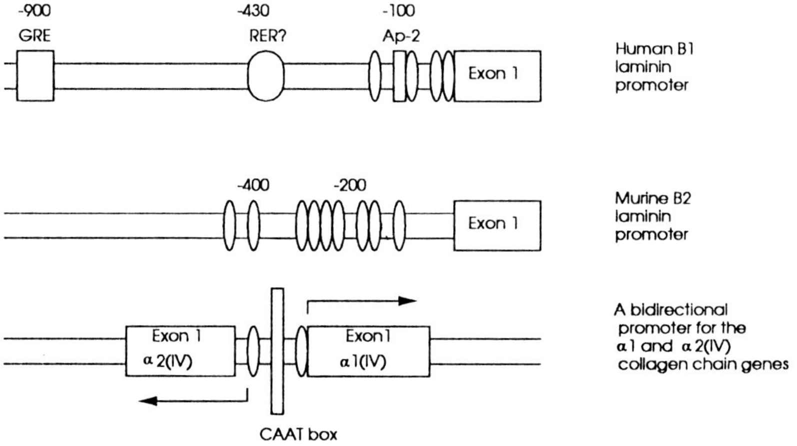

Fig. 1   The Promoters for Several Basement Membrane Components

A schematic is shown for the structure of several basement membrane promoters. The human B1 laminin promoter contains a potential retinoic acid responsive element and glucocorticoid element. The elliptical circles in the murine B2 promoter represent an 11 bp repeat found nine times. The bidirectional promoter for α1(IV) and α2(IV) collagen chain genes is 130 bp in size and contains a single CAAT box.

The genes for the α1(IV) and α2(IV) collagen chains exist in a head-to-head arrangement separated by an intergenic 130 bp bidirectional promoter region in both the human (Poschl et al., 1988; Soininen et al., 1988) and mouse (Burbelo et al.,1988; Kaytes et al., 1988). Although this region contains two GC boxes and no TATA box, transfection analysis using a CAT reporter system revealed low transcriptional activity (Killen et al., 1988; Poschl et al., 1988; Burbelo et al., 1988). However, inclusion of a DNA segment from the first intron, an enhancer, markedly stimulated transcriptional activity (See Table II). The enhancer activity within the first intron of the α1(IV) collagen gene appears to be required for transcription of both the α1(IV) and α2(IV) collagen chain genes, since both orientations of the bidirectional promoter together with the enhancer show similar activity (Burbelo et al., 1988). This enhancer appears to show cell specificity. For example, NIH-3T3 fibroblasts or dermal fibroblasts which produce very low levels of collagen IV, do not show activity with this enhancer construct. Rat hepatoma cells, which produce a small amount of collagen IV, show a low level of transcriptional activity with the collagen IV promoter-enhancer construct. The highest level of activity with the collagen IV promoter-enhancer construct is with both differentiated F9 cells and parietal yolk sack cells and these cells produce a high levels of collagen IV. These data suggest that in most cells the binding of cell-specific transcription factors to both the promoter and enhancer is responsible for cell-specific expression of collagen IV.

Table II Activity of Promoter/Enhancer Constructs For Collagen IV

Construct	Relative Activity	
	$F9^+$	NIH-3T3
Promoter	1	0.5
Promoter/Enhancer	10	0.5

A collagen IV promoter-CAT or collagen IV promoter/enhancer-CAT construct was tested in either F9 teratocarcinoma cells treated with both retinoic acid and cAMP or NIH-3T3 cells (Killen et al., 1988). Relative CAT activity is expressed relative to a positive transfection control β-actin-CAT. The promoter construct showed low activity in both $F9^+$ and NIH-3T3 cells. However, the collagen IV promoter/enhancer construct was active in the $F9^+$ but not in the NIH-3T3 cells.

Regulatory elements within the first intron enhancer fragment (5.0 kb) of the α1(IV) collagen gene have been identified by deletion analysis (Burbelo et al., 1991). Briefly,the intron enhancer fragment was digested with restriction enzymes or Bal-31 nuclease and the resulting fragments were subcloned in the CAT reporter plasmid and transfected into undifferentiated F9 cells. One region of approximately 210 bp was found with significant transcriptional activity. Protein-DNA interactions within this 210 bp piece were mapped more precisely by using DNAase I footprinting. Two regions, footprint A and B, showed protection of 15 and 14 bps, respectively. The role of the footprint A site was tested by creating a point mutation within one of the sites and was shown to decrease activity of the enhancer fragment. These results suggest that positive transcription factors interact with this site. Specific oligonucleotide affinity chromatography and Southwestern analysis using nuclear extracts from EHS tumor cells reveal two candidate transcription factors (Mr=94,000 and Mr=37,000) that interact with the Footprint A site. Present experiments are aimed at cloning both of these proteins to clarify their role in collagen IV transcription.

Sequence analysis of both the murine (Vasios et al., 1989; Yamada et al., 1990) and human laminin B1 gene (Vuolteenaho et al., 1990) reveal that there are no TATA or CAAT boxes but several Sp-1 binding sites (GC boxes). The murine B1 laminin chain gene promoter has been shown to respond to retinoic acid induction and a retinoic acid responsive element (RER) has been identified (Vasios et al., 1989). In vitro, gel retardation assays indicate that all three retinoic acid receptors can bind directly to the laminin B1 RER requiring three TGACC-like motifs for retinoic acid receptor binding (Vasios et al., 1991) Interestingly, the human laminin B1 gene may involve a regulatory mechanism different from the mouse, since it only contains one TGACC sequence (Vuolteenaho et al., 1990).

The murine (Ogawa et al.,1988) and human laminin B2 (Kallunki et al., 1991) promoters have also been isolated. Both the human and murine laminin B2 gene promoter do not contain a TATA or CAAT box. The human B2 promoter contains five GC boxes and three AP-2-like sites, while the murine promoter contains nine GC-boxes and two Ap-2-like sites. Interestingly, the AP-2 transcription factor is induced by retinoic acid (Williams et al., 1988) and may be responsible for the increased transcription of the laminin B2 gene when F9 cells are treated with retinoic acid. Transfection analysis of an 800 bp murine B2 promoter fragment showed significant transcriptional activity. This construct was active in NIH-3T3 cells and showed two-fold higher activity in differentiated F9 cells over undifferentiated F9 cells. Deletion analysis revealed that the first 100 bp of this promoter fragment showed full activity. DNA footprinting of this fragment revealed multiple protein binding sites including a potential AP-2 site (Kedar et al., unpublished). Current experiments using Southwestern screening of cDNA expression libraries and factor purification are aimed at identifying transcription factors that regulate the B2 gene.

LAMININ-INDUCED GENES

Certain cell types such as Sertoli cells (Hadley et al., 1985), mammary epithelial cells (Wicha,et al., 1982), embryonic mesenchymal cells (Klein et al., 1988), and neural cells (Baron van Evercooren et al., 1982) undergo differentiation when in contact with the basement membrane. Of all the basement membrane components, laminin appears to have the stongest biological activity including cell attachment, polarity, growth, migration, and differentiation. The mechanism of laminin induced-differentiation is poorly understood, but in many cases may involve the expression of new genes (Table III). For example, primary hepatocytes plated on collagen I exhibit a rapid loss of albumin production but can be transcriptionally activated by the addition of small amounts of laminin, but not by either collagen IV or perlecan (Caron, 1990).

Table III Genes Induced by Laminin

Cells	Induced Genes	Reference
Hepatocyte	albumin mRNA	Caron, 1990
Mammary Epithelial	β-casein mRNA	Li et al.1987
Mast cells	GMCSF mRNA	Thompson et al 1991
NG108-15	HSP-70	Weeks et al., 1991
NG108-15	Lilzip mRNA	Burbelo et al.1991

One method to detect new genes induced by laminin has been to use the subtractive hybridization approach (Burbelo et al., 1991). Briefly, a cDNA library from cells grown in the presence of laminin is constructed. This library is screened with a radioactive cDNA probe from cells grown in the presence of laminin plus the addition of cold RNA from cells grown in the absence of laminin. The strategy of this screen is to compete out genes in common between laminin-treated cells and untreated cells. Using this approach, several genes induced following laminin-mediated neurite outgrowth have been identified in NG108-15 neural cells. Several of the genes induced by laminin include mitochondrial genes, heat shock 70 and the protease tripeptidyl peptidase (Weeks et al., 1991).

A laminin-induced gene leucine zipper transcription factor (Lilzip) with similarity to c-jun and c-fos has been identified in NG108-15 cells (Burbelo et al., 1991). Lilzip-

1 codes for a protein which contains a basic amino acid DNA binding region and a large leucine zipper, and is a member of b-Zip family of transcription factors (Vinson et al., 1989). A second form of this protein also has been identified and contains an additional 25 amino acids, probably by alternative spilicing, in the amino terminus of the protein. Antibodies to the DNA binding region of Lilzip-1 stained the nucleus of NG108-15 cells. Western immunoblotting with this antibody detected a protein of Mr=46,000 found in a variety of tissues including brain, lung, liver and kidney. The Lilzip-1 fusion protein possesses DNA binding activity for AP-1 and CRE/ATF sites and the binding could be blocked in the gel shift assay by the antibody. The target genes for Lilzip are unknown but these genes may be responsible for laminin-induced gene expression in these cells.

```
RKIRNKRAAQESRKKKK-----L------Y------L------L------L------L------I    LILZIP

RLMKNREAARECRRKKK-----L------L------L------L------K                  CREB

KRMRNRIAASKCRKRKL-----L------L------L------L------L                  c-JUN

RKLKNRVAAQTARDRKK-----L------L------L------L------L                  HXBP-1

RRERNKMAAAKCRNRRR-----L------L------L------L------L                  FOS

BB-BN--AA-B-R-BB------L------L------L------L------L                  b-ZIP
                                                                     CONSENSUS
```

Fig. 2 Similarity of Lilzip to Other Members of the b-Zip Transcription Factor Family

The basic amino acid DNA binding region of Lilzip is similar to other members of the leucine zipper family of transcription factors

Transcription factors, such as c-jun and c-fos, have been shown to be induced as an immediate response to the presence of external stimuli and regulate a variety of genes. For example the transcription factors, NGF1A and HLH462, have been identified as genes induced by soluble growth factors such as nerve growth factor (Milbrandt, 1987) and fibroblast growth factor (Christy et al., 1991), respectively. The identification of a laminin-induced transcription factor suggests that laminin may induce specific transcription factors responsible for cell-specific gene regulation (ie. laminin induction of albumin synthesis in the hepatocyte). Thus,the basement membrane and laminin may induce both general transcription factors such as c-jun and c-fos, as well as those factors that regulate tissue-specific expression (Figure 5).

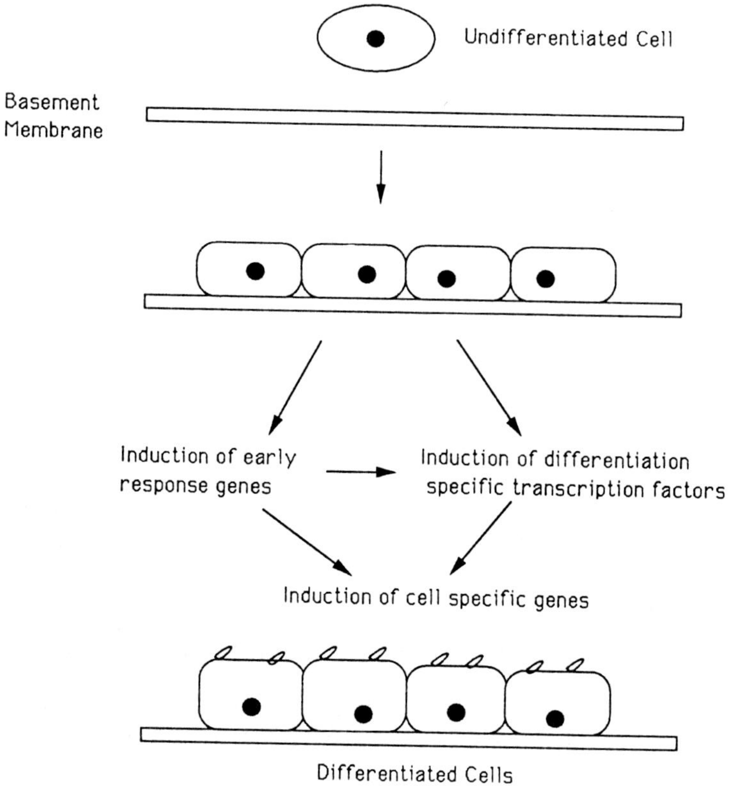

Fig. 3 Basement Membrane Induction of Cell-Specific Transcription Factors

CONCLUSIONS

The identification of regulatory elements for several of the genes for basement membrane components has begun. Identification of protein transcription factors which interact with these sites and regulate the synthesis of these basement membrane components during differentiation and development should increase our understanding of the control of these processes. Knowledge of the DNA elements and factors involved may also ellucidate the mechanisms involved in the overproduction of collagen IV and laminin in such diseases as glomerular nephritis, diabetes and liver cirrhosis. Furthermore, new information suggests that many of effects of basement membrane on cell differentiation are mediated by the induction of new gene expression. The discovery of a transcription factor induced by laminin in neural cells suggests that additional factors may be responsible for specific induction of gene expression in other cells types.

REFERENCES

Baron van Evercooren, A., Kleinman, H.K., Ohno, S., Marangos, P., Schwartz, J.P.a nd Dubois-Dalq, M.E. J.Neurosci. Res. 8: 179-194, 1982.

Burbelo, P.D, Bruggeman, L., Gabriel, G., Klotman, P. and Yamada, Y. J. Biol. Chem. 1991 (in press)

Burbelo, P.D., Martin, G.R., and Yamada, Y., Proc. Natl Acad. Sci. USA 85: 9679-9682, 1988.

Burbelo, P.D., Weeks, B., Gabriel, G., Kibbey, M., Yamada, Y. and Kleinman, H.K.1991 (submitted).

Caron, J.M. Mol. Cell. Biol. 10:1239-1243, 1990.

Christy, B.A., Sanders, L.K., Lau, L.F., Copeland, N.G., Jenkins, N.A. and Nathans, D. Proc. Natl. Acad. Sci. 88:1815-1819, 1991.

Hadley, M.A., Byers, S.W., Suarez-Quian, C.A., Kleinman, H.K., and Dym, M. J. Cell. Biol. 101:1511-1522, 1985.

Kallunki, T., Ikonen, J., Chow, L.T., Kallunki, P., and Tryggvason, K., J. Biol. Chem. 266: 221-228, 1991.

Killen, P.D.,Burbelo,P.D, Martin, G.R., and Yamada, Y., J. Biol. Chem. 263: 12310-12314, 1988.

Klein, G., Langegger, M., Timpl, R., and Ekbloom, P. Cell 55:331-341, 1988.

Li, M.L., Aggeler, J., Farson, D.A., Hatier, C., Hassell, J., and Bissell, M.J. Proc. Natl. Acad. Sci. 84: 136-140, 1987.

Martin, G.R. and Timpl, R. Ann. Rev. Cell. Biol. 3:57-85, 1987.

Milbrandt, J. Science 238:797-799, 1987.

Poschl,E., Pollner, and Kuhn,K.,EMBO 7:2687-2695, 1988

Soininen, R., Huotari, M.,Hoska,S.L.Prockop,D.J., and Tryggvason, K., J. Biol. Chem. 203: 17217-17220, 1989.

Thompson, H.L., Burbelo, P.D., Metcalf, D. and Yamada, Y. 1991 (manuscript in preparation).

Vasios, G.W., Gold, J.D., Petkovich, M., Chambon, P., and Gudas, L.J., Proc. Natl. Acad. Sci. USA 86: 9099-9103,1989.

Vinson, C.R., Sigler, P.B., and McKnight, S.L., Science 246,911-916, 1989.

Vuolteenaho, R., Chow, L.T., and Tryggvason, K. J. Biol. Chem., 265: 15611-15616.

Williams, T., Admon, A., Luscher, B., and Tijan, R. Genes and Dev. 2: 1557-1564, 1988.

Weeks, B.,Burbelo, P.D., Kleinman, H. (manuscript in preparation).

Wicha, M.S., Lowrie,G., Kohn, E., Bagavadose, P., and Mahn,T., Proc. Natl. Acad. Sci. USA 79, 3213-3217, 1982.

Yamada,Y., Graf, J., Iwamoto, J., Kato, S., Kleinman, H., Kohno, K., Martin, G.R., Ogawa, K., and Sasaki, M., Morphoregulatory Molecules. Edited by Edelman, Cunningham, and Thiery. 231-244, 1990.

Résumé

L'expression des gènes codant pour les protéines des lames basales est très importante au cours de la différenciation cellulaire, de la croissance et du développement. Les régions 5' des gènes codant pour les chaînes B1 et B2 de la laminine et les chaînes α_1 et α_2 du collagène IV ont été isolées afin de comprendre la régulation de ces gènes. Par des techniques de transfection, d'empreinte et de retardement sur gel, plusieurs éléments régulateurs ont été identifiés au niveau de l'ADN. Les travaux en cours permettront de caractériser les facteurs transcriptionnels qui interagissent avec ces éléments.

La laminine induit la différenciation cellulaire selon des mécanismes mal connus. Par criblage différentiel, un facteur de transcription induit par la laminine, "Lilzip-1", a été identifié dans les cellules neurales. Un ADN-c complet a été obtenu et caractérisé comme ayant un domaine riche en sérine, un domaine de liaison à l'ADN fortement basique et un domaine de dimérisation "leucine-zipper". Des anticorps anti-lilzip ont révélé une protéine de 46 kDa dans les tissus contenant des lames basales, tels que le cerveau, les reins et les poumons. Des expériences de liaison à l'ADN montrent que Lilzip a une forte affinité pour les séquences nucléotidiques AP-1 et CRE/ATF. Par conséquent, la différenciation induite par la laminine peut mettre en jeu l'induction de facteurs transcriptionnels spécifiques.

Cellular and Molecular Aspects of Cirrhosis. Eds B. Clément, A. Guillouzo. Colloque INSERM/John Libbey Eurotext Ltd. © 1992, Vol. 216, pp. 147-156

The regulation of hepatic matrix protein synthesis by cytokines

Francis R. Weiner [(1)], Silvia Degli Esposti [(2)], Mark J. Czaja [(1)] and Mark A. Zern [(2)]

[(1)] *Department of Medicine and the Marion Bessin Liver Research Center, Albert Einstein College of Medicine, Bronx, NY 10461, USA;* [(2)] *Department of Medicine, Brown University, Roger Williams Medical Center, Providence, RI 02908, USA*

INTRODUCTION

Liver extracellular matrix (ECM) consists of four major components: collagens, glycoproteins, such as fibronectin and laminin, proteoglycans, and elastin (Schuppan, 1990). Changes in ECM synthesis have a number of effects, including the alteration of hepatic cell behavior (Friedman et al., 1989a), as well as the development of hepatic fibrosis. Hence qualitative or quantitative changes of the hepatic ECM have substantial effects on liver function. This precisely regulated process involves a number of soluble factors which either increase or decrease ECM synthesis. Some of the potential mediators of hepatic ECM synthesis are now being elucidated. It is our contention that during hepatic fibrosis a shift occurs in the balance between those endogenous factors which normally inhibit ECM synthesis (e.g., retinoids, corticosteroids, and γ-interferon) and those factors which promote ECM synthesis either through a direct effect on ECM synthesis, (e.g. transforming growth factor-β1 (TGF-β1) or interleukin 1 (IL-1)) or indirectly through a pro-inflammatory or mitogenic effect (e.g. tumor necrosis factor-α (TNF-α), platelet derived growth factor, (PDGF), and colony stimulating factors (CSFs)). We postulate that it is the superabundance of fibrogenic factors which ultimately causes hepatic fibrogenesis. A simplified schema of the interactions between some of these factors is shown in Fig. 1. This schema obscures some of the complexity of the fibrotic process, because other modulating factors are probably also involved. For example, a low molecular weight cytoplasmic fraction found in animal models of hepatic fibrosis has been shown to stimulate collagen synthesis (Raghow et al., 1984). In addition, lipid peroxidation and oxygen-free radical formation may be stimulants for fibrogenesis. This chapter will focus on some cytokines that appear to play a role in hepatic fibrogenesis.

TRANSFORMING GROWTH FACTOR-β1

Transforming growth factor-β1 (TGF-β1) is a homodimer with a molecular weight of 25,000 daltons (Sporn et al., 1987). Many cell types are known to synthesize this peptide (Sporn et al., 1986); liver endothelial and Kupffer cells (Braun et al., 1988) as well as Ito cells (Weiner et al., 1990a) have been shown to contain TGF-β1 mRNA. In addition, essentially all cells have been demonstrated to have receptors for TGF-β1 (Sporn et al., 1986). While TGF-β1 is know to have numerous biologic effects including a role in embryogenesis and carcinogenesis (Roberts et al., 1988), the effect that is most germane to hepatic fibrosis is its ability to enhance extracellular matrix protein synthesis in in

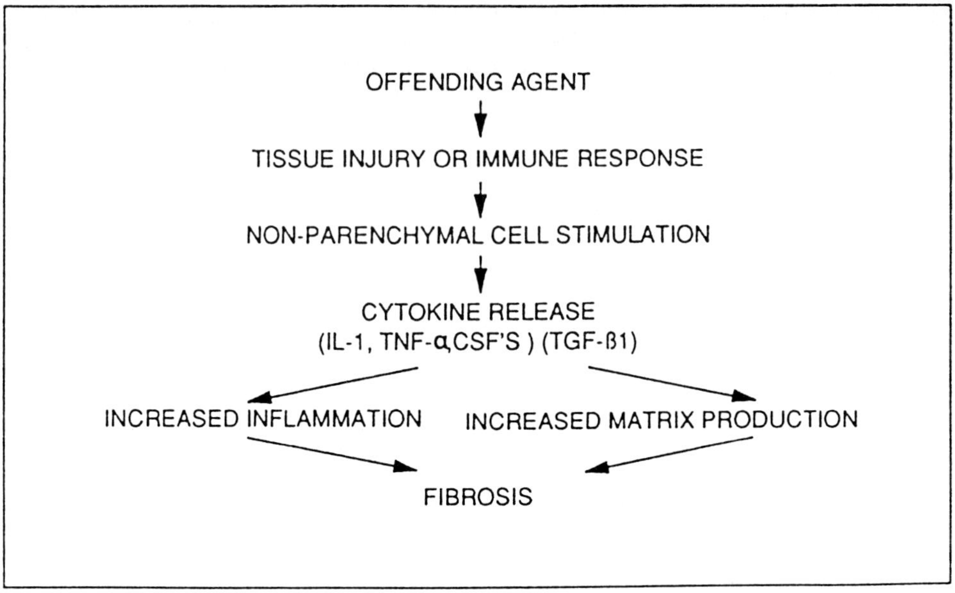

Figure 1. Schema of some of the postulated events in the initiation and progression of cirrhosis. Terms in parentheses are representative examples of a group of factors.

vitro and in vivo models (Graham et al., 1990; Matsuoka and Tsukamoto, 1990; Raghow et al., 1987; Falagana et al., 1987; and Roberts et al., 1987).

TGF-ß's has been shown to enhance the synthesis of extracellular matrix proteins (i.e., collagen, fibronectin, and proteoglycans) in many systems, including the liver (Sporn et al., 1987). TGF-ß1 increased Ito cell procollagen mRNA levels and collagen content (Matsuoka and Tsukamoto, 1990; and Weiner et al., 1990a), as well as Ito cell proteoglycan synthesis (Gressner and Bachem, 1990), and Ito cell fibronectin mRNA content (Weiner et al., 1989a). Davis (1988) has shown that the effect of TGF-ß1 on Ito cell ECM synthesis is influenced by the matrix on which the cells are cultured, thus suggesting a dynamic interaction between cytokines and the ECM environment.

In addition to TGF-ß1's stimulation of ECM synthesis, it appears to enhance fibrogenesis by inhibiting matrix degradation. It has been shown to decrease the synthesis of proteases (Sporn et al., 1987) and stromolysin (Matrisian et al., 1986) and to stimulate the synthesis of protease inhibitors such as plasminogen activator inhibitor (Keski-Oja et al., 1988). The stimulation of matrix synthesis as well as the inhibition of its degradation by TGF-ß1 suggest that this cytokine is an ideal candidate to serve as a modulator of liver fibrosis as well as other fibrotic processes. We, as well as other investigators, have undertaken a series of experiments in order to delineate the role TGF-ß1 plays in hepatic fibrogenesis (Czaja et al., 1989a; Weiner et al., 1990a; Weiner et al., 1990b; Annoni et al., 1988; Nakatsukasa et al., 1990, and Manthey et al., 1990).

Using two animal models of hepatic fibrosis, we investigated the relationship between the development of hepatic fibrosis and changes in TGF-ß1 expression (Czaja et al., 1989). Whereas the mechanisms of hepatic injury are different in the models, murine schistosomiasis and CCl_4-induced hepatic fibrosis in rats, the final common pathway is the development of liver fibrosis. The histologic development of hepatic fibrosis in both models was associated with an increase in both TGF-β1 and proα2 (I) collagen steady state mRNA levels, as well as collagen content. In hepatic schistosomiasis, immunohistochemical studies also demonstrated an increase in TGF-β1 protein in fibrotic livers. The increases in TGF-β1 and proα2 (I) collagen mRNA content in murine schistosomiasis were due to enhanced transcription of their respective genes. The steady state mRNA levels of two cytokines known to enhance inflammation and to act as mitogens for mesenchymal cells, TNF-α and IL-1, were shown to increase at an early stage of murine schistosomiasis, prior to the increase in TGF-β1. Other investigators have now confirmed the association of increased TGF-β1 expression in models of hepatic fibrosis (Nakatsuka et al., 1990; and Manthey et al., 1990). In streptococcal cell wall-induced granulomatous hepatic fibrosis, Manthey and co-workers showed that the development of liver fibrosis was associated with increased TGF-β1 mRNA content and increased histochemically detectable TGF-β1 in areas of active fibrogenesis. The streptococcal cell wall-induced granulomas were also demonstrated to release physiologically significant amounts of active TGF-β1 when they were cultured.

In order to further delineate the role of TGF-β1 in hepatic fibrosis, we examined the effect of TGF-β1 on Ito cells, the hepatic cell type thought to be the major source of extracellular matrix synthesis during liver fibrosis (Friedman, 1990; and Maher and McGuire, 1990). TGF-β1 treatment of cultured Ito cells enhanced their collagen content by 3.5-fold and this increase was associated with a similar increase in proα2 (I) collagen mRNA content (Weiner et al., 1990a). The increase in proα2(I) collagen mRNA content was due to both transcriptional and post-transcriptional mechanisms (Weiner et al., 1989a). TGF-β1 treatment also increased types III and IV procollagen, fibronectin, and proteoglycan mRNA levels in these cells by a post-transcriptional mechanism. Furthermore, TGFβ1 also increased Ito cell TGF-β1 mRNA content, suggesting an autocrine mechanism for perpetuating the fibrogenic process.

We have also examined the role of TGF-β1 in the development of hepatic fibrosis in man. Northern hybridization analysis revealed that patients with active liver disease had increased levels of type I procollagen mRNA which were significantly correlated with increases in their TGF-β1 mRNA levels (Annoni et al., 1988). These studies have subsequently been confirmed by Castilla et al., (1991). Given these findings **in vitro**, in **in vivo** models, and in man, there is strong evidence that TGF-β1 plays a significant role in hepatic fibrogenesis.

TUMOR NECROSIS FACTOR-α

Tumor necrosis factor-α(TNF-α) is a polypeptide of approximately 17 kilodaltons which is known to have several biologic effects. It has received considerable attention as the mediator of the wasting and cachexia associated with chronic disease as well as a mediator of shock associated with sepsis (Beutler and Cerami, 1986). It is also apparent that TNF-α affects inflammatory and reparative processes (Larrick and Kunkel, 1988). Many of the effects of TNF-α are exerted in concert with other cytokines, especially interleukin-1 and γ-interferon (Larrick and Kunkel, 1988; Kahari et al., 1991 and Ellias et al., 1990). However, in contrast to TGF-β1, little information is available as to the role TNF plays in hepatic fibrogenesis. **In vitro** studies using nonhepatic cells have shown TNF α to be active in acute inflammation (Larrick and Kunkel, 1988), in fibroblast chemotaxis (Postlethwaite and Seyer, 1990), in mesenchymal cell mitogenesis (Larrick and Kunkel, 1988), in fibroblast collagen synthesis (Elias et al., 1990) and in fibroblast proteoglycan synthesis (Elias et al., 1988). Certainly these findings would suggest that TNF-α may play a positive role in hepatic fibrogenesis. However, studies have reported contrasting findings as to the effect of TNF-α on collagen synthesis (Solis-Herruzo et al., 1988; Weiner et al., 1989b; Weiner et al., 1990a; and Matsuoka et al., 1989).

Solis-Herruzo and co-workers (1988), found that TNF-α had an inhibitory effect on collagen production in cultured hepatocytes and human fibroblasts. In contrast, we found that TNF-α increased collagen content in cultured Ito cells by three-fold (Weiner et al., 1990a). The discrepancies in these studies may reflect differences in the particular cell type examined, differences in the doses of TNF-α, and finally, differences in the methods used to evaluate collagen synthesis. Elias et al., (1990) have shown that the presence of other cytokines as well as changes in the matrix environment may ultimately influence the effect of a specific cytokine on collagen production. The differentiated state of a cell may also influence the effect of TNF-α on collagen gene expression. We found that while TNF-α treatment of differentiated 3T3-LI adipocytes increased their type I, III and IV procollagen mRNA expression, treatment of non-differentiated 3T3-LI preadipocytes was associated with a decrease in their procollagen mRNA expression (Weiner et al., 1989b). Whereas Matsuoka et al., (1989) found no stimulatory effect of TNF-α on Ito cell collagen synthesis they did find that TNF-α caused Ito cell proliferation, an event which is known to occur during hepatic fibrogenesis in vivo. Furthermore, TNF-α is known to stimulate the synthesis of other pro-inflammatory cytokines, such as interleukin-1 and granulocyte-macrophage colony stimulatory factor (Munker et al., 1986).

Although the findings regarding the effects of the cytokine in collagen synthesis are variable, there is abundant evidence that suggests a stimulatory role for TNF-α in the inflammatory response. In addition, TNF-α appears to serve as a mitogen for mesenchymal cells, including Ito cells. Therefore, given this function of TNF-α as an enhancer of inflammation, it would appear that the cytokine stimulates the fibrogenic process regardless of its direct effect on collagen synthesis.

INTERLEUKIN-1

Interleukin-1 (IL-1) appears to be one of the body's key effector molecules, and its synthesis is enhanced in response to infection, tissue injury, and inflammation (Dinarello,1988). It has become increasingly clear that the biological effects of TNF-α and IL-1 overlap and that this has contributed to the difficulties in sorting out the specific action of these cytokines. Adding to the complex interaction of these two cytokines is the fact that TNF-α and IL-1 often act in a synergistic manner (Dinarello, 1988; and Daireaux et al., 1990) and each induces IL-1 synthesis (Dinarello, 1988). There is considerable evidence that IL-1 can enhance collagen production (Cavalis, 1986; Heino and Heinoner 1990; and Daireaux et al., 1990); however, all studies do not demonstrate an IL-1-induced stimulation of collagen synthesis (Manriel et al., 1991).

Further evidence to suggest that IL-1 plays a role in hepatic fibrosis is provided by Zuccali et al., (1986). They demonstrated that IL-1 promoted the synthesis of tissue inhibition of metalloproteinase and thus prevented matrix degradation. Daireaux et al., (1990) have shown that IL-1 stimulated glycosaminoglycan production by cultured human synovial cells, and Matsuoka et al., (1989) showed that IL-1 caused Ito cell proliferation. Il-1 may also contribute to hepatic fibrogenesis by stimulating fibroblasts to increase their production of GM-CSF (Zuccali et al., 1986). Finally, we have shown an increase in IL-1 gene expression during the early stages of murine schistosomiasis, when inflammation occurs (Czaja et al., 1989). In summary, as with TNF-α, the primary role of IL-1 in the process of hepatic fibrosis may be through its stimulations of inflammation, not through any direct effect on the synthesis of matrix proteins.

COLONY STIMULATING FACTORS

Colony stimulating factors (CSF's) are a diverse group of glycoproteins that are essential for the growth and differentiation of hematopoietic progenitor cells. Considerable information is now accumulating about the regulation of CSF's, and their specific effects on hematopoietic cells. As with TNF-α and IL-1, it is now clear that a complex array of interactions occur between CSF's and other cytokines (Munker et al., 1986; Wing et al., 1989; Kaushansky et al., 1988; and Lindemann et al., 1988). Of particular interest to our laboratory has been macrophage-CSF (M-CSF, or CSF-1) which, in addition to stimulating the proliferation and differentiation of monocytes and neutrophils, can also activate macrophages, as exemplified by their enhanced cytotoxic potential (Ralph and Nakoinz, 1987). Since most forms of hepatic fibrosis are associated with increased numbers of activated macrophages, it is likely that CSF-1 may contribute to this pathologic process. Studies by Stanley and co-workers (1978) have demonstrated that CSF-1 treatment caused Kupffer cells to proliferate **in vitro**. Activated macrophages may in turn synthesize many of the cytokines involved in the initiation and progression of hepatic fibrosis.

In recent studies, we examined CSF-1 expression in murine schistosomiasis and in human liver disease (Shu-Ling et al., 1989; and Degli Esposti et al., 1990). In mice we demonstrated that CSF-1 mRNA and protein levels were elevated during the early stages of granuloma formation and peaked prior to maximal collagen synthesis. Analysis of the possible cellular source of CSF-1 revealed that Ito cells contained significant amounts of CSF-1 and that TNF-α treatment of these cells increased their CSF-1 mRNA levels 2 to 3-fold. Similarly, we found that patients with various forms of liver disease had significantly increased CSF-1 protein levels. These findings suggest that CSF-1 may play a role in the early stages of hepatic fibrogenesis. It would seem likely that other CSF's may also be crucial in initiating the inflammatory response that occurs in most forms of chronic liver disease, and it is possible that variation in the expression of the CSF's may determine the differences in the inflammatory infiltrate that is found. For example, the neutrophil infiltration of Laennec's cirrhosis may well be initiated by higher levels of GM-CSF or G-CSF than are present in the lymphocyte infiltration that occurs with chronic viral hepatitis.

PLATELET-DERIVED GROWTH FACTOR

Recently, considerable attention has focused on the mediators which induce quiescent Ito cells to proliferate, increase their collagen synthesis, and transform phenotypically in response to various fibrogenic stimuli **in vivo**. While several cytokines are probably involved in this process (Weiner et al., 1990a), several studies have now begun to examine the effect of platelet-derived growth factor (PDGF) on these cells. Pinzani et al., (1989) studied the effect of PDGF as well as other cytokines on Ito cell DNA synthesis. They found that PDGF could increase Ito cell DNA synthesis and growth, and that TGF enhanced this effect of PDGF. Friedman and Arthur (1989b) have suggested that increased expression of PDGF receptors is an early event associated with Ito cell proliferation. They also determined that Kupffer cells produced a factor that is required for the stimulatory effect of PDGF on Ito cells. Finally, Pencev et al., (1988) have shown immunoreactive peptides of the same molecular weight as PDGF in liver biopsies and ascitic fluid of patients with alcoholic hepatitis. In contrast, liver biopsies from normal patients did not contain any of this protein. These studies therefore suggest that PDGF may play a role in hepatic fibrogenesis through an effect on Ito cells.

GAMMA-INTERFERON

The previous sections of the chapter have described cytokines that act to increase matrix production directly or through an enhancement of the inflammatory reaction. This section describes the anti-fibrogenic effects of γ-interferon. While interferons are best known for their antiviral properties, their antifibrogenic actions have also received considerable attention (Jimenez et al., 1984; Goldring et al., 1986; and Stephenson et al., 1985). Studies of the effects of γ-interferon on liver fibrosis were first undertaken by Czaja et al., (1989a); they demonstrated that γ-interferon treatment markedly inhibited type I procollagen gene expression in cultured hepatic cells. These findings were then extended to an **in vivo** model of hepatic fibrosis. Interferon treatment of schistosoma-infected mice was found to decrease collagen deposition and to decrease types I and III procollagen mRNA levels compared to untreated, infected mice. These results suggest a potential role for interferon as an antifibrogenic agent **in vivo**.

ABSTRACT

In recent years it has become increasingly apparent that hepatic fibrogenesis results from a complex interaction of multiple factors. While this chapter has dealt with those cytokines which may be instrumental in the development of hepatic fibrosis, other factors will also be shown to be important in this process. Clearly if we are to develop more rational forms of therapy to treat or prevent liver fibrosis, further study will be required not only to delineate fibrogenic factors but also to determine the mechanisms by which they work.

The findings described in this chapter may be used to formulate a unifying, albeit oversimplified, hypothesis concerning the interplay of cytokines and hepatic fibrosis. The hepatocyte is injured by a toxin or by an immune response. This injury in turn initiates a complex interplay of cytokines which are synthesized by activated nonparenchymal cells. The earliest response appears to be the release of factors that stimulate the inflammatory response, such as the interleukins, TNF-α, PDGF, and colony stimulating factors. They enhance inflammation by increasing the proliferation of the lymphocytes, polymorphonuclear cells, and macrophages. In addition, these inflammatory cytokines act as mitogens for mesenchymal cells. The stimulation of the inflammatory response by this cascade of cytokines in the presence of continued liver injury allows for the perpetuation of further mononuclear cell activation and TGF-β1 release. This increased production of TGF-β1 then appears to enhance the synthesis of extracellular matrix by Ito cells and other matrix-producing cells.

To date much of the evidence for this cascade of cytokines that enhances hepatic fibrosis comes from **in vitro** studies and from animal models. Future studies must show that the cytokine interactions which appear to exist in the model systems also occur in man. The task for the coming years will be to define the kinetics of these cytokine interactions and to determine which of these factors are crucial for the pathogenesis of hepatic fibrosis and which are merely epiphenomena.

REFERENCES

Annoni, G., Czaja, M.J., Weiner, F.R., et al., (1988): Increased transforming growth factor-β1 (TGF-β1) gene expression in human liver disease. **Hepatology** 8,1227A.

Beutler, B., & Cerami, A. (1986): Cachectin and tumor necrosis factor as two sides of the same biological coin. **Nature** 320,584-588.

Braun, L., Mead, J.E., Panzica, M. et al. (1988): Transforming growth factor-β mRNA in creases during liver regeneration: A possible paracrine mechanism of growth regulation. **Proc. Natl. Acad. Sci.** USA 85,1539-1543.

Castilla, A., Pricto, J., & Fausto, N. (1991): Transforming growth factors-β1 and α in chronic liver disease: Effects of alpha interferon therapy. **N.Eng. J. Med.** 324,933-940.

Cavalis, E. (1986): Interleukin-1 has independent effects on DNA and collagen synthesis in cultures of rat calvariae. **Endocrinology** 118,74-81.

Czaja, M.J., Weiner, F.R., Flanders, K.C. et al. (1989a): **In vitro** and **in vivo** association of transforming growth factor-β1 with hepatic fibrosis. **J. Cell. Biol.** 108,2477-2482.

Czaja, M.J., Weiner, F.R., Takahashi, S., et al., (1989b): Gamma-interferon treatment inhibits collagen deposition in murine schistosomiasis. **Hepatology** 10,975-980.

Daireaux, M., Redini, F., Loyau, G., et al. (1990): Effects of associated cytokines (IL-1, TNF-alpha, IFN-gamma and TGF-beta) on collagen and glycosaminoglycan production by cultured human synovial cells. **Int. J. Tissue. React.** 12,21-31.

Davis, B.H. (1988): Transforming growth factor-β responsiveness is modulated by the extracellular collagen matrix during hepatic Ito cell culture. **J. Cell Physiol.** 136,547-553.

Degli Esposti, S., Stanley, R, & Zern, M.A. (1990): Macrophage colony stimulatory factor (CSF-1) content is markedly increased in human liver disease. **Hepatology** 12,908.

Dinarello, C.A. (1988): Interleukin-1, **Digestive Disease and Sciences** 33,25S-35S.

Elias, J.A., Krol, R.C., Freundlich, B., et al. (1988): Regulation of human lung fibroblast glycosaminoglycan production by recombinant interferons, tumor necrosis factor, and lymphotoxin. **J. Clin. Invest.** 81,325-333.

Elias, J.A., Freundlich, B., Adams, S., et al. (1990): Regulation of human lung fibroblast collagen production by recombinant interleukin-1, tumor necrosis factor, and interferon-gamma. **Ann. N.Y. Acad. Sci.** 580,233-244.

Falanga, V., Tiegs, S.L., Alstadt, S.P., et al. (1987): Transforming growth factor-beta: selective increase in glycosaminoglycan synthesis by cultures of fibroblasts from patients with progressive systemic sclerosis. **J. Invest. Dermatol.** 89,100-104.

Friedman, S.L., Roll, F.J., Boyles, J. et al. (1989a): Maintenance of differential phenotype of cultured hepatic lipocytes by basement membrane matrix. **J. Biol. Chem.** 264,10315-10320.

Friedman, S.L., & Arthur, M.J.P. (1989b): Activation of cultured rat hepatic lipocytes by Kupffer cell conditioned medium. **J. Clin. Invest.** 84,1780-1785.

Friedman, S.L. (1990): Cellular sources of collagen and regulation of collagen production in liver. **Sem. in Liver Dis.** 10,20-29.

Goldring, M.B., Sandell, L.J., Stephenson, M.L., et al. (1986): Immune interferon suppreses levels of procollagen mRNA and type II collagen synthesis in cultured human articular and costal chondrocytes. **J. Biol Chem.** 261,9049-9056.

Graham, M.F., Bryson, G.R., Diegelmann, R.F., et al., (1990): Transforming growth factor-beta 1 selectively augments collagen synthesis by human intestinal smooth muscle cells. **Gastroenterology** 99,447-453.

Gressner, A.M., & Bachem, M.G., (1990): Cellular sources of noncollagenous matrix proteins: Role of fat-storing cells in fibrogenesis. **Sem. in Liver Dis.** 10,30-46.

Heino, J., & Heinonen, T. (1990): Interleukin-1 beta prevents the stimulatory effect of transforming growth factor-beta on collagen gene expression in human skin fibroblasts. **Biochem. J.** 271,827-830.

Jimenez, S.A., Freudlich, B., & Rosenbloom, J. (1984): Selective inhibition of diploid fibroblast collagen synthesis by interferons. **J. Clin. Invest.** 74,1112-1116.

Kahari, V.M., Chen, Y.Q., Su, M.W., et al., (1990): Tumor necrosis factor-alpha and interferon gamma suppress the activation of human type I collagen gene expression by transforming growth factor-beta: Evidence of two distinct mechanisms of inhibition at the transcriptional and posttranscriptional levels. **J. Clin. Invest.** 86,1489-1495.

Kaushansky, K., Lin, N., & Adamson, J.W. (1988): Interleukin-1 stimulates fibroblasts to synthesize granulocyte-macrophage and granulocyte colony-stimulating factors. **J. Clin. Invest.** 81,92-97.

Keski-Oja, J., Raghow, R., & Sandey, M. (1988): Regulation of mRNAs for type-1 plasminogen activator inhibitor, fibronectin, and type I procollagen by transforming growth factor-β. **J. Biol. Chem.** 263,3111-3115.

Larrick, J.W., & Kunkel, S.L. (1988): The role of tumor necrosis factor and interleukin-1 in the immunoinflammatory response. **Pharm. Res.** 5,129-139.

Lindemann, A., Riedel, D, Oster, W., et al., (1988): Granulocyte-macrophage colony-stimulating factor induces interleukin-1 production by human polymorphonuclear neutrophils. **J. Immun.** 140,837-839.

Maher, J.J., & McGuire, R.F. (1990): Extracellular matrix gene expression increases preferentially in rat lipocytes and sinusoidal endothelial cells during hepatic fibrosis **in vivo. J. Clin. Invest.** 86,1641-1648.

Manthey, C.L., Allen, J.B., Ellingsworth, L.R., et al., (1990): In situ expression of transforming growth factor beta in streptococcal cell wall-induced granulomatous inflammation and hepatic fibrosis. **Growth Factors** 4,17-26.

Matrisian, L.M., Leroy, P., Ruhlmann, C., et al., (1986): Isolation of the oncogene and epidermal growth factor-induced transin gene: complex control in rat fibroblasts. **Mol. Cell. Biol.** 6,1679-1686.

Matsuoka, M., Pham, N-T., & Tsukamoto, H. (1989): Differential effects of interleukin-1 tumor necrosis factor-α and transforming growth factor-β 1 on cell proliferation and collagen formation by cultured fat-storing cells. **Liver** 9,71-78.

Matsuoka, M., & Tsukamoto, H. (1990): Stimulation of hepatic lipocyte collagen production by Kupffer cell-derived transforming growth factor-beta: implication for a pathogenetic role in alcohol liver fibrogenesis. **Hepatology** 11,599-605.

Mauviel, A., Heino, J., Kahari, V.M., et al., (1991): Comparative effects of interleukin-1 and tumor necrosis factor-alpha or collagen production and corresponding procollagen mRNA levels in human dernal fibroblasts. **J. Invest. Dermatol.** 96,243-249.

Munker, R., Gasson, J., Ogawa, M., et al., (1986): Recombinant human TNF induces production of granulocyte-monocyte colony-stimulating factor. **Nature** 323,79-82.

Nakatsukasa, H., Nagy, P., Evarts, R.P., et al., (1990): Cellular distribution of transforming growth factor-β1 and procollagen types I, III, and IV transcripts in carbon tetrachloride-induced rat liver fibrosis. **J. Clin. Invest.** 85,1883-1843.

Pencev, D., Lee, W.M., Kowalyk, K.K., et al., (1988): Increased levels of a PDGF-like factor in ascites in fibrotic liver from individuals with alcoholic liver disease. **Hepatology** 8,1228A.

Pinzani, M., Gesualdo, L., Sabbath, G.M., et al., (1989): Effects of platelet-derived growth factor and other polypeptide mitogens on DNA synthesis and growth of cultured rat liver fat-storing cells. **J. Clin. Invest.** 84,1786-1789.

Postlethwaite, A.E., & Seyer, J.M. (1990): Stimulation of fibroblast chemotaxis by human recombinant tumor necrosis factor-alpha (TNF-α) and a synthetic TNF-alpha 31-68 peptide. **J. Exp. Med.** 172,1749-1756.

Raghow, R., Gossage, D., Seyer, J., et al., (1984): Transcriptional regulation of type I collagen genes in cultured fibroblasts by a factor isolated from thioacetamide-induced fibrotic rat liver. **J. Biol. Chem.** 259,12718-12723.

Raghow, R., Postlethwaite, A.E., Keski-Oja, J., et al., (1987): Transforming growth factor- increases steady state levels of type I procollagen and fibronectin messenger RNAs posttranscriptionally in cultured human dermal fibroblasts. **J. Clin. Invest.** 79,1285-1289.

Ralph, P., & Nakoinz, I. (1987): Stimulation of macrophage tumoricidal activity by the growth and differentiation factor CSF-1. **Cell. Immunol.** 14,270-279.

Roberts, A.B., Sporn, M.B., Assoian, R.K., et al. (1987): Transforming growth factor-beta: Rapid induction of fibrosis and angiogenesis **in vivo** and stimulation of collagen formation **in vitro**. **Proc. Natl. Acad. Sci.** USA 83,4167-4171.

Roberts, A.B., Flanders, K.C., Kondaiah, P., et al., (1988): Transforming growth factor-β : Biochemistry and roles in embryogenesis, tissue repair and remodeling, and carcinogenesis. **Recent Progress in Hormone Research.** 44,157-197.

Schuppan, D. (1990): Structure of the extracellular matrix in normal and fibrotic liver: Collagens and glycoproteins. **Sem. in Liver Dis.** 10,1-10.

Shu-Ling, L., Degli Esposti, S., Bartocci, A., et al., (1989): Macrophage-colony stimulating factor (CSF-1) is produced by Ito cells **in vitro** and is elevated in an **in vivo** model of hepatic fibrosis. **Hepatology** 10,632A.

Solis-Herruzo, J.A., Brenner, D.A., & Chojkier, M. (1988): Tumor necrosis factor-α inhibits collagen gene transcription and collagen synthesis in cultured human fibroblasts. **J. Biol. Chem.** 263,5841-5845.

Sporn, M.B., Roberts, A.B., Wakefield, L.M., et al., (1986): Transforming growth factor-beta biological function and chemical structure. **Science.** 233,532-534.

Sporn, M., Roberts, A., Wakefield, L.M., et al., (1987): Some recent advances in the chemistry and biology and transforming growth factor-beta. **J. Cell. Biol.** 105,1039-1045.

Stanley, E.R., Chen, D-M., & Lin, H-S. (1978): Induction of macrophage production and proliferation by a purified colony stimulating factor. **Nature.** 274,168-170.

Stephenson, M.L., Krane, S.N., Amento, R.P., et al., (1985): Immune interferon inhibits collagen synthesis by rheumatoid synovial cells associated with decreased levels of procollagen mRNAs. **FEBS Lett.** 180,43-50.

Weiner, F.R., Shah, A., Czaja, M.J., et al., (1989a): Effect of transforming growth factor-β1 on Ito cell extracellular matrix gene expression. **Hepatology** 10,682A.

Weiner, F.R., Shah, A., Smith, P., et al., (1989b): Regulation of collagen gene expression in 3T3-L1 cells: Effects of adipocyte differentiation and tumor necrosis factor-α. **Biochemistry** 28,4094-4099.

Weiner, F.R., Giambrone, M-A., Czaja, M.J., et al., (1990a): Ito cell gene expression and collagen regulation. **Hepatology** 11,111-117.

Weiner, F.R., Shah, A., Biempica, L., et al., (1990b): Cellular sources of increased collagen and transforming growth factor-β1 gene expression in fibrotic liver. **Hepatology** 10,629A.

Wing, E.J., Magee, D.M., Whiteside, T.L., et al., (1989): Recombinant human granulocyte/macrophage colony-stimulating factors enhance monocyte cytotoxicity and secretion of tumor necrosis factor and interferon in cancer patients. **Blood** 73,643-646.

Zuccali, J.R., Dinarello, C.A., Oblon, D.J., et al., (1986): Interleukin-1 stimulates fibroblasts to produce granulocyte-macrophage colony-stimulating activity and prostaglandin E_2. J. **Clin. Invest.** 77,1857-1863.

Résumé

Au cours des dernières années, il est devenu de plus en plus évident que la fibrogénèse hépatique est le résultat de l'interaction complexe de multiples facteurs. A côté des cytokines décrites dans cette revue, d'autres facteurs sont également importants dans ce processus. Afin de développer des protocoles rationnels de traitement ou de prévention de la fibrose hépatique, des études sont nécessaires non seulement pour déterminer les facteurs fibrogènes mais aussi pour analyser les mécanismes par lesquels ils agissent.
Les résultats décrits dans cette revue permettent d'émettre une hypothèse, quoique simplifiée, sur les relations entre les cytokines et la fibrose hépatique. L'hépatocyte est lésé par une toxine ou par une réponse immunitaire. Cette agression produit, de ce fait, des interactions entre les cytokines synthétisées par des cellules parenchymateuses activées. Une des réponses précoces est la libération de facteurs qui stimulent la réponse inflammatoire, tels que les interleukines, le TNFα, le PDGF et les CSF. Ces cytokines augmentent l'inflammation en stimulant la prolifération des lymphocytes, des cellules polymorphonucléaires et des macrophages. De plus, elles agissent comme agents mitogènes pour les cellules mésenchymateuses. La stimulation de la réponse inflammatoire par cette cascade de cytokines, en cas d'agression continue du foie, permet une activation entretenue des cellules mononucléées et la libération de TGFβ1. La production accrue de TGFβ1 semble augmenter la synthèse de matrice extracellulaire par les cellules de Ito et les autres cellules impliquées dans cette synthèse.
A ce jour, la principale démonstration du rôle de cette cascade de cytokines dans la formation de la fibrose hépatique provient d'études *in vitro* ou chez l'animal. Des études devront démontrer que des interactions entre cytokines existent chez l'homme. Au cours des prochaines années, l'enjeu sera de définir les cinétiques de ces interactions et d'établir lesquels de ces facteurs sont déterminants dans la pathogénèse de la fibrose hépatique et lesquels sont principalement des épiphénomènes.

Cellular and Molecular Aspects of Cirrhosis. Eds B. Clément, A. Guillouzo. Colloque INSERM/John Libbey Eurotext Ltd. © 1992, Vol. 216, pp. 157-168

Parasinusoidal lipocytes : their contribution to hepatic connective tissue synthesis and to the mechanisms of matrix amplification in fibrogenesis

Axel M. Gressner and Max G. Bachem

Department of Clinical Chemistry and Central Laboratory, Philipps-University of Marburg, University Hospital, Baldingerstrasse, W-3550 Marburg, Germany

1. DEFINITION OF THE CHANGES OF EXTRACELLULAR MATRIX IN FIBROSIS AND FIBROGENESIS

Originally fibrosis has been defined as the "presence of excess collagen deposition due to new fibre formation" (Anthony et al., 1978), but data accumulated during last years clearly indicate the necessity of redefinition of "fibrosis" recognizing all the complexity of changes of the liver extracellular matrix (ECM) comprising (i) a 3 to 6-fold increase of the tissue concentrations of most of the extracellular matrix molecules including collagens, proteoglycans, structural glycoproteins, and hyaluronan, (ii) a disproportionate elevation of the various subtypes of individual extracellular matrix molecules, i.e. a preponderant increase of collagen types I and V, of proteodermatan sulfate and hyaluronan, and of certain structural glycoproteins like fibronectin, laminin and tenascin, (iii) subtle changes of the microcomposition of specific types of extracellular matrix molecules, e.g. concerning the degree of hydroxylation of the α-chains of collagen, the number, length and degree of sulfation (charge density) of glycosaminoglycans occupying the core proteins of proteoglycans, and (iv) the topographic redistribution of extracellular matrix in injured liver leading to an early and preponderant subendothelial accumulation of connective tissue in the space of Disse (perisinusoidal fibrosis) and to other forms of periportal, bridging, diffuse or focal deposition of connective tissue.

Fibrosis results from a disproportion of the rates of synthesis (= fibrogenesis) and degradation (= fibrolysis) of extracellular matrix molecules. It is now generally accepted that in tissue injury the disturbance of homeostasis leads primarily to an exaggerated matrix production, whereas the modulation of the catabolic pathways of matrix molecules might provide an auxiliary mechanism of ECM-accumulation. In the liver where a high regenerative capacity of parenchymal cells exists, stimulated matrix production forms an almost superfluous way of tissue repair. Fibrosis ensues when tissue injury and/or the inflammatory response is overexuberant and prolonged resulting in constant release of profibrogenic moieties and trophic factors to which certain target cells respond with increased production of ECM-components and/or multiplication. The central questions of the pathogenesis of liver fibrosis are concerned with (i) the identification of the cellular sources of individual ECM-components under normal and pathological conditions and (ii) the dissection of the molecular mechanisms leading to amplification of matrix production in areas of necroinflammation.

2. DESCRIPTION OF HEPATIC PARASINUSOIDAL LIPOCYTES

Based on a large number of cell culture studies and on in situ observations it is now evident that para-(peri-)sinusoidal lipocytes (PL, retinoid-storing cells, fat-storing cells, stellate cells, Ito-cells) are the principal connective tissue producing cell type in human and animal liver (Gressner, 1991a). These cells of mesenchymal origin (septum transversum) are distributed almost homogeneously throughout the different zones of the liver lobule. They are localized in the space of Disse (perisinusoidal space), the perikaryon embedded in recesses between adjacent hepatocytes. Normally, these cells display low mitotic activity and are engaged in the storage and metabolism of retinoids (Blomhoff et al., 1985; Hendriks et al., 1987). As much as 80% of total liver retinoids (mainly retinyl esters) might be stored in lipocytes (Blomhoff and Wake, 1991) which are characterized by large lipid droplets showing a greenish (vitamin A) fluorescence at 328 nm excitation-light and by cytoplasmic, dendritic processes along the endothelial tube (Geerts et al., 1990). In areas of tissue damage and necro-inflammation PL transform into smooth muscle iso-α-actin-positive and desmin-positive myofibro-blast-like cells (MFBIC) which actively synthesize a broad spectrum of ECM components. The transformation of PL occurs spontaneously under culture conditions on plastic surfaces. The phenotypic transition is associated with a number of typical morphological and biochemical changes (Fig. 1).

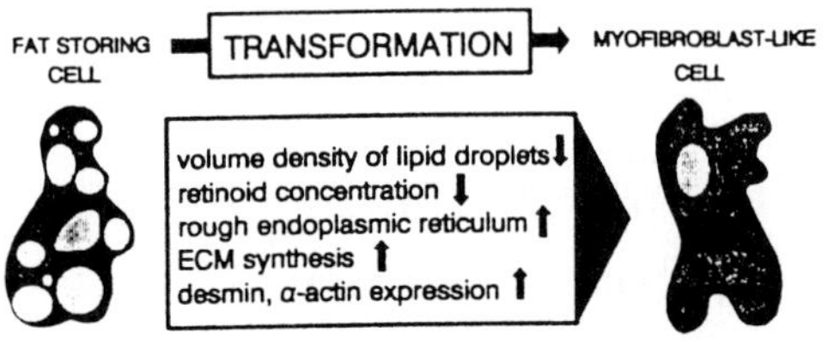

Fig. 1. Main phenotypic and biochemical changes of fat-storing cells during transition (transformation) to myofibroblast-like cells.

3. CONTRIBUTION OF LIPOCYTES TO MATRIX FORMATION IN RELATION TO OTHER CELL TYPES

3.1 Collagens

The capacity of PL to synthesize collagen has been studied in cultures of isolated cells and in vivo by in situ hybridization analyses. PL in primary culture on uncoated plastic were shown by immunofluorescence to express collagen type I, III, and IV, but type V collagen was not detectable. During the first week in culture the fractions of secreted type I collagen amount 0.8, of type III 0.5, and of type IV about 0.15 (Friedman et al., 1985). Five percent of total secreted protein was found to be collagen. The amount of collagen synthesized by PL per μg DNA is 10 fold greater than that produced by cultured hepatocytes and over 20 fold greater than that generated by endothelial cells. The latter cell type synthesizes mainly type IV collagen (Friedman et al., 1985). PL are the principal collagen producing cell type in liver, the rate of synthesis increases with progressive transformation towards myofibroblast-like cells. Culture of PL on a Engelbreth-Holm-Swarm (EHS) tumor matrix instead on uncoated plastic surfaces reduces by more than 70% synthesis/secretion of total collagen and, furthermore, changes the pattern from type I to III collagen (Friedman et al., 1989). In experimental fibrogenesis increases of the steady state levels of mRNAs of more than 30 fold of type I collagen and 5 fold of type III collagen relative to normal PL were measured whereas in endothelial cells an isolated increase of type I collagen mRNA was noticed. Type IV collagen mRNA in PL was only 2.5 fold increased (Maher and McGuire, 1990). A matter of controversy remains the potential of hepatocytes to contribute to collagen production in health and disease. Strong experimental data obtained with a dual label method designed to measure hepatocyte specific collagen synthesis in normal (Chojkier and Filip, 1986) and fibrotic (Chojkier et al., 1988) rat liver in vivo, Northern blottings of mRNAs from purified liver cells

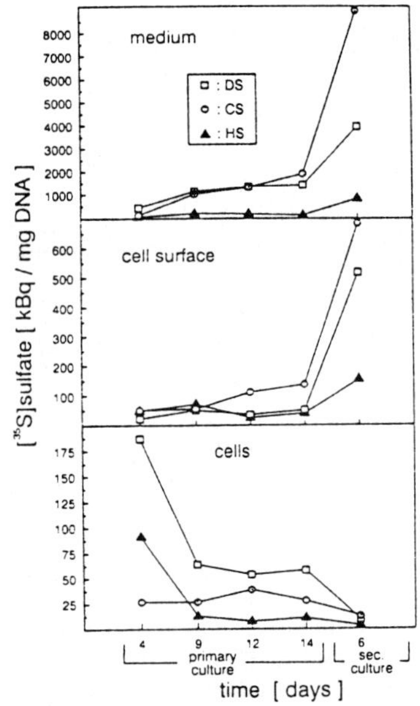

Fig. 2. Distribution of specific types of sulfated glycosaminoglycans in the medium, cell layer, and on the cell surface of fat-storing cells (PL) at various times of primary culture and at the sixth day of secondary culture. DS, dermatan sulfate; CS, chondroitin sulfate; HS, heparan sulfate.

(Brenner et al., 1990), and in situ hybridizations (Brenner et al., 1990, Yamada et al., 1989) suggest a major role of hepatocytes in liver collagen formation, but this conclusion is not supported by some other in situ hybridization studies which failed to detect procollagen mRNAs in normal and diseased human (Milani et al., 1990) and rat liver hepatocytes (Milani et al., 1989, Nakatsukasa et al., 1990). Without going into detail (cf review by Friedman, 1990) the important question on the role of hepatocytes in collagen production needs further experimental clarification.

3.2 Structural Glycoproteins

Recent data of immunoprecipitations, immunofluorescent stainings, Northern blottings, and partially of in situ hybridization studies provide evidence for a prominent role of PL in the production of fibronectin (Ramadori et al., 1987), tenascin (Ramadori et al., 1991), laminin (Maher et al., 1988), and of nidogen/entactin (Ramadori et al., 1990). However, as recently reviewed (Gressner and Bachem, 1990) Kupffer cells, endothelial cells and hepatocytes participate also in the production of certain structural glycoproteins. The contributions of cell types other than PL might be only minor ones.

3.3 Hyaluronan and Sulfated Proteoglycans

Hyaluronan, the only pure carbohydrate polymer in liver ECM, is synthesized in substantial amounts by PL in culture (Gressner and Haarmann, 1988a). The rate of synthesis (4.2 μg/mg DNA • h^{-1} at the 3rd culture day) increases significantly with culture time in parallel with ongoing transformation to myofibroblast-like cells (Gressner and Haarmann, 1988b) and is upregulated in transformed and nontransformed PL by the isoform BB of PDGF but not by PDGF-AA (Heldin et al., 1991). The fractional secretion rate of about 0.8 is not changed during culture. We did not detect any production of hyaluronan in hepatocytes, Kupffer cells, and endothelial cells, respectively which supports the view that PL are the primary (if not the exclusive) source of hyaluronan in liver.

In recent studies with PL in monolayer culture these cells were identified also as a major site of sulfated proteoglycan (PG) synthesis and secretion (Schäfer et al., 1987; Arenson et al., 1988). The predominant species of PG secreted in early cultures into the medium is dermatan sulfate followed by chondroitin sulfate whereas heparan sulfate constitutes only a minor fraction of PG in the medium. It should be emphasized that during culture total amount, profile and subcellular compartmentation of PG change significantly with a tendency that in advanced primary cultures and in secondary cultures chondroitin sulfate becomes the major type of PG in the medium and on cell surface of PL (Gressner, 1991b) (Fig. 2). When related to cellular DNA and protein content, PG synthesis in hepatocytes was only12 and 4%, respectively, of that of PL (Fig. 3). Furthermore, hepatocytes from normal and fibrotic livers (Meyer et al., 1990a) produce almost exclusively heparan sulfate which remains predominantly cell associated. Kupffer cells contained only 4 to 8% of PG when compared with PL (Gressner and Schäfer, 1989). Present studies are concentrated on the cellular idenfication of the expression of sulfated proteoglycans characterized by sequenced and cloned core proteins, of which the small chondroitin sulfate and dermatan sulfate bearing PG (decorin, biglycan) might be the most important ones with respect to collagen fibrillogenesis and TGFβ binding activity. In the medium of PL we identified in chondroitin ABC-lyase degraded PG at least 3 molecular size classes of core proteins having Mr of 101 kD, 51

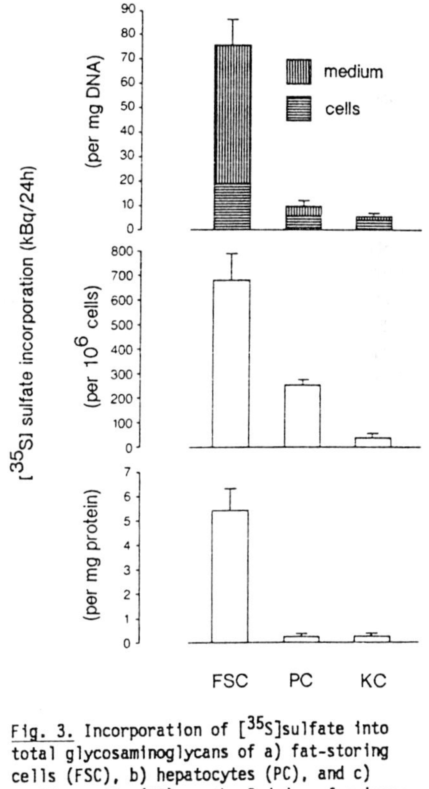

Fig. 3. Incorporation of [^{35}S]sulfate into total glycosaminoglycans of a) fat-storing cells (FSC), b) hepatocytes (PC), and c) Kupffer cells (KC) on the 3rd day of primary culture. Rates of incorpo-ration are referred to cellular DNA, protein, and cell number, respectively.

kD, and 46 kD, respectively (Witsch et al., 1989). The composition of secreted PG from 2 day old cultures was calculated to be 52% biglycan, 8% decorin, and 40% the novel PG with a core protein size of 101 kD. Northern blot hybridizations with cDNAs specific for the core proteins of decorin and biglycan have identified PL as the major (if not exclusive) site of expression of these PG in liver (unpublished). No transcripts could be detected in hepatocytes. In Kupffer cells there were also only trace amounts of the respective mRNAs detectable. All available data point clearly to PL as the major site of formation of sulfated proteoglycans, collagens, and structural glycoproteins of extracellular matrix of normal and fibrotic liver (Fig. 4).

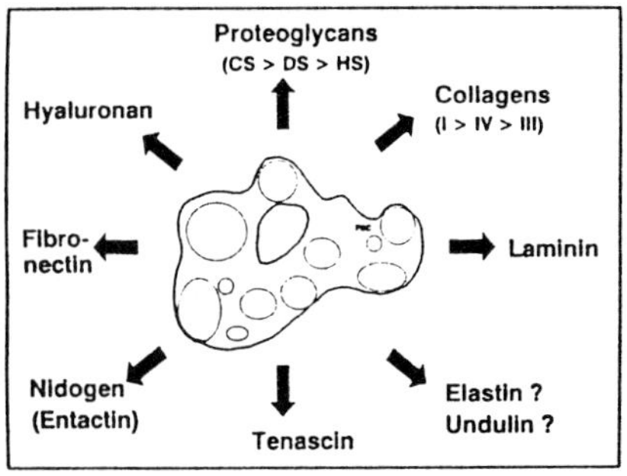

Fig. 4. Synopsis of components of the extracellular matrix synthesized by PL and their transformed counterpart, i.e. the myofibroblast-like cell.

4. UPREGULATION OF MATRIX SYNTHESIS INVOLVING ACTIVATION OF LIPOCYTES

In general upregulation of matrix synthesis in liver might be accomplished by several mechanisms: (i) stimulated proliferation of matrix producing cells, (ii) enhanced matrix synthesis per single cell, (iii) stimulated transition of resting PL into the highly synthetic myofibroblast-like cells. Studies using different cell types of the liver in highly purified culture systems have proven valuable not only for identifying the matrix producing cells but also for characterizing cell-cell interactions via soluble mediators or via direct cell-cell contact whereby proliferation/transition and matrix synthesis of PL is stimulated.

4.1 Paracrine activation/stimulation of parasinusoidal lipocytes involving Kupffer cells, platelets and myofibroblast-like cells.

Several previous studies have indicated that activation of PL plays a fundamental role in fibrogenesis since hereby via so called transitional cells (TC) highly active MFBIC are generated. The mechanisms leading to activated PL in culture but also in vivo during liver injury and inflammation are currently studied. The close proximity of liver macrophages (Kupffer cells [KC] and invaded monocytes), endothelial cells and platelet aggregates with PL and the observation that PL activation parallels KC proliferation, monocyte invasion and platelet aggregation (Ogawa et al., 1985) suggest that soluble factors released by these cells might influence activation, proliferation and connective tissue synthesis of PL and MFBIC. Using cell culture systems it was shown that secretions of KC change the phenotype (Friedman, 1990) and stimulate proliferation (Shiratori et al., 1986), collagen- (Friedman and Arthur, 1989), proteoglycan- (Gressner and Zerbe, 1987) and hyaluronan-synthesis (Gressner and Haarmann, 1988b) of PL. The stimulatory activity produced by activated KC (isolated from injured liver or activated in vitro by lipopolysacharide or zymosan) was higher compared to normal Kupffer cells. Using platelet lysates as stimulus an enhanced proliferation and PG synthesis was observed also (Bachem et al., 1989a). Conclusions drawn from these results suggest in liver injury a fibrogenic sequence from hepatocyte necrosis via platelet aggregation, invasion and activation of inflammatory cells (KC and monocytes) to the release of fibrogenic mediators which activate PL to change their phenotype from the resting retinoid- loaden cell to the highly proliferative and synthetic MFBIC. In coculture experiments using untransformed PL together with MFBIC a

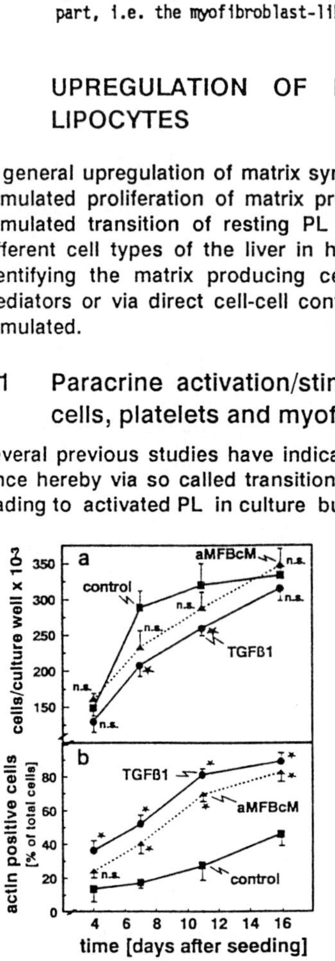

Fig. 5. Growth curve of PL in primary culture and expression of iso-α smooth muscle actin. (Control, 10% fetal calf serum; TGFβ1, 1ng/ml TGFβ1; aMFBcM, 20% transiently acidified medium conditioned by myofibroblast-like cells).

stimulated PL transformation (flat cell shape, accelerated reduction of number and size of fat droplets) was observed (data not shown). By monitoring the expression of smooth muscle iso-α-actin and the reduction of cellular retinyl palmitate at different time intervals after seeding PL activation was demonstrated. Medium conditioned by MFBlC (MFBcM) stimulated smooth muscle iso-α-actin expression (Fig.5). Compared to control, the difference was most pronounced 11 days after seeding. At that time interval, 70% of the PL treated with acidified MFBcM were iso-α smooth muscle actin positive; in controls only 27% of the cells were smooth muscle iso-α-actin positive. Total cell number was not significantly affected by 20% acidified MFBcM. Furthermore, as demonstrated in Fig. 6 transiently acidified MFBcM added to PL in primary culture stimulated the loss of cellular retinyl palmitate. The difference between MFBcM treated cultures and control was significant after 6 days in culture (Fig.6).

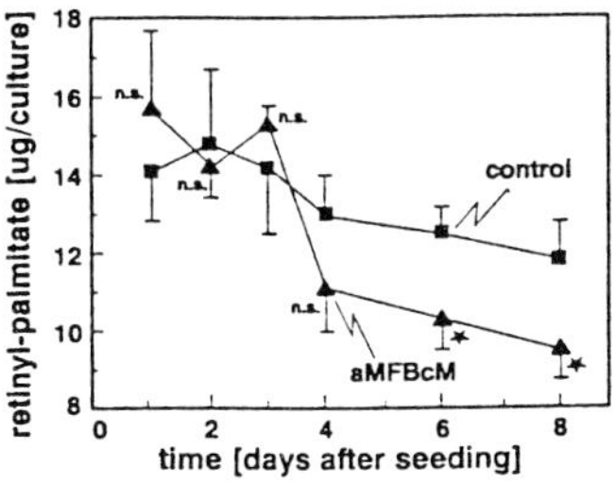

Fig. 6. Loss of cellular retinyl palmitate during primary culture (control, 0.5% fetal calf serum; aMFBcM, 40% transiently acidified medium conditioned by myofibro-blast-like cells).

Not only cell transformation but also matrix synthesis were stimulated by MFBcM. Transiently acidified MFBcM enhanced the synthesis of medium proteoglycans 2.2 fold above control and inhibited PL proliferation (Fig.7). However native MFBcM stimulated PL proliferation ([^{3}H]thymidine incorporation at 30% MFBcM 1.3 fold of control) suggesting that beside growth inhibitors also mitogens might be present in MFBcM.

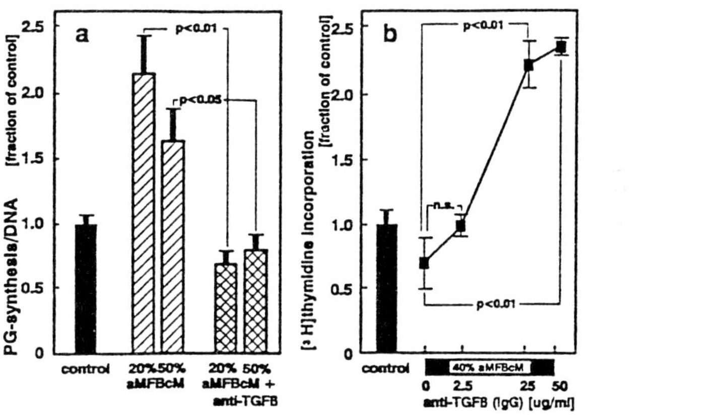

Fig. 7. Effect of neutralizing anti-TGFβ IgG on MFBlC-induced stimulation of PG synthesis (a) and inhibition of PL proliferation (b). Conditioned media were transiently acidified. Prior addition of the media to PL in culture anti-TGFβ IgG was added to the media and incubated for 1 h at 21°C on a rotating platform.

4.2 Identification of polypeptide growth regulators stimulating parasinusoidal lipocytes

Despite the central role of PL and in particular of MFBlC in hepatic fibrogenesis the factors modulating proliferation and/or matrix synthesis of these cells are incompletely understood. Using highly purified PL in primary culture we have shown recently that transforming growth factor (TGF) α, epidermal growth factor (EGF), and insulin-like growth factor (IGF1) stimulate PL proliferation (Bachem et al., 1989b) with only small effects on proteoglycan synthesis (Bachem et al., 1989c). Furthermore, we have shown that TGFβ1 inhibits the growth of early cultured PL but stimulates significantly matrix synthesis (Bachem, 1989b,c). In late primary cultures of PL and in MFBlC cultures TGFβ stimulates matrix synthesis without affecting proliferation of these cells (unpublished). Platelet derived growth factor was reported to influence only activated (transformed) PL (Friedman et al., 1989; Pinzani et al., 1989). These results demonstrate that polypeptide growth regulators modulate cell proliferation and proteoglycan synthesis depending strongly on the stage of cell activation/transformation. Recently, TGFβ was identified as the prominent mediator elaborated by Kupffer cells stimulating collagen (Matsuoka and Tsukamoto, 1990) and PG synthesis (Meyer et al., 1990b). Further potential candidates of the Kupffer cell and platelet derived fibrogenic activity seem to be TGFα/EGF (Meyer et al., 1990b), TNFα and PDGF. Since it was shown that (i) TGFβ stimulates collagen- (Davis, 1988) and proteoglycan-synthesis in PL (Bachem et al., 1989c), (ii) in acute CCl_4 induced liver injury the level of TGFβ-mRNA rises (Czaja et al., 1989), (iii) PL in culture express the TGFβ gene (Bachem et al., 1991) and, furthermore, (iv) TGFβ gene expression is significantly enhanced during active fibrogenesis associated with liver disease in man (Castilla et al., 1991) TGFβ is suggested to play a central role among the different polypeptide growth regulators in fibrogenesis. Using immunoperoxidase staining techniques TGFβ was demonstrated in activated Kupffer cells and together with collagens in liver granulomas (Manthey et al., 1990)). The important role of TGFβ in fibrogenesis is documented by two further properties of this polypeptide: TGFβ1 activates lipocytes to transdifferentiate into the fibrogenic MFBIC (see Fig.5) and TGFβ acts as a chemoattractant for fibroblasts and macrophages (Wahl et al., 1987). TGFα and TGFβ1 in combination (20ng/ml TGFα and 0.5ng/ml TGFβ1) elevated the synthesis of total medium glycosaminoglycans about 3fold. Determination of the specific glycosaminoglycans in media of early cultured PL indicated that TGFs enhanced chondroitin sulfate synthesis 15fold, whereas dermatan sulfate and heparan sulfate synthesis were slightly decreased (Fig.8). In MFBIC TGFs stimulated the synthesis of all the glycosaminoglycan subfractions (Fig.8). By fluorography after SDS-polyacrylamide-electrophoresis of [^{3}H]leucine labeled PG core proteins it was demonstrated that the enhanced [^{35}S] sulfate

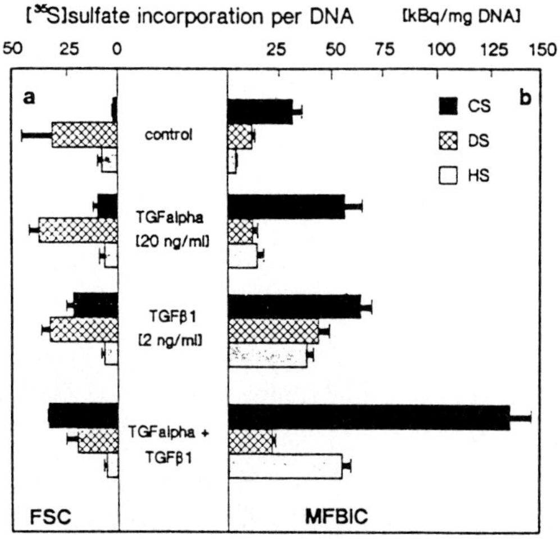

Fig. 8. Synthesis of sulfated PG by fat storing cells (FSC) and myofibroblast-like cells (MFBIC) stimulated by TGFα (20ng/ml), TGFβ1 (2ng/ml) or a combination of both (20ng/ml TGFα, 2ng/ml TGFβ1). CS, chondroitin sulfate; DS, dermatan sulfate; HS, heparan sulfate.

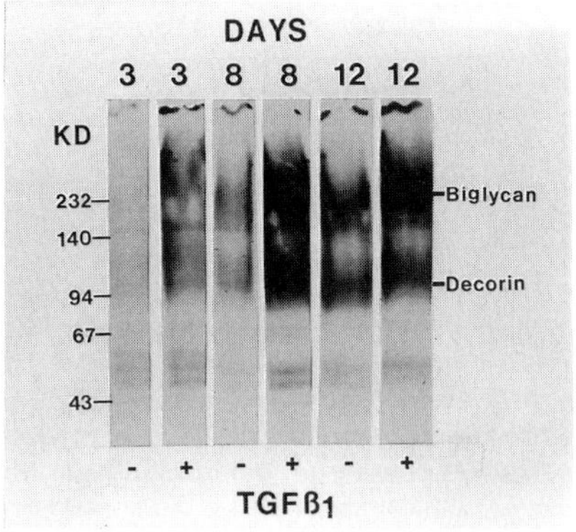

Fig. 9. Small proteoglycans (decorin and biglycan) from control (0.5% fetal calf serum) and TGFβ (1ng/ml) treated PL. SDS-PAGE and fluorography after [^{3}H]leucine label.

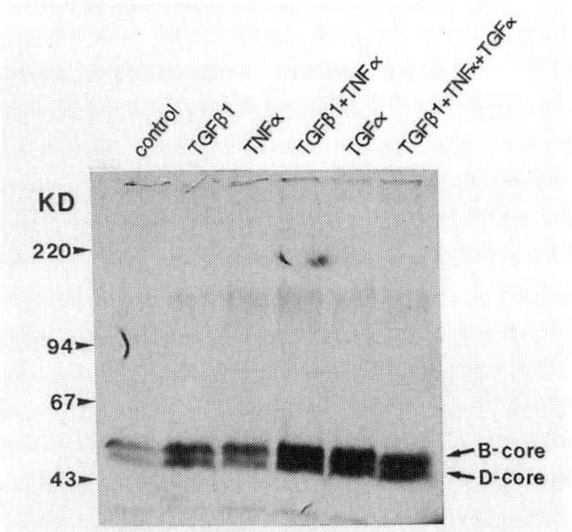

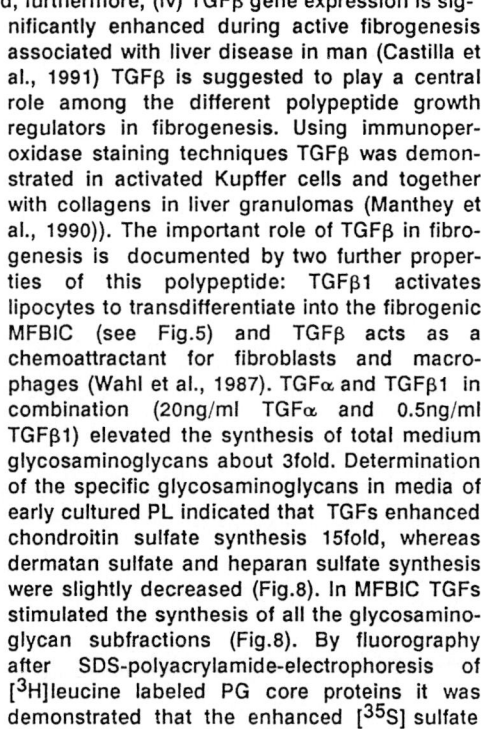

Fig. 10. Core proteins of decorin and biglycan from control (0.5% fetal calf serum) and stimulated PL. (1ng/ml TGFβ1, 5ng/ml TNFα, 20ng/ml TGFα).

incorporation into glycosaminoglycans of early cultured PL treated with TGFβ1 is caused by a stimulated biglycan and in particular decorin synthesis (Fig.9). Combinations of polypeptide growth regulators (TGFβ1, TGFα and TNFα) stimulate the synthesis of both small proteoglycans as demonstrated by the level of the [^{3}H]leucine labeled PG core proteins (Fig. 10). To demonstrate that TGFβ1 is responsible for the effects of MFBcM on PL the conditoned media were preincubated with TGFβ neutralizing antibodies before addition to PL. To verify the neutralizing potency of anti-TGFβ IgG 2ng/ml pure human TGFβ1 was incubated for 1 h at 22°C with increasing doses of anti-TGFβ (2.5-50μg/ml) before adding to PL monolayers. The growth inhibitory and PG synthesis stimulatory activity of 2 ng/ml TGFβ1 could be neutralized completely by 12.5 μg/ml anti-TGFβ (data not shown). As outlined in Fig.7 the PG synthesis stimulatory activity in the acidified MFBcM (2.1fold of control) was neutralized by preincubation of the medium with 12.5 μg/ml anti-TGFβ1. Furthermore, the growth inhibitory activity was abolished by preincubation of the acidified MFBcM with 2.5 μg/ml anti-TGFβ and even converted to a growth stimulation by higher concentrations of anti-TGFβ (Fig.7). These results not only confirm the presence of TGFβ in MFBcM, but also provide evidence for the presence of mitogens in MFBcM. Recently, TGFα (Bachem, et al. 1991) and IGF1 (Pinzani et al., 1990) were identified as mitogens produced by MFBIC. Kupffer cells synthesize beside TGFβ a great number of polypeptide growth regulators including PDGF, TGFα and TNFα which are suggested to be most important regarding paracrine stimulation of PL.

4.3 Autocrine stimulatory loops involved in proteoglycan synthesis of myofibroblast-like cells

TGFβ1 and TGFα mRNAs were demonstrated in PL and MFBIC. Increased levels of TGFα mRNA were found in PL on day 6 after seeding (relative amount 0.12) and predominantly in MFBIC (relative amount 0.84). TGFα transcripts were undetectable (relative amount <0.02) in PL at isolation and after 2 and 4 days in primary culture. The TGFβ1 transcripts were first detected in PL 2 days after seeding and increased gradually in primary culture. The strongest expression of TGFβ1 mRNA was found in MFBIC. Interestingly, TGFβ1 induced its own mRNA expression in PL (data not shown). TGFβ1 (1ng/ml) added at the second day after seeding to PL stimulated within 4 days its mRNA expression to a level 2-3 times higher than that in unstimulated cells.

The TGFα and TGFβ1 protein concentrations in media conditioned by PL and MFBcM were determined by competitive radioligand binding assays and calculated by comparison of dilution curves with those of standard curves. By sequential collections of medium at 24 h intervals from PL in primary culture during 10 days it was shown that TGFβ synthesis starts in parallel to transformation at day 5-6 after seeding, increased with culture time (transformation) and was highest in media conditioned by MFBIC. TGFα was only detected in media conditioned by transitional cells (10 days after seeding) and MFBIC. From these results we postulate that in the early stages of tissue response to injury, the release of TGFβ1 from platelets and activated macrophages results in an augmented trans-differentiation of PL to MFBIC. While PL and hepatocytes have been shown to be growth inhibited by TGFβ1 MFBIC have escaped the TGFβ induced growth inhibition. Furthermore, since MFBIC express elevated levels of TGFβ1 mRNA, secrete TGFβ1 in their media, respond to exogenous TGFβ1 by an enhanced matrix (proteoglycan) synthesis, and have escaped the growth inhibitory action of TGFβ1, autocrine positive loops in matrix synthesis via TGFβ1 are suggested. To prove autocrine regulation proteoglycan synthesis should be shown to be down regulated by eliminating the newly synthesized TGFβ1. The TGFβ1 neutralizing antiserum was used for this purpose. Addition of 20 μg anti-TGFβ1 to MFBIC 24h after seeding resulted in a 25% depressed proteoglycan synthesis per cell (Fig.11).

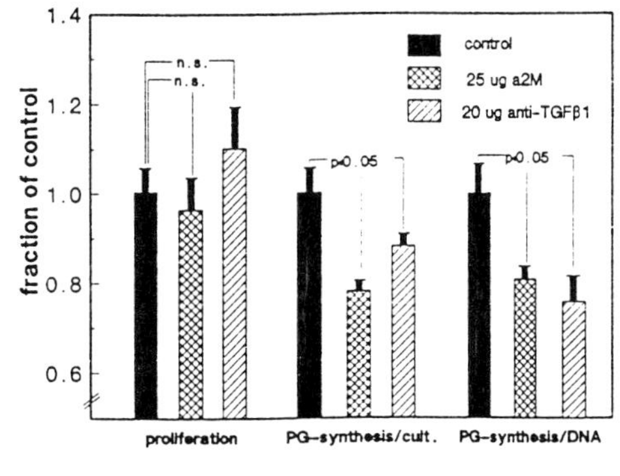

Fig. 11. Effects of Anti-TGFβ1 and α2-macroglobulin on proteoglycan synthesis of MFBIC.

4.4 Modifiers of PL activation and transforming growth factor activity

Since Kupffer cells, platelets and MFBIC produce predominantly the latent form of TGFβ, activation is required prior to receptor binding. In general, latent TGFβ may be activated by extreme, unphysiological pH (pH <2 or >12) (Wakefield et al., 1988), by several proteases (Lyons et al., 1988) and by glycosidases (Miyazono et al., 1989). The mechanisms of TGFβ activation in PL cultures and in injured liver remain to be established. The nature and magnitude of the TGFβ mediated PL stimulation may be regulated by (i) the TGFβ production rate, (ii) the balance of activation/inactivation, and (iii) by the expression of TGFβ receptors on cell surface. Since essentially all cell types of the liver seem to have receptors for TGFβ (unpublished) the activating and inactivating mechanisms are considered to be major regulatory steps.

Several proteoglycans function as modulators of growth factor activity. The role of the highly anionic heparan sulfate proteoglycans as binders and activators of fibroblast growth factors has been known for some time (Ruoslahti and Yamaguchi, 1991). Recently, it was shown that also the core protein of proteoglycans may bind TGFβ1. The type III TGFβ receptor was identified as a chondroitin-heparan sulfate proteoglycan (Andres et al., 1989). In contrast to type I and II TGFβ receptors the type III receptor called betaglycan has no function in signal transduction; its role is thought to be the binding of TGFβ for subsequent delivery to the true TGFβ receptors (Fig.12).

The core proteins of the extracellular small proteoglycans decorin and biglycan bind TGFβ also (Yamaguchi, 1990). Since TGFβ1 stimulates decorin and biglycan synthesis (Fig.9) a negative feedback loop of TGFβ activity in liver is suggested. Moreover, since the binding of TGFβ to decorin and biglycan is reversible these proteoglycans which exist in a soluble but also in a matrix bound form might act as reservoirs of TGFβ (Fig.12).

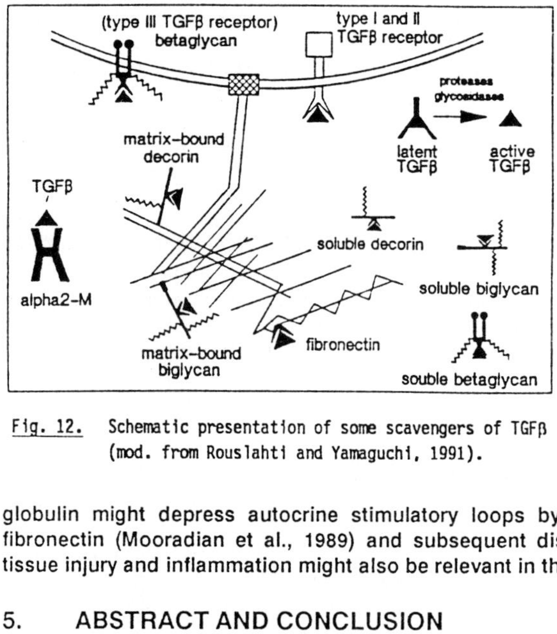

Fig. 12. Schematic presentation of some scavengers of TGFβ (mod. from Rouslahti and Yamaguchi, 1991).

Recently obtained results indicating that (i) α_2-macroglobulin is secreted by PL in increasing amounts beginning with the 5th day after seeding (Andus, 1987) and that (ii) α_2-macroglobulin may bind to and inactivate TGFβ (O'Connor-McCourt and Wakefield, 1987), suggest a potential role of α_2-macroglobulin as a scavenger for active TGFβ at sites of liver injury (Fig.12). Interestingly, heparin, which is structurally related to the PG heparan sulfate predominantly produced by parenchymal cells, may liberate active TGFβ from its complex with α_2-macroglobulin (McCaffrey et al., 1989). The pathobiochemical relevance of this mechanism is unclear. However, addition of purified α_2-macroglobulin to MFBIC in culture resulted in a depressed proteoglycan synthesis indicating that α_2-macroglobulin might depress autocrine stimulatory loops by binding active TGFβ1. Binding of TGFβ to fibronectin (Mooradian et al., 1989) and subsequent dissociation under acidic conditions at sites of tissue injury and inflammation might also be relevant in the development of liver fibrogenesis (Fig.12).

5. ABSTRACT AND CONCLUSION

Available data indicate that parasinusoidal lipocytes are qualitatively and quantitatively the principal site of connective tissue production in diseased liver. The activation of matrix synthesis is achieved by cytokine-mediated transformation of parasinusoidal lipocytes to myofibroblast-like cells, which are depleted of retinoid-loaden lipid droplets but produce a complex pattern of collagenous and noncollagenous matrix components. The initiation of transformation is mediated by a variety of polypeptide fibrogenic mediators but TGFβ might play a central role. In sustained inflammation an exaggerated production, release, and/or activation of latent TGFβ occurs. Furthermore, a diminished availibity of growth factor scavengers might also contribute to an increase of the fraction of active TGFβ, which results in an upregulation of matrix production. The balance of cytokine-regulated matrix synthesis by parasinusoidal lipocytes is modified by a complex network of intra- and extracellular activating and inactivating mechanisms.

REFERENCES

Andres, J.L., Stanley, K., Cheifetz, S., and Massagué, J. (1989): Membrane-anchored and soluble forms of betaglycan, a polymorphic proteoglycan that binds transforming growth factor-β. J. Cell. Biol. 109: 3137-3145.

Andus, T., Ramadori, G., and Heinrich, P.C. (1987): Cultured Ito cells of rat liver express the α_2-macroglobulin gene. Eur. J. Biochem. 168: 641-646.

Anthony, P.P, Ishak, K.G., Nayak, N.C., Poulsen, H.E., Scheuer, P.J., and Sobin, L.H. (1978): The morphology of cirrhosis. J. Clin. Pathol. 31: 395-414.

Arenson, D.M., Friedman, S.L., Bissell, D.M. (1988): Formation of extracellular matrix in normal rat liver: lipocytes as a major source of proteoglycan. Gastroenterology 95: 441-447.

Bachem, M.G., Melchior, R., and Gressner, A.M. (1989a): The role of thrombocytes in liver fibrogenesis: effects of platelet lysate and thrombocyte-derived growth factors on the mitogenic activity and glycosaminoglycan synthesis of cultured rat liver fat storing cells. J. Clin. Chem. Clin. Biochem. 27: 555-565.

Bachem, M.G., Riess, U., and Gressner, A.M. (1989b): Liver fat storing cell proliferation is stimulated by epidermal growth factor/transforming growth factor alpha and inhibited by transforming growth factor beta. Biochem. Biophys. Res. Commun. 162: 708-714.

Bachem, M.G., Riess, U., Melchior, R., Sell, K.M., and Gressner, A.M. (1989c): Transforming growth factors (TGF alpha and TGF beta 1) stimulate chondroitin sulfate and hyaluronate synthesis in cultured rat liver fat storing cells. FEBS Lett. 257: 134-137.

Bachem, M.G., Meyer, D., Melchior, R., Sell, K.M., and Gressner, A.M. (1991): Activation of rat liver perisinusoidal lipocytes by transforming growth factors derived from myofibroblast-like cells. A potential mechanism of self perpetuation in liver fibrogenesis. J. Clin. Invest., in press.

Blomhoff, R. and Wake, K. (1991): Perisinusoidal stellate cells of the liver: important roles in retinol metabolism and fibrosis. FASEB J. 5: 271-277.

Blomhoff, R., Rasmussen, M., Nilsson, A. et al. (1985): Hepatic retinol metabolism. J. Biol. Chem. 260: 13560-13565.

Brenner, D.A., Alcorn, J.M., Feitelberg, S.P., Leffert, H.L., and Chojkier, M. (1990): Expression of collagen genes in the liver. Mol. Biol. Med. 7: 105-115.

Castilla, A., Prieto, J., and Fausto, N. (1991): Transforming growth factors β1 and α in chronic liver disease - effects of interferon alpha therapy. New Engl. J. Med. 324: 933-940.

Chojkier, M. and Filip, M. (1986): Hepatocyte collagen production in vivo in normal rats. J. Clin. Invest. 78: 333-339.

Chojkier, M., Lyche, K.D., and Filip, M. (1988): Increased production of collagen in vivo by hepatocytes and nonparenchymal cells in rats with carbon tetrachloride-induced hepatic fibrosis. Hepatology 8: 808-814.

Czaja, M.J., Weiner, F.R., Flanders, K.C., Giambrone, M., Wind, R., Biempica, L., and Zern, M.A. (1989): In vitro and in vivo association of transforming growth factor-β1 with hepatic fibrosis. J. Cell. Biol. 108: 2477-2482.

Davis, B.H. (1988): Transforming growth factor β responsiveness is modulated by the extracellular collagen matrix during hepatic Ito cell culture. J. Cell. Physiol. 136: 547-553.

Friedman, S.L. (1990): Cellular sources of collagen and regulation of collagen production in liver. Sem. Liver Dis. 10: 20-29.

Friedman, S.L. and Arthur, M.J.P. (1989): Activation of cultured rat hepatic lipocytes by Kupffer cell conditioned medium. Direct enhancement of matrix synthesis and stimulation of cell proliferation via induction of platelet-derived growth factor receptors. J. Clin. Invest. 84 (6): 1780-1785.

Friedman, S.L., Roll, F.J., Boyles, J., and Bissell, D.M. (1985): Hepatic lipocytes: the principal collagen-producing cells of normal rat liver. Proc. Natl. Acad. Sci. USA 82: 8681-8685.

Friedman, S.L., Roll, F.J., Boyles, J., Arenson, D.M., and Bissell, D.M. (1989): Maintenace of differentiated phenotype of cultured rat hepatic lipocytes by basement membrane matrix. J. Biol. Chem. 264: 10756-10762.

Geerts, A., Bouwens, L., and Wisse, E. (1990): Ultrastructure and function of hepatic fat-storing and pit cells. J. Electr. Micros. Tech. 14: 247-256.

Gressner, A.M. (1991a): Liver fibrosis: perspectives in pathobiochemical research and clinical outlook. Eur. J. Clin. Chem. Clin. Biochem. 29: in press.

Gressner, A.M. (1991b): Time-related distribution profiles of sulfated glycosaminoglycans in cells, cell surfaces, and media of cultured rat liver fat-storing cells. Proc. Soc. Exp. Biol. Med. 196: 307-315.

Gressner, A.M. and Bachem, M.G. (1990): Cellular sources of noncollagenous matrix proteins: role of fat-storing cells in fibrogenesis. Sem. Liver Dis. 10: 30-46.

Gressner, A.M. and Haarmann, R. (1988a): Hyaluronic acid synthesis and secretion by rat liver fat-storing cells (perisinusoidal lipocytes) in culture. Biochem. Biophys. Res. Commun. 151: 222-229.

Gressner, A.M. and Haarmann, R. (1988b): Regulation of hyaluronate synthesis in rat liver fat-storing cell cultures by Kupffer cells. J. Hepatol. 7: 310-318.

Gressner, A.M. and Schäfer, S. (1989): Comparison of sulfated glycosaminoglycan and hyaluronate synthesis and secretion in cultured hepatocytes, fat-storing cells, and Kupffer cells. J. Clin. Chem. Clin. Biochem. 27: 141-149.

Gressner, A.M. and Zerbe, O. (1987): Kupffer cell-mediated induction of synthesis and secretion of proteoglycans by rat liver fat storing cells in culture. J. Hepatol. 5: 299-310.

Heldin, P., Pertoft, H., Nordlinder, H., Heldin, C.-H., and Laurent, T.C. (1991): Differential expression of platelet-derived growth factor α- and β-receptors on fat-storing cells and endothelial cells of rat liver. Exp. Cell Res. 193: 364-369.

Hendriks, H.F.J., Brouwer, A., and Knook D.L. (1987): The role of hepatic fat-storing (stellate) cells in retinoid metabolism. Hepatology 7: 1368-1371.

Lyons, R.M., Keski-Oja, J., and Moses, H.L. (1988): Proteolytic activation of latent transforming growth factor beta from fibroblast-conditioned medium. J. Cell. Biol. 106: 1659-1665.

Maher, J.J. and McGuire, R.F. (1990): Extracellular matrix gene expression increases preferentially in rat lipocytes and sinusoidal endothelial cells during hepatic fibrosis in vivo. J. Clin. Invest. 86: 1641-1648.

Maher, J.J., Friedman, S.L., Roll, J.F., and Bissell, D.M. (1988): Immunolocalization of laminin in normal rat liver and biosynthesis of laminin by hepatic lipocytes in primary culture. Gastroenterology 94: 1053-1062.

Manthey, C.L., Allen, J.B., Ellingsworth, L.R., and Wahl, S.M. (1990): In situ expression of transforming growth factor beta in streptococcal cell wall-induced granulomatous inflammation and hepatic fibrosis. Growth Factors 4: 17-26.

Matsuoka, M. and Tsukamoto, H. (1990): Stimulation of hepatic lipocyte collagen production by Kupffer cell-derived transforming growth factor β: implication for a pathogenetic role in alcoholic liver fibrogenesis. Hepatology 11: 599-605.

McCaffrey, T.A., Falcone, D.J., Brayton, C.F., Agarwal, L., Welt, F.G.P., and Weksler, B.B. (1989): Transforming growth factor-β activity is potentiated by heparin via dissociation of the transforming growth factor-β/alpha2-macroglobulin inactive complex. J. Cell Biol. 109: 441-448.

Meyer, D.H., Zimmermann, T., Müller, D., Franke, H., Dargel, R., and Gressner, A.M. (1990a): The synthesis of glycosaminoglycans in isolated hepatocytes during experimental liver fibrogenesis. Liver 10: 94-105.

Meyer, D.H., Bachem, M.G., and Gressner, A.M. (1990b): Modulation of hepatic lipocyte proteoglycan synthesis and proliferation by Kupffer cell-derived transforming growth factors type β1 and type α. Biochem. Biophys. Res. Commun. 171: 1122-1129.

Milani, S., Herbst, H., Schuppan, D., Surrenti, C., Riecken, E.O., and Stein, H. (1990): Cellular localization of type I, III and IV procollagen gene transcripts in normal and fibrotic human liver. Amer. J. Pathol. 137: 59-70.

Milani, S., Herbst, H., Schuppan, D., Hahn, E.G., and Stein, H. (1989): In situ hybridization for procollagen types I, III and IV mRNA in normal and fibrotic rat liver: Evidence for predominant expression in nonparenchymal liver cells. Hepatology 10: 84-92.

Miyazono, K. and Heldin, C.H. (1989): Role for carbohydrate structures in TGF-beta1 latency. Nature 338: 158-160.

Mooradian, D.L., Lucas, R.C., Weatherbee, J.A., and Furcht, L.T. (1989): Transforming growth factor-β1 binds to immobilized fibronectin. J. Cell. Biochem. 41: 189-200.

Nakatsukasa, H., Nagy, P., Evarts, R.P., Hsia, C.C., Marsden, E., and Thorgeirsson, S.S. (1990): Cellular distribution of transforming growth factor-β_1 and procollagen types I, III, and IV transcripts in carbon tetrachloride-induced rat liver fibrosis. J. Clin. Invest. 85: 1833-1843.

O'Connor-McCourt, M.D. and Wakefield, L.M. (1987): Latent transforming growth factor beta in serum. A specific complex with alpha 2-macroglobulin. J. Biol. Chem. 262: 14090-14099.
Ogawa, K., Suzuki, J.I., Narasaki, M., and Mori, M. (1985): Healing of focal injury in the rat liver. Am. J. Pathol. 119: 158-167.
Pinzani, M., Gesualdo, L., Sabbah, G.M., and Abboud, H.E. (1989): Effects of platelet-derived growth factor and other polypeptide mitogens on DNA synthesis and growth of cultured rat liver fat-storing cells. J. Clin. Invest. 84: 1786-1793.
Pinzani, M., Abboud, H.E., and Aron, D.C. (1990): Secretion of insulin-like growth factor-I and binding proteins by rat liver fat-storing cells: Regulatory role of platelet-derived growth factor. Endocrinology 127: 2343-2349.
Ramadori, G., Rieder, H., Knittel, Th., Dienes, H.P., and Meyer zum Büschenfelde, K.-H. (1987): Fat-storing cells (FSC) of rat liver synthesize and secrete fibronectin. J. Hepatol. 4: 190-197.
Ramadori, G., Schwögler, S., Veit, Th., Rieder, H., and Meyer zum Büschenfelde, K.-H. (1990): Fettspeicherzellen (Ito-Zellen) der Rattenleber synthetisieren und sezernieren Entactin (Nidogen). Vergleich mit anderen Leberzellen. Z. Gastroenterol. XXVIII: p. 56 (Abstract).
Ramadori, G., Schwögler, S., Veit, Th., Rieder, H., Chiquet-Ehrismann, R., Mackie, E.J., and Meyer zum Büschenfelde, K.-H. (1991): Tenascin gene expression in rat liver and in rat liver cells. Virchows Archiv B Cell Pathol. 60: 145-154.
Ruoslahti, E. and Yamaguchi, Y. (1991): Proteoglycans as modulators of growth factor activities. Cell 64: 867-869.
Schäfer, S., Zerbe, O., Gressner, A.M. (1987): The synthesis of proteoglycans in fat-storing cells of rat liver. Hepatology 7: 680-687.
Shiratori, Y., Geerts, A., Ichida, T., Kawase, T., and Wisse, E. (1986): Kupffer cells from CCl_4-induced fibrotic livers stimulate proliferation of fat-storing cells. J. Hepatol. 3: 294-303.
Wahl, S.M., Hunt, D.A., Wakefield, L.M., McCartney-Francis, N., Wahl, L.M., Roberts, A.B., and Sporn, M.B. (1987): Transforming growth factor beta (TGF-beta) induces monocyte chemotaxis and growth factor production. Proc. Natl. Acad. Sci. USA 84: 5788-5792.
Wakefield, L.M., Smith, D.M., Flanders, K.C., and Sporn, M.B. (1988): Latent transforming growth factor beta from human platelets. A high molecular weight complex containing precursor sequences. J. Biol. Chem. 263: 7646-7654.
Witsch, P., Kresse, H., and Gressner, A.M. (1989): Biosynthesis of small proteoglycans by hepatic lipocytes in primary culture. FEBS Lett. 2: 233-235.
Yamada, H., Aida, T., Taguchi, K., and Asano, G. (1989): Localization of type III procollagen mRNA in areas of liver fibrosis by in situ hybridization. Acta Pathol. Jap. 39: 719-724.
Yamaguchi, Y., Mann, D.M., and Ruoslahti, E. (1990): Negative regulation of transforming growth factor-β by the proteoglycan decorin. Nature 346: 281-284.

Résumé

Les données actuellement disponibles indiquent que les lipocytes parasinusoïdaux sont le site principal de la production du tissu conjonctif dans le foie pathologique tant au point de vue qualitatif que quantitatif. L'activation de la synthèse de matrice extracellulaire est obtenue par la transformation, médiée par les cytokines, des lipocytes parasinusoïdaux en cellules de type fibroblastique qui sont dépourvues de gouttelettes lipidiques riches en rétinoïdes mais produisent un ensemble complexe de composants matriciels collagéniques et non collagéniques. Le début de la transformation est induit par une variété de médiateurs polypeptidiques fibrogènes parmi lesquels le TGFβ pourrait jouer un rôle primordial. Au cours de l'inflammation continue, une production accrue, un relargage et/ou une activation du TGFβ latent surviennent.
De plus, une diminution de la disponibilité des produits de dégradation des facteurs de croissance pourrait également contribuer à l'augmentation de la fraction active du TGFβ, qui aboutit à une régulation positive de la production de matrice extracellulaire. La balance de la synthèse de matrice extracellulaire par les lipocytes parasinusoïdaux, régulée par les cytokines, est modifiée par un réseau complexe de mécanismes activateurs et inactivateurs intra- et extracellulaires.

Cellular and Molecular Aspects of Cirrhosis. Eds B. Clément, A. Guillouzo. Colloque INSERM/John Libbey Eurotext Ltd. © 1992, Vol. 216, pp. 169-176

Kupffer cells and fibrogenesis

G. Ramadori

I. Department of Internal Medicine, University of Mainz, Langenbeckstrasse 1, 6500 Mainz, Germany

SUMMARY

The process of inflammation and repair which involves both fibrosis and angiogenesis is characterized by an ordered accumulation of inflammatory cells followed by an activation of mesenchymal cells responsible for the synthesis of connective tissue components. In chronic liver diseases inflammation and repair mechanisms take place throughout the organ and lead to the development of fibrosis and cirrhosis.
Tissue macrophages of the different organs are phenotypically and functionally different. They also differ from their progenitor cell, the blood monocyte. The main function of Kupffer cells (Kc), the liver macrophages, is phagocytosis of soluble and particulate material. However, it is supposed that Kc secrete mediators and growth factors responsible for activation of Ito-cells and for their increased synthesis of different matrix proteins.
In order to explore whether recruited blood mononuclear leucocytes or liver tissue macrophages are the effector cells during liver injury, we analysed the phenotype of the mononuclear cells present in acutely or chronically (CCl_4 induced) damaged rat liver. Cells present in the necrotic areas were characterized by using the two monoclonal antibodies ED 1 and ED 2 and then also studied for the expression of the Ia-antigen.

This work was supported by the Deutsche Forschungsgemeinschaft (Grants SFB 311 A7 and Ra 362/6-2), Giuliano Ramadori holds a Hermann and Lilly Schilling professorship.

Acknowledgement:

The author greatfully acknowledges the help of Dr. Thomas Knittel, Thomas Armbruster and Thomas Veit. The author is very thankful to Dr. Dijkstra for the monoclonal antibodies ED 1 and ED 2.

Three days after the first CCl_4-administration the number of ED 1 + ve cells present in the necrotic pericentral area was comparable with the number of ED 2 + ve cells. Enlarged ED 1 and ED 2 + ve cells were detected along the sinusoids.
Ia-positivity was detectable only in the pericentral, necrotic areas. All the ED 1 + ve and ED 2 + ve cells expressed the Ia-antigen.
The results suggest that mainly recruited Ia + ve mononuclear leucocytes and not the liver tissue macrophages are the effector cells in experimental liver fibrosis.

INTRODUCTION

Since the beginning of the seventies it has become clear, that liver fibrosis during chronic liver disease is not due to the collaps of preexisting connective tissue because of liver cell necrosis, but it is the result of increased synthesis of matrix components. Patrick and Mc Gee first hypothesized an important role of fat storing (Ito-) cells in liver fibrosis (Patrick & MacGee, 1972). This hypothesis was confirmed by Kent and coworkers (Kent et al., 1976) and later by several other authors (Enzan, 1985, Burt et al., 1986). Major advances in the knowledge about the role of Ito-cells in the synthesis of connective tissue proteins have been achieved since a method for isolation and culture of this cell population has been made available (De Leeuw et al., 1984). In vitro Ito-cells dedifferentiate into myofibroblasts like cells loosing the fat droplets and vitamin A and begin to divide. This behaviour resembles the situation observed in vivo after acute or chronic liver damage (Ramadori et al., 1989).
Ito-cell-dedifferentiation is not a self-induced process, but it is induced by growth factors and other cytokines released by platelets and inflammatory mononuclear cells. Infact, pathophysiology of liver fibrosis resembles more and more that of the wound healing process. To investigate whether the liver tissue macrophages, namely the Kupffer cells or newly recruited blood monocytes are mainly involved in liver fibrosis we performed phenotypic differentiations of the mononuclear cells of the inflammatory infiltrate induced in the rat by acute and chronic administration of carbon tetrachloride. As immunological mechanisms were also suggested to be involved in certain models of liver fibrosis (Jezequel et al., 1989) we also studied the expression of the Ia-antigen.

MATERIAL AND METHODS

Animals

Wistar rats (200-250 gm body weight) were maintained under 12 h light/dark cycles with food and water ad libitum. In conducting the research described in this report we adhered to the National Institute of Health guidelines for the care and use of laboratory animals.

Reagents

Chemicals were obtained from the following sources: RPMI Gey's balanced salt solution (GBSS) and fetal calf serum (FCS) from Flow Laboratories (Bonn, Germany), phosphate buffered saline (PBS) from Seromed (Biochrom, Berlin, Germany), pronase E from Merck (Darmstadt, Germany) and Nycodenz from Nyegaard (Oslo, Norway). Diaminobenzidine, H_2O_2, Histopaque (Ficoll and collagenase from Sigma (Munich, Germany).

Antisera and antibodies

The monoclonal antibodies ED 1 and ED 2 were kindly provided by Dr. Dijkstra (Dept. of Histology, University of Amsterdam, Netherlands; Dijkstra et al., 1985). Monoclonal antibodies directed against smooth muscle alpha-actin and FITC-conjugated anti mouse IgG were from Sigma. The monoclonal antibody against desmin and peroxidase labeled anti mouse immunoglobulins were from Dako (Copenhagen, Denmark).

ISOLATION AND PHENOTYPIC IDENTIFICATION OF BLOOD MONOCYTES AND TISSUE MACROPHAGES IN VITRO

a) Blood monocytes

15 ml of heparinized rat blood were diluted in 20 ml of culture medium (RPMI) and peripheral blood leucocytes were separated by density gradient (Ficoll). Cells were washed three times and plated onto 24 well Falcon plates containing glass cover slips. Two hours after plating non adherent cells were washed three times and new cells were plated. This procedure was repeated three times.

b) Peritoneal macrophages

Normal Wistar rats were anesthesized with ether and 50 ml of culture medium were injected into the abdominal cavity. The fluid of the animal was then shaken several times and the fluid was aspirated from the abdominal cavity. After centrifugation and washing procedures cells were resuspended in culture medium and plated as described for blood leucocytes.

c) Kupffer cells

Kupffer cells were isolated according to Knook and coworkers (Knook et al., 1977) as described elsewhere (Ramadori et al., 1986). Cells were plated onto 24 well Falcon plates containing cover slips.

d) Immunocytochemistry

Cells were fixed one day after plating with methanol (5 min) and acetone (10 sec at 20°C), washed three times and covered with the corresponding monoclonal antibody (ED 1, ED 2 or anti-Ia) and incubated for 1 h at 37°C in a humid chamber. Cells were then washed again and incubated with peroxidase labeled anti IgG mouse. Cells were then washed and incubated with a diaminobenzidine (0,5 mg/ml) and H_2O_2 (0,01%) contaning solution, washed, counterstained in Meyer's hemalaun and rinsed before covering with a coverslip.

INDUCTION OF ACUTE LIVER DAMAGE AND OF FIBROSIS

Acute liver damage was induced in rats according to Enzan (1985) as described elsewhere (Ramadori et al., 1990). For induction of fibrosis rats were treated by oral administration of carbon tetrachloride according to Proctor and Chatamra (1982) as already described (Ramadori et al, 1990). For acute liver damage animals were sacrificed 48 h after the first treatment. Chronic liver damage was achieved after the fourth, sixth and tenth administration of CCl_4 at weekly intervals. Two animal were sacrificed three weeks after the tenth administration of carbon tetrachloride. Liver was taken from all animals snap frozen in liquid nitrogen and stored at - 80°C.

IMMUNOHISTOCHEMISTRY

Cryostat sections (6 μm thick) of rat liver tissue were dried and fixed with cold acetone (-20°C). Immunohisto-chemical studies were performed by means of the peroxi-dase technique as described above. In some cases the immunofluorecence technique was prefered.

RESULTS

Immunocytochemical phenotyping of mononuclear cells

The results of phenotyping of monocytes, peritoneal macrophages and Kupffer cells are listed in Table 1. Monocytes, peritoneal macrophages and Kupffer cells were ED 1 positive. Monocytes were ED 2 negative, about 50% of the peritoneal macrophages were ED 2 positive and Kupffer cells were all ED 2 positive. All cells were Ia positive. The results indicate that peritoneal macrophages, which also belong to the tissue macrophages are slightly different from Kupffer cells. They could be somewhat between blood monocytes and Kupffer cells.

Cells	ED 1	ED 2	Ia
MONO	+	-	+
MAC	+	(+)	+
Kc	+	+	+

Table 1: Phenotypical differences of rat blood monocytes (MONO), peritoneal macrophages (MAC) and Kupffer cells (Kc) in vitro (+: 100% positivity, (+): 50% positive cells, -: negative)

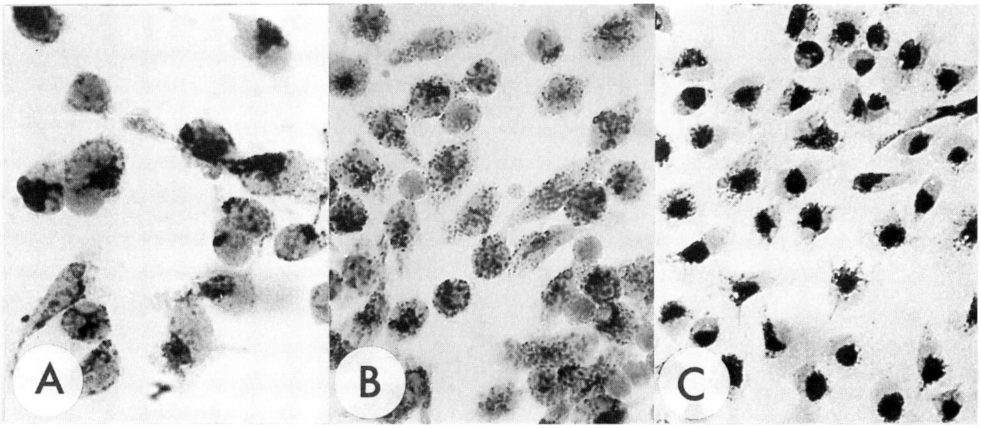

Figure 1: Immunohistochemical detection of ED 1 positive cells within monocytes (A), peritoneal macrophages (B) and Kupffer cells (C). Rat blood monocytes (A), rat peritoneal macrophages (B) and rat liver Kupffer cells (C) were isolated as stated under material and methods. At day 1 after seeding cells were fixed and examined for ED 1 positive cells by indirect peroxidase technique using the monoclonal antibody ED 1 and anti mouse immunoglobuline (magnification: A: 400, B, C: 200 x).

HISTOPATHOLOGY AND IMMUNHISTOCHEMISTRY

a) Histopathology

Massive liver necrosis was observed after a single dose of carbon tetrachloride. The necrosis was prominent in the pericentral area. Repeated administration of the drug lead first to a confluence of the necrotic areas and then to septa formation, increase of connective tissue and finally to cirrhosis. Three weeks after the last CCl_4-administration fibrotic septa were not detectable and a few mononuclear cells were detected in the areas of the previous septa.

b) Immunohistochemistry

In normal rat liver ED 1 and ED 2 + cells were found in the sinusoids and some ED 1 and ED 2 positive cells were detectable around the portal area. Only few Ia+ cells were detectable in the sinusoid. Two days after the administration of a large dose of CCl_4 numerous ED 1+ ve, Ia + ve, ED 2 negative cells were detectable in the pericentral necrotic areas. The pattern outside of this area was comparable to that of the normal liver. Desmin positivity was also increased around the pericentral area. These results indicate that monocytes were recruited from the blood. The increased desmin expression could be due to an increased number or to a initiated dedifferentiation process of the Ito-cells.

The Ia-expression in absence of T-lymphocytes clearly show that it can be induced without the need of an immunological reaction. After the fourth administration mainly ED 1 + Ia + and only a few ED 2 positive cells were detected within the septa. The cells were in contact to desmin and alpha-smooth-muscle-actin positive cells, which lined in contact with hepatocytes. After the tenth CCl_4 administration, mononuclear cells in the fibrous septa were again in contact with desmin and alpha-smooth-muscle-actin positive cells. T-lymphocytes were only seldom detectable. Three weeks after the last CCl_4 administration ED 1 + Ia + but ED 2 negative cells were detectable in the area of the former fibrotic septa. The pattern in the rest of the liver resembled that of the normal liver.

DISCUSSION

In this study we demonstrate, that stimulated (Ia+) blood monocytes are recruited into the necrotic pericentral area of the rat liver after a single dose of carbon tetrachloride. ED 1 positive cells are prominent in the early septa where they seem to start to express the ED 2 antigen. According to the in vitro findings e.g. in peritoneal macrophages a subpopulation of the infiltrating blood monocytes could maturate to tissue macrophages. The contact of the cells of the monocyte/macrophage lineage with desmin- as well as alpha-smooth-muscle-actin-positive cells might be responsible for the activation of Ito-cells. The expression of the Ia-antigens in absence of T-lymphocytes confirms the data obtained in vitro (own unpublished data) indicating that Ia expression can be induced by unspecific stimulation and not only by immunological activation.

At the stage of cirrhosis (after the tenth) administration all the cells inside of the septa seem to be mature macrophage as they are all ED 1, ED 2 and Ia-positive. During the recovery-phase (three weeks after the last CCl_4-administration) again ED 1 + but ED 2- cells in the areas of the former septa could represent a phenotypic change from mature macrophages back to the monocytes. Our experiments could represent an in vivo model for studying phenotypical and functional changes of blood monocytes to tissue macrophages. Isolation of mononuclear inflammatory cells from damaged livers and their phenotypical and functional analysis are underway in our laboratory.

LITERATURE

Burt, A.D., Robertson, J.L., Heir, J., Roderick A., Mc Sween N.M. (1986): Desmin containing stellate cells in rat liver, distribution in normal animals and response to experimental acute liver injury. J Pathol 150, 29-35

De Leeuw, A.H., Mc Carthy, S.B., Geerts, A., Knook. D.L. (1984): Purified rat liver fat storing cells in culture divide and contain collagen. Hepatology 4, 392-403

Dijkstra, C.D., Döpp, E.A., Joling, P., Kraal, G. (1985): The heterogeneity of mononuclear phagocytes un lymphoid organs: Distinct macrophage subpopulation in the rat recognized by monoclonal antibodies ED 1, ED 2 and ED 3. Immunology 54, 589-599

Enzan, H. (1985): Proliferation of Ito-cells (fat storing cells) in acute carbon tetrachloride liver injury. A light and electron microscopic autoradiographic study. Acta Pathol Jpn 35, 1301-1308

Jezequel, A.M., Mancini. R., Rinaldesi, M,L,, Ballardini, G., Failani, M., Bianchi, F., Orlandi, F. (1989): Dimethylnitrosamine-induced cirrhosis. Evidence for an immunological mechanism. J Hepatol 8, 42-52

Kent, G., Gay, S., Inouyem T., Bahum R., Minick, D.T., Popper, H. (1976): Vitamin A containing lipocytes and formation of type III collagen in liver injury. Proc Natl Acad Sci USA 73, 3719-3722

Knook, D.L., Blansjaar, N., Sleyster, C.H. (1977): Isolation and characterization of Kupffer and endo-thelial cells from the rat liver. Exp Cell Res 109, 317-329

Mc Gee, J.O, Patrick, R.S. (1972): The role of peri-sinusoidal cells in hepatic fibrogenesis. An electron microscopic study of acute carbon tetrachloride liver injury. Lab Invest 26, 429-440

Proctor, E., Chatamra K. (1982): High yield micronodular cirrhosis in the rat. Gastroenterology 83, 1183-1190

Ramadori, G., Rieder, H., Theiss, F., Meyer zum Büschenfelde, K.H. (1989): Fat storing (Ito)-cells of rat liver synthesize and secrete apolipoproteins: Comparison with hepatocytes. Gastroenterology 97, 63-72

Ramadori, G., Dienes, H.P., Burger, R., Meuer, S., Rieder, H., Meyer zum Büschenfelde, K.H. (1986): Expression of Ia-antigens in guinea pig Kupffer cells. Studies with monoclonal antibodies. J Hepatol 2, 208-217

Ramadori, G., Veit, T., Schwögler, S., Dienes, H.P., Knittel, T., Rieder, H., Meyer zum Büschenfelde, K.H. (1990): Expression of the gene of the alpha-smooth-muscle-actin isoform in rat liver and in rat fat storing (Ito) cells. Virchows Arch B Cell Pathol 59, 349-357

Résumé

Les processus inflammatoire et de réparation qui mettent en jeu une fibrogénèse et une angiogénèse, sont caractérisés par une accumulation organisée de cellules inflammatoires suivie d'une activation de cellules mésenchymateuses responsables de la synthèse de composants du tissu conjonctif. Dans les maladies chroniques du foie, les mécanismes d'inflammation et de réparation ont lieu dans l'ensemble de l'organe et aboutissent à la formation d'une fibrose puis d'une cirrhose.

Les macrophages présents dans les différents organes sont phénoty-piquement et fonctionnellement différents. Ils diffèrent également de leurs cellules souches, les monocytes sanguins. La principale fonction des cellules de Kupffer (Kc), les macrophages hépatiques, est la phagocytose de particules et de substances solubles. Cependant, on pense que les Kc sécrètent des médiateurs et des facteurs de croissance responsables de l'activation des cellules de Ito et de la synthèse de protéines matricielles par ces cellules. Afin de déterminer si les leucocytes mononucléés sanguins ou les macrophages hépatiques sont les cellules effectrices au cours de l'atteinte hépatique, nous avons étudié le phénotype des cellules mononucléées présentes dans des foies de rat après traitement aigu ou chronique au CCl_4. Les cellules présentes dans les zones de nécrose ont été caractérisées à l'aide de deux anticorps monoclonaux ED1 et ED2 puis étudiées quant à l'expression de l'antigène Ia. Trois jours après le premier traitement au CCl_4, le nombre de cellules positives pour ED1 dans les zones de nécrose centrolobulaires était comparable au nombre de cellules positives pour ED2. De grosses cellules positives pour ED1 et ED2 étaient détectées dans les sinusoïdes. L'antigène Ia était détectable uniquement dans les zones de nécrose centrolobulaires. Toutes les cellules positives pour ED1 et ED2 étaient également positives pour l'antigène Ia. Ces résultats suggèrent que ce sont principalement les leucocytes mononucléés périphériques exprimant l'antigène Ia et non les macrophages hépatiques qui sont les cellules effectrices au cours de la fibrose expérimentale.

Cellular and Molecular Aspects of Cirrhosis. Eds B. Clément, A. Guillouzo. Colloque INSERM/John Libbey Eurotext Ltd. © 1992, Vol. 216, pp. 177-186

Hepatocyte-matrix interactions

Bruno Clément, Pierre-Yves Rescan, Olivier Loréal, Françoise Levavasseur and André Guillouzo

Unité de Recherches Hépatologiques, INSERM U 49, Hôpital Pontchaillou, 35033 Rennes, France

ABSTRACT

Most normal cells require attachment to extracellular matrix for survival, growth, migration and differentiation. In the liver, hepatocytes interact with a complex set of macromolecules, including interstitial and basement membrane components. Interactions of hepatocytes with extracellular matrix components occur throughout cell surface receptors that specifically recognize these proteins. These receptors include both integrins and non-integrin membrane-associated proteins. Integrins that belong to the β1 family are involved in the binding of hepatocytes to collagens, fibronectin, laminin and perlecan. Non-integrin receptors include the 32/67 kD laminin receptor, the 38/36 kD perlecan receptor and other versatile plasma membrane-associated proteins. Recently, it has been shown that these receptors may bind specific sites within matrix macromolecules. It may be hypothesized that both the composition of the extracellular matrix and the molecular structure of each component, modulate the behavior of hepatocytes in normal liver and in the course of hepatic fibrosis.

INTRODUCTION

Cell-matrix interactions are involved in most, if not all, of the key-events of cell life. Embryonic development, maintenance of tissue architecture, tissue repair, inflammation and tumor metastasis are some examples of biological processes in which extracellular matrix plays an important role. During the last ten years, this field has been intensively explored, leading to the discovery of cell surfaces receptors as mediators between extracellular macromolecules and the intracellular machinery. The molecular mechanisms involved in signal transduction are currently being investigated.

The liver is composed of several cell types which are organized within the hepatic lobule in a precise architecture. Hepatocytes, the major liver cell type which performs most hepatic functions, interact with both non-parenchymal cells and the extracellular matrix. Besides soluble factors, e.g. hormones and cytokines, structural requirements are involved in the stability and modulation of liver specific functions.

Personal works were supported by the Institut National de la Santé et de la Recherche Médicale and by grants from the International Coordinating Council for Cancer Research and The Philippe Foundation. F.L. is a recipient of a fellowship from La Ligue Française contre le Cancer.

At least three groups of specialized cell surface proteins maintain specific relationships between cells and either neighboring cells or extracellular matrix. These include cell adhesion molecules (CAMs), junction molecules and extracellular matrix receptors, i.e. integrins and non-integrin receptors.
This review will summarize our current knowledge on extracellular matrix receptors in the normal liver. Integrins, basement membrane structure and functions, laminin receptors, as well as the effects of extracellular matrix on hepatocyte behavior have been recently reviewed elsewhere (Abelda and Buck, 1990 ; Buck, 1987 ; Martin and Timpl, 1987 ; Mecham, 1991 ; Ruoslahti, 1991 ; and reviews by Schuppan et al. and Bissell in this book).

THE HEPATIC EXTRACELLULAR MATRIX

Normal adult liver contains only small amounts of extracellular matrix components. However, both immunofluorescent and immunoelectron studies have shown that hepatocytes interact with almost all the essential components of both interstitial extracellular matrix, e.g. collagens I, III, V and VI, and fibronectin, and basement membranes, e.g. collagen IV, laminin, entactin and the heparan sulfate proteoglycan, perlecan (Bianchi et al., 1984 ; Clément et al., 1984 ; Grimaud et al., 1980 ; Hahn et al., 1980 ; Martinez-Hernandez, 1984 ; Rescan et al. submitted). Furthermore, dramatic changes in both the amount and composition of the extracellular matrix occur in a variety of liver diseases leading to the development of hepatic fibrosis. For example during the "capillarization" process laminin, collagen IV and probably perlecan accumulate, thus forming a continuous basement membrane in the space of Disse. Recent immunoelectron studies have shown, in addition, that basement membrane components are much more abundant in fetal than in adult liver, particularly at the contact of hepatocyte microvilli (Rescan et al., 1989). Thus, the hepatic extracellular matrix must be considered not as a static network but rather as a dynamic structure which may change during the various physiopathological stages of the liver.
For a long time the origin of the hepatic extracellular matrix has been a matter of debate. Indeed, *in vitro* studies have shown that most liver cells, including hepatocytes (Diegelmann, 1986) and Ito cells (Friedman et al., 1985 ; Schafer et al., 1987 ; Weiner et al., 1990), may express matrix proteins when put in culture. During the last few years, it

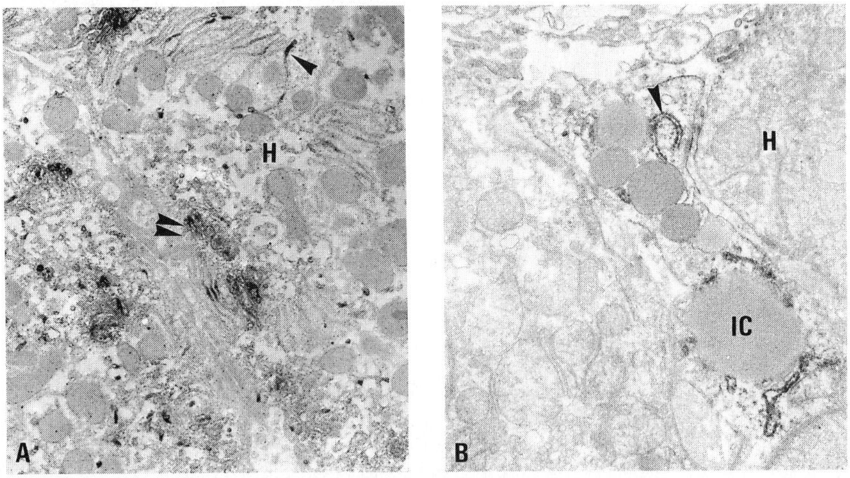

Figure 1 : Electron microscopy. Immunoperoxidase localization of fibronectin (A) and collagen IV (B) in normal adult rat liver. Fibronectin is abundant in the rough endoplasmic reticulum (arrowheads) and Golgi apparatus (double arrowheads) of hepatocytes (H), and collagen IV in the rough endoplasmic reticulum of an Ito cell (IC). (A : x 5,200; B : x 11,600)

became clear that the expression of matrix proteins at high levels by cultured liver cells are related to an adaptative process to survive *in vitro*. Accordingly, these findings indicate that liver cells have the capacity to express matrix genes in certain conditions, particularly when their environment is altered. Immunoelectron studies and more recently *in situ* hybridization have somewhat clarified the respective participation of each liver cell type in the formation of the hepatic extracellular matrix *in vivo* (Clément et al., 1984 ; 1986 ; 1988 ; Geerts et al., 1986 ; Milani et al., 1989a ; 1989b ; Takahara et al., 1989). Except for fibronectin adult normal hepatocytes are not a major source of extracellular matrix components (Figure 1). Rather, both endothelial and Ito cells have been shown to contain precursors of matrix proteins or their corresponding mRNAs. Interestingly, hepatocytes, in addition to sinusoidal cells, were found to produce extracellular matrix proteins, particularly basement membrane components, in alcoholic human livers (Clément et al., 1986) and in cholestatic rat livers (Abdel-Aziz et al., 1991), as well as during the perinatal period in both species (Rescan et al., 1989).

CELL SURFACE RECEPTORS FOR EXTRACELLULAR MATRIX

Adhesion molecules mediate interactions between cells and the extracellular milieu. Among these molecules, specific receptors allow cells to recognize extracellular matrix proteins. During the last few years the molecular mechanisms by which hepatocytes interact with extracellular matrix located in the space of Disse have been investigated. First lines of evidence that hepatocytes specifically bind individual extracellular matrix proteins came from *in vitro* studies (Rubin et al., 1981 ; Bissell et al., 1986). After their isolation from rat liver, hepatocytes can be set up on various substrata made of purified extracellular matrix components. As shown in figure 2, hepatocytes differently attach and spread on these substrata. Interestingly, the most efficient matrix molecules for

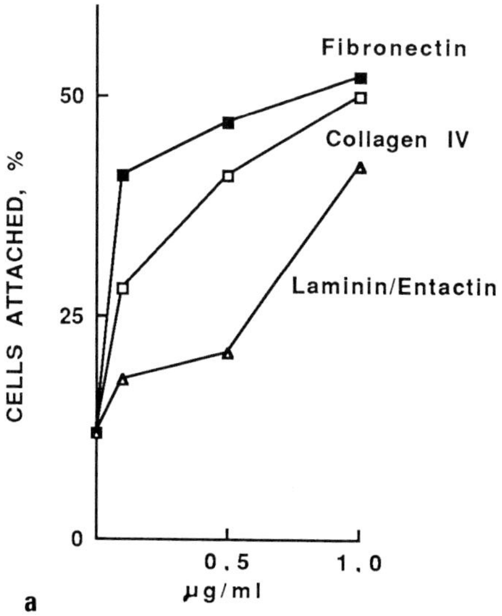

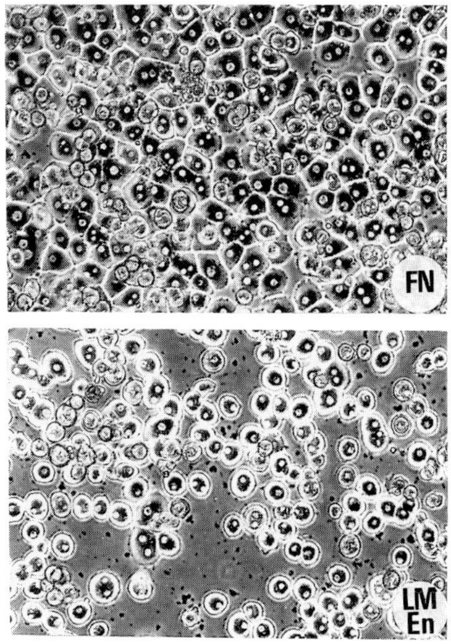

Figure 2 : Cell attachment of hepatocytes to various extracellular matrix components.
(a) : Various amounts of fibronectin, collagen IV and laminin/entactin complex were coated on 0.32-cm2 well tissue-culture plates. Then, freshly isolated hepatocytes (60,000 cells) were added in serum-free medium. After 30 min, plates were gently washed with phosphate buffer. The percentage of attached cells was determined using a lactacte dehydrogenase assay.
(b) : Phase-contrast microscopy. Hepatocytes were cultured on dishes coated with either fibronectin (FN) or laminin/entactin complex (LM/En) for 4 h. (x140)

attachment and spreading appear to be the less effective for maintenance of liver-specific functions, i.e. fibronectin and collagens vs laminin. These findings suggest that specific membrane proteins mediate hepatocyte interaction to distinct components of the hepatic extracellular matrix.

Integrins

Integrins are heterodimers consisting of noncovalently associated α and β subunits that mediate both cell-substratum and cell-cell adhesion. The integrin family is divided in at least three groups according to their common β chain. Most of integrins interacting with extracellular matrix components belong to the $\beta 1$ - or VLA - subfamily. $\beta 1$ integrins serve as receptors for fibronectin ($\alpha 1\beta 1$; $\alpha 3\beta 1$; $\alpha 5\beta 1$; $\alpha v\beta 1$), collagens ($\alpha 1\beta 1$; $\alpha 2\beta 1$; $\alpha 3\beta 1$), and laminin ($\alpha 1\beta 1$; $\alpha 2\beta 1$; $\alpha 3\beta 1$; $\alpha 6\beta 1$). In addition, other integrins from the $\beta 3$ (e.g. $\alpha v\beta 3$) $\beta 4$ (e.g. $\alpha 6\beta 4$) and $\beta 5$ subfamilies (e.g. $\alpha v\beta 5$) have been shown to interact with matrix proteins. Since integrins were found to be present in every tissue or cells so far studied, it was expected to find integrins in the liver. Recently, Volpes et al (1991) have studied by immuno-histochemistry the distribution of the $\beta 1$ chain and the variable α chain -1 to 6- of the VLA subfamily in normal, inflammatory and cholestatic human livers. The common $\beta 1$ chain was always detected in portal spaces and in the sinusoids, while the pattern of staining for the α chains was different according to the structure analyzed and/or the pathological state of the liver. Specifically, only $\alpha 1$ and $\alpha 5$ chains were evidenced on both hepatocytes and sinusoidal cells in normal liver. By contrast, hepatocytes became positive for $\alpha 2$, $\alpha 3$, $\alpha 5$ and $\alpha 6$ chains in inflammatory and/or cholestatic livers.

Another strategy to identify integrins is to isolate these proteins from purified cell populations. The first identified integrin in hepatocytes was the fibronectin receptor. Johansson et al. (1987), have isolated a fibronectin receptor which specifically bound cell-binding fibronectin domain in a R-G-D-dependent manner. It appeared to consist of a $\beta 1$ chain associated with an α chain distinct from that in fibroblastic cell lines. $\beta 1$ integrins are also involved in the interactions of hepatocytes with perlecan (Rescan et al. submitted) and laminin, particularly the $\alpha 1\beta 1$ integrin (see below).

Non-integrin matrix receptors

Extracellular matrix binding proteins that do not belong to the integrin family have been identified in hepatocytes. Rubin et al. (1986) have isolated rat liver glycoproteins with affinity for collagen I. They found that antibodies against the purified glycoproteins - Mr= 105 Kd, 115 Kd and 130 Kd- inhibited attachment of hepatocytes to collagen I, but not to either fibronectin or collagen IV. In chick liver, a major Mr=47,000 collagen binding protein that binds gelatin and native collagens I, III and IV has been localized in smooth muscle cells of the arterial wall and in perisinusoidal cells, but not in the hepatocyte (Saga et al., 1987). This glycoprotein is not likely to be a receptor surface protein, but may play a role in intracellular protein processing or translocation. More recently we have identified a Mr=80,000 protein on the surface of hepatocytes that binds collagen IV and also other basement membrane components, including laminin and perlecan (Clément and Yamada, 1990). The core protein of perlecan has been shown to directly interact with freshly isolated rat hepatocytes (Clément et al., 1989). A major Mr=36/38,000 and a Mr = 26,000 membrane proteins have been purified from cell surface iodinated hepatocytes using affinity chromatography column made with the core protein of perlecan. The 36/38 kD protein(s) was found on a variety of cells that contact basement membrane, including MDCK and NRK-52E kidney cells, mouse melanoma M2 cells and EHS tumor cells. Laminin binding protein(s) can be isolated from cell membranes by affinity chromatography on laminin-Sepharose. Thus, a major Mr=67,000 protein has been identified on a variety of cells, including tumor cells, muscle cells, macrophages, endothelial and epithelial cells and neuronal cells (for review, see Mecham, 1991). Wewer et al. (1986) have reported a partial cDNA for the human 67 kDa laminin binding protein. Subsequently, several groups have isolated full-length cDNA having a coding capacity for a 32 kDa, but not 67 kDa protein (Yow et al., 1988 ; Segui-Real et al., 1989). Recently, various proteins from isolated membranes of cell-surface iodinated hepatocytes were identified using a laminin affinity column, including Mr=67,000 ; 45,000 ; and 32,000 proteins (Clément et al., 1990). These cell-surface proteins were recognized by antibodies made against a bacterial fusion protein coded for by the ß-galactosidase gene plus the 0.9 kb cDNA sequence encoding the nearly entire 32 kD laminin binding protein molecule (LBP-32). Northern-blot analysis revealed that hepatocytes contain 1.1 kb LBP-32 mRNAs (Rescan et al., 1990). Interestingly, the steady state LBP-32 mRNA level was much more higher in fetal and neoplastic hepatocytes as well as in hepatoma cell lines and in cultured adult hepatocytes, than in the normal adult liver (Rescan et al., 1990 ; 1991). This overexpression paralleled with the expression of B1 and/or B2 laminin chains. These findings suggest that the expression of both laminin chains and receptors in hepatocytes is related to changes of the normal phenotype and/or the pericellular environment.

INVOLVEMENT OF THE STRUCTURE OF LAMININ IN SPECIFIC INTERACTIONS WITH HEPATOCYTES

Laminin, the major component in basement membranes, was found to be composed of three genetically distinct chains, i.e. A (Mr=440,000), B1 (Mr=220,000) and B2 (Mr= 210,000) in murine Engelbreth-Holm-Swarm (EHS) tumor. Laminin of non-neoplastic origin may differ in either the A, B1 and B2 ratio or the presence of different chain(s). Thus, a variety of cells express A chain at very low level, if any. In addition, several normal tissues, including placenta, heart and neuromuscular junctions were found to contain laminin formed by the assembly of homologous but genetically distinct chains.
In the liver, although abundant in neighboring laminin-producing cells, i.e. sinusoidal endothelial and Ito cells, this glycoprotein is only sparsely deposited at the contact of hepatocytes (Clément et al., 1988 ; Hahn et al., 1980). Laminin extracted from the EHS tumor is a potent regulator of hepatocyte morphology and functions *in vitro* (Bissell et al., 1987). However, the relevance of these findings may depend on the actual structure of laminin in the space of Disse. Indeed, since this glycoprotein is a very large molecule it can be expected that several different cellular receptors on hepatocytes will bind to multiple cell adhesion sites on laminin, thus inducing specific regulatory signals.

Structure of laminin interacting with hepatocytes

Immunoelectron studies have clearly shown that in the normal adult liver, Ito cells is a major source of laminin that is deposited in the space of Disse (Clément et al., 1988). Recently, we have investigated the expression of the three chains of laminin in isolated rat lipocytes (Loréal et al., 1991). Both B1 and B2 chains, but not A were found in the medium of 5-day-old lipocyte primary cultures by western blotting and immunoprecipitation of radiolabeled proteins. An additional Mr=380,000 protein was found by immunoprecipitation only, while only one Mr=900,000 band was found under non-reducing conditions, thereby suggesting that lipocytes produce a variant form of laminin composed by the assembly of B1, B2 and the 380 kD polypeptide. Northern blots confirmed these data and showed that only B2 mRNAs were clearly detectable in freshly isolated lipocytes. Although both A and B1 genes could be transcribed at low levels and/or mRNAs rapidly processed, it is likely that Ito cells produce a variant form of laminin *in vivo*. Interestingly, Maher and MacGuire (1990) have recently shown that, in addition to Ito cells, endothelial cells isolated from normal adult rat liver contained high B2 chain mRNA levels.
Although not producing detectable laminin in the normal adult liver, hepatocytes have the capacity to express laminin genes (Clément et al., 1988 ; Rescan et al., 1989 ; 1990 ; 1991). By immunoelectron microscopy in both liver and cultured cells, immunoblotting and/or immunoprecipitation of proteins from media of cultured cells and Northern blotting, we have shown that hepatocytes express B1 chain of laminin in fetal liver, and both B1 and B2 chains in neoplastic hepatocytes from diethylnitrosamine-treated rat livers as well as in hepatoma cell lines. Interestingly, both rat and human hepatoma cells were found to synthesize a Mr=380,000 polypetide, not related to the A chain of laminin (Rescan et al., 1991). Finally, in normal adult hepatocyte primary cultures, B2 chain mRNAs were present as early as 4 hours after cell seeding, while the steady state B1

mRNA level remained very low during the first day in culture. Both B1 and B2 mRNA levels dramatically increased during the following 2 days. These findings clearly indicate that the expression of laminin chains by hepatocytes is not coordinated, depends on the maturation of the cells, and is related to changes of the normal phenotype and/or the pericellular environment.
Taken together, these data suggest that laminin probably exists in the space of Disse in a different form compared to that originally characterized from the EHS tumor.

Specific binding domains on laminin chains

Two complementary approaches have been designed to map laminin regions involved in biological activities, including proteolytic cleavage of the EHS laminin and synthetic peptides deduced from the cloned sequence of its three chains (Figure 3).

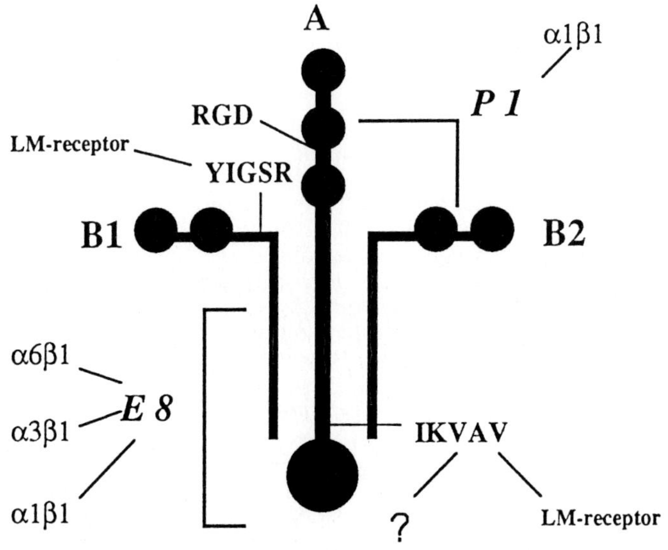

Figure 3 : Interactions of receptors with specific binding domains on EHS laminin chains

At least five active sites for cell adhesion have been identified using synthetic peptides, including YIGSR, PDGSR and F9 on the B1 chain (residues 929-933, 902-906 and 641-660, respectively) and CQFALRGDNP and CSRARKQAASIKVAVSADR on the A chain (residues 1115-1124 and 2091-2108, respectively). Interestingly, it has been shown that YIGSR and the sequence RYVVLPR within the F9 peptide inhibit metastasis (Graf et al., 1987 ; Skubitz et al., 1990), while SIKVAV-containing peptide promotes tumor cell invasion (Kanemoto et al., 1990). Rat hepatocytes bind to three different sites within the B1 and A chains of the EHS laminin, including YIGSR and RGD- and SIKVAV-containing peptides (Clément et al., 1990; Tashiro et al., 1989). SIKVAV-containing peptide was the most potent peptide, reaching 70% of the activity of laminin for hepatocyte adhesion. Affinity chromatography on peptide columns revealed that the SIKVAV-containing peptide specifically bound LBP-32 and related cell membrane proteins, as well as other minor membrane-associated proteins.

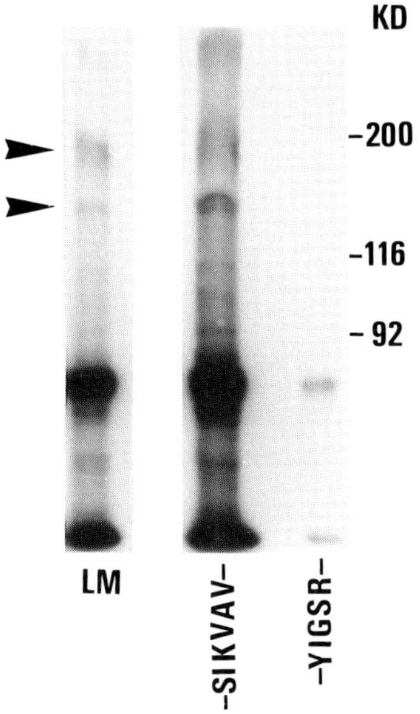

Figure 4 : Identification of cell surface proteins that bind laminin and related peptides in a divalent cation-dependent manner

^{125}I-labeled purified cell membranes of normal adult hepatocytes were prepared in the presence of $MnCl_2$ and passed over columns made with either laminin (LM), SIKVAV or YIGSR. EDTA eluted a major Mr = 80,000 protein from these columns. In addition, Mr = 200,000 and 150,000 proteins (arrows) were eluted from laminin and SIKVAV columns but not from a YIGSR column.

Cell surface proteins that bind this peptide in a divalent cation-dependent manner were also identified (Figure 4). Although these proteins were not easily detectable, it is likely that proteins that belong to the integrin family may mediate the interaction of hepatocytes with this biologically active site. Other cell surface proteins were also identified interacting with YIGSR and RGD-containing peptides. This group of proteins (Mr = 80, 55, 38 and 36 kD) bound these peptides with lower activity than the others. In addition, YIGSR peptide elutes a Mr = 67 kD protein (LBP-32) from affinity column (Graf et al., 1987). It is noteworthy that polymeric and cyclic forms of YIGSR are required for activity, thus suggesting that tertiary structure may be critical for its recognition by receptor(s).

Another strategy to identify specific domains of laminin interacting with receptors consists in preparing proteolytic fragments of the molecule. Four different fragments of the EHS laminin -E5, E6, E8 and P1- may interact with hepatocytes (Timpl et al., 1983 ; Forsberg et al., 1990). Recently, $\alpha 1\beta 1$ integrins were found to recognize both the E8 and P1 fragments of laminin on hepatocytes (Forsberg et al., 1990). Also $\alpha 3\beta 1$ and $\alpha 6\beta 1$ integrins have been shown to interact with the E8 fragment (Gehlsen et al., 1989 ; Hall et al., 1990). Taken together these findings show that a specific domain of laminin may recognize different receptors and, on the other hand a same receptor may recognize different domains of laminin.

As above discussed, is likely that in any case normal hepatocytes do not interact with laminin formed by the assembly of A, B1 and B2 chains in a stochiometric complex. Whether analogues of laminin chains, e.g. S-laminin or merosin, might be present in the space of Disse remain to be elucidated. Since attachment of hepatocytes to a substratum made of EHS laminin in culture occurs, at least in part, via active sites within the A chain (Clément et al., 1990), conclusions from *in vitro* studies might be unrelevant compared to the normal situation *in vivo*. The presence of multiple binding proteins on the surface of hepatocytes which interact with active sites on laminin emphasizes the concept that the specificity of interactions of cells with extracellular matrix involves both specialized receptors and key-domains of macromolecules.

REFERENCES

Abdel-Aziz, G., Rescan, P.Y., Clément, B., Lebeau, G., Rissel, M., Grimaud, J.A., Campion, J.P. & Guillouzo, A. (1991): Cellular sources of matrix proteins in experimentally induced cholestatic rat liver. *J. Pathol.* 164, 167-174.

Abelda, S.M. & Buck, C.A. (1990): Integrins and other cell adhesion molecules. *FASEB J.* 4, 2868-2880.

Bianchi, F.B., Fiagini, G., Ballardini, G., Genacchi, G., Faccani, A., Pisi, E., Laschi, R., Liotta, L. & Garbisa, S. (1984): Basement membrane production by hepatocytes in chronic liver disease. *Hepatology* 4, 1167-1172.

Bissell, D.M., Arenson, D.M., Maher, J.J. & Roll, F.J. (1987): Support of cultured hepatocytes by a laminin-rich gel. Evidence for a functionally significant subendothelial matrix in normal liver. *J. Clin. Invest.* 79, 801-812.

Bissell, D.M., Stomatoglou, S.C., Nermut, M.V. & Hughes, R.C. (1986): Interactions of rat hepatocytes with type IV collagen, fibronectin and laminin matrices. Distinct matrix-controlled modes of attachment and spreading. *Eur. J. Cell. Biol.* 40, 72-78.

Buck, C.A. (1987): Cell surface receptors for extracellular matrix molecules. *Ann. Rev. Cell Biol.* 3, 179-205.

Clément, B., Emonard, M., Rissel, M., Druguet, M., Grimaud, J.A., Herbage, D., Bourel, M. & Guillouzo, A. (1984): Cellular origin of collagen and fibronectin in the liver. *Cell. Mol. Biol.* 30, 489-496.

Clément, B., Grimaud, J.A., Campion, J.P., Deugnier, Y. & Guillouzo, A. (1986): Cell types involved in the production of collagen and fibronectin in normal and fibrotic human liver. *Hepatology,* 6, 225-234.

Clément, B., Rescan, P.Y., Baffet, G., Loréal, O., Lehry, D., Campion, J.P. & Guillouzo, A. (1988): Hepatocytes may produce laminin in fibrotic liver and in primary culture. *Hepatology* 8, 794-803.

Clément, B., Segui-Real, B., Hassell, J.R., Martin, G.R. & Yamada, Y. (1989): Identification of a cell surface-binding protein for the core protein of the basement membrane proteoglycan. *J. Biol. Chem.* 264, 12467-12471.

Clément, B., Segui-Real, B., Savagner, P., Kleinman, H.K. & Yamada, Y. (1990a): Hepatocyte attachment to laminin is mediated through multiple receptors. *J. Cell. Biol.* 110, 185-192.

Clément, B. & Yamada, Y. (1990b): A Mr 80K hepatocyte surface protein(s) interacts with basement membrane components. *Exp. Cell Res.* 187, 320-323.

Diegelman, R.F. (1986): Synthesis of extracellular matrix components by cultured hepatocytes. In *Isolated and Cultured Hepatocytes,* eds. A. Guillouzo & C. Guguen-Guillouzo, pp. 209-224. Paris: Les Editions INSERM & London: John Libbey.

Forsberg, E., Paulsson, M., Timpl, R. & Johansson, S. (1990): Characterization of a laminin receptor on rat hepatocytes. *J. Biol. Chem.* 265, 6376-6381.

Friedman, S.L., Roll, F.J., Boyles, J. & Bissell, D.M. (1985) : Hepatic lipocytes : the principal collagen-producing cells of normal rat liver. *Proc. Natl. Acad. Sci. USA,* 82, 8681-8685.

Geerts, A., Geuze, H.J., Slot, J.W., Voss, B., Schuppan, D., Schellinck, P. & Wisse, E. (1986) : Immunogold localization of procollagen I, fibronectin and heparan sulfate proteoglycan on ultrathin frozen sections of the normal rat liver. *Histochemistry,* 84, 355-362.

Gehlsen, K., Dickerson, K., Argraves, W.S., Engvall, E. & Ruoslahti, E. (1989) : Subunit structure of a laminin-binding integrin and localization of its binding site on laminin. *J. Biol. Chem.* 264, 19034-19038.

Graf, J., Iwamoto, M., Martin, G.R., Kleinman, H.K., Robey, F.A. & Yamada, Y. (1987) : Identification of an amino acid sequence in laminin mediating cell attachment, chemotaxis, and receptor binding. *Cell* 48, 989-996.

Grimaud, J.A., Druguet, M., Peyrol, S., Chevalier, O., Herbage, D. & El Badrawy, N. (1980) : Collagen immunotyping in human liver : light and electron microscope study. *J. Histochem. Cytochem.* 28, 1145-1156.

Hahn, E., Wick, G., Pencev, D. & Timpl, R. (1980): Distribution of basement membrane proteins in normal and fibrotic human liver : collagen type IV, laminin, and fibronectin. *Gut* 21, 63-71.

Hall, D.E., Reicherdt, L.F., Crowley, E., Holley, B., Moezzi, H., Sonnenberg, A. & Damsky, C.H. (1990): The $\alpha1/\beta1$ and $\alpha6/\beta1$ integrin heterodimers mediate cell attachment to distinct sites on laminin. *J. Cell Biol.* 110, 2175-2184.

Johansson, S., Forsberg, E. & Lundgren, B. (1987): Comparison of fibronectin receptors from rat hepatocytes and fibroblasts. *J. Biol. Chem.* 262, 7919-7824.

Kanemoto, T., Reich, R., Greatorex, D., Adler, S.H., Shiraishi, N., Martin, G.R., Yamada, Y. & Kleinman, H.K. (1990): Identification of an amino acid sequence from the laminin A chain that stimulates metastasis and collagenase IV production. *Proc. Natl. Acad. Sci. USA* 87, 2279-2283.

Loréal, O., Levavasseur, F., Rescan, P.Y., Yamada, Y., Guillouzo, A. & Clément, B. (1991): Differential expression of laminin chains in hepatic lipocytes. *FEBS Lett.* 290, 9-12.

Maher, J.J. & McGuire, R.F. (1991): Cellular matrix gene expression increases preferentially in rat lipocytes and sinusoidal endothelial cells during hepatic fibrosis in vivo. *J. Clin. Invest.* 86, 1641-1648.

Martin, G.R. & Timpl, R. (1987): Laminin and other basement membrane components. *Ann. Rev. Cell Biol.* 3, 57-85.

Martinez-Hernandez, A. (1984): The hepatic extracellular matrix. I. Electron immunohistochemical studies in normal rat liver. *Lab. Invest.* 51, 57-74.

Mecham, R.P. (1991): Receptors for laminin on mammalian cells. *FASEB J.* 5, 2538-2546.

Milani, S., Herbst, H., Schuppan, D., Hahn, E.G. & Stein, H. (1989a): In situ hybridization for procollagen types I, III and IV mRNA in normal and fibrotic rat liver : evidence for predominant expression in nonparenchymal liver cells. *Hepatology* 10, 84-92.

Milani, S., Herbst, H., Schuppan, D., Riecken, E.O. & Stein, H. (1989b): Cellular localization of laminin gene transcripts in normal and fibrotic human liver. *Am. J. Pathol.* 134, 1175-1182.

Rescan, P.Y., Clément, B., Grimaud, J.A., Guillois, B., Strain, A. & Guillouzo, A. (1989): Participation of hepatocytes in the production of basement membrane components in human and rat liver during the perinatal period. *Cell Diff. Dev.* 26, 131-144.

Rescan, P.Y., Clément, B., Yamada, Y., Segui-Real, B., Baffet, G., Guguen-Guillouzo, C. & Guillouzo, A. (1990): Differential expression of laminin chains and receptor (LBP-32) in fetal and neoplastic hepatocytes compared to normal adult hepatocytes in vivo and in culture. *Am. J. Pathol.* 137, 701-709.

Rescan, P.Y., Clément, B., Yamada, Y., Segui-Real, B., Glaise, D., Guguen-Guillouzo, C. & Guillouzo A. (1991): Expression of laminin and its receptor LBP-32 in human and rat hepatoma cells. *Hepatology* 13, 289-296.

Rubin, K., Hook, M., Obrink, B. & Timpl, R. (1981): Substrate adhesion of rat hepatocytes : Mechanism of attachment to collagen substrates. *Cell* 24, 463-470.

Rubin, K., Gullberg, D., Borg, T.K., & Obrink, B. (1986): Hepatocyte adhesion to collagen. Isolation of membrane glycoproteins involved in adhesion to collagen. *Exp. Cell Res.* 164, 127-138.

Ruoslahti, E. (1991): Integrins. *J. Clin. Invest.* 87, 1-5.

Saga, S., Nagata, K., Chen, W.T. & Yamada, K.M. (1987): pH-dependent function, purification and intracellular location of a major collagen-binding glycoprotein. *J. Cell Biol.* 105, 517-527.

Schafer, S., Zerbe, O. & Gressner, A.M. (1987): The synthesis of proteoglycans in fat-storing cells of rat liver. *Hepatology* 7, 680-687.

Segui-Real, B., Rhodes, C., & Yamada, Y. (1989): The human genome contains a pseudogene for the Mr = 32 000 laminin binding protein. *Nucleic Acids Res.* 17, 1257.

Skubitz, A.P.N., McCarthy, J.B., Zhao, Q., Yi, X.Y. & Furcht, L.T. (1990): Definition of a sequence, RYVVLPR, within laminin peptide F-9 that mediates metastatic fibrosarcoma cell adhesion and spreading. *Cancer Res.* 50, 7612-7622.

Takahara, T., Kojima, T., Miyabayashi, C., Inoue, K., Sasaki, H., Muragaki, Y. & Ooshima, A. (1989): Collagen production in fat-storing cells after carbon tetrachloride intoxication in the rat. Immunoelectron microscopic observation of type I, type III collagens, and prolyl hydroxylase. *Lab. Invest.* 59, 509-521.

Tashiro, K.I., Sephel, G.C., Weeks, B., Sasaki, M., Martin, G.R., Kleinman, H.K. & Yamada, Y. (1989): A synthetic peptide containing the IKVAV sequence from the A chain of laminin mediates cell attachment, migration, and neurite outgrowth. *J. Biol. Chem.* 264, 16174-16182.

Timpl, R., Johansson, S., Van Delden, V., Oberbaümer, I. & Hook, M. (1983): Characterization of protease-resistant fragments of laminin mediating attachment and spreading of rat hepatocytes. *J. Biol. Chem.* 258, 8922-8927.

Volpes, R., Van Den Oord, J.J. & Desmet, V.J. (1991): Distribution of the VLA family of integrins in normal and pathological human liver tissue. *Gastroenterology* 101, 200-206.

Weiner, F.R., Giambrone, M.A., Czaja, M.J., Shah, A., Annoni, G., Takahashi, S., Eghbali, M. & Zern, M. (1990): Ito-cell gene expression and collagen regulation. *Hepatology* 11, 111-117.

Wewer, U.M., Liotta, L.A., Jaye, M., Ricca, G.A., Drohan, W.N., Claysmith, A.P., Rao, C.N., Wirth, P., Coligan, J.E., Albrechtsen, R., Mudryj, M. & Sobel, M.E. (1986): Altered levels of laminin receptor mRNA in various human carcinoma cells that have different abilities to bind laminin. *Proc. Natl. Acad. Sci. USA* 83, 7137-7141.

Yow, H., Wong, J.M., Chen, H.S., Lee, C., Steele, G.D. & Chen, LB (1988): Increased mRNA expression of a laminin binding protein in human colon carcinoma : complete sequence of a full length cDNA encoding the protein. *Proc. Natl. Acad. Sci. USA* 85, 6394-6398.

Résumé

La plupart des cellules normales doivent s'attacher à une matrice extracellulaire pour leur survie, leur croissance, leur migration et leur différenciation. Dans le foie, les hépatocytes interagissent avec un assemblage complexe de macromolécules extracellulaires de type intersticiel ou de composants des lames basales. L'interaction des hépatocytes avec la matrice extracellulaire est possible grâce à des récepteurs membranaires qui reconnaissent spécifiquement chacune des protéines extracellulaires. Ces récepteurs sont des intégrines ou d'autres protéines associées aux membranes plasmiques. Les intégrines de la famille β_1 sont responsables des liaisons de l'hépatocyte avec les collagènes, la fibronectine, la laminine et le perlecan. Parmi les récepteurs n'appartenant pas à la super-famille des intégrines on trouve le récepteur à la laminine de 32/67 kD et le récepteur au perlecan de 38/36 kD. Récemment, il a été démontré que ces récepteurs interagissent avec les protéines extracellulaires via des sites spécifiques. Il est possible que, aussi bien la composition de la matrice extracellulaire hépatique que la structure de chacune des macromolécules qui la compose module le fonctionnement des hépatocytes dans le foie normal et cirrthotique.

Cellular and Molecular Aspects of Cirrhosis. Eds B. Clément, A. Guillouzo. Colloque INSERM/John Libbey Eurotext Ltd. © 1992, Vol. 216, pp. 187-197

Effects of extracellular matrix on hepatocyte behavior

D. Montgomery Bissell

Liver Center Laboratory, University of California, Building 40, Room 4102, San Francisco General Hospital, San Francisco, CA 94110, USA

SUMMARY

Immunohistological studies have characterized the ECM in normal liver as a basement membrane-like structure. Culture systems incorporating a substratum of similar composition demonstrate a striking dependence of normal adult hepatocytes on contact with ECM. Taken together, these findings are persuasive with respect to a central role for ECM in normal liver. Current work focuses on ECM receptors expressed by hepatocytes and on ECM-regulated transcription of liver-specific genes. An expanding new area concerns the role of ECM in binding and presenting cytokines and growth factors to the cell. The work to date suggests that alteration of this ECM may underlie hepatocellular dysfunction in fibrosing liver diseases.

HISTORICAL BACKGROUND

The unusual structure of the liver subserves the specialized metabolic role of this tissue. Conversely, the integrity and function of hepatocytes may depend on this unique environment. The latter view is reflected in work that dates from Carrel and the development of in vitro cultivation techniques (Bang & Warwick, 1965). Indeed, many of the currently used culture models, including collagenous substrata and co-culture approaches, were explored by investigators working thirty years ago (Bang & Warwick, 1965). Current progress reflects two major developments: the introduction of methods to quantitatively disperse the liver with recovery of viable hepatocytes (Berry & Friend, 1969); and elucidation of the composition and structure of the extracellular matrix (ECM) (Burgeson, 1988). The first enabled the preparation of mass primary cultures, with sufficient material for the examination of liver-specific function in culture (Bissell et al, 1973). The second has stimulated a detailed investigation of hepatocyte interaction with specific kinds of ECM, as will be discussed.

Appreciation of the role of extracellular matrix (ECM) in liver was slow to emerge, despite striking evidence of its biological importance for other cell types. A thin layer of fibrillar (type I) collagen on plastic was shown to mediate the maturation in culture of myoblasts to myotubes (Haushka & Konigsberg, 1966). It was reported also that thyroid cells form "acini" and exhibit secretory activity within a collagen gel, in contrast to conventional cultures on uncoated plastic (Elsdale & Bard, 1972). Similar studies with human fetal hepatocytes showed little or no effect of a collagen gel (Bissell & Tilles, 1971), although adult rat hepatocytes maintained on floating gels exhibited slightly (but significantly) higher levels of cytochrome P-450 than did parallel cultures on plastic (Michalopoulos et al, 1976). The latter system was adopted for mammary cells in culture and appeared to have substantially greater effects on these cells than on hepatocytes (Emerman et al, 1977; Bissell MJ, 1981).

The limited effect of collagen on hepatocytes implied either a minimal interaction of these cells with ECM or, alternatively, a requirement for a specific type of ECM. Present evidence favors the latter possibility. Although electron microscopic examination of young rat liver (the tissue usually studied) fails to reveal a morphologically distinct basement membrane, "reticulin" staining material is regularly associated with the hepatic sinusoids. Pathologic hepatic fibrosis within the space of Disse correlates with clinically severe disease (Bissell & Roll, 1990) suggesting that hepatocytes respond negatively to replacement of the normal ECM.

THE EXTRACELLULAR MATRIX OF THE LIVER

The development of monospecific antibodies for individual ECM proteins and the use of immunohistology has brought new insight to the composition and distribution of hepatic ECM. While the data from various studies are not entirely consonant, they confirm the presence of perisinusoidal ECM and, qualitatively, suggest a structure that resembles a basement membrane (Martinez-Hernandez, 1984; Hahn et al, 1980). Type IV collagen clearly is present in a sinusoidal distribution (Clement et al, 1986). Laminin is associated with lipocytes (Clement et al, 1988; Maher et al, 1988) as is heparan sulfate proteoglycan (Arenson et al, 1988) and tenascin (Van Eyken et al, 1989). The perisinusoidal ECM has been visualized also by alkali maceration, a technique which removes cellular material but leaves the ECM in its original location and configuration (Ohtani, 1988). By scanning electron microscopy, the ECM of young rat liver and human liver appear similar, although the density of the ECM in the rat clearly is less than in the human liver. While it is unknown whether this low-density ECM in fact constitutes a basement membrane, this is suggested by both its composition and, as will be discussed, by the biologic effects of "basement membrane" on hepatocytes in culture.

CELL CULTURE EVIDENCE FOR HEPATOCYTE-ECM INTERACTION

Freshly isolated adult rat hepatocytes in serum-free medium attach poorly to culture plastic, possibly reflecting the fact that their production of ECM proteins appears to be limited to plasma fibronectin and heparan sulfate proteoglycan (Stamatoglou et al, 1987). They produce little or no collagen (Maher & McGuire, 1990). By contrast, when the culture substratum consists of plastic coated with fibrillar collagen (generally type I collagen prepared from rat tail tendon), the cells attach with high efficiency and spread rapidly. An interaction with the helical portion of the collagen molecule has been postulated (Rubin et al, 1981) and specific receptors partially characterized (Gullberg et al, 1989). Hepatocytes attach also to fibronectin on plastic (Johansson & Hook, 1984), and specific fibronectin receptors have been described (Johansson et al, 1987). Attachment to laminin occurs but differs kinetically from binding to collagen or fibronectin (Bissell et al, 1986),consistent with the presence of discrete receptors for this protein (Clement et al, 1990). Heparan sulfate proteoglycan on plastic does not bind hepatocytes efficiently but reportedly mediates the formation of multicellular floating aggregates (Koide et al, 1989). A receptor for the core protein of this proteoglycan has been described (Clement et al, 1989).

The rapid attachment of hepatocytes and the evidence for specific receptors suggest that the observed interactions are physiologic. However, monitoring of liver-specific functions indicates marked differences in the biologic effect of individual ECM-protein complexes on hepatocytes. In general, in spreading cells the expression of liver-specific function declines and, for some functions, declines dramatically. Changes can occur within hours of plating, exemplified by the loss of total cytochrome P-450 (Bissell & Guzelian, 1975); or the change may appear after 4-6 days only, as for albumin secretion (Guguen-Guillouzo & Guillouzo, 1983). For the albumin gene, this involves an early decrease in transcription, with stabilization of residual mRNA (Jefferson et al, 1984). Other functions have not been examined in detail.

As noted above, the perisinusoidal ECM of the normal liver comprises basement membrane proteins rather than fibrillar collagen. Thus, basement membrane ECM in culture may more nearly mimic the normal liver than does fibrillar collagen alone. This postulate has been widely tested and verified with culture substrata that resemble basement membrane. A substratum currently in widespread use is derived from the Engelbreth-Holm-Swarm (EHS) sarcoma, which is a transplantable solid tumor maintained in C57B or Swiss-Webster mice. The tumor elaborates impressive amounts of an extracellular matrix rich in laminin. A relatively simple extraction with 2 M urea yields an extract of basement membrane proteins, which is soluble at 4°C but rapidly forms a clear gel upon warming (Kleinman et al, 1985). The preparation is termed EHS gel here; it is available commercially as Matrigel® (Collaborative Research Inc., Bedford, MA). With respect to the total protein in the gel, the material is about 90% laminin and 4% type IV collagen, the remainder being heparan sulfate proteoglycan, entactin and minor proteins (Bissell et al, 1987). Although relatively little analysis has been published, differences between native basement membrane and the EHS gel are evident. The high proportion of laminin in the EHS extract appears to be atypical (Grant et al, 1985). Another difference concerns the type of laminin present in the extract. Laminin was first purified from the EHS tumor and shown to consist of 3 subunits termed A, B_1, and B_2, respectively (Timpl, 1989). Subsequent work with normal tissue has demonstrated that laminin is heterogeneous, with 4 types currently recognized (Table 1).

Table 1. Laminin subunit variation

Name	Subunit composition	Reference
Laminin	A, B_1, B_2	Timpl et al, 1989
S-Laminin	A, S, B_2	Sanes et al, 1990
Merosin	M, B_1, B_2	Leivo & Engvall, 1988
S-Merosin	M, S, B_2	Engvall et al, 1990

In normal rat liver, only the B chains are detectable as protein (Maher et al, 1988). It remains to be demonstrated whether the predominance of laminin in the EHS gel and the cell-binding activity of the A chain are significant with respect to the use of EHS gel for hepatocyte culture.

Cultures of hepatocytes on the EHS gel contrast with those on type I collagen both morphologically and functionally. While cells attach rapidly to both substrata, little or no flattening occurs on the EHS gel (Bissell et al, 1987). Rather, aggregates or columns appear; in prolonged culture (greater than 10 days) the cellular groups may become multilayered. The effects of the EHS gel on hepatocyte function are broad and include support of both constitutively expressed functions such as albumin secretion (Bissell et al, 1987) and inducible genes such as the liver-specific forms of cytochrome P-450 (Scheutz et al, 1988). With respect to DNA synthesis also, the normal resting (G_0) state of the cells is better preserved on EHS gel than on type I collagen, with low expression of cytoskeletal genes associated with movement through the cell cycle (Ben-Ze'ev et al, 1988). Ultrastructural studies reveal well-preserved endoplasmic reticulum and Golgi membrane, relative to comparison cultures on collagen only (Bissell et al, 1987). While the effects of a basement membrane-like substratum are remarkable, they do not extend across the entire spectrum of liver-specific function (Schuetz et al, 1988). Moreover, the ability to support liver-specific functions in culture is not unique to the EHS gel. Extending the earlier work of Michalopoulos (1976), Ben-Ze'ev and colleagues (1988) showed that a gel of type I collagen supports an intermediate level of function: greater than that of a thin layer of collagen applied to plastic but quantitatively less than that of an EHS gel. Lindblad et al (1991) have reported that hepatocytes respond to the physical properties of a gel as well as to its protein composition, a point made also by Opas (1989). On the other hand, some hepatocyte functions clearly do not require a solid collagenous substratum. Albumin production is elicited by addition of diluted soluble EHS extract or laminin alone to cultures on a conventional substratum that have undergone flattening and exhibit minimal albumin production (Caron, 1990). Addition of soluble type I collagen has a similar effect (Dunn et al, 1989). Hepatocyte morphology, by phase-contrast microscopy, is unaffected by the addition of soluble ECM protein (Caron, 1990), although subtle changes in cell shape and cytoskeletal structure have not been excluded. These findings, while limited as yet, suggest that the regulatory effect of ECM has several mechanisms, which may vary in importance for individual liver-specific genes.

REGULATION OF LIVER-SPECIFIC GENE TRANSCRIPTION BY ECM

Recent work in this area has focused on the EHS gel system and indicates that the effect of the culture substratum for at least some genes is exerted at the level of transcription (Caron, 1990). The nuclear events involved in this response are under study, initial efforts being directed at elucidating the DNA elements involved in the response to ECM. The albumin gene is controlled by a large (ca. 12 Kb) segment of DNA upstream of the transcriptional start site (Johnson, 1990). In general, elements and factors within the initial 160 bp of this segment confer liver-specificity of transcription (Gorski et al, 1986); another region at approximately -9.5 to -10.5 Kb includes a powerful enhancer (Pinkert et al, 1987). To date, the findings suggest that the ECM-response element(s) is not in the proximal 440 bp of this region (Bissell et al, 1990) but may be present in the far-upstream enhancer (Zaret et al, 1988). The latter work was carried out with SV40-transformed hepatocytes and awaits confirmation with normal (nontransformed) hepatocytes.

BINDING OF CYTOKINES AND GROWTH FACTORS TO ECM

Among ECM-associated proteins are cytokines, growth factors and other soluble regulators of biologic responses. Several growth factors bind to the heparan sulfate constituent of basement membrane (Table 2).

Table 2. Binding of Cytokines to Extracellular Matrix

Cytokine	ECM Binder	Activity of Bound Form	Reference
GM-CSF	heparan sulfate	active	Roberts et al, 1988
aFGF	heparan sulfate	active	Thompson et al, 1989
bFGF	heparan sulfate	? inactive	Folkman et al, 1988
INFγ	heparan sulfate	active	Lortat-Jacob et al, 1991
PDGF	collagen	active	Smith et al, 1982
TGFβ1	collagen IV	active	Paralkar et al, 1991
TGFβ1	decorin	inactive	Yamaguchi et al, 1990

Abbreviations: GM-CSF, granulocyte/macrophage colony stimulating factor
aFGF, acidic fibroblast growth factor
bFGF, basic fibroblast growth factor
INFγ, interferon-gamma
PDGF, platelet-derived growth factor
TGFβ, transforming growth factor-beta, type 1

For some factors, the ECM appears to serve as a repository, the bound factors becoming active only upon their release from the ECM. For others, formation of an ECM complex may lead to enhanced or prolonged action; an example of the latter is TGFβ bound to type IV collagen (Paralkar et al, 1991). The EHS gel, as routinely prepared, contains active TGFβ1 which raises the problem of whether effects of the gel are mediated by the growth factor or by direct cell-ECM interactions. Given recent evidence that ECM-associated TGFβ is biologically active, its role in modulating the behavior of cells cultured on EHS gel clearly must be examined for each function under study. Experiments with cytokine-free substrata will be important, and a method for stripping TGFβ from EHS extract has been described (Taub et al, 1990).

TURNOVER OF ECM

Another aspect of cell-ECM interaction of growing interest is ECM degradation and remodelling. There has been substantial progress in characterizing collagenases, gelatinases, stromelysins and elastase, which partially overlap in terms of genetic relatedness and/or substrate specificity (Woessner, 1991). Matrix proteinases in liver have been a subject of study for many years, under the assumption that their main role is the removal of excess collagen in fibrotic injury. Current studies suggest a substantially broader and more complex role.

Matrix proteinases may mediate alteration of the normal ECM during the initial stages of injury, and they may regulate the effect of ECM-bound cytokines and growth factors. The best documented activity is a 65 kD type IV collagenase (gelatinase) produced by lipocytes; a 92 kD gelatinase is produced by Kupffer cells (Arthur et al, 1989). It will be important to examine the expression of these activities and their extracellular regulation in normal growth and disease states: such studies are in the offing.

REFERENCES

Arenson, D.M., Friedman, S.L., & Bissell, D.M. (1988): Formation of extracellular matrix in normal rat liver: lipocytes as a major source of proteoglycan. Gastroenterology 95, 441-447.

Arthur, M.J.P., Friedman, S.L., Roll, F.J., & Bissell, D.M. (1989): Lipocytes from normal rat liver release a neutral metalloproteinase that degrades basement membrane (type IV) collagen. J Clin Invest 84, 1076-1085.

Bang, F.B. & Warwick, A.C. (1965): Liver. In Willmer, E.N. (ed): Cells and Tissues in Culture. Methods, Biology and Physiology. New York: Academic Press, pp. 607-630.

Ben-Ze'ev, A., Robinson, G.S., Bucher, N.L.R., & Farmer, S.R. (1988): Cell-cell and cell-matrix interactions differentially regulate the expression of hepatic and cytoskeletal genes in primary cultures of rat hepatocytes. Proc Natl Acad Sci USA 85, 2161-2165.

Berry, M.N. & Friend, D.S. (1969): High-yield preparation of isolated rat liver parenchymal cells. J Cell Biol 43, 506-520.

Bissell, D.M., Arenson, D.M., Maher, J.J., & Roll, F.J. (1987): Support of cultured hepatocytes by a laminin-rich gel. Evidence for a functionally significant subendothelial matrix in normal rat liver. J Clin Invest 79, 801-812.

Bissell, D.M., Caron, J.M., Babiss, L.E., & Friedman, J.M. (1990): Transcriptional regulation of the albumin gene in cultured rat hepatocytes. Mol Biol Med 7, 187-197.

Bissell, D.M. & Guzelian, P.S. (1975): Microsomal functions and phenotypic change in adult rat hepatocytes in primary monolayer culture. In Gerschenson, L.E. and Thompson, E.B. (eds): Gene expression and carcinogenesis in cultured liver. New York: Academic Press Inc., pp. 119-136.

Bissell, D.M., Hammaker, L.E., & Meyer, U.A. (1973): Parenchymal cells from adult rat liver in nonproliferating monolayer culture. J Cell Biol 59, 722-734.

Bissell, D.M. & Roll, F.J. (1990): Connective tissue metabolism and hepatic fibrosis. In Zakim, D. and Boyer, T.D. (eds): Hepatology, 2nd Edition. New York: W.B. Saunders Co., pp. 424-444.

Bissell, D.M., Stamatoglou, S., Nermut, M., & Hughes, C. (1986): Interactions of rat hepatocytes with type IV collagen fibronectin and laminin matrices. Distinct matrix-controlled modes of attachment and spreading. Eur J Cell Biol 40, 72-78.

Bissell, D.M. & Tilles, J.G. (1971): Morphology and function of cells of human embryonic liver in monolayer culture. J Cell Biol 50, 222-231.
Bissell, M.J. (1981): The differentiated state of normal and malignant cells or how to define a "normal" cell in culture. International Review of Cytology 70, 27-100.
Burgeson, R.E. (1988): New collagens, new concepts. Ann Rev Cell Biol 4, 551-577.
Caron, J.M. (1990): Induction of albumin gene transcription in hepatocytes by extracellular matrix proteins. Mol Cell Biol 10, 1239-1243.
Clement, B., Grimaud, J.-.A., Campion, J.-.P., Deugnier, Y., & Guillouzo, A. (1986): Cell types involved in collagen and fibronectin production in normal and fibrotic human liver. Hepatology 6, 225-234.
Clement, B., Rescan, P.Y., Baffet, G., Loreal, O., Lehry, D., Campion, J.P., & Guillouzo, A. (1988): Hepatocytes may produce laminin in fibrotic liver and in primary culture. Hepatology 8, 794-803.
Clement, B., Segui-Real, B., Hassell, J.R., Martin, G.R., & Yamada, Y. (1989): Identification of a cell surface-binding protein for the core protein of the basement membrane proteoglycan. J Biol Chem 264, 12467-12471.
Clement, B., Segui-Real, B., Savagner, P., Kleinman, H.K., & Yamada, Y. (1990): Hepatocyte attachment to laminin is mediated through multiple receptors. J Cell Biol 110, 185-192.
Dunn, J.C., Yarmugh, M.L., Koche, H.G., & Tompkins, R.G. (1989): Hepatocyte function and extracellular matrix geometry: long-term culture in a sandwich configuration. FASEB J 3(2), 174-7.
Elsdale, T. & Bard, J. (1972): Collagen substrata for studies on cell behavior. J Cell Biol 54, 626-637.
Emerman, J.T., Enami, J., Pitelka, D., & Nandi, S. (1977): Hormonal effects on intracellular and secreted casein in cultures of mouse mammary epithelial cells on floating collagen membranes. Proc Natl Acad Sci USA 74, 4466.
Engvall, E., Earwicker, D., Haaparanta, T., Ruoslahti, E., & Sanes, J.R.(1990): Distribution and isolation of four laminin variants; tissue restricted distribution of heterotrimers assembled from five different subunits. Cell Regulation 1, 731-740.
Folkman, J., Klagsbrun, M., Sasse, J., Wadzinski, M., Ingber, D., & Vlodavsky, I. (1988): A heparin-binding angiogenic protein - basic fibroblast growth factor - is stored within basement membrane. Am J Pathol 130, 393-400.
Gorski, K., Carneiro, M., & Schibler, U. (1986): Tissue-specific in vitro transcription from the mouse albumin promoter. Cell 47, 767-776.
Grant, D.S., Kleinman, H.K., Leblond, C.P., Inoue, S., Chung, A.E., & Martin,G.R. (1985): The basement-membrane-like matrix of the mouse EHS tumor: II.Immunohistochemical quantitation of six of its components. Amer J Anat 174, 387-398.
Guguen-Guillouzo, C. & Guillouzo, A. (1983): Modulation of

functional activities in cultured rat hepatocytes. Mol Cell Biochem 53/54, 35-56.
Gullberg, D., Terracio, L., Borg, T.K., & Rubin, K. (1989): Identification of integrin-like matrix receptors with affinity for interstitial collagens. J Biol Chem 264, 12686-12694.
Hahn, E., Wick, G., Pencev, D., & Timpl, R. (1980): Distribution of basement membrane proteins in normal and fibrotic human liver: collagen type IV, laminin, and fibronectin. Gut 21, 63-71.
Hauschka, S.D. & Konigsberg, I.R. (1966): The influence of collagen on the development of muscle clones. Proc Natl Acad Sci USA 55, 119-126.
Jefferson, D.M., Clayton, D.F., Darnell, J.E., & Reid, L.M. (1984): Posttranscriptional modulation of gene expression in cultured rat hepatocytes. Mol Cell Biol 4, 1929-1934.
Johansson, S., Forsberg, E., & Lundgren, B. (1987): Comparison of fibronectin receptors from rat hepatocytes and fibroblasts. J Biol Chem 262, 7819-7824.
Johansson, S. & Hook, M. (1984): Substrate adhesion of rat hepatocytes: on the mechanism of attachment to fibronectin. J Cell Biol 98, 810-817.
Johnson, P.F. (1990): Transcriptional activators in hepatocytes. Cell Growth & Differentiation 1, 47-52.
Kleinman, H.K., McGarvey, M.L., Hassell, J.R., Star, V., Cannon, F.B., Laurie, G.W., & Martin, G.R. (1985): Basement membrane complexes with biological activity. Biochemistry 25, 312-318.
Koide, N., Shinji, T., Tanabe, T., Asano, K., Kawaguchi, M., Sakaguchi, K., Koide, Y., & Masayasu, M. (1989): Continued high albumin production by multicellular spheroids of adult rat hepatocytes formed in the presence of liver-derived proteoglycans. Biochem Biophys Res Commun 161, 385-391.
Leivo, I. & Engvall, E. (1988): Merosin, a protein specific for basement membranes of Schwann cells, striated muscle, and trophoblast, is expressed late in nerve and muscle development. Proc Natl Acad Sci USA 85,1544-1548.
Lindblad, W.J., Schuetz, E.G., Redford, K.S., & Guzelian, P.S. (1991): Hepatocellular phenotype in vitro is influenced by biophysical features of the collagenous substratum. Hepatology 13, 282-288.
Lortat-Jacob, H., Kleinman, H.K., & Grimaud, J.-.A. (1991): High-affinity binding of interferon-gamma to a basement membrane complex (Matrigel). J Clin Invest 87, 878-883.
Maher, J.J. & McGuire, RF (1990): Extracellular matrix gene expression increases preferentially in rat lipocytes and sinusoidal endothelial cells during hepatic fibrosis in vivo. J Clin Invest 86, 1641-1648.
Maher, J.J., Friedman, S.L., Roll, F.J., & Bissell, D.M. (1988): Immunolocalization of laminin in normal rat liver and biosynthesis of laminin by hepatic lipocytes in primary culture. Gastroenterology 94, 1053-1062.
Martinez-Hernandez, A. (1984): The hepatic extracellular matrix. I. Electron immunohistochemical studies in normal rat liver. Lab Invest 51, 57-74.

Michalopoulos, G., Sattler, C.A., Sattler, G.L., & Pitot, H.C. (1976): Cytochrome P-450 induction by phenobarbital and 3-methylcholanthrene in primary cultures of hepatocytes. Science 193, 907-909.

Ohtani, O. (1988): Three-dimensional organization of the collagen fibrillar framework of the human and rat livers. Arch Histol Cytol 51, 473-488.

Opas, M. (1989): Expression of the differentiated phenotype by epithelial cells in vitro is regulated by both biochemistry and mechanics of the substratum. Developmental Biology 131, 281-293.

Paralkar, V.M., Vukicevic, S., & Reddi, A.H. (1991): Transforming growth factor beta type 1 binds to collagen IV of basement membrane matrix:implications for development. Developmental Biology 143, 303-308. Peng, H., Armentano, D.,

Pinkert, C.A., Ornitz, D.M., Brinster, R.L., & Palmiter, R.D. (1987): An albumin enhancer located 10 kb upstream functions along with its promoter to direct efficient, liver-specific expression in transgenic mice. Genes Devel 1, 268-276.

Roberts, R., Gallagher, J., Spooncer, E., Allen, T.D., Bloomfield, F., & Dexter, T.M. (1988) Heparan sulphate bound growth factors: a mechanism for stromal cell mediated haemopoiesis. Nature 332, 376-378.

Rubin, K., Hook, M., Obrink, B., & Timpl, R. (1981): Substrate adhesion of rat hepatocytes: mechanism of attachment to collagen substrates. Cell 24, 463-470.

Sanes, J., Engvall, E., Butkowski, R., & Hunter, D.D. (1990): Molecular heterogeneity of basal laminae: isoforms of laminin and collagen IV at the neuromuscular junction and elsewhere. J Cell Biol 111, 1685-1699.

Sasaki, M., Kleinman, H.K., Huber, H., Deutzmann, R., & Yamada, Y. (1988): Laminin, a multidomain protein. J Biol Chem 263, 16536-16544.

Schuetz, E.G., Li, D., Omiecinski, C.J., Muller-Eberhard, U., Kleinman, H.K., Elswick, B., & Guzelian, P.S. (1988): Regulation of gene expression in adult rat hepatocytes cultured on a basement membrane matrix. J Cell Physiol 134, 309-323.

Smith, J.C., Singh, J.P., Lillquist, J.S., Goon, D.S., & Stiles, C.D. (1982): Growth factors adherent to cell substrate are mitogenically active in situ. Nature 296, 154-156.

Stamatoglou, S.C., Hughes, R.C., & Lindahl, U. (1987): Rat hepatocytes in serum-free primary culture elaborate an extensive extracellular matrix containing fibrin and fibronectin. J Cell Biol 105, 2417-2425.

Taub, M., Wang, Y., Szczesny, T.M., & Kleinman, H.K. (1990): Epidermal growth factor or transforming growth factor alpha is required for kidney tubulogenesis in matrigel cultures in serum-free medium. Proc Natl Acad Sci USA 87, 4002-4006.

Thompson, J.A., Haudenschild, C.C., Anderson, K.D., DiPietro, J.M., Anderson, W. F., & Maciag, T. (1989): Heparin-binding growth factor 1 induces the formation of organoid neovascular structures in vivo. Proc Natl Acad Sci USA 86, 7928-7932.

Timpl, R. (1989) Structure and biological activity of basement

membrane proteins. Eur J Biochem 180, 487-502.
Van Eyken, P., Sciot, R., & Desmet, V.J. (1989): Distribution of a novel extracellular matrix glycoprotein tenascin in normal and pathological human liver: an immunohistochemical study. Hepatology 10, 632.
Woessner, J.F. (1991): Matrix metalloproteinases and their inhibitors in connective tissue remodeling. FASEB J 5, 2145-2154.
Yamaguchi, Y., Mann, D.M., & Ruoslahti, E. (1990): Negative regulation of transforming growth factor-beta by the proteoglycan decorin. Nature 346, 281-284.
Zaret, K.S., DiPersio, C.M., Jackson, D.A., Montigny, W.J., & Weinstat, D.L. (1988): Conditional enhancement of liver-specific gene transcription. Proc Natl Acad Sci USA 85, 9076-9080.

Résumé

L'étude immunohistochimique de la matrice extracellulaire (MEC) du foie conduit à la définir comme une structure de type lame basale. Cultivés sur un support de composition comparable, les hépatocytes adultes normaux montrent une étroite dépendance vis à vis de la MEC. Toutes ces données suggèrent fortement que la MEC joue un rôle capital dans le foie normal. Les recherches actuelles portent sur les récepteurs à la MEC exprimés par les hépatocytes et sur la régulation de la transcription de gènes hépatiques spécifiques par la MEC. Une autre voie de recherche actuellement en plein développement concerne le rôle de la MEC dans la fixation de facteurs de croissance et la livraison de ceux-ci à la cellule. Les résultats actuels suggèrent qu'une altération de la MEC peut indiquer un dysfonctionnement hépatocellulaire au cours des maladies fibrotiques.

Cellular and Molecular Aspects of Cirrhosis. Eds B. Clément, A. Guillouzo. Colloque INSERM/John Libbey Eurotext Ltd. © 1992, Vol. 216, pp. 199-209

Progressive renal failure : role of extracellular matrix protein deposition in the renal mesangium

Leslie A. Bruggeman, Jeffrey B. Kopp and Paul E. Klotman *

Molecular Medicine Section, Laboratory of Developmental Biology, National Institute of Dental Research, National Institutes of Health, Bethesda, MD, USA

* *Corresponding author*

ABSTRACT

Glomerulosclerosis is a scarring process similar to liver cirrhosis which is characterized by an excessive deposition of matrix. The matrix is synthesized by a unique pericyte in the renal glomerulus, the mesangial cell, which plays a similar role as the Ito cell in hepatic fibrosis. The sclerotic process in the kidney is caused, at least in part, by an activation of gene expression of the normal matrix constituents such as laminin, type IV collagen and fibronectin, and interstitial collagens, types I and III. The activation of matrix gene expression and mesangial cell proliferation is initiated by 1) a mesangial cell response to various cytokines, growth factors and immune mediators produced by infiltrating immune cells, mesangial cells, or other resident cells in the kidney; and by 2) direct interactions of the mesangial cells with the various matrix components. In diabetic nephropathy, the sclerosis is characterized by an expansion of the mesangial matrix and a thickening of the glomerular and tubular basement membranes. The stimulatory mechanism for matrix deposition may involve products of arachidonic acid metabolism, particularly, the vasoconstrictor thromboxane. It is possible therapies against thromboxane and other mediators of the inflammatory response may help ameliorate the scarring process in the kidney that progresses to end-stage renal failure.

Glomerulosclerosis is an indolent scarring process, caused by diseases of various etiologies (Table 1), which usually results in end-stage renal failure. Similar to liver cirrhosis, glomerulosclerosis is characterized by an abnormal deposition of matrix proteins, cellular proliferation, and a loss of renal function. The fibrotic process is believed to be due, in part, to an inflammatory response to tissue injury resulting in infiltration of immune cells and remodeling of the extracellular matrix. In both diseases, the key modulator of this tissue injury has been identified as a specialized pericyte, which participates in many complex cell-cell and cell-matrix interactions. The specialized pericyte in the kidney, the glomerular mesangial cell, and in the

Leslie Bruggeman is a post doctoral fellow supported by the Arthritis Foundation.

TABLE 1
Causes of End-Stage Glomerulosclerosis

Primary Renal Diseases	Secondary Renal Diseases
Focal Segmental Glomerulosclerosis	Amyloid Nephropathy
Crescentic Glomerulonephritis	Connective Tissue Disorders
Mesangial Proliferative Glomerulonephritis	Lupus Nephritis
IgA Nephritis	Scleroderma
Post-streptococcal Glomerulonephritis	Chronic Allograft Rejection
Other Post-infectious Glomerulonephritis	Diabetes Mellitus
Idiopathic	Hypertensive Nephrosclerosis
Membranous Nephropathy	Obesity
Congenital Nephropathy	Heroin Nephropathy
Alport's Syndrome	Interstitial Nephritis
Membranoproliferative Glomerulonephritis	Analgesic Nephropathy
	Reflux Nephropathy
	Heavy Metal Toxic Nephropathy

liver, the Ito cell, both have the potential to convert to a "fibrotic phenotype" and are primarily responsible for the excessive deposition of matrix.

The Ito cell is a pericyte and functions as a reservoir for vitamin A (Blumhoff & Wake, 1991; Bissell et al., 1990). In normal liver tissue the Ito cells are adjacent to hepatocytes and sinusoidal endothelial cells, and are separated by a basement membrane (Space of Disse). In liver cirrhosis, the Ito cell differentiates to a myofibroblast and deposits additional matrix, thus destroying the normal tissue architecture. The myofibroblastic state is maintained and the cells proliferate in response both to mitogens and to the altered extracellular matrix. The differentiation of the Ito cell to the myofibroblast is believed to be initiated in response to various cytokines produced by Kupffer cells. The progression of fibrosis is enhanced by production of inflammatory mediators from infiltrating macrophages and leukocytes attracted to hepatic cell injury and death.

THE MESANGIAL CELL AND THE MESANGIAL MATRIX

Similar to the Ito cell, the renal mesangial cell is also a specialized pericyte (Schlondorff, 1987). The mesangial cell has characteristics of both smooth muscle cells and of macrophages. Alternatively, mesangial cells may actually represent two populations of cells, one that resembles a smooth muscle cell and the other that resembles a bone marrow-derived resident macrophage (Schreiner and Unanue, 1984). The mesangial cell is located centrally in the glomerulus, which is a vascular lobule of capillaries branching from one afferent arteriole. The mesangial cells are situated at the hilum and within the glomerular tuft, and function to support the capillaries (Fig. 1). Because of its unique location and its contractile properties, mesangial cells can constrict and dilate the glomerular capillaries and thus, may affect the intraglomerular filtration area by controlling plasma flow through the capillary loops and/or the capillary surface area available for ultrafiltration. The mesangial cell sits in an extracellular matrix, the mesangial matrix, which it presumably has synthesized. The mesangial matrix surrounds the mesangial cells and extends to the glomerular basement membrane and the endothelial cell

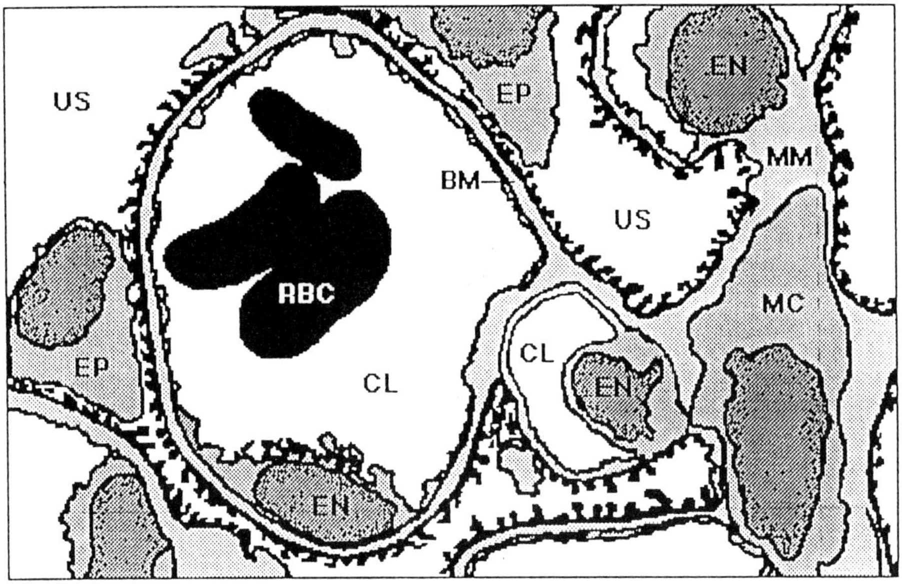

Fig. 1. Cellular boundaries of a glomerular capillary. US, urinary space; EP, epithelial cell; EN, endothelial cell; MC, mesangial cell; CL, capillary lumen; RBC, red blood cell; BM, basement membrane; MM, mesangial matrix. Digitized from an electron micrograph from Antonovych and Mostofi (1980); used with permission.

membrane. The mesangial matrix is separated from the bloodstream only by a "leaky" endothelium, without an intervening basement membrane, and is in constant contact with plasma. Another extracellular matrix structure present in the glomerulus, the glomerular basement membrane, is presumably deposited by both glomerular endothelial and epithelial cells. It surrounds the glomerular capillaries and is an integral part of the filtration apparatus.

The constituent proteins of the glomerular basement membrane and mesangial matrix are similar to the basement membrane structure of the Space of Disse (Martin et al., 1988; Brazy et al., 1991). The glomerular basement membrane contains type IV collagen, heparan sulfate proteoglycan, entactin, laminin and some fibronectin. The mesangial matrix is similar in composition but does not form the unique structure morphologically characteristic of a basement membrane. The mesangial matrix contains a greater amount of fibronectin, several chondroitin sulfate proteoglycans, thrombospondin and biglycan. In general, the sclerotic lesions in glomeruli contain all of the normal components of the glomerular basement membrane and mesangium only in greater amounts, as well as different isoforms of collagen including types I, III, V, and VI and decorin, a small chondroitin sulfate proteoglycan. Expression of matrix proteins and interstitial collagens I and III in normal adult kidney is very low (Laurie et al., 1989; Swazcuk et al., 1989). The change in matrix expression in glomerulosclerosis resembles a pattern of expression seen in the mesangial cell during glomerular development. During nephrogenesis, abundant matrix is deposited including collagen types I and III as mesenchyme differentiates into its glomerular components. Although the mesangial cell does not undergo the same dramatic differentiation as the Ito cell in cirrhosis, the increased matrix production and the expression of collagen types I and III implies a de-differentiation of the mesangial cell to a more fetal-like state.

The increase in deposition of matrix could arise from several different mechanisms, including; 1) an increase in the transcriptional rate or an increase in the lifetime of messenger RNA (mRNA) for the genes coding for the matrix proteins, 2) an increase in the translational efficiency or post-translational processing and secretion of the proteins, or 3) a decrease in the extracellular degradation of the matrix proteins. Presently, very little is known about these various mechanisms, however, several recent investigations indicate changes in the steady-state mRNA levels for the basement membrane genes may be a significant factor to the development of sclerotic lesions. In a model of lupus nephritis, the NZB/W F1 mouse, the mRNA levels of collagens I, III, IV, laminin chains B1, B2 and heparan sulfate proteoglycan are elevated by 50% in animals exhibiting proteinuria (Nakamura et al., 1991a). Immunolocalization reveals excess matrix deposition in peripheral capillary loops and mesangial matrix. In a mouse model of minimal change nephritis created by treatment with puromycin aminoglycoside ("PAN" nephritis), the mRNA levels of type IV collagen, laminin A, B1 and B2 are increased and the mRNA level of heparan sulfate proteoglycan is decreased as compared to control animals (Nakamura et al., 1991b). These alterations in extracellular matrix proteins are associated with a decreased number of anionic sites in the basement membrane, altered charge barrier to macromolecules, and proteinuria. In two models of diabetic nephropathy, the streptozotocin-induced diabetic rat (Poulsum et al., 1988) and the spontaneously occurring diabetic KKay mouse (Ledbetter et al., 1990), sclerotic kidneys have increased mRNA levels for laminin B1 and type IV collagen respectively. In a transgenic mouse models for growth hormone which develops glomerulosclerosis, mRNA levels for type IV collagen, laminin B2 and heparan sulfate proteoglycan are increased in the sclerotic kidneys (Doi et al., 1991). And, in a transgenic model of HIV-associated nephropathy, kidney mRNA levels for type IV collagen but not laminin B2 are increased in animals with glomerulosclerosis (Adler et al., 1990; Kopp, unpublished). In conclusion, these studies suggest that transcriptional activation of matrix genes expression contributes to matrix deposition in glomerulosclerosis although the quantity of matrix present is obviously the result of a balance between the synthetic and degradative processes.

Degradation of the mesangial matrix and glomerular basement membrane occurs through the action of several proteases. Mesangial cells and isolated glomeruli in culture secrete several proteolytic enzymes including interstitial collagenases, type IV and type V-specific gelatinases and stromelysin (Woessner, 1991). These proteases are also produced by other cells in the kidney including epithelial cells and infiltrating immune cells such as neutrophils and macrophages. For example, in an animal model of glomerulonephritis, the *in vivo* administration of a protease inhibitor reduces proteinuria (Baricos et al., 1988). Also, in an animal model of Heymann nephritis, isolated glomeruli produce greater amounts of gelatinase, and gelatinase activity can be stimulated by treatment with interleukin-1 or tumor necrosis factor α (Watanabe et al., 1990). Although one might assume that reduced proteinase activity is more consistent with the sclerotic process, proteinase activity could contribute to glomerulosclerosis in a manner different from simply degrading the matrix proteins present in the mesangium. Some of the matrix proteins, laminin and fibronectin in particular, have numerous biological effects on cell function, and these biological activities have been mapped to specific epitopes on the molecules (Timpl, 1989). Proteolytic degradation of the matrix may expose different matrix proteins or specific epitopes not usually presented to the mesangial cell and thus alter mesangial cell behavior.

Mesangial cell behavior may be altered in response to "injury" of the glomerular basement membrane or mesangial matrix such that the expression of matrix proteins is enhanced or mesangial cell proliferation occurs. For example, mesangial cells grown *in vitro* on laminin or type IV collagen substrate produce greater amounts of laminin, fibronectin, and collagen types III and IV when compared with cells grown on fibronectin substrate (Ishimura et al., 1989). In addition, mesangial cells will proliferate when grown on fibronectin or on interstitial collagen substrates (I and III), but proliferation is inhibited when grown on laminin or collagen IV substrates (Kitamura et al., 1990). Mesangial cells interact with the matrix through specific cell surface receptors, including those belonging to the integrin family of matrix receptors (Akiyama et al., 1990). The interaction of these matrix receptors is specific to distinct epitopes on matrix proteins and can have different effects on the mesangial cell. *In vitro*, mesangial cells adhere and spread on laminin substrate. Adherence is specific to two distinct epitopes on laminin, RGD and CIKVAV as determined by competition experiments with synthetic peptides. Mesangial cells express non-integrin laminin receptors which are differentially regulated in development (Weeks et al., 1991). The 32kDa laminin receptor is predominantly expressed on mesangial cells isolated from fetal tissue, and the 67kDa and 110kDa laminin receptors predominate on adult cells. To spread along the glomerular basement membrane and extend into the peripheral capillary loops in mesangial sclerotic diseases, mesangial cells must also migrate. Migration, like attachment, involves the use of integrins and other matrix receptors for cell movement along the matrix. The stimulus for initiation of cell migration is unknown but two recent reports suggest fibronectin and platelet-derived growth factor are chemotactic for mesangial cells (Barnes & Hevey, 1990; Barnes & Hevey, 1991). Based on these findings, it appears that various matrix substrates and specific cytokines and growth factors might influence mesangial cell migration, redistribution, and proliferation in glomerulosclerosis.

The complex changes in mesangial cell behavior and in the mesangial matrix during glomerulosclerosis appear to be critically dependent upon cytokines, growth factors, and inflammatory mediators produced by mesangial cells and infiltrating immune cells. Within the last year, there have been numerous reports of cytokine stimulation of cellular proliferation, activation of signal transduction pathways, and alterations in gene expression in renal mesangial and epithelial cells *in vitro*. There have also been several studies which suggest cytokines and growth factors alter the expression of matrix genes in both renal and non-renal tissues. For example, tumor necrosis factor-α and interferon-γ decrease collagen synthesis by mesenchymal cells *in vitro* (Czaja et al., 1989; Nanes et al., 1989; Solis-Herruzo et al., 1988). Interleukin-1α and β increase type I collagen synthesis by cultured skin fibroblasts but decrease type I collagen synthesis by cultured synovial fibroblasts (Goldring & Krane, 1987; Kähäri et al., 1987; Postlethwaite et al., 1988). Thus, cytokines and immune mediators appear to be important modulators of gene expression and mesangial cell function and are particularly relevant in diseases characterized by progressive glomerulosclerosis such as diabetic nephropathy.

DIABETIC NEPHROPATHY

Diabetes mellitus is a small vessel disease involving, among other microvessel systems, the glomerular capillaries (Brazy et al., 1991). The pathological features (Fig. 2) of human diabetic nephropathy include 1) glomerulosclerosis which is both diffuse (all glomeruli affected) and global (all lobules of each glomerulus affected); 2) nodular glomerulosclerosis, characterized by acellular aggregates of extracellular matrix material within capillary lobules; this lesion has been termed the Kimmelstiel-Wilson lesion and is nearly pathognomic for diabetes, although it is seen in only a minority of patients with diabetic nephropathy; 3) thickening of the glomerular capillary basement membrane, Bowman's capsule which surrounds the glomerulus and lies in continuity with the glomerular basement membrane, and the tubular basement membranes; and 4) the hyaline lesion, which consists of homogeneous eosinophilic material lying either within the capillary loop or in Bowman's space; this material stains positively for lipid and has a similar appearance to hyaline material occupying the lumens of arterioles in the kidney and other organs from diabetic patients.

Human diabetic glomeruli with sclerosis manifest increased laminin, fibronectin and types IV and V collagen as shown by immunolocalization studies (Falk et al., 1983; Bruneval et al., 1985; Karttunen et al., 1986). Furthermore, type IV collagen is increased in the glomeruli obtained from streptozotocin-diabetic rats, and insulin treatment normalizes type IV collagen expression and abrogates the appearance of type III collagen in the mesangium (Cohen & Khalifa, 1977; Abrass et al., 1988). Whether an increase in type III collagen is a feature of other models of diabetic nephropathy remains to be determined, and further studies, particularly with human material, will be of interest. The glomerular mesangium of obese, insulin-treated diabetic rhesus monkeys expresses increased amounts of type IV collagen, laminin, and fibronectin (Kopp et al., 1990 & unpublished data). Recently, differential expression of type IV collagen chains has been reported in human patients with insulin-dependent diabetes and nephropathy. The thickened glomerular basement membrane reacts strongly with antibodies directed against α3(IV) and α4(IV), and reacts to a much lesser degree with antibodies against classical type IV collagen, including α1(IV) and α2(IV). By contrast, the expanded mesangium contains mainly classical type IV collagen. Obsolescent glomeruli contain exclusively α3(IV) and α4(IV) chains (Kim et al., 1991). These intriguing findings suggest differential regulation of type IV collagen isoforms in diabetes.

The mechanisms responsible for stimulating extracellular matrix deposition in the diabetic kidney are unknown, but recent evidence supports an important role for the products of arachidonic acid metabolism. In the streptozotocin-induced rodent model and in human disease, there is increased renal thromboxane production and reduced renal prostacyclin production (Cravin & DeRubertis, 1989). Thromboxane, a vasoactive lipid which induces vasoconstriction and platelet aggregation, is

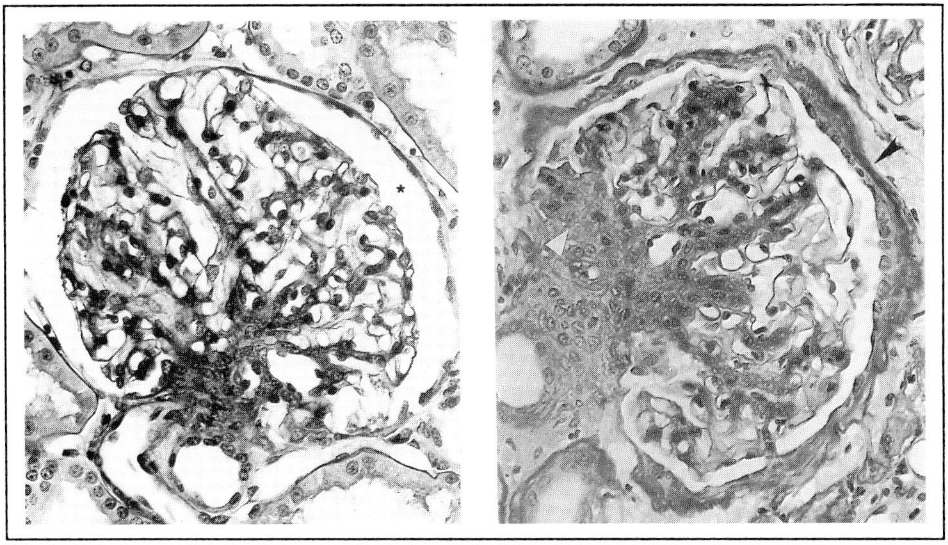

Fig. 2. PAS-stained kidney sections from rhesus monkeys with non-insulin-dependent diabetes mellitus, original magnification 100X. Left panel: kidney from normal monkey, with normal glomerular architecture. Asterisk lies within Bowman's space. Right panel: kidney from monkey with diabetes of 4 years duration. White triangle lies within a capillary lobule which has been replaced by accumulated extracellular matrix components. Black arrowhead indicates thickened Bowman's capsule.

produced in the kidney by renal mesangial and epithelial cells and infiltrating immune cells. *In vitro*, thromboxane analogs stimulate mesangial cell contraction and, as a result, may lower the capillary ultrafiltration coefficient. *In vivo* administration of thromboxane analogs reduces renal blood flow and glomerular filtration rate, and infusion of thromboxane analogs into isolated kidneys results in a dose-dependent increase in vascular tone (Collins et al., 1991). High protein diets have been well-documented to accelerate the development of proteinuria and glomerulosclerosis and the renal production of thromboxane is also increased in both humans and rodents fed high protein diets. When streptozotocin-induced diabetic rats are fed a high protein diet, renal thromboxane production is increased and mesangial sclerosis is exacerbated (Collins et al., 1989). Many of these changes have been attributed to renal injury resulting from perturbations in renal hemodynamic function and transglomerular pressure.

Recently, we explored the direct effects of thromboxane and prostacyclin on mesangial matrix gene expression in cell culture, independent of the hemodynamic effects of these eicosanoids (Bruggeman et al., 1991). *In vitro*, treatment of mesangial cells with a stable thromboxane analog increased the steady state mRNA level of laminin, fibronectin, and type IV collagen and decreased the expression of heparan sulfate proteoglycan. Treatment with prostacyclin had the opposite effects, in general. These data suggest that alterations in renal eicosanoid metabolism may directly affect the composition of the mesangial matrix. In a recent study by Ledbetter et al., (1990) the administration of a thromboxane synthetase inhibitor prevented the increase in type IV collagen mRNA in kidneys from spontaneously occurring diabetic mice (KKay model). In combination, these findings suggest a potential novel therapeutic approach to diabetic nephropathy as well as other mesangial sclerotic diseases.

In summary, glomerulosclerosis, much like liver cirrhosis, is a progressive scarring process controlled by a unique pericyte, the renal mesangial cell. The mesangial cell produces increased amounts of matrix proteins as it responds to its surrounding matrix, other cells, or locally active cytokines, growth factors and immune mediators. These same factors can influence mesangial cell migration and stimulation mesangial cell proliferation. A fundamental understanding of the mesangial cell and its contribution to sclerosis will aid design of therapies directed to the prevention of end-stage renal failure.

REFERENCES

Abrass, C.K., Peterson, C.V. & Rauji, G.J. (1988): Phenotypic expression of collagen types in mesangial matrix of diabetic and non-diabetic rats. *Diabetes* 37, 1695-1702.

Adler, S.H., Kopp, J.B., Dickie, P., Marinos, N.M., Bryant, J.L., Felser, J.M., Notkins, A.L. & Klotman, P.E. (1990): Enhanced renal extracellular matrix protein accumulation in mice transgenic for HIV genes. *J. Am. Soc. Neph.* 1, 523.

Akiyama, S.K., Nagata, K. & Yamada, K.M. (1990): Cell surface receptors for extracellular matrix components. *Biochem. Biophys. Acta* 1031, 91-110.

Antonovych, T.T. & Mostofi, F.K. (1980): in *Atlas of Kidney Biopsies*. p. 7. Washington, D.C., Armed Forces Institute of Pathology.

Baricos, W.H., O'Connor, S.E., Cortez, S.L., Wu, L.-T. & Shah, S.V. (1988): The cysteine proteinase inhibitor, E-64, reduces proteinuria in an experimental model of glomerulonephritis. *Biochem. Biophys. Res. Comm.* 155, 1318-1323.

Barnes, J.L. & Hevey, K.A. (1990): Glomerular mesangial cell migration in response to platelet-derived growth factor. *Lab. Invest.* 62, 379-382.

Barnes, J.L. & Hevey, K.A. (1991): Glomerular mesangial cell migration: Response to platelet secretory products. *Am. J. Pathol.* 138, 859-866.

Bissel, D.M., Friedman, SL., Maher, J.J. & Roll, F.J. (1990): Connective tissue biology and hepatic fibrosis: Report of a conference. *Hepatology* 11, 488-498.

Blumhoff, R. & Wake, K. (1991): Perisinusoidal stellate cells of the liver: Important roles in retinol metabolism and fibrosis. *FASEB J.* 5, 271-277.

Brazy, P.C., Kopp, J.B. & Klotman, P.E. (1991): Glomerulosclerosis and progressive renal disease. in *Contemporary Issues In Nephrology*, New York: Churchill Livingstone. (In press).

Bruggeman, L.A., Horigan, E.A., Horikoshi, S., Ray, P.E. & Klotman, P.E. (1991): Thromboxane stimulates synthesis of extracellular matrix proteins *in vitro*. *Am. J. Physiol.* (In press).

Bruneval, P., Foidart, J.M., Nochy, D., Camilleri, J.P. & Bariety, J. (1985): Glomerular matrix proteins in nodular glomerulosclerosis in association with light chain deposition disease and diabetes mellitus. *Hum. Pathol.* 16, 477-484.

Cohen, M.P. & Khalifa, A. (1977): Renal glomerular collagen synthesis in streptozotocin diabetes. *Biochem. Biophys. Acta.* 500, 395-404.

Collins, D. M., Coffman, T.M. & Klotman, P.E. (1991): The role of thromboxane in the pathogenesis of acute renal failure. in *Acute Renal Failure*, ed. K. Solez & L.C. Racusen, pp. 13-48. New York: Marcel Dekker, Inc.

Collins, D.M., Coffman, T.M., Ruiz, P. & Klotman, P.E. (1989): High-protein feeding stimulates renal thromboxane production in rats with streptozocin-induced diabetes. *J. Lab. Clin. Med.* 114, 545-553.

Craven, P.A. & DeRubertis, F.R. (1989): Role for local prostaglandin and thromboxane production in the regulation of glomerular filtration rate in the rat with streptozotocin-induced diabetes. *J. Lab. Clin. Med.* 113, 674-681.

Czaja, M.J., Weiner, F.R., Takahasi, S., Giambrone, M.A., van der Meide, P.H., Schellekens, H., Biempica, L. & Zern, M.A. (1989): γ-Interferon treatment inhibits collagen deposition in murine schistosomiasis. *Hepatology* 10, 795-800.

Doi, T., Striker, L.J., Kimata, K., Peten, E.P., Yamada, Y. & Striker, G.E. (1991): Glomerulosclerosis in mice transgenic for growth hormone. Increased mesangial extracellular matrix is correlated with kidney mRNA levels. *J. Exp. Med.* 173, 1287-1290.

Falk, R.J., Scheinman, J.I., Mauer, S.M. & Michael, A.F. (1983): Polyantigenic expansion of basement membrane constituents in diabetic nephropathy. *Diabetes* 32 (Suppl. 2), 34-39.

Goldring, M.B. & Krane, S.M. (1987): Modulation by recombinant interleukin-1 of synthesis of types I and III collagens and associated procollagen mRNA levels in cultured human cells. *J. Biol. Chem.* 262, 16724-16729.

Ishimura, E., Sterzel, R.B., Budde, K. & Kashgarian, M. (1989): Formation of extracellular matrix by cultured rat mesangial cells. *Am. J. Pathol.* 134, 843-855.

Kähäri, V-M., Heino, J. & Vuorio, E. (1987): Interleukin-1 increases collagen production and mRNA levels in cultured skin fibroblasts. *Biochem. Biophys. Acta* 929, 142-147.

Karttunen, T., Risteli, J., Autio-Harmainen, H. & Risteli, L. (1986): Effect of age and diabetes on type IV collagen and laminin in human kidney cortex. *Kidney Int.* 30, 586-591.

Kim Y., Kleppel, M.M., Butkowski, R., Mauer, S.M., Wieslander, J. & Michael, A.F. (1991): Differential expression of basement membrane collagen chains in diabetic nephropathy. *Am. J. Path.* 138, 413-420.

Kitamura, M., Yoshida, H., Nagasawa, R., Mitarai, T., Maruyama, N. & Sakai, O. (1990): Three-dimensional environment of extracellular matrix modulates the behaviors of cultured mesangial cells: Possible role of mesangial matrix constituents. *J. Am. Soc. Neph.* 1, 551.

Kopp, J.B., Marinos, N.J., Bodkin, N.L., Hansen, B.C. & Klotman, P.E. (1990): Increased laminin in nodular glomerulosclerosis affecting rhesus monkeys with non-insulin dependent diabetes mellitus (NIDDM). *J. Am. Soc. Neph.* 1, 551.

Laurie, G.W., Horikoshi, S., Killen, P.D., Sequi-Real, B. & Yamada, Y. (1989): In situ hybridization reveals temporal and spatial changes in cellular expression of mRNA for a laminin receptor, laminin, and basement membrane (type IV) collagen in the developing kidney. *J. Cell Biol.* 109, 1351-1362.

Ledbetter, S., Copeland, E.J., Noonan, D., Vogeli, G. & Hassell, J. R. (1990): Altered steady-state mRNA levels of basement membrane proteins in diabetic mouse kidneys and thromboxane synthase inhibition. *Diabetes* 39, 196-203.

Martin, G.R., Timpl, R. & Kühn, K. (1988): Basement membrane proteins: Molecular structure and function. *Adv. Prot. Chem.* 39, 1-50.

Nakamura, T., Ebihara, I., Shirato, I., Tomino, Y. & Koide, H. (1991a): Increased steady-state levels of mRNA coding for extracellular matrix components in kidneys of NZB/W F1 mice. *Am. J. Physiol.* (In press).

Nakamura, T., Ebihara, I., Shirato, I., Tomino, Y. & Koide, H. (1991b): Modulation of basement membrane component gene expression in glomeruli of aminonucleoside nephrosis. *Lab. Invest.* 64, 640-647.

Nanes, M. S., McKoy, W.M. & Marx, S.J. (1989): Inhibitory effects of tumor necrosis factor-α and interferon-γ on deoxyribonucleic acid and collagen synthesis by rat osteosarcoma cells (ROS17/2.8). *Endocrinology* 124, 339-345.

Postlethwaite, A.E., Raghow, R., Stricklin, G.P., Poppleton, H., Seyer, J.M. & Kang, A.H. (1988): Modulation of fibroblast functions by interleukin-1: Increased steady-state accumulation of type I procollagen messenger RNAs and stimulation of other functions but not chemotaxis by human recombinant interleukin 1α and β. *J. Cell Biol.* 106, 311-318.

Poulsom, R., Kurkinen M., Prockop D.J. & Boot-Handford, R.P. (1988): Increased steady-state levels of laminin B_1 mRNA in kidneys of long-term streptozotocin-diabetic rats. *J. Biol. Chem.* 263, 10072-10076.

Sawczuk, I.S., Olsson, C.A., Buttyan, R., Nguyen-Huu, M.C., Zimmerman, K.A., Alt, F.W., Zakeri, Z., Wolgemuth, D. & Reitelman, C. (1989): Gene expression in renal growth and regrowth. *J. Urology* 140, 1145-1148.

Schlondorff, D. (1987): The glomerular mesangial cell: An expanding role for a specialized pericyte. *FASEB J.* 1, 272-281.

Schreiner, G.F. & Unanue, E.R. (1984): Origin of the rat mesangial phagocyte and its expression of the leukocyte common antigen. *Lab. Invest.* 51, 515-523.

Solis-Herruzo, J.A., Brenner, D.A. & Chojkier, M. (1988): Tumor necrosis factor α inhibits collagen gene transcription and collagen synthesis in cultured human fibroblasts. *J. Biol. Chem.* 263, 5841-5845.

Timpl, R. (1989): Structure and biological activity of basement membrane proteins. *Eur. J. Biochem.* 180, 487-502.

Watanabe, K., Kinoshita, S. & Nakagawa, H. (1990): Gelatinase secretion by glomerular epithelial cells. *Nephron* 56, 405-409.

Weeks, B.S., Kopp, J.B., Horikoshi, S., Cannon, F.B., Garrett, M., Kleinman, H.K. & Klotman, P.E. (1991): Adult and fetal human mesangial cells interact with specific laminin domains. *J. Cell Biol.* (In press).

Résumé

La sclérose du glomérule rénal est un processus de cicatrisation comparable à la cirrhose du foie, caractérisée par un dépôt excessif de matrice extracellulaire. La matrice extracellulaire est synthétisée par un péricyte particulier dans le glomérule rénal, la cellule mésangiale, qui joue un rôle comparable à la cellule de Ito dans la fibrose hépatique. Le processus de sclérose dans le rein est dû, au moins en partie, à une activation de l'expression des gènes codants pour les constituants de la matrice extracellulaire normale, tels que la laminine, le collagène IV et la fibronectine, et les collagènes intersticiels de types I et III. L'activation de l'expression de ces gènes ainsi que la prolifération des cellules mésangiales sont initiées par : 1) une réponse des cellules mésangiales aux différents cytokines, facteurs de croissance et médiateurs produits par les cellules immunitaires infiltrées, par les cellules mésangiales ou par d'autres cellules résidentes dans le rein ; 2) les interactions directes des cellules mésangiales avec différents composants de la matrice extracellulaire. Dans les néphropathies diabétiques, la sclérose est caractérisée par une expansion de la matrice associée aux cellules mésangiales et par un épaississement des lames basales glomérulaires et tubulaires. Le mécanisme de stimulation du dépôt de la matrice extracellulaire peut mettre en jeu les produits du métabolisme de l'acide arachidonique, particulièrement le thromboxane vasoconstricteur. Il est possible que les traitements dirigées contre le thromboxane et les médiateurs de l'inflammation pourraient améliorer le processus de cicatrisation dans le rein, processus qui conduit à l'insuffisance rénale.

Cellular and Molecular Aspects of Cirrhosis. Eds B. Clément, A. Guillouzo. Colloque INSERM/John Libbey Eurotext Ltd. © 1992, Vol. 216, pp. 211-213

Collagen fibrillar framework of rat liver with carbon tetrachloride-induced fibrosis demonstrated by cell-maceration/scanning electron microscope method

Yoshihide Nakayama, Chiharu Miyabayashi, Terumi Takahara, Hiroyuki Itoh, Akiharu Watanabe, Osamu Ohtani * and Hiroshi Sasaki **

*Third Department of Internal Medicine, First Department of Anatomy *, University Hospital **, Toyama Medical and Pharmaceutical University, 2630 Sugitani, Toyama, 930-01 Japan*

INTRODUCTION

The extracellular matrix (ECM) is indispensable to organ strucure and function. Collagen, the most abandant ECM component, plays an important role in maintaining the mechanical structure of the liver (Rojkind & Ponce-Noyola, 1982). Electron microscopic and immuno-histochemical studies have revealed that the amount of this component is increased in the fibrotic liver (Schaffner & Popper, 1963; Gay et al., 1975; Grimaud et al., 1980). However, three-dimensional collagen network has not been observed in liver fibrosis. Recently, we were able to demonstrate the collagen fibrillar framework by cell maceration/scanning electron microscope (SEM) method (Ohtani, 1987; Ohtani et al., 1988). In the present report, we describe the three-dimensional collagen fibrillar framework of the cirrhotic liver demonstrated by this method.

MATERIALS AND METHODS

Forty-three male Wistar rats were administered CCl_4 as a model of liver fibrosis (Takahara et al., 1988). For induction of acute CCl_4 intoxication, 8 rats were administrated a single dose of 50% CCl_4 in olive oil (0.2ml/100gm) through a gastric tube. For induction of chronic intoxication, 30 rats received 50% CCl_4 subcutaneously twice a week, these were sacrificed at 2-week intervals. Five control rats received either olive oil alone injected subcutaneously or were left untreated. Small liver specimens were fixed in 2.5% glutar-aldehyde for more than 24 hours, macerated in 2N NaOH for 3-7 days at room temperature, then rinsed in distilled water for a few days until the pieces became transparent. They were then immerted in 1% aqueous tannic acid for 2-3 hours for conductive staining, rinsed in ditilled water, and postfixed in 1% aqueous solution of OsO_4 for 1-2 hours. The specimens were dehydrated in graded ethanol series and critical point-dried using liquid CO_2. They were mounted, coated with gold, and observed under a SEM (Hitachi H-200).

RESULTS

This cell-maceration method revealed the three-dimensional collagen fibrillar network under SEM. The network consists of thread-like units of collagen fibrils, which are about 60 nm in diameter. In control livers, condensation of collagen fibrils was observed in the portal tract and central vein (Fig. 1a). The ECM in the vessels and bile duct consisted of thick bundles interlaced with collagen fibrils. The collagen fibrillar framework was much sparser in Disse's space, but the network was connected with that in the portal tract and central vein. In livers of rats with acute CCl_4 intoxication, the number of collagen fibrils in the sinusoids in the area of hepatic necrosis adjacent to the central vein was decreased (Fig. 1b). In livers of rats with chronic intoxication, the network of collagen fibrils in the portal tract was more condensed than that in controls, and disarrangement of collagen fibrils in the hepatic lobule was noted prior to formation of a central septum (Fig. 1c). The network became rigid, but the diameter of the collagen fibrils themselves remained unchanged (Fig. 1d).

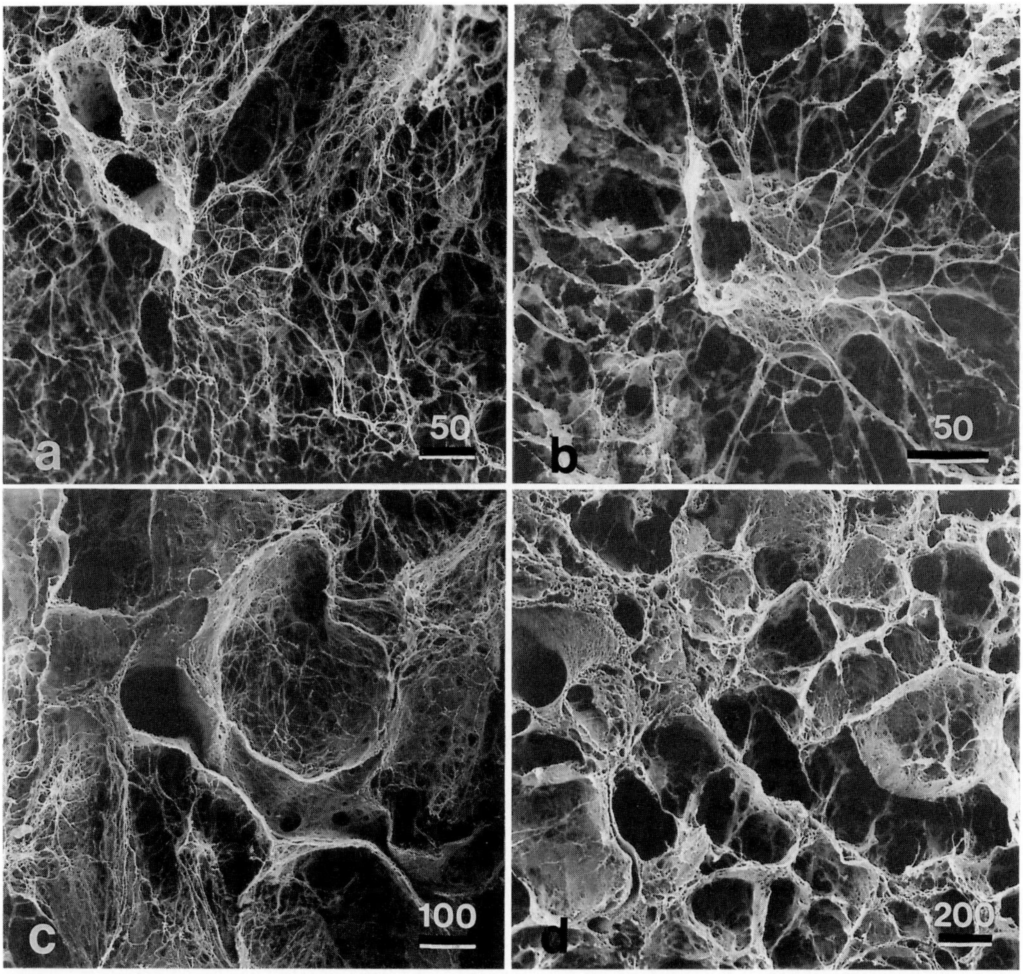

Fig. 1. Collagen fibrollar framework of rat liver demonstrated by the cell-maceration/SEM method. (a) Control liver. (b) Acute CCl_4 intoxication. Collagen fibrillar frameworkin the lobule was decreased. (c) Chronic intoxication after 4-week administration of CCl_4. (d) Fibrotic liver after 8-week administration of CCl_4. Note the honeycomb-like lobular architecture.

CONCLUSION

The cell-maceration/SEM method revealed the morphology of the collagen fiber network in control and CCl_4-injured livers and clealy demonstrated the qualitative and quantitative changes of collagen fibrils. The alteration of the collagen network may change the microcirculation of the liver and restrict free exchange of macromolecules between hepatocytes and the sinusoid.

ACKOWLEDGEMENT

We wish to acknowledge the expert technical assistance of Miss Hiromi Gamada and Mr. Masahiko Kawahara.

REFERENCES

Gay, S., et al. (1975): Liver cirrhosis: Immunofluorescence and biochemical studies demonstrate two types of collagen. Klin. Wochenschr. 53, 205-208.

Grimaud, J. A., et al. (1980): Collagen immunotyping in human liver. Light and electron microscopic study. J. Histochem. Cytochem. 28, 1145-1156.

Ohtani, O. (1987): Three-dimensional organization of the connective tissue fibers of the human pancreas: A scanning electron microscopic study of NaOH treated tissues. Arch. Histol. Jap. 50, 557-566.

Ohtani, O., et al. (1988): Collagen fibrillar frameworks as skeletal frameworks: A demonstration by cell-maceration/scanning electron microscope method. Arch. Histol. Cytol. 51, 249-261.

Rojkind, M. & Ponce-Noyola, P. (1982): The extracellular matrix of the liver. Collagen Relat. Res. 2, 151-175.

Schaffner, F & Popper H. (1963): Capillarization of hepatic sinusoids in man. Gastroenterology 44, 239-242.

Takahara, T., et al. (1988): Collagen production in fat-storing cells after carbon tetrachloride intoxication in the rat. Immunoelectron microscopic observation of type Ⅰ, type Ⅲ collagens, and prolyl hydroxylase. Lab. Invest. 59, 509-521.

Cellular and Molecular Aspects of Cirrhosis. Eds B. Clément, A. Guillouzo. Colloque INSERM/John Libbey Eurotext Ltd. © 1992, Vol. 216, pp. 215-218

Identification of collagen, fibronectin and laminin gene transcripts in freshly isolated liver cells

Albert Geerts (1), Patricia Greenwel (2), Mike Cunningham (2), Pieter De Bleser (1), Vera Rogiers (3), Eddie Wisse (1) and Marcos Rojkind (2)

(1) Laboratory for Cell Biology and Histology and (3) Laboratory for Toxicology, Free University Brussels (V.U.B.), 1090 Brussels-Jette, Belgium; (2) Liver Research Center, Albert Einstein College of Medicine, 10461 Bronx, New York, USA

The cellular origin of the extracellular matrix in normal liver is still under investigation. In the present study, we have isolated and purified parenchymal, endothelial, Kupffer and fat-storing (Ito) cells, extracted RNA, and examined the presence of collagen α1(I), collagen α1(III), collagen α1(IV), fibronectin and laminin B1 gene transcripts by Northern hybridization.

Materials and methods

Cells were obtained from adult male Wistar rats, weighing 300 - 400 grams. Parenchymal cells were isolated and purified as described [Rogiers et al, 1984]. Kupffer and endothelial cells were isolated and purified using centrifugal elutriation [Van Bossuyt et al, 1988]. Fat-storing cells were isolated and purified by centrifugation through 13 and 11 % (w/v) Nicodenz [De Bleser et al, 1991].

RNA was extracted as described [Chomszynski and Sacchi, 1987]. The amount of RNA extractable from each sample was determined by $A_{260\ nm}$ spectrophotometry. Poly(A)$^+$ enriched RNA was extracted using oligo-dT columns. Specific RNA species were visualized by Northern hybridization [Sambrook et al, 1989]. Ten µg total RNA, or 4 µg poly(A)$^+$ enriched RNA were electrophoresed in 1 % agarose/3 % formaldehyde gel, stained with ethydium bromide and transferred to GeneScreen. The filters were baked for 2 hrs at 80 ^{o}C. After a 2 hrs prehybridization, the filters were hybridized overnight at 42 ^{o}C with the following cDNA probes : rat α1(I) procollagen [Genovese et al, 1984], rat α1(III) procollagen [Vuorio et al, 1989], mouse α1(IV) procollagen [Ebihara et al, 1988], rat fibronectin [Schwarzbauer et al, 1983] and mouse laminin B1 chain [Ebihara et al, 1988]. cDNA probes were labeled with ^{32}P-dCTP using a multiprime extension kit (Amersham). After hybridization, the filters were washed at 65°C under stringent conditions. Filters were then exposed to Kodak XAR-5 film.

For each cell type, three representative cell isolates were examined by transmission electron microscopy. Cells were resuspended in 1.5 % glutaraldehyde, and centrifuged for 4 min at 9000 x g. The pellet was further fixed in 1 % OsO_4, dehydrated and embedded in Epon. For each cell preparation, at least 500 cells were counted in randomly selected fields.

---

1. We thank to Dr. D. Rowe, Dr. E. Vuorio, Dr. Y. Yamada, and Dr. R. Hynes for having provided us with the necessary plasmids, and Drs. R. De Zanger for assisting A.G. to edit this manuscript.

2. This work was supported by FGWO grants 30.028.86 and 30.078.90, OZR-VUB grant 1903220550, grant DK 41918 from NIH and a grant from Alcoholic Beverage Medical Research Foudation. Part of this study was performed while A.G. was a beneficiary of Fulbright and NATO travel fellowships.

Results

Freshly isolated parenchymal cells contained 29.6 μg RNA per 10^6 cells, endothelial cells 1.4 μg, Kupffer cells 2.5 μg and fat-storing cells 2.0 μg. These differences should be taken into account when interpreting the Northern data.

With the molecular probe to collagen α1(I) mRNA, no signal was observed in total RNA of freshly isolated liver cells. When poly(A)$^+$ enriched RNA of parenchymal cells was used, we found a weak signal (Fig. 1a). Freshly isolated sinusoidal cells did not contain sufficient total RNA to prepare poly(A)$^+$ enriched RNA. Collagen α1(III) mRNA was strongly expressed in freshly isolated fat-storing cells (Fig. 1b). In freshly isolated endothelial and parenchymal, but not in Kupffer cells, this transcript was also present. Scanning densitometry indicated that the signal registered in freshly isolated fat-storing cells was 65 times stronger than the signal found in parenchymal cells and 21 times stronger than in endothelial cells. In freshly isolated fat-storing and endothelial cells, collagen a1(IV) transcripts were present (Fig. 1c). In fat-storing cells, we observed a signal which was 5-fold stronger than in endothelial cells. Fibronectin mRNA transcripts were found in freshly isolated parenchymal cells. In contrast, freshly isolated endothelial, Kupffer and fat-storing cells were negative (Fig. 1d). Laminin B1 chain transcripts were observed in freshly isolated fat-storing cells. The other cells were negative (Fig. 1e).

Figure 1. Hybridization signals in poly(A)$^+$ enriched or total RNA extracted from freshly isolated liver cells

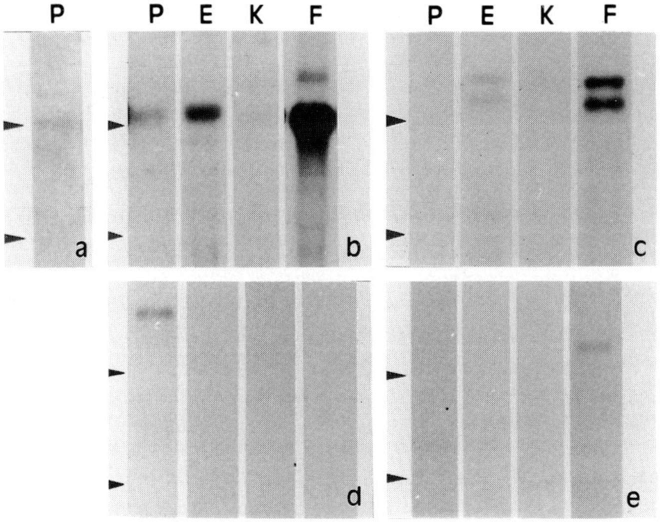

Steady state levels of connective tissue protein mRNAs in freshly isolated parenchymal (P), endothelial (E), Kupffer (K) and fat-storing cells (F). **(a)**: *low levels of collagen α1(I) mRNA were observed in parenchymal cells.* **(b)**: *in fat-storing cells (lane 4), an intense hybridization signal for collagen α1(III) was found. In endothelial cells and parenchymal cells, but not in Kupffer cells, the transcript was also present. The hybridization signal in endothelial cells was due to fat-storing cell contamination. The hybridization signal in parenchymal cells was genuine.* **(c)**: *In fat-storing and endothelial cells, collagen α1(IV) transcripts were present.* **(d)**: *fibronectin mRNA levels. Transcripts were found only in freshly isolated parenchymal cells.* **(e)**: *laminin B1 chain mRNA levels. Transcripts were observed only in freshly isolated fat-storing cells. Arrowheads : 18S and 28S ribosomal RNA.*

The ultrastructural characteristics and purity of isolated and purified parenchymal, endothelial, Kupffer and fat-storing cells were studied by transmission electron microscopy. Parenchymal cells were 86.8 % pure. The most frequently occurring contaminating cells were endothelial cells (8.9 %). Fat-storing cell contamination of parenchymal cells was less than 1 %. Endothelial cell preparations were 87.5 % pure with Kupffer cells contaminating this cell preparation for 7.3 % and fat-storing cells for 2.9 %. Kupffer cell isolates were 87.4 % pure with endothelial cells accounting for some 9.1 %; fat-storing cells represented less than 1 % of the total number of cells. Fat-storing cell preparations were 69.1 % pure, with endothelial and Kupffer cells contaminating these cells for 14.5 % and 12.3 % respectively.

Discussion

Ten µg RNA of freshly isolated liver cells did not contain sufficient collagen α1(I) mRNA to allow detection by Northern hybridization, which is in keeping with recent in situ hybridization studies [Nakatsukasa et al, 1990a ; Nakatsukasa et al, 1990b]. However, when using poly(A)$^+$ RNA of freshly isolated parenchymal cells, detection of low levels of collagen α1(I) mRNA was possible. The signal for collagen α1(I) in parenchymal cells is genuine and cannot be explained by the presence of contaminating fat-storing cells or other sinusoidal cells. Total RNA of fat-storing, endothelial and parenchymal cells contained gene transcripts for collagen α1(III). The strongest signal was present in fat-storing cells, indicating that under unstimulated conditions these cells expressed collagen α1(III) to a much higher level than collagen α1(I). The hybridization signal observed in endothelial cells was 21 times less intense than the signal observed in fat-storing cells. Taking into account that fat-storing cells contaminated endothelial cell preparations for 2.9 %, and that fat-storing cells contain 1.6-fold more RNA per 10^6 cells than endothelial cells, we calculated that the hybridization signal in endothelial cell preparations was due to contamination. If endothelial cells express collagen type III, as was reported previously [Clement et al, 1984 ; Maher and McGuire, 1990], our data indicate that the level of expression is low in comparison to the level of expression in fat-storing cells. Collagen α1(III) mRNA was also observed in parenchymal cells. Taking into account the level of fat-storing cell contamination, the expression of collagen α1(III) by parenchymal cells was shown to be genuine. This observation is in agreement with immunocytochemical data that parenchymal cells contain small amounts of collagen type III [Geerts et al, 1986], and with synthesis of collagen type III by parenchymal cells in early primary culture [Moshage et al, 1990]. Although the amount of collagen α1(III) mRNA per 10 µg total RNA is 75 times lower in parenchymal cells than in fat-storing cells, the total amount of collagen α1(III) message in the parenchymal cell compartment is of the same magnitude as the amount of specific mRNA in the fat-storing cell compartment. Collagen α1(IV) mRNA was detected in freshly isolated fat-storing cells and endothelial cells. After correction for contamination, the intensity of the hybridization signal was approximately 6 times stronger in fat-storing cells than in endothelial cells. Since fat-storing cells contain 1.6 times more RNA per 10^6 cells than endothelial cells, and are 1.2-fold less numerous than the latter cells, fat-storing cells are clearly the predominant source of collagen type IV in normal liver. Fibronectin mRNA was found only in parenchymal cells. Therefore, in normal liver, parenchymal cells are the principal source of this protein. In freshly isolated fat-storing cells, laminin B1 mRNA was detected. This observation is consistent with previous studies that reported laminin synthesis by quiescent fat-storing cells [Clement et al, 1988 ; Maher et al, 1988].

References

Chomszynski, P. and Sacchi, N. (1987): Single-step method of RNA isolation by acid guanidinium thiocyanate - phenol - chloroform extraction. Anal. Biochem. 162 : 156-159.

Clement, B., Emonard, H., Rissel, M., Druguet, M., Grimaud, J., Herbage, D., Bourel, M. and Guillouzo, A. (1984): Cellular origin of collagen and fibronectin in the liver. Cell. Molec. Biol. 30 : 489-496.

Clement, B., Rescan, P., Baffet, G., Loreal, O., Lehry, D., Campion, J. and Guillouzo, A. (1988): Hepatocytes may produce laminin in fibrotic liver and in primary culture. Hepatology 8 : 794-803.

De Bleser, P., Geerts, A., Van Eyken, P., Vrijsen, R., Lazou, J., Desmet, V. and Wisse, E. (1991): Tenascin synthesis in cultured rat liver fat-storing cells. In Cells of the Hepatic Sinusoid , eds. E. Wisse, D. Knook and R. McCuskey, p. in press. Rijswijk (The Netherlands): Kupffer Cell Foundation.

Ebihara, I., Killen, P., Laurie, G., Huang, T., Yamada, Y., Martin, G. and Brown, K. (1988): Altered mRNA expression of basement membrane components in a murine model of polycyctic kidney disease. Lab. Invest. 58 : 262-269.

Geerts, A., Geuze, H., Slot, J., Voss, B., Schuppan, D., Schellinck, P. and Wisse, E. (1986): Immunogold localization of procollagen type III, fibronectin and heparan sulfate proteoglycan on ultrathin frozen sections of the normal rat liver. Histochemistry 84 : 355-362.

Genovese, C., Rowe, D. and Kream, B. (1984): Construction of DNA sequences complementary to rat α1 and α2 collagen mRNA and their use in studying the regulation of type I collagen synthesis by 1,25-dihydroxyvitamin D. Biochemistry 23 : 6210-6216.

Maher, J., Friedman, S., Roll, J. and Bissell, D. (1988): Immunolocalization of laminin in normal rat liver and biosynthesis of laminin by hepatic lipocytes in primary culture. Gastroenterology 94 : 1053-1062.

Maher, J. and McGuire, R. (1990): Extracellular matrix gene expression increases preferentially in rat lipocytes and sinusoidal endothelial cells during hepatic fibrosis in vivo. J. Clin. Invest. 86 : 1641-1648.

Moshage, H., Casini, A. and Lieber, C. (1990): Acetaldehyde selectively stimulates collagen production in cultured rat liver fat-storing cells but not in hepatocytes. Hepatology 12 : 511-518.

Nakatsukasa, H., Nagy, P., Evarts, R., Hsia, C., Marsden, E. and Thorgeirsson, S. (1990): Cellular distribution of transforming growth factor β1 and procollagens types I, III and IV transcripts in carbon tetrachloride-induced rat liver fibrosis. J. Clin. Invest. 85 : 1833-1843.

Nakatsukasa, H., Evarts, R. P., Hsia, C. and Thorgeirsson, S. (1990): Transforming growth factor-β1 and type I procollagen transcripts during regeneration and early fibrosis of rat liver. Lab. Invest. 63 : 171-180.

Rogiers, V., Paeme, G., Vercruysse, A. and Bouwens, L. (1984): Procyclidine metabolism in isolated rat liver cells. In Pharmacological, morphological and physiological aspects of liver ageing , ed. C. Van Bezooyen, pp. 121-126. Rijswijk (The Netherlands): Eurage.

Sambrook, J., Fritsch, E. and Maniatis, T. (1989): Extraction, purification and analysis of messenger RNA from eukaryotic cells. In Molecular cloning. A laboratory manual. 2nd Edition , eds. J. Sambrook, E. Fritsch and T. Maniatis, pp. 7.37-7.52. Cold Spring Harbor (USA): Cold Spring Harbor Laboratory Press.

Schwarzbauer, J., Tamkun, J., Lemischka, I. and Hynes, R. (1983): Three different fibronectin mRNAs arise by alternative splicing within the coding region. Cell 35 : 421-431.

Van Bossuyt, H., Bouwens, L. and Wisse, E. (1988): Isolation, purification and culture of sinusoidal liver cells. In Sinusoids in human liver : health ans disease , eds. P. Bioulac-Sage and C. Balabaud, pp. 1-16. Rijswijk (The Netherlands): Kupffer Cell Foundation.

Vuorio, E., Makela, J., Vuorio, T., Poole, A. and Wagner, J. (1989): Characterization of excessive collagen production during development of pulmonary fibrosis induced by chronic silica inhalation in rats. Br. J. Exp. Path. 70 : 305-315.

Cellular and Molecular Aspects of Cirrhosis. Eds B. Clément, A. Guillouzo. Colloque INSERM/John Libbey Eurotext Ltd. © 1992, Vol. 216, pp. 219-222

Proliferation and phenotypic modulation of perisinusoidal (Ito) cells following acute liver injury: temporal relationship with TGFβ1 expression

S.J. Johnson, K.J. Hillan *, J.E. Hines, R. Ferrier * and A.D. Burt **

*Division of Pathology, School of Pathological Sciences, University of Newcastle upon Tyne, Royal Victoria Infirmary, Newcastle upon Tyne, NE1 4LP, UK; * University Department of Pathology, Western Infirmary, Glasgow, G11 6NT, UK*

*** Corresponding author*

ABSTRACT

We have examined the temporal relationship between the responses of perisinusoidal cells (PSCs), monocytes and Kupffer cells (KCs), and expression of transforming growth factor β1 (TGFβ1) following acute carbon tetrachloride-induced injury in rats. PSCs were identified in tissue sections by immunolocalization of desmin; blood monocytes and KCs were demonstrated using the monoclonal antibody ED1; KCs alone were detected using the monoclonal antibody ED2. Proliferation within these cell populations was studied using a 5-bromo-2'-deoxyuridine (BrdU) double-labelling method. Evidence of PSC activation was sought by demonstration of α-(smooth muscle) actin (α-SMA) expression. TGFβ1 mRNA was identified in tissue sections using a non-isotopic digoxigenin-labelled method for *in situ* hybridisation (ISH).

Increased numbers of desmin-positive and α-SMA-positive PSCs were found in perivenular zones of treated animals. Maximal numbers were noted at days 3 and 4 following administration of the toxin with the peak in PSC proliferation occurring at day 2. Expansion of the KC population was also noted in perivenular zones, maximal numbers were reached at day 3. Expansion of the KC population was contributed to by local proliferation, the peak of proliferative activity occurring at day 1, and by influx of blood monocytes, maximal expansion of the ED1-positive cell population occurring at day 2. The peak in TGFβ1 expression as assessed by ISH was seen at day 2; signal was identified in cells with morphological features of monocytes and KCs. These results indicate that the monocyte/KC response to acute liver injury precedes that of the PSCs. Furthermore, the results are in keeping with the hypothesis that monocyte and KC-derived TGFβ1 may mediate PSC activation.

INTRODUCTION

Perisinusoidal (Ito) cells are considered to play a major role in the production of extracellular matrix proteins during hepatic fibrogenesis (Friedman, 1990). The exact cellular mechanisms underlying their response to liver injury, however, remain unclear. It has been proposed (Gressner and Bachem, 1990) that parenchymal cell damage leads to stimulation of Kupffer cells (KCs) which then secrete peptide growth factors, including transforming growth factor β1 (TGFβ1) and platelet-derived growth factor (PDGF). These in turn mediate PSC proliferation and activation towards myofibroblast(MFB)-like cells with resultant increased synthesis of matrix proteins. Previous studies of the effects of peptide growth factors on PSCs *in vitro* have shown that TGFβ1 preferentially stimulates matrix protein production (Matsuoka *et al* 1989), whereas PDGF has potent mitogenic activity (Pinzani *et al*, 1989). Similar effects have been produced by the addition of KC-conditioned medium to PSCs in culture (Pinzani *et al* 1989; Matsuoka and Tsukamoto, 1990), and it has been shown *in vitro* that KCs produce TGFβ1 (Matsuoka and Tsukamoto, 1990).

In the present study we have examined the *in vivo* response of KCs and PSCs to acute liver injury induced by a single sub-lethal bolus of the toxin carbon tetrachloride. Proliferation within these cell populations was studied using a BrdU double-labelling method (Johnson *et al*, 1991) and evidence of PSC activation was sought using an antibody to α-SMA. In addition, TGFβ1 expression was investigated using a non-isotopic method for ISH. The temporal relationship between the KC and PSC responses and TGFβ1 expression was examined.

MATERIALS AND METHODS

Animals: Twenty one male Wistar rats (200-225g) were used for this study. Acute liver injury was induced in 18 animals by a single intragastric bolus of 1ml 40 per cent carbon tetrachloride in liquid paraffin, 1, 2, 3, 4, 7 and 10 days before death (n=3 per time point); untreated day 0 animals served as controls (n=3). A standard laboratory diet and water were available *ad libitum* throughout the study. BrdU (50mg/kg) was administered intraperitoneally to each animal one hour prior to death. Wedges of liver tissue were fixed in (i) formal sublimate or (ii) Bouin's fixative, and then processed according to normal histological procedures.

Immunohistochemical identification of PSCs and KCs: Three micron sections of dewaxed, formal sublimate-fixed liver tissue were used in all immunohistochemical studies. PSCs were identified using the monoclonal anti-desmin antibody D33 (1:300; Dako), activated PSCs (or MFB-like cells) using the anti-α-SMA antibody 1A4 (1:500; Sigma) and monocytes and KCs using the monoclonal antibodies ED1 and ED2 (1:600 and 1:60; Serotec). An indirect immunoperoxidase method was used with 3,3'-diaminobenzidine (DAB) as chromagen; trypsinization was required prior to incubation with the antibodies ED1 and ED2. Cell numbers were assessed using a Leitz Laborlux microscope fitted with an eyepiece graticule at a magnification of x400. Three sections were examined from each animal and the results expressed as a mean ± SEM per unit area ($0.635mm^2$) for three animals at each time point. Values were obtained using random fields or fields selected to include perivenular or periportal zones; results presented here relate to perivenular zones.

Cell proliferation was demonstrated by simultaneous detection of desmin and incorporated BrdU (PSCs) or ED2 and BrdU (KCs) (Johnson *et al*, 1991). In these experiments nuclear incorporated BrdU was visualized, following acid DNA denaturation, using the monoclonal anti-BrdU antibody B44 (1:250; Becton Dickinson) with nickel/cobalt enhanced DAB as chromagen. The number of double-labelled cells was expressed as a percentage of total desmin-positive or ED2-positive cells to obtain labelling indices.

In situ hybridization (ISH) for TGFβ1: A non-isotopic method of ISH using a digoxigenin-labelled antisense RNA probe to TGFβ1 mRNA was performed on paraffin-embedded Bouin's-fixed liver tissue. The probe was derived from pGEM4 plasmid (kindly provided by Dr. Snorri Thorgeirsson) containing the 582 base pair SmaI fragment from the human TGFβ1 gene.

Sections were dewaxed and hydrated. A series of pretreatments, including digestion with 300μg/ml of protease VIII (Sigma) for 30 minutes at 37°C, were carried out prior to hybridization. Sections were prehybridized in 50 per cent formamide/2xSSC (0.15M sodium chloride, 0.015M sodium citrate) for 2 hours at 37°C. Hybridization was carried out overnight at 37°C using probes diluted (1:20) in 20μl hybridization buffer (0.01M Tris HCl pH7.5, 12.5 per cent Denhardt's solution, 2xSSC, 50 per cent formamide, 0.5 per cent sodium dodecyl sulphate, 10 per cent dextran sulphate, 250μg/ml salmon sperm DNA, 5mg/ml sodium pyrophosphate). After hybridization sections were washed in SSC buffers and then incubated with alkaline phosphatase conjugated anti-digoxigenin antisera (1:500) for 2 hours at room temperature. Antibody was detected using nitroblue tetrazolium chloride/5-bromo-4-chloro-3-indolylphosphate as substrate. Negative (no probe added) and positive (poly dT probe) controls were performed. Sections were counterstained with haematoxylin and mounted with glycergel.

RESULTS

PSC response: In carbon tetrachloride-treated animals there was a significant increase in numbers of both desmin-positive and α-SMA-positive PSCs compared to controls, this being limited principally to the damaged perivenular zones (fig. 1). The increase was first seen at day 1 and reached peak values at days 3 and 4 (desmin: day 0 - 0.9 ± 0.7 cells/$0.635mm^2$, day 3 - 277.7 ± 30.8 cells/$0.635mm^2$; α-SMA: day 0 - 4.9 ± 0.8 cells/$0.635mm^2$, day 3 - 226.1 ± 8.2 cells/$0.635mm^2$); cell numbers then returned to control values (data not shown). The labelling index for BrdU-positive proliferating desmin-positive cells reached a significant peak at day 2 (day 0 - 1.7 ± 1.7 per cent; day 2 - 20.3 ± 1.4 per cent).

KC response: In carbon tetrachloride-treated animals there was a significant increase in ED1-positive cells, representing monocytes and KCs, principally within the perivenular zones (fig. 2). This increase began at day 1 and reached a peak at day 2 (day 0 - 188.7 ± 9.9 cells/$0.635mm^2$; day 2 - 799.0 ± 44.8 cells/$0.635mm^2$); cell numbers then returned to control values by day 7 (data not shown). There was also a significant expansion of the ED2-positive KC population in perivenular zones first seen at day 1 and reaching a peak at day 3 (day 0 - 51.7 ± 5.2 cells/$0.635mm^2$; day 3 - 258.1 ± 12.0 cells/$0.635mm^2$). The labelling index for KC proliferation reached a peak value at day 1 (day 0 - 0 ± 0 per cent; day 1 - 13.6 ± 5.2 per cent).

TGFβ1 expression: In control animals weak signal was noted within stellate non-parenchymal cells in portal tracts as well as in occasional periportal hepatocytes. Within the acini, signal was present in a few stellate non-parenchymal cells. No signal was seen in negative control sections.

In carbon tetrachloride-treated animals, there was a dramatic increase in signal for TGFβ1 mRNA, predominantly within the damaged perivenular zones (fig. 3a), although some increase in the number of labelled cells was also seen elsewhere in the acini. Increased signal began at day 1 and appeared maximal at day 2; from day 3 onwards there was a reduction in the number of labelled cells and control levels were reached by day 10.

The majority of the signal for TGFβ1 mRNA was noted within non-parenchymal cells, many of these cells being large stellate cells with broad cytoplasmic processes. In addition, on days 1 and 2 some of the positive cells were smaller and rounded in shape, and often clustered within hepatic vein lumina; these appearances are more characteristic of blood monocytes. Signal was seen within occasional hepatocytes (fig. 3a and b).

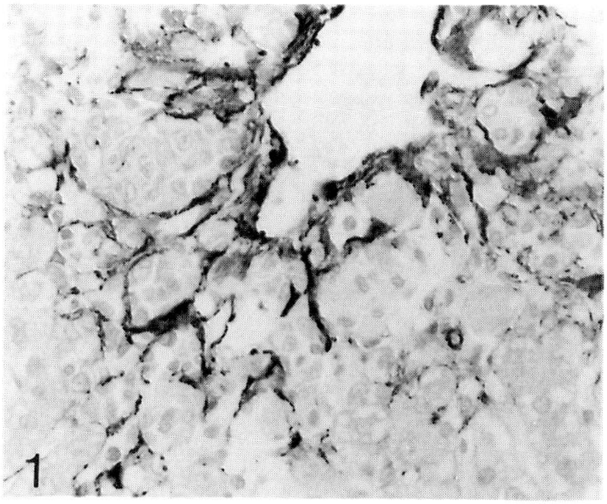

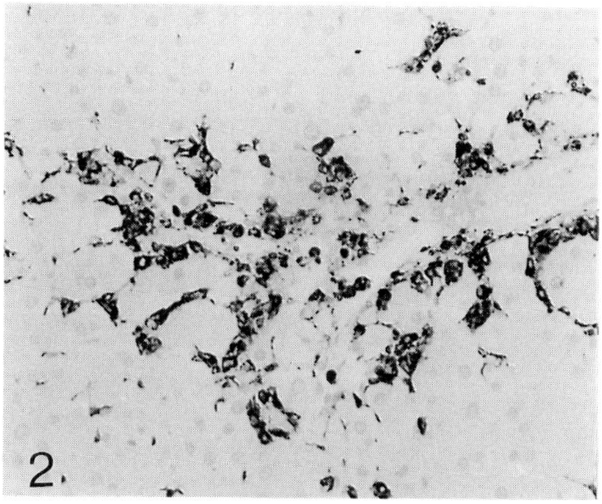

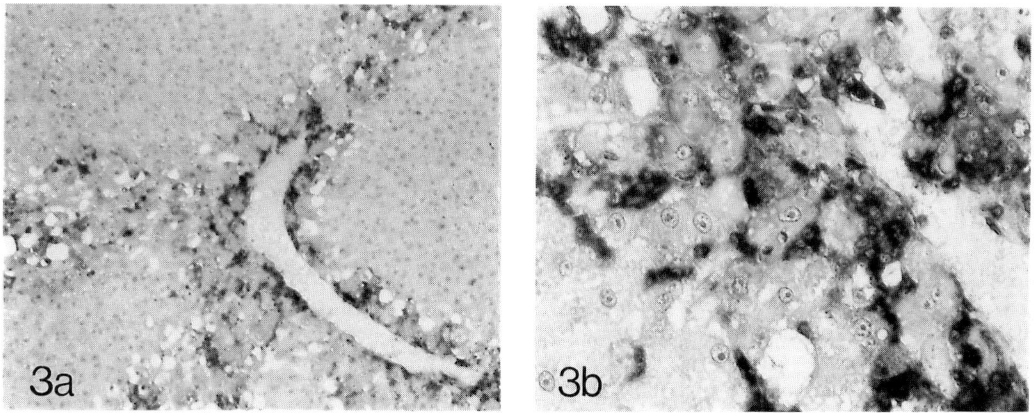

Fig. 1: α-SMA-positive cells in a perivenular zone of a day 3 animal. Fig. 2: ED1-positive cells (monocytes and KCs) in a day 2 animal. Fig. 3: *In situ* hybridization for TGFβ1 mRNA in a day 2 animal: (a) signal can be seen principally within perivenular zones; (b) positivity is predominantly present in nonparenchymal cells with features of KCs and monocytes.

DISCUSSION

These results confirm previous reports (Ramadori *et al*, 1990) that there is expansion of the PSC population following acute liver injury, and demonstrate that this in part results from local cell proliferation. Demonstration of increased numbers of α-SMA-positive cells in perivenular zones is in keeping with the suggestion that PSCs undergo phenotypic modulation to MFB-like cells in the response to injury; the kinetics of the α-SMA-positive cell response was similar to that of the desmin-positive cell population although the absolute numbers were lower. The findings also demonstrate expansion of the KC population following acute liver damage, this expansion resulting in part from local KC proliferation and in part from influx of blood monocytes into the areas of hepatic injury. The peak in desmin-positive and α-SMA-positive cell numbers occurred at days 3 and 4, with a peak in proliferative activity at day 2. This was preceded by the responses of the ED1- and ED2-positive cell populations, which reached maximal numbers at days 2 and 3 respectively, with a peak in KC proliferation at day 1.

Increased signal for TGFβ1 mRNA was noted following carbon tetrachloride administration in rats compared to control animals. This occurred predominantly within the damaged perivenular zones and appeared to be maximal at day 2, before returning to control levels by day 10. Positivity could be seen to be principally within non-parenchymal cells, especially large cells resembling KCs with broad cytoplasmic processes and also smaller rounder cells resembling monocytes. This finding is in keeping with the results of Nakatsukasa *et al* (1990) who observed a peak in TGFβ1 mRNA, as assessed by Northern blotting, on day 2 following carbon tetrachloride administration. In their study, using an isotopic method of ISH, TGFβ1 mRNA was localized first to mononuclear inflammatory cells in the damaged perivenular areas, and then to desmin-positive PSCs. In contrast, Czaja *et al* (1989) localized TGFβ1 mRNA almost exclusively to hepatocytes following chronic carbon tetrachloride administration. In our study, on morphological assessment the TGFβ1 transcripts appeared to be expressed principally by cells of the monocyte/macrophage series, although some expression by activated PSCs cannot be excluded; expression by hepatocytes was not prominent. The time of maximal expression of TGFβ1 mRNA coincided with the peak of expansion of the monocyte/KC population (day 2), and preceded the time of maximal α-SMA expression by the PSC population (day 3).

These findings are in keeping with the hypothesis that TGFβ1, produced by macrophages and monocytes following liver damage, plays an important role in mediating the response of the perisinusoidal cell population to hepatic injury.

ACKNOWLEDGEMENTS

This work was supported by grants from the Newcastle Health Authority Research Committee and the University of Newcastle upon Tyne Research Committee.

REFERENCES

Czaja, M.J., Weiner, F.R., Flanders, K.C., Giambrone, M-A., Wind, R. Biempica, L. & Zern, M.A. (1989): *In vitro* and *in vivo* association of transforming growth factor β1 with hepatic fibrosis. *J. Cell. Biol.* 108, 2477-2482.

Friedman, S. (1990): Cellular sources of collagen and regulation of collagen production in liver. *Semin. Liver Dis.* 10, 20-29.

Gressner, A.M. & Bachem, M.G. (1990): Cellular sources of noncollagenous matrix proteins: role of fat-storing cells in fibrogenesis. *Semin. Liver Dis.* 10, 30-46.

Johnson, S.J., Hines, J.E. & Burt, A.D. (1991): Immunolocalisation of proliferating perisinusoidal (Ito) cells in rat liver. *Histochem. J.* (in press).

Matsuoka, M., Pham, N-T. & Tsukamoto, H. (1989): Differential effects of interleukin-1α, tumor necrosis factor α, and transforming growth factor β1 on cell proliferation and collagen formation by cultured fat-storing cells. *Liver* 9, 71-78.

Matsuoka, M. & Tsukamoto, H. (1990): Stimulation of hepatic lipocyte collagen production by Kupffer cell-derived transforming growth factor β: implication for a pathogenetic role in alcoholic liver fibrosis. *Hepatology* 11, 599-605.

Nakatsukasa, H., Evarts, R.P., Hsia, C-C. & Thorgeirsson, S.S. (1990): Transforming growth factor β1 and type I procollagen transcripts during regeneration and early fibrosis of rat liver. *Lab. Invest.* 63, 171-180.

Pinzani, M., Gesualdo, L., Sabbah, G.M. & Abboud, H.E. (1989): Effects of platelet-derived growth factor and other polypeptide mitogens on DNA synthesis and growth of cultured rat liver fat-storing cells. *J. Clin. Invest.* 84, 1786-1793.

Ramadori, G., Veit, S., Schwögler, S. Dienes, H.P., Knittel, T., Reider, H. & Meyer zum Buschenfelde, K.-H. (1990) Expression of the gene of the α-smooth muscle-actin isoform in rat liver and in rat fat-storing (Ito) cells. *Virchows Archiv. B Cell Pathol.* 59, 349-357.

Cellular and Molecular Aspects of Cirrhosis. Eds B. Clément, A. Guillouzo. Colloque INSERM/John Libbey Eurotext Ltd. © 1992, Vol. 216, pp. 223-226

The response of rat liver perisinusoidal lipocytes to polypeptide growth regulators changes with cell transdifferentiation into myofibroblast-like cells

Max G. Bachem, Dieter H. Meyer, Wolfgang Schäfer, Uwe Riess, Ralph Melchior, Klaus-Martin Sell and Axel M. Gressner

Department of Clinical Chemistry, Philipps-University, Baldingerstraße, W-3550 Marburg, Germany

SUMMARY

Perisinusoidal lipocytes (PL) transdifferentiate in culture on uncoated plastic to myofibroblast-like cells (MFBIC). Whereas in early cultured PL (untransformed) mitotic activity was stimulated by TGFα/EGF and inhibited by TGFβ, these cytokines were without effect on the growth activity of MFBIC. Opposite effects were obtained with PDGF which only stimulated growth of MFBIC. Insulin-like growth factor (IGF1) was mitogenic in both cell types. Whereas TGFβ1 stimulated proteoglycan (PG) synthesis of PL, addition of TGFα stimulated PG synthesis of MFBIC. IGF1 and PDGF, respectively, neither stimulated PG synthesis in PL nor in MFBIC significantly. The obtained results demonstrate that the effects of the polypeptide growth regulators depend on the cell phenotype (stage of cell activation) and may be completely different in PL and MFBIC.

INTRODUCTION

In experimental (Mak et al. 1984) and in human alcoholic liver injury (Horn et al. 1986) but also in culture on uncoated plastic PL lose their differentiated phenotype and transform to highly activated MFBIC. PL and to an even higher capacity their transformed counterpart produce the majority of the extracellular matrix found in fibrotic liver (for rev. see Gressner & Bachem 1990; Friedman 1990). Despite the central role of PL and in particular of MFBIC in fibrogenesis the factors modulating proliferation and/or matrix synthesis by these cells are incompletely understood. Recently, we have shown that transforming growth factor (TGF) alpha, epidermal growth factor (EGF) and insulin-like growth factor (IGF1) stimulate PL proliferation with little effect on PG synthesis whereas TGFβ1 inhibits the growth of early cultured PL but significantly stimulates matrix synthesis (Bachem et al. 1989 a-c). Using late primarily cultured PL or secondarily cultured PL (in vitro transformed to MFBIC) it was shown that TGFβ stimulates matrix synthesis without affecting proliferation of these cells (Czaja et al. 1989; Matsuoka et al. 1989). Platelet derived growth factor (PDGF) (Friedman & Arthur 1989) and acetaldehyde (Savolainen et al. 1984) were reported to influence only activated (transformed) PL. These results suggest that the response of rat liver PL to fibrogenic mediators depends on the degree of cell activation/transformation. In order to evaluate this hypothesis the known fibrogenic mediators TGFα, TGFβ, PDGF, FGF and IGF1 were added alone and in combination to early (untransformed) and late (partially transformed) primarily cultured PL and to secondarily cultured MFBIC (completely transformed) and the effects of these cytokines on proliferation and PG synthesis were measured. Our results demonstrate that the cytokines modulate cell proliferation and proteoglycan synthesis differently depending strongly on the stage of cell activation/transformation.

METHODS

The detailed procedure of the isolation and culture of PL from rats has been published previously from this laboratory (Schäfer et al. 1987). To obtain MFBIC confluent PL in primary culture (6-7 days after seeding) were passaged using trypsin and EDTA. In general the cytokines (TGFα, TGFβ1, IGF1, FGF and PDGF) were added in the presence of 0.5% fetal calf serum (to PL 44h after seeding and to MFBIC

72h after seeding). Twentyfour hours later the cytokines were added again during a further medium change whereby cultures were labeled with radionuclide.

Determination of cell proliferation was performed by DNA measurement, [^{3}H]thymidine incorporation and cell count.

The synthesis of total medium proteoglycans was determined by the incorporation of [^{35}S]sulfate (20μCi/ml medium) during a labeling period of 24 h (details described by Schäfer et al. 1987). Proteoglycan synthesis was expressed as radioactivity on the basis of DNA.

RESULTS

Within the first 3 days after seeding the cells (untransformed PL) appeared homogenous and showed a characteristic morphology with lipid droplets surrounding the nucleus. At this stage a bright intracellular staining was observed with the anti-vimentin antibody, but only part of the cells (50-60%) were labeled for the intermediate filament desmin and obviously none of these early cultured cells was positive for iso-α smooth muscle actin. During the next several days the cells transdifferentiated spontaneously into MFBIC showing long cytoplasmic extensions, loss of fat droplets and expression of desmin and iso α-smooth muscle actin (Fig.1). While TGFα stimulated and TGFβ1 inhibited the mitotic activity of early cultured PL dose dependently, both cytokines were without effect on the growth of secondary cultured MFBIC as measured by DNA (Fig.2) and [^{3}H]thymidine incorporation (data not shown). In contrast to TGFs PDGF(AB) acted as a mitogen only in MFBIC and only in the absence of fetal calf serum (Fig.3). The growth of early cultured PL was unaffected by PDGF(AB) (data not shown). IGF1 stimulated the proliferation of early cultured PL and MFBIC (Fig.3). bFGF neither stimulated the proliferation of PL nor MFBIC significantly (data not shown). Furthermore, single cell GAG synthesis of PL was stimulated to a maximum of about 2fold by 2.5 ng/ml TGFβ1 and to about 1.4fold of control by 5ng/ml TGFα (data not shown). However, since TGFα stimulated proliferation too, GAG synthesis per culture well was stimulated to a maximum of 1.9fold by 5 ng/ml TGFα. The effects of the cytokines TGFα, TGFβ1, PDGF and IGF1 on proliferation and proteoglycan synthesis of PL and MFBIC are summarized in Tab.1.

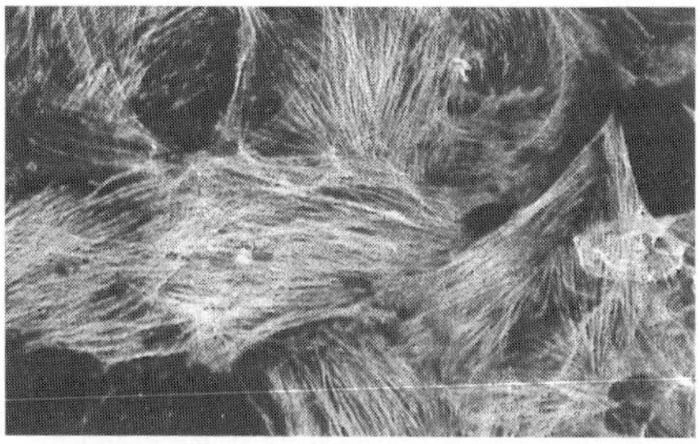

Fig.1 Demonstration of iso-α smooth muscle actin in MFBIC (indirect immunofluorescence).

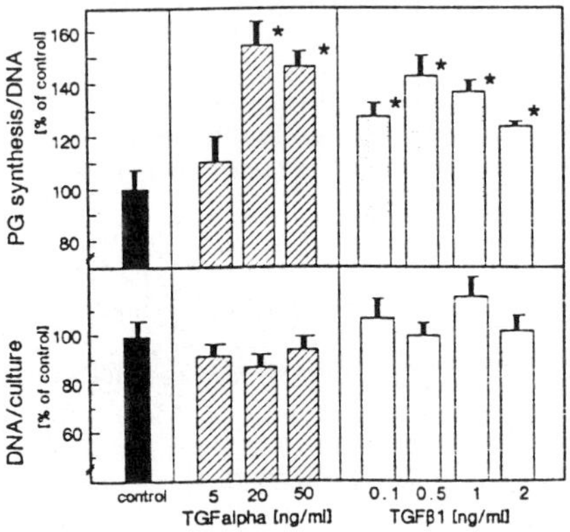

Fig.2 Effects of TGFs on proliferation and proteoglycan synthesis of myofibroblast-like cells.

	PL		MFBIC	
	prolif.	PG synth.	prolif.	PG synth.
TGFα	+	(+)	0-(-)	++
TGFβ1	-	++	0	+
PDGF(AB)	0	0	+	0
IGF1	+	0	+	0

Table 1: Effects of the polypeptide growth regulators on proliferation and proteoglycan synthesis of PL (4 days after seeding) and MFBIC (passaged cells, 4 days after seeding). (0, no effect; -, inhibition; +, stimulation; ++, strong stimulation).

Both TGFs in combination (20ng/ml TGFα and 0.5ng/ml TGFβ1) elevated the synthesis of total medium GAG about 3fold. Determination of the specific GAGs in media of early cultured PL indicated that in controls (DMEM with 0.5% fetal calf serum) most (70-80%) of the incorporated [^{35}S]sulfate was found in the fraction of dermatan sulfate whereas heparan sulfate and chondroitin sulfate together represented the remaining 20-30%. Addition of 20ng/ml TGFα to early cultured PL resulted in an 3fold increase of the chondroitin sulfate synthesis. TGFβ1 (2ng/ml) caused a 8fold increase of the chondroitin sulfate synthesis. The combination of both TGFs enhanced chondroitin sulfate synthesis 15fold, whereas dermatan sulfate and heparan sulfate synthesis slightly decreased. In MFBIC GAG synthesis was stimulated to a maximum of 1.5fold of control by 20ng/ml TGFα and to a maximum of 1.4fold by 0.5ng/ml TGFβ1, respectively. Both mitogens PDGF and IGF1 caused no significant enhancement of the GAG synthesis in early cultured PL and in MFBIC.
To investigate why PL and MFBIC show differences in their response to growth factors the expression of the cell surface receptors was studied by binding of radiolabeled growth factors ([^{125}I]TGFα, [^{125}I]TGFβ1, [^{125}I]PDGF and [^{125}I]IGF1) to PL (1 and 4 days after seeding) and MFBIC (passaged cells). In contrast to the TGFα-, TGFβ1- and IGF1 receptor the PDGF receptor is expressed only in activated cells (Pl 4 days after seeding and MFBIC) (see Fig.4).

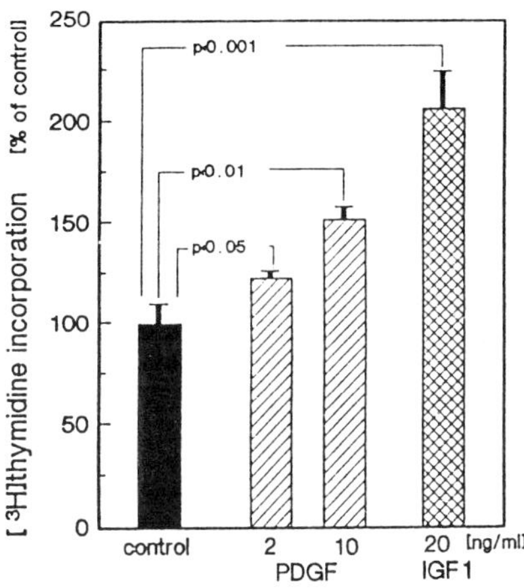

Fig.3 PDGF and IGF1 stimulated proliferation of myofibroblast-like cells.
(mean ± SD of 3 experiments each with n = 3).

DISCUSSION

It is suggested that in liver injury the sequence from hepatocyte necrosis via platelet aggregation, invasion and activation of inflammatory cells (KC and monocytes) and release of fibrogenic mediators which activate PL to change their phenotype from the resting retinoid storing cell into the highly proliferative and synthetic MFBIC might be keysteps of hepatic fibrosis (Friedman 1990; Gressner & Bachem 1990; Bachem et al. 1991). Despite the central role of PL and in particular of MFBIC in hepatic fibrogenesis the factors modulating proliferation and/or matrix synthesis by these cells are incompletely understood. In vitro several pure cytokines were shown to be capable of modulating perisinusoidal lipocyte proliferation and/or stimulating extracellular matrix synthesis (Pinzani et al. 1989; Bachem et al. 1989a-c; Matsuoka et al. 1989; Czaja et al. 1989). Since in vivo PL are exposed to several cytokines simultaneously and/or sequentially, it was relevant to determine (i) the effects of combinations of polypeptide growth regulators on PL proliferation and activation and (ii) the effects of polypeptide growth regulators on PL matrix synthesis sequentially during activation to MFBIC.

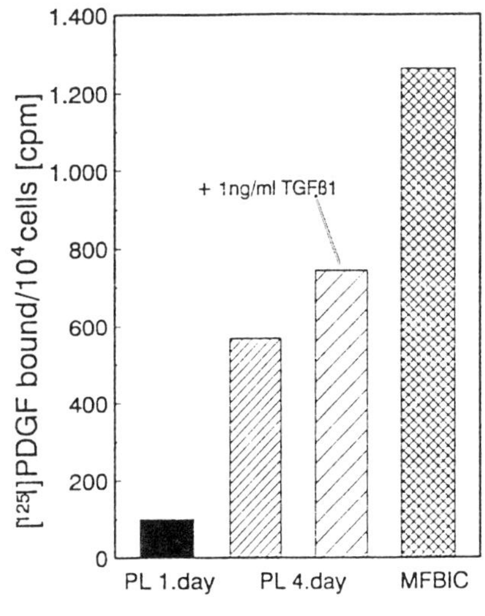

Fig.4 PDGF receptor expression in PL and MFBIC.

Using highly purified PL in primary culture we have shown recently that TGFα, EGF and IGF1 stimulate PL proliferation (Bachem et al. 1989a, 1989b) with little effect on proteoglycan synthesis (Bachem et al. 1989c). Furthermore we have shown that TGFβ1 inhibits the growth of early culture PL but stimulates significantly its matrix synthesis (Bachem et al. 1989b, 1989c). In late primary cultured PL and MFBIC TGFβ stimulates matrix synthesis without inhibiting proliferation of these cells (Matsuoka et al. 1989; Czaja et al. 1989; Pinzani et al. 1989). Obviously MFBIC have escaped the growth inhibitory action of TGFβ. This result seems very important since: (1) MFBIC express the mRNA of TGFβ1 and secrete the corresponding protein (Bachem et al. 1991); (2) via TGFβ1 autocrine positive loops in matrix synthesis

of MFBIC are suggested (Bachem et al. in preparation). PDGF was reported to stimulate late primarily cultured PL and passaged cells (Pinzani et al. 1989) or cells which had been activated by Kupffer cell conditioned media (Friedman & Arthur, 1989). In contrast to the report of Heldin et al. (1991) in our experiments PDGF was shown to stimulate only transformed PL. Furthermore our results suggest that resting PL (1st day after seeding, iso-α smooth muscle actin negative) lack the PDGF receptor and that during transdifferentiation the PDGF receptor is expressed. Interestingly factors synthesized by Kupffer cells induced PDGF receptor expression in PL too (Friedman & Arthur 1989).
Since polypeptide growth regulators modulate cell proliferation and proteoglycan synthesis depending on the cells phenotype the stage of cell activation/transformation has to be defined in the different studies evaluating the effects of growth factors. This has to be recognized in particular when data of different studies are compared. The underlying mechanisms of the phenomena that the cells phenotype affects the response to growth factors are not yet entirely understood but may include differences in growth factor activation/inactivation, differences in the expression of growth factor receptors (e.g. PDGF), post receptor events (second messenger mechanisms), and autocrine stimulatory loops (TGFβ1 and TGFα).

REFERENCES

Bachem, M.G., Meyer, D., Schäfer, W., and Gressner, A.M. (1989a): Evaluation of fibrogenic polypeptide mediators stimulating fat storing cell proliferation and/or proteoglycan synthesis. In The liver, metabolism and aging, eds K.W. Woodhouse, C. Yelland and O.F.W. James, Vol.13, pp. 169-178. Rijswijk: Eurage.

Bachem, M.G., Riess, U., and Gressner, A.M. (1989b): Liver fat storing cell proliferation is stimulated by epidermal growth factor/transforming growth factor alpha and inhibited by transforming growth factor beta. Biochem. Biophys. Res. Commun. 162: 708-714.

Bachem, M.G., Riess, U., Melchior, R., Sell, K.M., and Gressner, A.M. (1989c): Transforming growth factors (TGF alpha and TGF beta 1) stimulate chondroitin sulfate and hyaluronate synthesis in cultured rat liver fat storing cells. FEBS Lett. 257: 134-137.

Bachem, M.G, Meyer, D., Melchior R., Sell, K.M., and Gressner A.M. (1991) J. Clin. Invest. 86: in press.

Czaja, M.J., Weiner, F.R., Flanders, K.C., Giambrone, M., Wind, R., Biempica, L., and Zern M.A. (1989): In vitro and in vivo association of transforming growth factor-β1 with hepatic fibrosis. J. Cell Biol. 108: 2477-2482.

Friedman, S.L. (1990): Cellular sources of collagen and regulation of collagen production in liver. Sem. Liv. Dis. 10: 20-29.

Friedman, S.L., and Arthur, M.J.P. (1989): Activation of cultured rat hepatic lipocytes by Kupffer cell conditioned medium. Direct enhancement of matrix synthesis and stimulation of cell proliferation via induction of platelet-derived growth factor receptors. J. Clin. Invest. 84 (6): 1780-1785.

Gressner, A.M., and Bachem, M.G. (1990): Cellular sources of noncollagenous matrix proteins: Role of fat-storing cells in fibrogenesis. Sem. Liv. Dis. 10: 30-46.

Heldin, P., Pertoft, H., Nordlinder, H., Heldin, C.H., and Laurent, T.C. (1991): Differential expression of platelet-derived growth factor α- and β-receptors on fat-storing cells and endothelial cells of rat liver. Exp. Cell Res. 193: 364-369.

Horn, T., Junge, J., and Christoffersen, P. (1986): Early alcoholic liver injury. Activation of lipocytes in acinar zone 3 and correlation to degree of collagen formation in Disse space. J. Hepatol. 3: 333-340.

Mak, K., Leo, M.A. and Lieber, C.S. (1984): Alcoholic liver injury in baboons: transformation of lipocytes to transitional cells. Gastroenterology 87: 188-200.

Matsuoka, M., Pham, N.T., and Tsukamoto, H. (1989): Differential effects of interleukin-1 alpha, tumor necrosis factor alpha, and transforming growth factor beta 1 on cell proliferation and collagen formation by cultured fat-storing cells. Liver 9: 71-78.

Pinzani, M., Gesualdo, L., Sabbah, G.M., Abboud, H.E. (1989) Effects of platelet-derived growth factor and other polypeptide mitogens on DNA synthesis and growth of cultured rat liver fat-storing cells. J. Clin. Invest. 84: 1786-1793.

Savolainen, E.R., Leo, M.A., Timpl, R., and Lieber, C.S. (1984): Acetaldehyde and lactate stimulate collagen synthesis of cultured baboon liver myofibroblasts. Gastroenterology 87: 777-787.

Schäfer, S., Zerbe, O., and Gressner, A.M. (1987): The synthesis of proteoglycans in fat storing cells of rat liver. Hepatology 7: 680-687.

Cellular and Molecular Aspects of Cirrhosis. Eds B. Clément, A. Guillouzo. Colloque INSERM/John Libbey Eurotext Ltd. © 1992, Vol. 216, pp. 227-232

Influence of various polysaccharides on morphology and function of adult rat hepatocytes in primary culture

Ivan Diakonov [1,2], Alain Fautrel [1] and André Guillouzo [1]

[1] INSERM U 49, Unité de Recherches Hépatologiques, Hôpital Pontchaillou, 35033 Rennes Cedex, France and [2] Institute of Cytology, St Petersbourg, USSR

INTRODUCTION

The extracellular matrix (ECM) promotes tissue morphogenesis and the differentiation of a variety of cell types. Its molecular components, which include collagens, noncollagenous glycoproteins and proteoglycans, are interconnected with the cytoskeleton via transmembrane receptors. The functions of proteoglycans are the least known. Recently some unexpected functions have been attributed to these components such as modulation of growth factor activity (Ruoslahti and Yamaguchi, 1991) and a role in protein recycling. Polysaccharide residues appear to play some important roles ; recently they have been reported to act as cell regulators e.g. heparin for smooth muscle cells (Castellot et al., 1986) and carrageenans for immune cells (Palanivel, 1987).
Since the liver is richly endowed with proteoglycans located in basement membranes and in plasma membranes, we decided to evaluate the influence of various polysaccharides on morphology and function of the hepatocytes. Primary hepatocyte cultures which have been proved to be a useful system for investigating the effects of ECM on cell differentiation were used as an experimental model in this study.

MATERIALS AND METHODS

1 - Source of polysaccharides

The different polysaccharides used in this study are listed in Table I. Heparin purified from bovine intestinal mucosa, lung heparin, alginate, lambda-carrageenan, cartilage chondroitin-6-sulfate, dextran-sulfate and pullulan were obtained from Sigma. Carboxymethyl-cellulose was purchased from Fluka. Zosterin, kappa- and iota-carrageenans and chitosan were provided from the Pacific Ocean Institute of Bioorganic Chemistry (Vladivostok, USSR). Chemically substituted carboxymethyl-chitosan and chitosan-sulfate were a gift from the Technologic Institute of Textile Industries (Moscow). Purified fungal polysaccharides were kindly provided from the Chemico-pharmaceutical Institute (St Petersbourg).

2 - Hepatocyte isolation and culture

Liver parenchymal cells were isolated from Sprague-Dawley rats as previously described (Guguen-Guillouzo and Guillouzo, 1986). Cells were plated at a density of 3 x 10^4 cells per well in 96-well plates in serum-free Williams E medium containing 10 µg/ml bovine insulin and 3.4×10^{-6} M hydrocortisone hemisuccinate. Polysaccharides were added 4 hr later and every two days thereafter at the concentration of either 25 or 250 µg/ml and cultures were maintained for 2, 4 or 8 days.

Polysaccharide group	Name	Designation	Degree of inhibition of hepatocyte spreading
Anionic gel-forming	Alginate	A	++
	Zosterin	Z	++
Anionic sulfated	Chitosan-sulfate	CS	+
	Rodexman-sulfate	RS	+++
	Dextran-sulfate	DS	++++
	Lambda-carrageenan	LC	++++
	Kappa-carrageenan	KC	+++
	Iota-carrageenan	JC	+++
Anionic carboxy-methylated	CM-cellulose	CCE	+
	CM-dextran	CMD	0
	CM-chitosan	CCH	+
Fungal neutral	SP-50	SP	+++
	B-678	B	+
	Rodexman	R	+
	Crilan	CR	++
	Aubasidan	AU	0
	Pullulan	PU	0
Mammalian glycosaminoglycans	Intestinal heparin	HM	+
	Lung heparin	HL	0
	Cartilage chondroitin-6-sulfate	CIS	0

TABLE 1 : **Test polysaccharides and their inhibitory effects on cell spreading.**
The extent of spreading inhibition is graded from 0 (no effect) to +++ (major effect) by comparison with control cultures.

3 - Cell viability measurement

Cells in 96-well plates were incubated with 50 µg/ml of neutral red in culture medium for 2 hr, then washed with PBS and fixed by a formol (4 %) - $CaCl_2$ (1 %) solution. The dye was extracted by a alcohol-acetic acid solution and optical density was measured at 540 nm using a multiscan MCC spectrophotometer (Labsystems, Les Ulis, France).

4 - Biochemical assays

7-Ethoxyresorufin O-dealkylase (EROD) and pentoxyresorufin O-dealkylase (PROD) activities were measured in intact cells by spectrofluorimetry. Ethoxyresorufin and pentoxyresorufin, both at 5×10^{-6} M, were used as substrates and subsequent conjugation was prevented by addition of 1.5 mM salicylamide. Glutathione S-transferase (GST) activity was determined by spectrophotometry after addition of 1 mM of glutathione and 1 mM 1-chloro-2,4 dinitrobenzene to sonicated cells in phosphate buffer pH 6.5. A unit activity was defined as the enzyme amount required to form 1 mmol of product/min at 25°C. Total cellular proteins were estimated using the Bio-Rad protein assay and rat albumin as a standard.

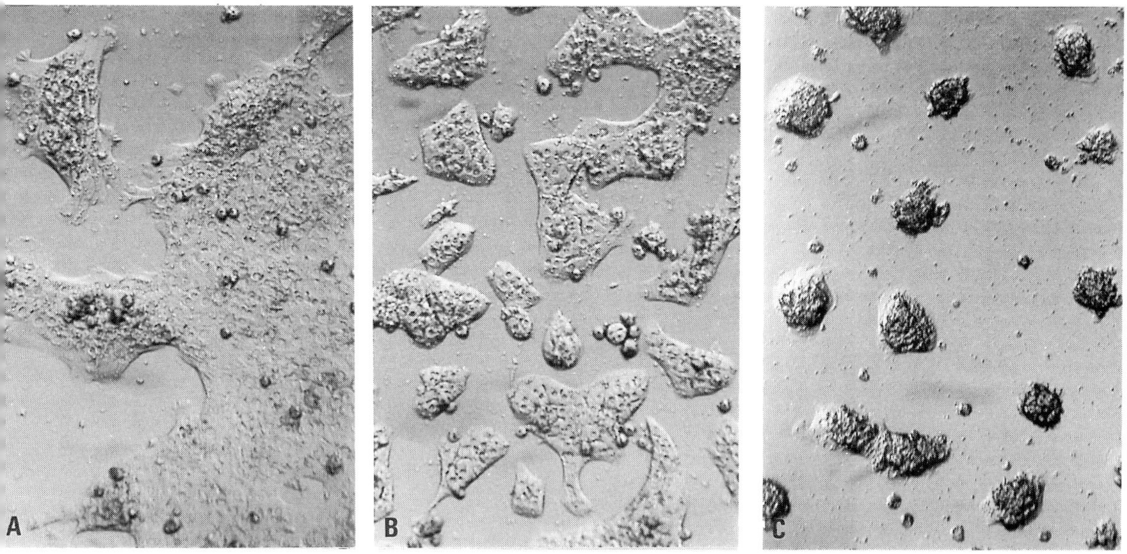

Figure 1 : **Light microscopic appearance of rat hepatocytes cultured in the absence or presence of polysaccharides for 2 days.**
Intestinal heparin (B) and dextran-sulfate (C), both added at the concentration of 250 µg/ml, have an inhibitory effect on cell spreading ; A : control cultures.

RESULTS

Whatever the polysaccharide tested, either at 25 or 250 µg/ml, no cytotoxicity effect was observed on the basis of the neutral red uptake assay (not shown). However, the polysaccharides differently affected cell morphology (Figure 1). Most of them strongly reduced cell spreading, compared to control cells (Table I). The most potent inhibitors of cell spreading were dextran sulfate and carrageenans which were effective at the lowest concentration (2.5 µg/ml), inducing cell rounding and formation of aggregates. Some fungal galactomannans were also effective in maintaining the globular shape of hepatocytes but at a concentration of 250 µg/ml or more. Sulfated polysaccharides including chitosan-sulfate, rodexman sulfate and heparin blocked extensive cell spreading with lamella and protusion formation at 25 µg/ml. Carboxy-methyl-substituted polysaccharides had no influence on cell morphology up to 250 µg/ml. At this high concentration they had a slight inhibitory effect on cell spreading. The last group of polysaccharides composed of calcium chelators bearing carboxy residues has little effect on cell morphology at a concentration lower than 250 µg/ml and were stronger inhibitors than carboxy-methyl-substituted polysaccharides at this high concentration.
As shown in figure 2 marked variations occurred in both EROD and PROD activities in control cultures as a function of time. While EROD levels were increased PROD activity was strongly decreased after 4 days of culture. Most polysaccharides enhanced EROD activity ; some of them were effective as soon as day 2. Huge differences were observed, compared to control cells. In the presence of polysaccharides except for alginate and the fungal polysaccharide b-678 a 2- to 6-fold increase was found after 4-8 days. PROD activity was also modulated by most of the polysaccharides. Only alginate at 25 µg/ml, and crilan at

250 µg/ml were not effective, and b-678 at 250 µg/ml, had in inhibitory effect. Dextran sulfate and intestinal heparin (Figures 2A and 2B) were the most stimulating polysaccharides on both enzymes.
By contrast, only a few polysaccharides affected GST activity. The increase in GST levels did not exceed 1.5- to 2.5- fold and was not obvious before 8 days of culture (Figure 3). However dextran-sulfate and heparin were the most the stimulating molecules as well. Alginate and SP-50 had a negative effect.

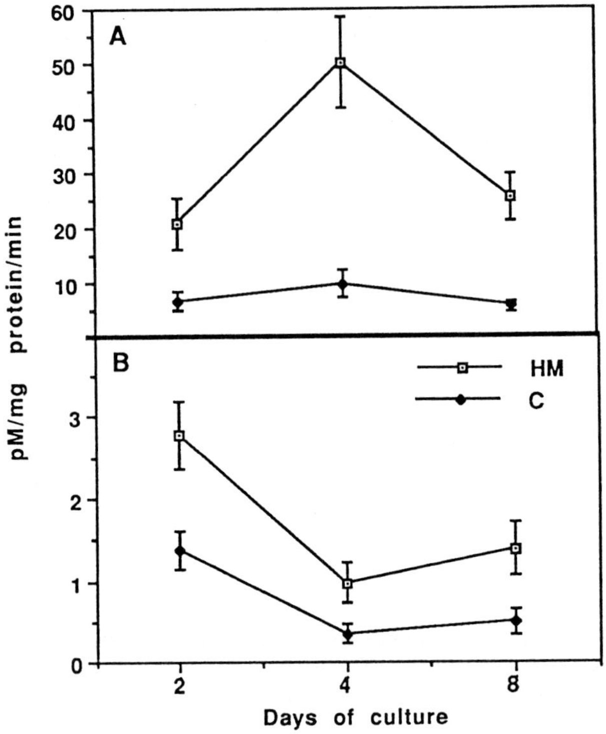

Figure 2 : **Influence of heparin (HM) on ethoxyresorufin deethylase (A) and pentoxyresorufin deethylase (B) activities in rat hepatocytes as a function of culture time.**
C : Control cultures. The values are expressed as mean ± SD of 5 cultures.

DISCUSSION

A number of studies have shown that both cell shape and liver-specific functions are affected by ECM in primary hepatocyte cultures. When the cells are cultured on an ECM-derived gel, termed matrigel, both the globular shape and various specific functions are preserved for at least several days (Bissell et al., 1987). This gel is mainly composed of type IV collagen, laminin and proteoglycans. However, growth factors and cytokines have been reported to be associated with ECM, making it possible their implication in matrix-cell interactions (Lortat-Jacob et al., 1991). Most of the polysaccharides used in

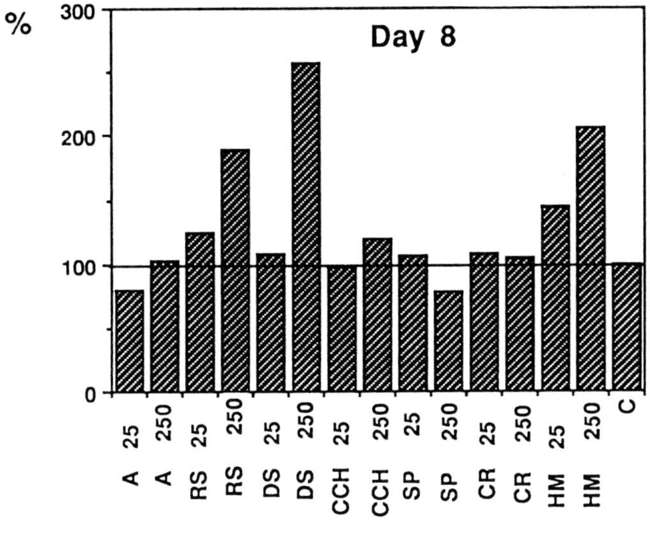

Figure 3 : Glutathione S-transferase activity in rat hepatocytes cultured in absence or presence of various polysaccharides for 8 days.
The names of polysaccharides are given in Table I. These were used either at 25 or 250 µg/ml. The values are expressed as percentages of control cultures (C).

this study were of non animal origin, making unlikely the presence of growth factors and/or cytokines capable of perturbing their effects.

Several polysaccharides were found to inhibit hepatocyte spreading, in agreement with a previous report from Spray et al. (1987). Dextran-sulfate, lambda- and iota-carrageenans were demonstrated as potent inhibitors in both studies. However, kappa-carrageenans were much more effective and heparins much less in our study. These discrepancies could be related either to the source or the test concentrations of polysaccharides or to the time of addition. In the protocol devised by Spray et al. (1987) polysaccharides were added only after 24 h of culture ; consequently, cell contraction rather spreading inhibition was estimated.

The functional capacities of rat hepatocytes were evaluated over a 8 days period and were not found to be directly related to the cell shape. Indeed, heparin which was the most effective polysaccharides on drug metabolizing enzymes failed to prevent cell spreading. By contrast fungal polysaccharides, such as SP and B-678, inhibited cell spreading without enhancing drug metabolizing enzyme activities. Only dextran-sulfate was able to affect both cell shape and enzyme activities. Interestingly the most abundant glycans in the extracellular matrix in contact with hepatocytes are heparins and dextran-sulfate is also present. Since their composition varies with tissular and species sources, variable quantitative effects may be expected.

Most effects were only transient and no major changes were also found in the levels of secreted albumin (not shown) ; therefore it may be wondered whether polysaccharides alone can act as potent effectors on long-term regulation of liver-specific functions *in vitro*. Further studies should allow to answer.

ACKNOWLEGDMENTS.

Ivan Diakonov's stay in Rennes was supported by the French Foreign Ministery.

REFERENCES

Bissell, D.M., Arenson, D.M., Maher, J.J., and Roll, F.J. (1987). Support of cultured hepatocytes by a laminin-rich gel. *J. Clin. Invest.* 79, 801-812.

Castellot, J.J., Choay, J., Lormeau, J.C., Petitou, M., Sache, E. & Karnovsky, M.J. (1986). Structural determinants of the capacity of heparin to inhibit the proliferation of vascular smooth muscle cells. II. Evidence for a pentasaccharide sequence that contains a 3-O sulfate group. *J. Cell Biol.* 102, 1979-1984.

Guguen-Guillouzo, C. & Guillouzo, A. (1986): Methods for preparation of adult and fetal hepatocytes. In *Isolated and Cultured Hepatocytes*, eds. A. Guillouzo & C. Guguen-Guillouzo, pp. 1-12. Paris: Les Editions INSERM & London: John Libbey Eurotext.

Lortat-Jacob, H., Kleinman, H.K. & Grimaud, J.A. (1991): High affinity binding of interferon-gamma to a basement membrane-like complex (matrigel). *J. Clin. Invest.* 87, 878-883.

Palanivel, V. (1987). Modulation of murine anti-SRBC response by carrageenan : possible mechanism. *Immunol. Lett.* 15, 335-339.

Ruoslahti, E. & Yamaguchi, Y. (1991). Proteoglycans as modulators of growth factor activities. *Cell* 64, 867-869.

Spray, D.C., Fujita, M., Saez, J.C., Choi, H., Watanabe, T., Hertzberg, E., Rosenberg, L.C. & Reid, L.M. (1987): Proteoglycans and glycosaminoglycans induce gap junction synthesis and function in primary liver cultures. *J. Cell Biol.* 105,541-551.

Dynamics in cirrhosis : remodeling, regeneration, hepatocarcinogenesis

Dynamique de la cirrhose : remodelage, régénération, hépatocarcinogenèse

Cellular and Molecular Aspects of Cirrhosis. Eds B. Clément, A. Guillouzo. Colloque INSERM/John Libbey Eurotext Ltd. © 1992, Vol. 216, pp. 235-244

The metalloproteinases

Michael J.P. Arthur

Medicine II, University of Southampton, Southampton General Hospital, Tremona Road, Southampton, Hampshire SO9 4XY, UK

SUMMARY

Liver fibrosis is a dynamic process potentially involving changes in both the synthesis and degradation of matrix proteins. The role of matrix degradation in liver fibrosis is poorly understood, but recent advances indicate that several of the matrix metalloproteinases may be involved.

The matrix metalloproteinases are divided into three broad groups according to their substrate profile; collagenases which degrade interstitial collagens (types I, II and III), stromelysins which degrade a broad range of substrates including proteoglycans, laminin, gelatins and fibronectin, and type IV collagenases/gelatinases which degrade basement membrane (type IV) collagen and gelatins. Regulation of matrix metalloproteinases occurs at three levels; alterations in gene transcription, activation of secreted proenzymes, and inhibition of activated metalloproteinases by TIMP (tissue inhibitor of metalloproteinases) or alpha-2- macroglobulin.

In liver, current evidence indicates that hepatic lipocytes (fat-storing or Ito cells) and Kupffer cells play a central role in synthesis and regulation of matrix metalloproteinases. Activated hepatic lipocytes synthesize 72kD type IV collagenase/gelatinase and possibly interstitial collagenase. Recent work from our laboratory indicates that they also secrete TIMP. Kupffer cells synthesize 92kD type IV collagenase/gelatinase and may also synthesize interstitial collagenase and a wide array of cytokines involved in metalloproteinase regulation. Thus sinusoidal liver cells have the ability to degrade - and regulate degradation of - both the normal liver matrix and the interstitial fibrillar collagens laid down during liver fibrosis. As yet, an important role for metalloproteinases and their inhibitors in liver fibrosis remains speculative but theoretically compelling.

THE FAMILY OF MATRIX METALLOPROTEINASES

Matrix metalloproteinases are the products of a family of closely related genes. They possess several well conserved domains in their primary sequence (for review see Matrisian 1990). The properties of individual enzymes are summarized in Table 1.

TABLE 1 THE MATRIX METALLOPROTEINASES

	Enzyme	Substrate Profile
1)	Collagenases	
	Interstitial collagenase	COLL III > I > II
	Neutrophil collagenase	COLL I > II > III
2)	Stromelysins	
	Stromelysin-1	PG, FN, LM, GEL, COLL III, IV, V, CAS
	Stromelysin-2	FN, GEL, COLL III,IV,V
	Stromelysin-3	ND
	PUMP-1	FN, LM, GEL, CAS, COLL IV
3)	Type IV Collagenases/Gelatinases	
	72 kD	COLL IV, ?V, VII, X, GEL
	92 kD	COLL IV, V, GEL

Abbreviations used: COLL - Collagen subtype, PG - Proteoglycans, FN - Fibronectin GEL - Gelatins, CAS - Casein, LM - Laminin, ND - No data available.

METALLOPROTEINASE REGULATION

Regulation of matrix metalloproteinases is mediated by three mechanisms; changes in gene transcription, activation of secreted proenzymes, and inhibition of activated enzymes. Many of these regulatory mechanisms are common to all members of the metalloproteinase family, but some are more specific to individual metalloproteinases.

Regulation of metalloproteinase gene transcription

Many different factors alter metalloproteinase gene transcription but of those described, growth factors and cytokines are particularly important. Expression of most metalloproteinase genes is increased by interleukin-1, tumour necrosis factor-α (TNF-α), platelet derived growth factor (PDGF), epidermal growth factor (EGF) and basic fibroblast growth factor (b-FGF) (Murphy et al, 1985a; Brenner et al, 1989; Chua et al, 1985; Edwards et al, 1987). The effects of transforming growth factor-beta (TGF-beta) are particularly interesting as this growth factor has differing effects on expression of different members of the matrix metalloproteinase gene family; interstitial collagenase and stromelysin expression are inhibited whereas 72kD type IV collagenase/gelatinase expression is increased (Edwards et al, 1987; Overall, 1989). Metalloproteinase gene expression is also inhibited by corticosteroids and retinoic acid (Clark et al, 1987). These regulatory effects on metalloproteinase gene expression are mediated via stimulation - or inhibition - of expression of the proto-oncogene products c-Fos and C-Jun (for review see Matrisian, 1990). These act as transactivating factors which bind to the activator protein-1 (AP-1) binding site in the promotor region of some metalloproteinase genes and enhance their transcription. In contrast, other factors, e.g. TGF-β and retinoic acid may have either a direct inhibitory effect on the promoter region of metalloproteinase genes or act via inhibition of C-Fos expression.

In macrophages, matrix metalloproteinase synthesis is stimulated by endotoxin or by mixed lymphokines (Wahl et al, 1974; 1975), but inhibited by gamma-interferon (Shapiro, 1990). This effect of endotoxin is mediated via stimulation of PGE_2 synthesis which increases intracellular cyclic AMP levels and can be inhibited by corticosteroids or prostaglandin synthetase inhibitors (Wahl et al, 1977; McCarthy et al, 1980; Werb 1978).

Activation of prometalloproteinases

Matrix metalloproteinases are secreted as latent proenzymes which are activated by disruption of the interaction between the zinc atom at the catalytic site and a cysteine residue in the propeptide domain (Van Wart, 1990). This leads to autoproteolysis with cleavage of the propiece (~80 amino acids) and permanent conversion to an active metalloproteinase. In vivo, this may be initiated by a proteolytic cascade involving conversion of plasminogen to plasmin by the action of urokinase (plasminogen activator). Plasmin can partially activate both procollagenase and prostromelysin, but active stromelysin then leads to further activation of interstitial collagenase (Murphy et al, 1987; He 1989). Plasminogen-activator inhibitor-1 (PAI-1) can also be produced by cells that synthesize metalloproteinases (He, 1989) and this may be important in regulating this pathway of proenzyme activation.

Other candidate mechanisms of metalloproteinase activation have implicated mast cell tryptase (Gruber, 1989), neutrophil elastase, cathepsin G (Okada, 1989) and hydroxyl radicals formed during the oxidative burst of neutrophils (Saari, 1990).

Inhibition of active Metalloproteinases

The activity of metalloproteinases is further regulated by inhibitors, including the tissue inhibitors of metalloproteinases (TIMPs), TIMP-1 and TIMP-2, and general proteinase scavengers e.g. α2-macroglobulin. The balance between local concentrations of active metalloproteinases and these inhibitors will determine the extent of local matrix degradation.

TIMP-1 is a 28 kD glycoprotein which binds irreversibly to - and inhibits - active metalloproteinases including interstitial collagenase, neutrophil collagenase, stromelysin, and both 92 kD and 72 kD type IV collagenase/gelatinase (Murphy et al, 1981). Studies of TIMP gene expression have shown that it is regulated by many of the same growth factors and cytokines involved in metalloproteinase gene regulation. Expression can be coregulated, e.g. EGF and b-FGF increase both TIMP-1 and metalloproteinase expression, or inversely coregulated e.g. TGF-β increases expression of TIMP-1 but decreases expression of interstitial collagenase and stromelysin (Edwards et al, 1987). TGF-β is consequently very effective at reducing matrix degradation within tissues. Other factors can have similar effects; retinoids increase expression of TIMP-1 but inhibit expression of interstitial collagenase whereas corticosteroids inhibit both (Clark et al, 1987).

TIMP-2 is a 21 kD protein which demonstrates significant amino acid sequence homology with, and similar properties to TIMP-1 (Stetler-Stevenson, 1989b). Its primary action is to inhibit the active form of 72 kD type IV collagenase/gelatinase (Goldberg, 1989). TIMP-2 gene expression can be regulated independently of TIMP-1, e.g. expression of TIMP-2 is decreased by TGF-β whereas TIMP-1 is increased (Stetler-Stevenson, 1990).

Alpha-2-macroglobulin is an important metalloproteinase scavenger which is synthesized in the liver and is able to bind and inhibit interstitial collagenase, stromelysin and other metalloproteinases (Enghild, 1990).

MATRIX METALLOPROTEINASES, METALLOPROTEINASE INHIBITORS AND THE LIVER

Matrix metalloproteinases have the potential to play an important role in liver fibrosis through degradation of either normal liver matrix components or newly deposited interstitial collagens, but relatively little is known about these enzymes - or their inhibitors - in liver. Recent advances suggest that much of the earlier work on matrix metalloproteinases in liver fibrosis should now be re-evaluated. Improvements in methods of cell isolation and matrix protein biochemistry, together with the application of molecular techniques have facilitated some progress in the study of matrix metalloproteinases in liver.

Interstitial Collagenase

Interstitial collagenase was first characterised in studies of tissue explants obtained from tadpole tails undergoing morphogenesis (Gross et al, 1962). It is now clear that this enzyme is secreted by many different cell types including fibroblasts, other connective tissue cells and macrophages. Human fibroblast interstitial collagenase has been cloned and sequenced (Goldberg et al, 1986) and the biosynthetic pathway for the enzyme defined (Nagase et al, 1981; 1983). It is synthesized as a prepro-enzyme, Mr 54 kD, with a signal peptide of 19 amino acids. The primary secretion products are procollagenases, Mr 57 kD (glycosalated), and Mr 52 kD (unmodified). Proteolytic cleavage of the N-terminal 81 amino acid residues gives rise to activated forms of interstitial collagenase, Mr 47 kD and Mr 42 kD respectively, the properties of which are summarised in Table 1.

Because of the potential importance of this enzyme in liver fibrosis, much effort has been directed towards defining the cellular origin and regulation of interstitial collagenase in liver. No clear picture has emerged; several different cell types have been reported as the source of this enzyme and various regulatory mechanisms have emerged.

Previous studies have suggested that Kupffer cells are the cellular source of interstitial collagenase in liver, with release regulated by PGE_2 (Fujiwara et al, 1973; Bhatnagar et al, EJB 1982). However, these cultures usually contain an outgrowth of hepatic lipocytes which are a potential source of the reported collagenase activity. Similar criticism may be levelled at a previous report of interstitial collagenase release from 8 day-old hepatocyte cultures (Nagai et al, 1982), which also contain lipocytes (Maher et al, 1988). Other groups have described release of interstitial collagenase by co-cultures of hepatocytes and mixed sinusoidal liver cells, but the cellular source of the enzyme was not defined further (Maruyama et al, 1983; Kashiwazaki et al, 1986). A soluble factor released by CCl_4 or endotoxin-treated hepatocytes stimulated release of interstitial collagenase activity by mixed sinusoidal liver cell cultures (Kashiwazaki et al, 1986). This is a potentially important regulatory mechanism for collagenase expression in diseased liver.

Hepatic lipocytes are central to the pathogenesis of liver fibrosis and are an important candidate source of interstitial collagenase. In a recent study of passaged fibroblasts - prepared by outgrowth from a single human liver sample - mRNA for interstitial collagenase and release of collagenase activity was demonstrated in cells exposed to IL-1 or TNF-α (Emonard, 1990). The origin of these cells and their relationship to hepatic lipocytes is unknown, but they may represent lipocytes which have transformed into a myofibroblastic phenotype.

There have been many attempts to define the role of interstitial collagenase in the pathogenesis of liver fibrosis. This followed the initial observation that liver explants obtained from CCl_4-treated rats degrade a type I collagen substratum more readily than explants from normal liver (Okazaki et al, 1974). Many subsequent studies have investigated interstitial collagenase activity in whole liver homogenates prepared from fibrotic liver, but results are widely divergent. In the early stages of CCl_4-induced rat liver fibrosis, both an increase (Carter et al, 1982) and no change (Rojkind 1978) in interstitial collagenase activity have been reported. A further study has reported a progressive decrease in interstitial collagenase activity relative to hepatic collagen content with increasing liver fibrosis (Perez-Tamayo et al, 1987). In contrast, studies of alcoholic liver disease in man or baboons have demonstrated increased hepatic interstitial collagenase activity in homogenates prepared from fatty liver, with a greater increase in fibrotic liver, but decreased activity in advanced alcoholic cirrhosis (Maruyama et al, 1981; 1982).

The information obtained with studies of whole liver homogenates is at best restricted to measurements of net interstitial collagenase activity, which may reflect changes in synthesis and release not only of interstitial collagenase, but also TIMP or $\alpha 2$ macroglobulin. Studies of murine schistosomiasis have shed some light on the interactions that can occur between these factors in a diseased liver (Takahashi 1980, 1981, 1984). Eight weeks after experimental infection, hepatic interstitial collagenase activity was maximal with increased release of interstitial collagenase confirmed by radioimmunoassay. As infection progressed beyond 8 weeks, interstitial collagenase activity fell, in part due to decreased collagenase synthesis, but also due to increased synthesis of alpha-2 macroglobulin which binds interstitial collagenase and forms inactive enzyme-inhibitor complexes (Truden, 1988).

Type IV Collagenases/Gelatinases (Mr 72kD and 92 kD)

These enzymes are particularly interesting in liver because they have the ability to degrade the normal liver matrix. This may be of physiological importance in matrix modelling during organogenesis, but degradation of normal liver matrix may also be an important aspect of liver injury and fibrosis. Interaction between normal liver matrix and hepatocytes is important for maintenance of their specific gene functions e.g. albumin expression (Bissell, 1987) and current evidence indicates that normal liver matrix maintains hepatic lipocytes in a quiescent non-proliferative, non-fibrogenic phenotype (Friedman et al, 1989). Degradation of the normal liver matrix may therefore disturb hepatocyte function and promote proliferation of fibrogenic hepatic lipocytes. There are two distinct members of the metalloproteinase gene family with degradative activity against type IV collagen.

72 kD Type IV Collagenase/Gelatinase was initially described both as a type IV collagenase released by a metastatic murine tumour (Liotta et al, 1979) and as a gelatinase released by rabbit bone cultures (Murphy et al, 1985b). The cDNA sequence has been determined (Collier et al, 1988) and it is now evident that this enzyme is synthesized and released by a wide variety of neoplastic cells, fibroblasts and other connective tissue cells. It is secreted as a latent proenzyme, Mr 72 kD, and is activated by cleavage of the N-terminal 80 amino acids (Stetler-Stevenson, 1989a) to give an active form, Mr 66 kD. The properties of the active enzyme are summarised in Table 1.

Current evidence indicates that hepatic lipocytes are the cellular source of 72 kD type IV collagenase/gelatinase in liver. Rat hepatic lipocytes in primary culture release an enzyme which has degradative activity against type IV collagen and gelatins, (Arthur et al, 1989). Moreover, human hepatic lipocytes in primary culture contain mRNA for 72 kD type IV collagenase/gelatinase and immunoreactive enzyme has been localised to these cells and detected in culture media (Arthur et al, 1991). Preliminary data suggest that 72 kD type IV collagenase/gelatinase expression is minimal in early cultures but increases as lipocytes adopt a myofibroblast-like phenotype, (unpublished observations).

92kD Type IV collagenase/gelatinase is released predominantly by neutrophils and macrophages. The cDNA sequence has recently been described (Wilhelm, 1990) and the biosynthetic pathway defined (Mainardi 1990). It is synthesized as a proenzyme (Mr 78-82 kD) which is glycosylated before secretion as a 92 kD species. Cleavage of the N-terminal 73 amino acids yields an active form of the enzyme, Mr 84 kD, the properties of which are summarised in Table 1.

Preliminary evidence suggests that Kupffer cells are the cellular source of this enzyme in liver. A 92 kD metalloproteinase with degradative activity against gelatin is released by cultured Kupffer cells prepared from normal rat liver and its release appears to be related to the state of Kupffer cell activation (Winwood et al, 1991).

These studies indicate that 'activated' hepatic lipocytes and Kupffer cells secrete 72 kD and 92 kD type IV collagenases/gelatinases respectively, but it is not known whether these enzymes are synthesized by these cells in intact normal or diseased liver. It is speculated that they could make a significant contribution to the early stages of liver fibrosis.

Stromelysin-1

The cDNA sequence and biosynthetic pathway for human fibroblast stromelysin-1 has now been described (Wilhelm et al, 1987). It is synthesized as two proenzyme species, Mr 57 kD (unmodified) and Mr 60 kD (glycosylated); cleavage of the N-terminal 84 amino acids results in active stromelysin, Mr 45 kD, the properties of which are summarised in Table 1.

The cellular origin of stromelysin-1 in liver is unknown. An enzyme with similar properties is released by fibroblast-like cells derived originally from murine Schistosoma granuloma explants (Takahashi et al, 1981). By immunohistochemistry we have been unable to detect stromelysin-1 in primary cultures of human hepatic lipocytes. There is no published information about the synthesis of this enzyme in either intact normal or diseased human liver.

Other Metalloproteinases

There are several other metalloproteinases described (see Table 1) for which there is no information relevant to liver; these include neutrophil collagenase, stromelysins 2 and 3 and Pump-1. Of these, neutrophil collagenase is potentially interesting, particularly as neutrophil infiltrates are common in liver disease, e.g. alcoholic hepatitis.

Metalloproteinase Inhibitors

The properties of metalloproteinase inhibitors (TIMP-1 and TIMP-2) and α2-macroglobulin are described above (see Metalloproteinase Regulation). In liver, α2-macroglobulin is synthesized predominantly by hepatocytes, but rat hepatic lipocytes in primary culture also contain mRNA for, and synthesize, this proteinase scavenger (Andus et al, 1987). We have recently demonstrated that primary cultures of human hepatic lipocytes also contain mRNA for, and synthesize, TIMP-1 (unpublished observations). Regulatory signals for expression of α2-macroglobulin and TIMP-1 by hepatic lipocytes are currently unknown, but this is likely to be of major importance in regulating matrix degradation in liver.

CONCLUSIONS

The role of metalloproteinases and their inhibitors in liver fibrosis remains speculative. Recent data suggest that sinusoidal liver cells, particularly hepatic lipocytes and Kupffer cells, synthesize some, if not all, of the metalloproteinases and their inhibitors. Detailed future analysis of their expression in normal and diseased liver and investigation of the factors involved in regulating their synthesis by sinusoidal liver cell cultures may improve our understanding of the role of matrix metalloproteinases in liver fibrosis.

ACKNOWLEDGEMENTS

My thanks are extended to the Wellcome Trust and the Wessex Medical Trust for their support and to Mrs Barbara Thomas for preparation of this manuscript.

REFERENCES

Andus, T., Ramadori, G., Heinrich, P.C., Knittel, T. & Meyer Zum Buschenfelde, K.H. (1987): Cultured Ito cells of rat liver express the alpha2-macroglobulin gene. European Journal of Biochemistry, 168: 641-646.

Arthur, M.J.P, Friedman, S.L., Roll, F.J. and Bissell, D.M. (1989): Lipocytes from normal rat liver release a neutral metalloproteinase that degrades basement membrane (type IV) collagen. Journal of Clinical Investigation, 84: 1076-1085.

Arthur, M.J.P., Stanley, A.P., Iredale, J.P., Murphy, G., Hembry, R. and Friedman, S.L. (1991): Release of type IV collagenase by cultured human lipocytes; analysis of gene expression, protein synthesis and proteinase activity. Gastroenterology (Abstract). In press.

Bhatnagar, R., Schade, U., Rietschel, E.T. and Decker, K. (1982): Involvement of prostaglandin E and adenosine 3'5' - monophosphate in lipopolysaccharide-stimulated collagenase release by rat Kupffer cells. European Journal of Biochemistry, 124: 2405-2409.

Bissell, D.M., Arenson, D.M., Maher, J.J. & Roll, F.J. (1987): Support of cultured hepatocytes by a laminin-rich gel: evidence for a functionally significant subendothelial matrix in normal rat liver. Journal of Clinical Investigation, 79: 801-812.

Brenner, D.A., O'Hara, M., Angel, P., et al. (1989): Prolonged activation of jun and collagenase genes by tumour necrosis factor-alpha. Nature, 337: 661-663.

Carter, E.A., McCarron, M.J., Alpert, E. and Isselbacher, K.J. (1982): Lysyl oxidase and collagenase in experimental acute and chronic liver injury. Gastroenterology, 82: 526-534.

Chua, C.C., Geiman, D.E., Keller, G.H. and Ladda, R.L. (1985): Induction of collagenase secretion in human fibroblast cultures by growth promoting factors. Journal of Biological Chemistry, 260: 5213-5216.

Clark, S.D., Kobayashi, D.K. & Welgus, H.G. (1987): Regulation of the expression of tissue inhibitor of metalloproteinases and collagenase by retinoids and glucocorticoids in human fibroblasts. Journal of Clinical Investigation, 80: 1280-1288.

Collier, I.E., Wilhelm, S.M., Eisen, A.Z., et al. (1988): H-ras oncogene-transformed human bronchial epithelial cells (TBE-1) secrete a single metalloprotease capable of degrading basement membrane collagen. Journal of Biological Chemistry, 263: 6579-6587.

Edwards, D.R., Murphy, G., Reynolds, J.J., et al. (1987): Transforming growth factor beta modulates the expression of collagenase and metalloproteinase inhibitor. EMBO Journal, 6: 1899-1904.

Emonard, H., Guillouzo, A., Lapiere, Ch.M. and Grimaud, J.A. (1990): Human liver fibroblast capacity for synthesizing interstitial collagenase in vitro. Cellular and Molecular Biology, 36: 461-467.

Enghild, J.J., Salvesen, G., Brew K. and Nagase, H. (1989): Interaction of human rheumatoid synovial collagenase (matrix metalloproteinase 1) and stromelysin (matrix metalloproteinase 3) with human alpha-2-macroglobulin and chicken ovostatin. Journal of Biological Chemistry, 264: 8779-8785.

Friedman, S.L., Roll, F.J., Boyles, J., Arenson, D.M. and Bissell, D.M. (1989): Maintenance of differentiated phenotype of cultured rat hepatic lipocytes by basement membrane matrix. Journal of Biological Chemistry, 264: 10756-10762.

Fujiwara, K., Sakai, T., Oda, T., Igarashi, S. (1973): The presence of collagenase in Kupffer cells of the rat liver. Biochemical and Biophysical Research Communications, 54: 531-536.

Goldberg, G.I., Wilhelm, S.M., Kronberger, A., et al. (1986): Human fibroblast collagenase. Complete primary structure and homology to an oncogene transformation-induced rat protein. Journal of Biological Chemistry, 261: 6600-6605.

Goldberg, G.I., Marmer, B.L., Grant, G.A., Eisen, A.Z., Wilhelm, S. and He, C. (1989): Human 72-kilodalton type IV collagenase forms a complex with a tissue inhibitor of metalloproteases designated TIMP-2. Proceedings of the National Academy of Sciences, USA, 86: 8207-8211.

Gross, J. and Lapiere, C.M. (1962): Collagenolytic activity in amphibian tissues: a tissue culture assay. Proceedings of the National Academcy of Sciences, (USA), 48: 1014-1022.

Gruber, B.L., Marchese, M.J., Suzuki, K., Schwartz, L.B., Okada, Y., Nagase, H. and Ramamurthy, N.S. (1989): Synovial procollagenase activation by human mast cell tryptase dependence upon matrix metalloproteinase 3 activation. Journal of Clinical Investigation, 84: 1657-1662.

He, C., Wilhelm, S.M., Pentland, A.P., Marmer, B.L., Grant, G.A., Eisen, A.Z. and Goldberg, G.I. (1989): Tissue cooperation in a proteolytic cascade activating human interstitial collagenase. Proceedings of the National Academy of Sciences, USA, 86: 2632-2636.

Kashiwazaki, K., Hibbs, M.S., Seyer, J.M., et al. (1986): Stimulation of interstitial collagenase in co-cultures of rat hepatocytes and sinusoidal cells. Gastroenterology, 90: 829-36.

Liotta, L.A., Abe, S., Gehron-Robey, P. and Martin, G.R. (1979): Preferential digestion of basement membrane collagen by an enzyme derived from a metastatic murine tumour. Proceedings of the National Academy of Sciences, USA, 76: 2268-2272.

Maher, J.J., Bissell, D.M., Friedman, S.L. & Roll, F.J. (1988): Collagen measured in primary cultures of normal rat hepatocytes derives from lipocytes within the monolayer. Journal of Clinical Investigation, 82: 450-459.

Maruyama, K., Feinman, L., Okazaki, I., Lieber, C.S. (1981): Direct measurement of neutral collagenase activity in homogenates from baboon and human liver. Biochimica et Biophysica Acta, 658: 121-131.

Maruyama, K., Feinman, L., Fainsilber, Z., et al. (1982): Mammalian collagenase increases in early alcoholic liver disease and decreases with cirrhosis. Life Science, 30: 1379-1384.

Maruyama, K., Okazaki, I., Kobayashi, T., et al. (1983): Collagenase production by rabbit liver cells in monolayer culture. Journal of Laboratory and Clinical Medicine, 102: 543-550.

Matrisian, L.M. (1990): Metalloproteinases and their inhibitors in matrix remodelling. Trends in Genetics, 6: 121-125.

McCarthy, J.B., Wahl, S.M., Rees, J.C., et al. (1980): Mediation of macrophage collagenase production by 3'-5' cyclic adenosine monophosphate. Journal of Immunology, 124: 2405-2409.

Murphy, G., Cawston, T.E. and Reynolds, J.J. (1981): An inhibitor of collagenase from human amniotic fluid. Purification, characterisation and action on metalloproteinases. Biochemical Journal, 195: 167-170.

Murphy, G., Reynolds, J.J. and Werb, Z. (1985a): Biosynthesis of tissue inhibitor of metalloproteinases by human fibroblasts in tissue culture. Stimulation by 12-0-tetradecanoylphorbol-13-acetate and interleukin 1 in parallel with collagenase. Journal of Biological Chemistry, 260: 3079-3083.

Murphy, G., McAlpine, C.G., Poll, C.T. and Reynolds, J.J. (1985b): Purification and characterisation of a bone metalloproteinase that degrades gelatin and types IV and V collagen. Biochimica et Biophysica Acta, 831: 49-58.

Murphy, G., Lockett, M.I., Stephens, P.E., et al. (1987): Stromelysin is an activator of procollagenase. A study with natural and recombinant enzymes. Biochemical Journal, 248: 265-268.

Nagai, Y., Hori, H., Hata, R.I., et al. (1982): Collagenase production by adult rat hepatocytes in primary culture. Biomedical Research, 3: 345-349.

Nagase, H., Jackson, R.C., Brinckerhoff, C.E., et al. (1981): A precursor form of latent collagenase produced in a cell free system with mRNA from rabbit synovial cells. Journal of Biological Chemistry, 256: 11951-11954.

Nagase, H., Brinckerhoff, C.E., Vater, C.A. and Harris, E.D. (1983): Biosynthesis and secretion of procollagenase by rabbit synovial fibroblasts. Inhibition of procollagenase secretion by monensin and evidence for glycosallation of procollagenase. Biochemical Journal, 214: 281-288.

Okada, Y. and Nakanishi I. (1989): Activation of matrix metalloproteinase 3 (stromelysin) and matrix metalloproteinase 2 ('gelatinase') by human neutrophil elastase and cathepsin G. FEBS Letters, 249: 353-356.

Okazaki, I., Maruyama, K. (1974): Collagenase activity in experimental hepatic fibrosis. Nature, 252: 49-50.

Overall, C.M., Wrana, J.L. and Sodek, J. (1989): Independent regulation of collagenase, 72-kDa progelatinase and metalloproteinase inhibitor expression in human fibroblasts by transforming growth factor-beta. Journal of Biological Chemistry, 264: 1860-1869.

Perez-Tamayo, R., Montfort, I. and Gonzalez, E. (1987): Collagenolytic activity in experimental cirrhosis of the liver. Experimental and Molecular Pathology, 47: 300-308.

Rojkind, M., Takahashi, S. and Giambrone, M.A. (1978): Collagenase and reversible hepatic fibrosis in the rat. (Abstr) Gastroenterology, 75: 984.

Saari, H., Suomalainen, K., Lindy, O., Konttinen, Y.T. and Sorsa, T. (1990): Activation of latent human neutrophil collagenase by reactive oxygen species and serine proteases. Biochemical and Biophysical Research, 171: 979-987.

Shapiro, S.D., Campbell, E.J., Kobayashi, D.K. and Welgus, H.G. (1990): Immune modulation of metalloproteinase production in human macrophages. Selective pretranslational suppression of interstitial collagenase and stromelysin biosynthesis by interferon-gamma. Journal of Clinical Investigation, 86: 1204-1210.

Stetler-Stevenson, W.G., Krutzsch, H.C., Wacher, M.P., Margulies, I.M.K. and Liotta, L.A. (1989a): The activation of human type IV collagenase proenzyme. Sequence identification of the major conversion product following organomercurial activation. Journal of Biological Chemistry, 264: 1353-1356.

Stetler-Stevenson, W.G., Krutzsch, H.C. and Liotta, L.A. (1989b): Tissue inhibitor of metalloproteinase (TIMP-2). Journal of Biological Chemistry, 264: 17374-17378.

Stetler-Stevenson, W.G., Brown, P.D., Onisto, M., Levy, A.T. and Liotta, L.A. (1990): Tissue inhibitor of metalloproteinases-2 (TIMP-2) mRNA expression in tumor cell lines and human tumor tissues. Journal of Biological Chemistry, 265: 13933-13938.

Takahashi, S., Dunn, M.A. and Seifter, S. (1980): Liver collagenase in murine schistosomiasis. Gastroenterology, 78: 1425-1431.

Takahashi, S. and Simpser, E. (1981): Granuloma collagenase and EDTA-sensitive neutral protease production in hepatic murine schistosomiasis. Hepatology, 1: 211-220.

Takahashi, S. and Koda, K. (1984): Radioimmunoassay of soluble and insoluble collageanses in fibrotic liver. Biochemical Journal, 220: 157-164.

Truden, J.L. and Boros, D.L. (1988): Detection of alpha2-macroglobulin, alpha1-protease inhibitor, and neutral protease-antiprotease complexes with liver granulomas of Schistosoma mansoni-infected mice. American Journal of Pathology, 130: 281-288.

Van Wart, H.E. and Birkedal-Hansen H. (1990): The cysteine switch: A principle of regulation of metalloproteinase activity with potential applicability to the entire matrix metalloproteinase gene family. Proceedings of the National Academy of Sciences, USA, 87: 5578-5582.

Wahl, L.M., Wahl, S.M., Mergenhagen, S.E. and Martin, G.R. (1974): Collagenase production by endotoxin-activated macrophages. Proceedings of the National Academy of Sciences, USA, 71: 3598-3601.

Wahl, L.M., Wahl, S.M., Mergenhagen, S.E. and Martin, G.R. (1975): Collagenase production by lymphokine-activated macrophages. Science, 187: 261-263.

Wahl, L.M., Olsen, C.E., Sandberg, A.L. and Mergenhagen, S.E. (1977): Prostaglandin regulation of macrophage collagenase production. Proceedings of the National Academy of Sciences, USA, 74: 4955-4958.

Werb, Z. (1978): Biochemical actions of glucocorticoids on macrophages in culture. Specific inhibition of elastase, collagenase and plasminogen activator secretion, and effects on other metabolic functions. Journal of Experimental Medicine, 147: 1695-1712.

Wilhelm, S.M., Collier, I.E., Kronberger, A., et al. (1987): Human skin fibroblast stromelysin; structure, glycosylation, substrate specificity, and differential expression in normal and tumorigenic cells. Proceedings of the National Academy of Sciences, USA, 84: 6725-6729.

Wilhelm, S.M., Collier, I.E., Marmer, B.L., Eisen, A.Z., Grant, G.A., Goldberg, G.I. (1989): SV40-transformed human lung fibroblasts secrete a 92kD Da type IV collagenase which is identical to that secreted by normal human macrophages. Journal of Biological Chemistry, 264: 17213-17221.

Winwood, P.J., Kowalski-Saunders, P.S., Arthur, M.J.P. (1991): Kupffer cells release a 92 kD metalloproteinase with degradative activity against gelatin. Gut (Abstract). In press.

Résumé

La fibrose hépatique est un processus dynamique qui peut impliquer des altérations de la synthèse et de la dégradation des protéines matricielles. Le rôle de la dégradation de la matrice au cours de la fibrose hépatique est mal connu mais des données récentes montrent que plusieurs métalloprotéinases matricielles peuvent être concernées.

Les métalloprotéinases matricielles sont classées en 3 grands groupes selon le type de substrat : les collagénases qui dégradent les collagènes intersticiels (types I, II et III), les stromélysines qui dégradent un large spectre de substrats qui incluent des protéoglycanes, la laminine, des gélatines et la fibronectine, et les collagénases/gélatinases de type IV qui dégradent le collagène des lames basales (type IV) et des gélatines. La régulation des métalloprotéinases peut se situer à 3 niveaux : altérations de la transcription génique, activation des proenzymes sécrétées et inhibition des métalloprotéinases par le TIMP (l'inhibiteur tissulaire des métallo-protéinases) ou l'α_2-macroglobuline.

Dans le foie il est admis que les lipocytes (fat-storing cells ou cellules de Ito) et les cellules de Kupffer jouent un rôle primordial dans la synthèse et la régulation des métalloprotéinases matricielles. Les lipocytes activés produisent une collagénase/gélatinase de type IV de 72 KD et probablement une collagénase intersticielle. Des travaux récents réalisés dans notre laboratoire montrent qu'ils secrétent également le TIMP. Les cellules de Kupffer, quant à elles, synthétisent une collagénase/gélatinase de type IV de 92 KD et peuvent en outre produire une collagénase intersticielle et une variété de cytokines impliquées dans la régulation des métalloprotéinases. Les cellules sinusoïdales hépatiques ont donc la capacité de dégrader et de réguler la dégradation de non seulement la matrice extracellulaire normale mais également les collagènes intersticiels fibrillaires qui sont déposés au cours de la fibrose. Au total, si un rôle important des métalloprotéinases est encore spéculatif, des arguments théoriques s'accumulent néanmoins.

Cellular and Molecular Aspects of Cirrhosis. Eds B. Clément, A. Guillouzo. Colloque INSERM/John Libbey Eurotext Ltd. © 1992, Vol. 216, pp. 245-254

Regulatory signals in liver regeneration

Reza Zarnegar

Department of Pathology, University of Pittsburgh Medical Center, Pittsburgh, PA 15261, USA

A central challenge in modern cell biology is understanding cell growth and differentiation at the molecular level. A spectacular example of controlled tissue growth is regeneration of the liver. This can be induced experimentally by chemical treatment or by surgical removal of the liver in intact animals. *In vitro*, isolated hepatocytes have been used to identify and study different regulatory substances for hepatocyte growth. Using this system, several polypeptide growth factors such as Epidermal Growth Factor (EGF), Transforming Growth Factor α (TGFα), Hepatocyte Growth Factor (HGF, also known as Hepatopoietin A--HPTA), acidic and basic Fibroblast Growth Factors (FGFs), Transforming Growth Factor β, (TGFβ), and cytokines like Interleukin 1 and 6 have been identified as either potent mitogenic or mitoinhibitory substances for hepatocytes. Our studies have focused on Hepatocyte Growth Factor (HGF) and its role in liver regeneration. Using HGF-specific molecular probes such as antibodies and a cDNA clone, we have analyzed temporal expression of HGF in normal and regenerating rat livers. Levels of immunoreactive HGF rapidly increase and peak within 2 to 6 hr in the plasma of rats treated with carbon tetrachloride (CCl_4) or in the plasma of rats that have undergone partial hepatectomy. This release of HGF in the plasma is followed by a marked increase in the HGF mRNA in the liver of treated animals which gradually peaks by 12 hr post-treatment and returns to the background levels by 72 hr. Immunohistological analyses of liver sections from these animals reveal that there are no apparent differences between the livers of partially hepatectomized and normal animals immunostained for HGF. Meanwhile, in CCl_4 animals, a marked increase in the immunoreactive HGF is noted in liver sections of animals 24 hr post-administration. HGF immunostaining is localized to the damaged or necrotic hepatocytes surrounding the central veins. This may suggest an autocrine role for HGF in liver regeneration after hepatotoxin injury.

We have recently shown that HGF exerts its mitogenic effect on hepatocytes through a specific cell-surface receptor with Mr of 160,000 which may be the proto-oncogene product c-MET. Abnormal or lack of functional HGF receptor may result in the inability of the liver to regenerate or may contribute to malignancy. In this context, we are currently analyzing the expression of c-MET in regenerating liver. How HGF, its receptor and other polypeptide growth factors affect liver regeneration is further presented.

INTRODUCTION

During the last several years, investigators including ourselves have reported the presence of a large molecular weight hepatomitogenic substance in the serum and plasma of rats and humans and have consequently attempted to isolate and characterize this factor. It has been referred to by different names such as Hepatotropin (Nakamura, *et al*, 1984; Selden, *et al*, 1989) and Hepatopoietin A (Michalopoulos, *et al*, 1984; Zarnegar, *et al*, 1989); however, the name that is most used is Hepatocyte Growth Factor--HGF (Nakamura, *et al*, 1987). Recent advances in techniques such as protein purification and microsequencing combined with advances in molecular biology techniques like cDNA cloning and DNA sequencing have facilitated the characterization of HGF. At the present time, HGF has been purified to homogeneity while its primary structure has been deduced from its cDNA nucleotide sequence by several laboratories (Miyazawa, *et al*,1989; Nakamura, *et al*, 1989). The expression of HGF in normal rabbit and rat tissues as well as tissues from hepatectomized or hepatotoxin-treated rats have been studied (Kinoshita, *et al*, 1989; Zarnegar, *et al*, 1990; Noji, *et al*, 1990; Selden, *et al*, 1990; Okajima, *et al*, 1990; Zarnegar, *et al*, 1991). In addition, HGF has been found in the sera of patients with various liver diseases such as fulminant hepatic failure suggesting a role for HGF in hepatic regeneration (Tsubouchi, *et al*, 1991). Within the past year, it also became clear that HGF is mitogenic for cells other than hepatocytes (Kan, *et al*, 1991; Rubin, *et al*, 1991) and that it has additional biological activities such as promoting the migration of epithelial cells (Gherardi and Stoker, 1990). Therefore, recent studies have focussed on determining the physiological role of HGF, especially in liver growth and regeneration.

Biochemical Properties of HGF Hepatocyte growth factor (HGF) also known as Hepatopoietin-A is a heparin-binding glycoprotein with Mr of 100,000 as determined by SDS-PAGE. HGF's affinity for heparin has facilitated its purification from various sources by heparin affinity chromatography (Nakamura, *et al*, 1987; Zarnegar, *et al*, 1989a). Comparison of the partial amino acid sequence of rabbit Hepatopoietin A (Zarnegar, *et al*, 1989b) with that of human HGF (Miyazawa, *et al*, 1989) confirmed that these two growth factors are indeed the same molecular species; thus, HPTA is now referred to as HGF. Purified HGF isolated from plasma, serum or platelets migrates as a heterodimer with Mr of 65,000 (heavy chain) and 35,000 (light chain) on SDS-PAGE under reducing conditions (Nakamura, *et al*, 1987; Gohda, *et al*,1988; Zarnegar, *et al*, 1989a). However, HGF purified from human placenta mainly consists of single chain HGF (Hernandez, *et al*, 1991). The primary structure of HGF as deduced by Nakamura, *et al* (1989) from HGF's cDNA nucleotide sequence indicates that both heavy and light chains of HGF are encoded in a single open reading frame. Proteolytic cleavage at the Arg-Val site located at the end of the heavy chain and at the beginning of the light chain is believed to be responsible for the generation of the mature heterodimeric form of HGF. Our preliminary results have indicated that neither tissue plasminogen activator nor urokinase which specifically cleave proteins at Arg-Val sites are able to cleave single chain HGF purified from placenta. Identification of an enzyme which cleaves HGF at the Arg-Val site and the enzyme's possible role in the activation of HGF may provide valuable insight into the mechanism(s) by which HGF functions. For further information on the biochemical and molecular properties of HGF, see Nakamura, *et al* (1989).

Biological effects of HGF Addition of HGF at nanogram concentrations to primary cultures of hepatocytes in chemically defined medium and in the absence of serum and insulin stimulates DNA synthesis (up to 80% labeling index). The addition of EGF and insulin or norepinephrine and insulin to HGF-containing hepatocyte cultures results in an even greater labeling index. Twenty-four hours after incubation of hepatocytes with HGF, a drastic change in the morphological appearance of the hepatocytes is noted which is probably due to rearrangement of cytoskeletal elements. As with EGF-stimulated hepatocyte cultures, DNA synthesis begins 24 hours after the addition of HGF to freshly isolated hepatocytes and peaks at 36-48 hr. Recently, we have shown that HGF is mitogenic for cells such as mouse keratinocytes, human melanoma cells, non-parenchymal liver epithelial cells, and rat proximal tubule epithelial cells. Human foreskin fibroblasts and umbilical vein endothelial cells, meanwhile, were unresponsive. HGF can also induce anchorage-independent growth of a SV40 transformed rat proximal tubule epithelial cells and can induce a transformed phenotype in these cells (Kan, *et al*, 1991; Rubin, *et al*, 1991). We have also shown that, in addition to stimulating DNA synthesis, HGF stimulates protein synthesis in hepatocytes. Both of these activities are suppressed in the presence of TGFß; however, DNA synthesis is suppressed to a much greater extent than protein synthesis (Zarnegar, *et al*, 1989a; Hernandez, *et al*, 1991).

Distribution of HGF in tissues and cells The development of an HGF-specific polyclonal antibody in a chicken has enabled us to study the tissue distribution of HGF by immunohistochemistry. We demonstrated strong cytoplasmic HGF immunoreactivity in most surface epithelia, large neurons, distal tubules and collecting ducts of the kidney, salivary glands, thyroid glands, prostate gland, epididymis, trophoblast, megakaryocytes, granulocytes, macrophages, small intestine, exocrine pancreas, endothelial cells and Kupffer's cells. In addition, considerable amounts of HGF can be purified from most of the tissues that stain positive for HGF. On the other hand, parathyroid, adrenal medulla, hepatocytes, lymphocytes, myocytes, glial cells, and most fibroblasts were negative for HGF staining (Zarnegar, *et al*, 1990a; Wolf, *et al*, 1991). The expression of HGF mRNA in other normal tissues such as kidney, lung, brain and spleen using northern blot analysis has been reported (Tashiro, *et al*, 1990; Okajima, *et al*, 1990).

The HGF receptor and signal transduction In earlier studies, we demonstrated that HGF does not compete with radiolabeled EGF or aFGF for binding to hepatocytes indicating that the receptor for HGF is distinct. Our recent investigations using ^{125}I-HGF and intact hepatocytes in culture showed that HGF binds to hepatocytes through a specific cell-surface receptor (Zarnegar, *et al*, 1990b). One binding site with a relatively low affinity is apparently the result of HGF binding to heparin or heparin-like molecules on the cell surface while a second specific site with high affinity is most likely the actual receptor for HGF. Scatchard analysis revealed an apparent Kd of 3.5 nM with 120,000 sites per cell for the latter, specific cell-surface receptor. The importance of the low affinity heparin-like site in the modulation of HGF activity or as a possible storage site for HGF deserves further investigation. [As it has recently been shown by Masumoto, *et al* (1991), a large amount of bioactive HGF-like molecule is present in the extracellular matrix of the liver. The HGF-like substance associated with the liver matrix was eluted with 1 M NaCl by *in situ* perfusion. This suggests an additional storage location for HGF.] When the affinity cross-linked radio-labeled HGF/receptor complex was analyzed by SDS-PAGE, the Mr of the receptor was estimated to be 150,000. It is of interest to note that in the presence of heparin, biological activity of HGF as well as its binding to hepatocytes is drastically reduced as opposed to the biological activity of aFGF which requires heparin for activation. Since HGF is also present in the plasma, it is reasonable to postulate that it may exist complexed in an inactive form with heparin or another carrier protein [Under physiological conditions, the Mr of HGF is greater than 200,000 as determined by gel filtration HPLC (Zarnegar, *et al*, 1989a).] In a collaborative work with Dr. P. Comoglio at the University of Torino in Italy, we found that HGF stimulates the tyrosine kinase activity of the c-MET proto-oncogene. This proto-oncogene encodes a heterodimeric transmembrane protein with an Mr of 190,000 which has the structural features of a tyrosine kinase receptor. No other growth factor or ligand is known to activate this receptor (Naldini, *et al*, 1991). Similar studies by Bottaro, *et al* (1991) have indicated that HGF does indeed activate the kinase of the c-MET proto-oncogene, and a smaller form of HGF which was referred to as "P28 HGF" was affinity cross-linked to c-MET (Bottaro, *et al*, 1991). Based on these results, Bottaro, *et al*, concluded that c-MET is the receptor for HGF. The possibility of other receptors existing for HGF, however, is still questioned. The lack of functional HGF receptors may result in liver diseases such as fulminant hepatic failure since plasma HGF levels in most of the patients suffering from this disease are substantially greater than normal individuals which may suggest that HGF is not being removed from circulation by its receptor on hepatocytes. Therefore, identification and characterization of the HGF receptor(s) may increase our understanding of liver regeneration and liver diseases. Neither the exact fate of the HGF/receptor complex nor the pathway by which HGF transduce its mitogenic signal to the nucleus is known at the present time. Most likely, some early events such as Ca^{++} mobilization and activation of cell-cycle dependent genes such as c-FOS, c-JUN, and c-MYC proto-oncogenes occurs. These studies, as well as studies exploring the temporal expression of HGF receptor during liver regeneration, are currently under investigation in our laboratory.

Role of HGF in liver regeneration Earlier studies have shown that liver regeneration is associated with the appearance of hepatocyte mitogen(s) in the peripheral blood (Grisham, *et al*, 1964; Fisher *et al*, 1971). To date, only one such substance, namely HGF, has been identified; it has been purified to homogeneity and characterized in detail. Despite the significant progress in the biochemical characterization of HGF, its direct role as a physiological mediator of liver regeneration remains to be conclusively established. Studies in our laboratory as well as in others using HGF-specific antibodies or cDNA probes on tissues of animals with damaged livers indicate a temporal change in the HGF protein and its mRNA expression. We showed that the amount of immunoreactive HGF in the plasma of rats markedly increases within 2 hr post-hepatectomy or post-administration of the hepatotoxin, carbon tetrachloride (CCl_4). The elevation of HGF slowly returns to normal levels after 72 hr (Lindroos, *et al*, 1991). Immunohistological staining of the CCl_4-treated rat liver sections taken 24 hr post treatment indicates strong immunoreactivity in damaged hepatocytes with anti-HGF antiserum. Whether this is due to an enhanced uptake of HGF by damaged hepatocytes or actual HGF expression remains to be defined. The rapid elevation of HGF in the plasma (1-6 hr) may be due to the release of this growth factor already present in the liver extracellular matrix (Masumoto and Yamamoto, 1991) or due to the release from other tissues mentioned earlier which are known to contain substantial amounts of HGF (Zarnegar, *et al*, 1990a). These include the pancreas, salivary glands, small intestine, thyroid, and brain. In fact, Okajima, *et al* (1990) reported a substantial increase in HGF mRNA expression in the liver and spleen of hepatotoxin-treated rats. Therefore, it is conceivable that HGF from these tissues (in an endocrine fashion) as well as HGF synthesized by the liver (non-parenchymal cells such as endothelial cells and Kupffer's cells [Noji et al, 1990] in a paracrine fashion) triggers hepatocyte proliferation.

We have also examined the expression of HGF mRNA in hepatectomized rats. We found that HGF mRNA levels in liver remnants dramatically rise 3 to 6 hr post-operation, peak at 12 hr (more than 20 fold) and gradually return to undetectable levels by 72 to 96 hr post hepatectomy (Zarnegar, *et al*, 1991). We also measured DNA synthesis activity (*in vivo*) in the liver remnants of rats that underwent partial hepatectomy. It is of interest to note that hepatic DNA synthesis peaks at 24 hours post-hepatectomy, 12 hours after the peak of HGF mRNA synthesis (and/or its stabilization). Our results confirm the findings of Selden, *et al.* (1990), who also detected a significant rise in HGF mRNA levels in liver remnants which peak by 10 hours post hepatectomy. Two separate laboratories have reported an increase in the HGF mRNA in the liver of *hepatotoxin-treated* rats by 10 hr post treatment, but they did not see a significant change in HGF mRNA levels in the livers of *hepatectomized* rats (Kinoshita, *et al*, 1989; Okajima, *et al*, 1990). Perhaps, it is possible that Okajima, *et al.*, were unable to detect changes in HGF mRNA levels after hepatectomy due to the fact that they analyzed HGF mRNA starting 24 hours after surgery, a time when HGF mRNA levels are already declining. As previously mentioned, the levels of HGF also rise in the sera of patients with fulminant hepatic failure or other liver diseases such as acute and chronic hepatitis and cirrhosis (Tsubouchi, *et al*, 1991). Taken together, these results indicate an *in vivo* role for HGF in maintaining hepatocyte proliferation and viability.

Other growth factors possibly involved in liver regeneration Although a comprehensive discussion of other regulatory molecules (such as Insulin, Glucagon, Norepinephrine, Vasopressin, Angiotensin, and Estrogen) and signals involved in hepatocyte proliferation and liver regeneration is beyond the scope of this article, interested individuals are referred to a recent review by Michalopoulos, 1990 and Koch et al, 1990. Instead, only three of the well-known polypeptide mitogens, namely TGFα , EGF and aFGF, will be discussed.

In addition to HGF, EGF/TGFα, and FGFs (acidic and basic) are also potent inducers of hepatocyte DNA synthesis in serum-free chemically defined medium (McGowan, *et al*, 1981; Mead and Fausto, 1989; Kan, *et al*, 1989). Indeed, a combination of EGF and insulin when injected into intact animals can induce liver DNA synthesis (Bucher, *et al*, 1982). Unlike HGF, these growth factors are not known to be circulating in substantial amounts in the blood and are believed to act locally at the site of action. This is especially noted with EGF; the level of EGF in the serum of hepatectomized rats does not change, and EGF is not produced by the liver. However, TGFα which is a potent hepatomitogen and shares the same receptor with EGF is known to be made by hepatocytes. The levels of TGFα mRNA in liver also increase by 8 hr and peak at 24 hr post-hepatectomy. This peak coincides with the peak of hepatocyte DNA synthesis (Mead and Fausto, 1989). Based on these kinetic data, it seems unlikely that TGFα per se is responsible for the transition of hepatocytes from the static state, G_0, to the G_1 phase of the cell cycle. We previously showed that aFGF in the presence of heparin is a potent hepatocyte mitogen (Houck, *et al*, 1990). A detailed study by Kan, *et al* (1989) demonstrated that aFGF protein and its mRNA are expressed in hepatocytes and in non-parenchymal cells after partial hepatectomy. The elevation of FGF mRNA reached 80% of the maximum level by 4 hr post operation, peaked by 24 hr and persisted up to 7 days in the liver (Kan, *et al*, 1989). Based on these findings, we suggest that the following events occur during liver regeneration in animal models with hepatic injury:

(1) An initial rise in the plasma HGF levels (2-6 hr post-treatment) originating from hepatic (bound to extracellular matrix) and extrahepatic sources such as the pancreas and the small intestine induce hepatocytes in a paracrine/endocrine fashion through an HGF-specific receptor to enter the cell cycle. It is possible that HGF may be chemotactic attracting macrophages to the site of injury. These macrophages (Kupffer's cells) in turn may produce HGF and possibly aFGF.

(2) A second wave of HGF synthesis occurs as indicated by a marked increase in HGF mRNA in the liver which peaks 12 hr post-treatment. This HGF further sustains the stimulation of hepatocyte DNA synthesis and hepatocyte expansion. The source of HGF may be the non-parenchymal cells such as Kupffer's cells and endothelial cells as reported by Noji, *et al* (1990) who used *in situ* hybridization to detect HGF mRNA in the liver sections of CCl_4 treated rats. It is not yet clear whether hepatocytes are also synthesizing HGF.

(3) Other growth factors such as TGFα, aFGF and possibly bFGF and which are produced locally by hepatocytes or non-parenchymal cells may also act in an autocrine/paracrine fashion to transmit mitogenic stimuli to hepatocytes and to non-parenchymal cells such as bile duct epithelial cells, Ito cells, endothelial cells, and Kupffer's cells whose peak of DNA synthesis is 48 hr post-hepatectomy. Whether the initial increase in plasma HGF levels enhance the expression of these growth factors and/or their receptors, or its own expression in the liver remains to be investigated. As mentioned above, TGFß is a potent inhibitor of HGF-,

EGF/TGFα-, and FGF-induced mitogenesis in hepatocytes, and TGFß's mRNA expression peaks at 72 hr post hepatectomy; therefore, it is conceivable that TGFß may be involved in tempering or terminating liver regeneration. It should be emphasized that no growth or tropic factor alone can be responsible for liver regeneration; rather, several factors are most likely involved in creating a cascade of events that lead to restoration of liver mass.

CONCLUSION

Studies that have focused on liver regeneration have brought insight to the integrated mechanisms of growth factors, their receptors and other related cytokines that influence cell growth. One polypeptide growth factor in particular, Hepatocyte Growth Factor, appears to be intrinsically involved in hepatocyte proliferation. Future studies using HGF transgenic mice (including gene targeting by which the HGF gene is deliberately destroyed) may provide models for understanding the role of this growth factor in normal adult and embryonic development and its pathobiology in liver growth and neoplasia.

ACKNOWLEDGEMENTS

Special thanks should be given to George Michalopoulos, Marie C. DeFrances, Bryon Petersen, and Pamela Lindroos for their critical and technical support during the preparation of this work. This project was supported by National Institutes of Health Grants CA43632, CA35373, and CA30241.

REFERENCES

Bottaro, DP, Rubin, JS, Faletto, DL, Chan, A M-L, Kmiecik, TE, Vande Woude, GF, and Aaronson, SA (1991): Identification of the Hepatocyte Growth Factor Receptor as the c-MET proto-oncogene product *Science* 251: 802-804

Bucher, NLR (1972) Thirty years of liver regeneration: a distillate. In *Cold Spring Harbor Conferences on Cell Proliferation* Vol. 9 Growth of cell in chemically defined media, p. 15-26

Gherardi, E, and Stoker, M (1990): Hepatocytes and Scatter Factor. *Nature* 346: 228

Gohda, E., Tsubouchi, H., Nakayama, H., Hirono, S., Takahashi, K., Koura, M., Hoshomoto, M., and Dikuhara, Y. (1986): Human Hepatocyte Growth Factor in plasma from patients with hepatic failure. *Exp. Cell Res.* 166: 139-150.

Gohda, E., Tsubouchi, H., Nakayama, H., Hirono, S., Takahashi, K., and Myazaki, K., (1988): Partial purification and characterization of hepatocyte growth factor from plasma of patients with fulminant hepatic failure. *J. Clin. Invest.* 81: 414-419.

Grisham, J.W. (1962): A morphological study of deoxyribonucleic acid synthesis and cell proliferation in regenerating liver, autoradiography with ^{3}H-thymidine. *Cancer Res.* 22: 842-849.

Grisham, J.W., Leong, G.F., and Hole, B.V. (1964): Heterotropic partial autotransplantation of rat liver. Technique and demonstration of structure and function of the graft. *Cancer Res.* 24: 1474-1501.

Hernandez, J, Zarnegar, R, Strom, S, and Michalopoulos, GK: Characterization of the effects of human placental HGF/HPTA on hepatocytes from rat (normal and regenerating) and human liver. Submitted

Houck, K, Zarnegar, R, Muga, S, and Michalopoulos, GK (1990): Acidic Fibroblast Growth Factor (HBGF-1) stimulates DNA synthesis in primary rat hepatocyte cultures *J. of Cell Phys.* 143: 129-132

Jirtle, R.L., and Michalopoulos, G.K. (1982): Effects of partial hepatectomy on transplanted hepatocytes. *Cancer Res.* 42: 3000-3004.

Kan, M., Huang, J., Mansson, P., Yasumitsu, H., Carr, B., and McKeehan, W (1989): Heparin-binding growth factor type 1: A potential biphasic autocrine and paracrine regulator of hepatocyte regeneration. *Proc. Natl. Acad. Sci., USA* 86: 7434-7436.

Kan, M., Zhang, Zarnegar, R., Michalopoulos, G.K., Myoken, Y., McKeehan, W and Stevens, J.L. (1991): Hepatocyte growth factor/Hepatopoietin A stimulates the growth of rat kidney proximal tubule epithelial cells, rat non-parenchymal liver cells, human melanoma cells, mouse keratinocytes and stimulates anchorage independent growth of SV-40 transformed rat liver epithelial cells. *Biochem. Biophys. Res. Commun.* 174: 331-337.

Kinoshita, T., Tashiro, K., and Nakamura, T. (1989): Marked increase of HGF mRNA in non-parenchymal liver cells of rats treated with hepatotoxins *Biochem. Biophys. Res. Commun.* 165, 1229-1234.

Koch, K.S., Lu, X.P., Brenner, D.A., Fey, G.H., Martinez-Conde, A., and Leffert, H.L. (1990): Mitogens and hepatocyte growth control *in vivo* and *in vitro*. *In Vitro Cell. Dev.* 26: 1011-1023.

Lindroos, P., Zarnegar, R. and Michalopoulos, G.K. (1991): Hepatocyte Growth Factor (Hepatopoietin A) rapidly increases in plasma before DNA synthesis and liver regeneration stimulated by partial hepatectomy and carbon tetrachloride administration *Hepatology* 13: 743-750.

Masumoto, A, and Yamamoto, N. (1991): Sequestration of a hepatocyte growth factor in extracellular matrix in normal adult rat liver. *Biochem.Biophys.Res. Commun.* 174: 90-95.

McGowan, JA, Strain, AJ, and Bucher, NLR (1981): DNA synthesis in primary cultures of adult rat hepatocytes in a defined medium: effects of epidermal growth factor, insulin, glucagon, and cyclic-AMP *J. Cell. Phys* 180: 353-363

Mead, J.E., and Fausto, N. (1989): Transforming growth factor type α (TGFα) may be a physiological regulator of liver regeneration. *Proced. Natl. Acad Sci., USA* 86: 1558-1562.

Michalopoulos, G.K., Houck, K.A., Dolan, M., and Luetteke, N. (1984): Control of hepatocyte proliferation by two serum factors. *Cancer Res.* 44: 4414-4419.

Michalopoulos, G. (1990): Liver regeneration: Molecular mechanisms of growth control. *FASEB J.* 4: 176-187.

Miyazawa, K., Tsubouchi, H., Naka, D., Takahashi, K., Okigaki, M., Arakaki,, H., Hirono, S., Sakiyama, O., Gohda, E., Daikuhara, Y., and Kitamura, N. (1989): Molecular cloning and sequence analysis of cDNA for human hepatocyte growth factor *Bioch. Biophys. Res. Commun.* 163: 967-973.

Moolten, C.G. and Bucher, N.R. (1971): Regeneration of rat liver: Transfer of a humoral agent across circulation. *Science* 158: 272-274.

Nakamura, T., Nawa, K., and Ichihara, A. (1984): Partial purification and characterization of hepatocyte growth factor from serum of hepatectomized rats. *Biochem. Biophys. Res. Commun.* 122: 1450-1459.

Nakamura, T., Nawa, K., Ichihara, A., Kasie, A., and Nishino, T. (1987): Subunit structure of hepatocyte growth factor from rat platelets *FEBS. Lett.* 224: 311-318.

Nakamura, T., Nishizawa, T., Hagiya, M., Seki, T., Shimonish, M., Sugimura, A., Tashiro, K., and Shimizu, T. (1989): Molecular cloning and expression of hepatocyte growth factor *Nature* 342: 440-443.

Naldini, L, Vigna, E, Narsimhan, R, Guadino, G, Zarnegar, R, Michalopoulos, G, and Comoglio, P. (1991): Hepatocyte Growth Factor stimulates the tyrosine kinase activity of the receptor encoded by the proto-oncogene, c-MET *Oncogene* In press

Noji, S., Tashiro, K., Koyama, E., Nohno, T., Ohyama, K., Taniguchi, S., and Nakamura, T. (1990): Expression of Hepatocyte Growth Factor gene in endothelial and Kupffer's cells of damaged rat livers as revealed by *in situ* hybridization *Biochem. Biophys. Res. Commun.* 173: 42-47.

Okajima, A., Miyazawa, K., and Kitamura, N (1990): Primary structure of rat Hepatocyte Growth Factor and induction of its mRNA during liver regeneration following hepatic injury *Eur. J. Biochem.* 193: 375-381.

Rubin, J.S., Chan, M.L., Bottaro, D., Burgess, W., Taylor,W.J., Cech, A.C., Hirschfield D.W.,Wong, J., Miki, T., Finch, P., and Aaronson, T. (1991): A broad -spectrum human lung fibroblast-derived mitogen is a variant of hepatocyte growth factor *Proc. Natl. Acad. Sci., USA* 88: 415-419.

Selden, C., and Hodgson H.J.F (1989): Further characterization of hepatotropin, a high molecular weight hepatotrophic factor in rat serum. *J. of Hepatology* 9: 167-176.

Selden, C., Jones, M., Wade, D., and Hudgson, M. (1990): Hepatotropin mRNA expression in foetal liver development and in liver regeneration *FEBS Lett.* 270: 81-84.

Tashiro, K., Hagiya, M., Hishizawa, T., Seki, T.,Shimonishi, M., Shimizu, S., and Nakamura , T. (1990): Deduced primary structure of rat hepatocyte growth factor and expression of the mRNA in rat tissues. *Proc. Natl. Acad. Sci., USA* 87, 3200-3204

Tsubouchi, H, Hirono, S, Gohda, E, Nakayama, H, Takahashi, K, Sakiyama, O, Miyazaki, H, Sugihara, J, Tomita, E, Muto, Y, Daikuhara, Y, and Hashimoto, S (1989): Clinical significance of human Hepatocyte Growth Factor in blood from patients with fulminant hepatic failure *Hepatology* 9(6): 875-881

Tsubouchi, H., Niitani, Y., Hirono, S., Nakayama., H., Gohda, E., Arakaki, N., Sakiyama, N., Takahashi, K., Kimoto, M., Kawakami, S., Setoguch, M., Tachkawa, T., Shin, S., Arima, T., and Daikuhara, Y. (1991): Levels of the Human Hepatocyte Growth Factor in serum of patients with various liver diseases determined by an Enzyme-linked Immunosorbent Assay *Hepatology* 13: 1-5.

Wolf, H., Zarnegar, R., Oliver., L., and Michalopoulos, G.K. (1991): Hepatocyte growth factor in human placenta and trophoblastic disease. *Am. J. Path.* 138: 1035-1043.

Wolf, H, Zarnegar, R, and Michalopoulos, GK (1991): Localization of Hepatocyte Growth Factor in human and rat tissues. *Hepatology* In Press.

Zarnegar, R., and Michalopoulos, G. (1989a): Purification and biological characterization of human Hepatopoietin A: A polypeptide growth factor for hepatocytes. *Cancer Research* 49: 3314-3320.

Zarnegar, R., Muga, S., Enghild, J., and Michalopoulos, G. (1989b): NH_2-terminal amino acid sequence of rabbit Hepatopoietin A: A heparin-binding polypeptide growth factor for hepatocytes *Biochem. Biophys.Res. Commun.* 163: 1370-1376.

Zarnegar, R., Muga, S., Rahija, R., and Michalopoulos, G. (1990a): Tissue distribution of Hepatopoietin A: A heparin binding polypeptide growth factor for hepatocytes. *Proc. Natl. Acad. Sci.USA* 87: 1252-1256.

Zarnegar, R., DeFrances, M.C., Oliver, L., and Michalopoulos, G.K. (1990b): Identification and partial characterization of receptor binding sites for HGF on rat hepatocytes. *Biochem. Biophys. Res. Commun.* 173: 1179-1185.

Zarnegar, R, DeFrances, MC, Kost, D, Lindroos, P, and Michalopoulos, GK (1991): Expression of Hepatocyte Growth Factor (HGF) in regenerating rat liver after partial hepatectomy. *Biochem Biophys Res Commun* 177: 559-565.

Résumé

Un des buts majeurs de la biologie moderne est la compréhension de la croissance cellulaire et de la différenciation au niveau moléculaire. Un exemple spectaculaire d'une croissance tissulaire contrôlée est la régénération du foie. Celle-ci peut être induite expérimentalement par un traitement chimique ou par résection du foie chez des animaux normaux. *In vitro*, les hépatocytes isolés ont été utilisés pour identifier et étudier les différents facteurs de régulation de la croissance hépatocytaire. Ce modèle a permis de découvrir comme agents mitogènes ou inhibiteurs de la prolifération des hépatocytes plusieurs facteurs de croissance polypeptidiques tels que le facteur de croissance épidermique (EGF), le facteur de croissance transformant α (TGFα), le facteur de croissance hépatocytaire (HGF) appelé également hépatopoïétine A (HPTA), les facteurs de croissance fibroblastiques acide et basique (FGFs), le facteur de croissance transformant β (TGFβ) et des cytokines telles que les interleukines 1 et 6. Nos études ont été concentrées sur le facteur de croissance hépatocytaire (HGF) et son rôle dans la régénération hépatique. L'expression au cours du temps de l'HGF dans le foie de rat normal et en régénération a été analysée à l'aide d'outils moléculaires spécifiques d'HGF tels que des anticorps et un clone d'ADNc. Les taux plasmatiques d'HGF immunoréactif s'élèvent rapidement et atteignent un pic entre 2 et 6 heures chez des rats traités par le CCl_4 ou ayant subi une hépatectomie partielle. Cette libération d'HGF dans le plasma est suivie d'une forte augmentation de l'ARNm correspondant dans le foie des animaux traités qui atteint progressivement un pic après 12 hr et revient aux valeurs basales après 72 hr. L'examen immunohistologique des coupes de foie de ces animaux montre qu'il n'existe apparemment aucune différence entre les foies d'animaux partiellement hépatectomisés et normaux dans l'immunolocalisation de l'HGF. Par contre, chez les animaux traités par le CCl_4 une nette augmentation de l'HGF immunoréactif est constatée dans les coupes de foies examinées après 24 hr de traitement. Par immunolocalisation l'HGF est détectée dans les hépatocytes lésés ou nécrotiques entourant les veines centrolobulaires. Ceci pourrait indiquer un rôle autocrine d'HGF au cours de la régénération hépatique après les dommages causés par un agent hépatotoxique.

Nous avons récemment montré qu'HGF exerce un effet mitogène sur l'hépatocyte par l'intermédiaire d'un récepteur membranaire spécifique de 160 kD qui pourrait être le produit du protooncogène c-MET. L'absence d'un récepteur fonctionnel ou un récepteur anormal pourrait conduire à l'incapacité du foie à régénérer et pourrait contribuer à la transformation maligne. Aussi, nous étudions actuellement l'expression du c-MET au cours de la régénération hépatique. Comment le HGF, son récepteur et d'autres facteurs polypeptidiques affectent la régénération hépatique est également présenté.

Cellular and Molecular Aspects of Cirrhosis. Eds B. Clément, A. Guillouzo. Colloque INSERM/John Libbey Eurotext Ltd. © 1992, Vol. 216, pp. 255-264

Hepatocyte growth factor (HGF) : molecular structure and liver regeneration

Kunio Matsumoto and Toshikazu Nakamura

Department of Biology, Faculty of Science, Kyushu University, Fukuoka 812, Japan

INTRODUCTION

Studies on the molecular mechanism of liver regeneration are of importance not only in clinically, but also for understanding regulations of cell growth, differentiation, and tissue repair. After removal of 70% of the liver of rats, the cells in the residual liver stump rapidly proliferate, and the original liver weight and liver specific functions are restored in about 10 days after resection. Liver cell growth can also be induced in animals by treatment with hepatotoxins such as carbon tetrachloride (CCl_4) and D-galactosamine or by ischemia.

The existence of a blood borne factor (hepatotrophic factor) that initiates liver regeneration was postulated from experiments on parabiotic rats and from transplantation experiments in the 1950s and 1960s (Bucher, 1963). But despites many attempts to isolate this factor, its chemical nature remained unknown for a long period. In the 1980s, we and others found that adult rat hepatocytes in primary culture proliferate in appropriate culture media containing epidermal growth factor (EGF) and proline at low cell density (Tomita et al., 1981; Nakamura et al., 1983a; Nakamura et al., 1984a). Thus, primary cultures of adult rat hepatocytes provided a suitable assay system for the identification and purification of hepatotrophic factor.

The first convincing evidence for the presence of hepatotrophic factor in the blood of partially hepatectomized rats was obtained in 1984 (Nakamura et al., 1984b), and the factor was named hepatocyte growth factor (HGF) or hepatotropin, and we purified HGF to homogeneity from rat platelets (Nakamura et al., 1986; Nakamura et al., 1987). In 1989, we achieved molecular cloning of both human and rat HGF cDNAs and from its deduced primary structure, HGF was found to be a novel growth factor with no homology to other known growth factors (Nakamura et al., 1989; Tashiro et al., 1990).

MOLECULAR STRUCTURE OF HGF

Purified rat HGF gives a single band corresponding to a molecular weight of 82kD under non-reducing condition on SDS-PAGE, while in reducing conditions it gives two bands with molecular weights of 69kD (α-subunit) and 34kD (β-subunit), respectively (Nakamura et al., 1987).

We cloned human HGF cDNA derived from cDNA libraries of the liver (Nakamura et al., 1989) and leukocytes (Seki et al., 1990), and rat HGF cDNA from cDNA library of the liver (Tashiro et al., 1990). The sequence of the full length 6 kb cDNA consisted of a 5' non-coding region of 134 nucleotides, a single open reading frame of 2,184 nucleotides, and a 3' non-coding region of 3,580 nucleotides. The 3' non-coding region contained an many A+U-rich sequence, which is known to be the recognition signal for an mRNA processing pathway for specific degradation of the mRNA. A polypeptide of 728 amino acids, which include both the α- and β-chain, is encoded by a single open reading frame of human HGF cDNA. The alignment of the amino acid sequences of human and rat HGF are shown in Fig. 1. The amino acid sequence of rat HGF is >90% identical with that of human HGF. This would explain why these HGFs show no species specificity in biological activity. The sequences of the liver-derived cDNA clone and the leukocyte-derived clone showed differences in 14 amino acid residues. The sequence of the other leukocyte-derived cDNA clone had an in-frame deletion of 15 base-pairs within the first kringle region. The difference in the sequence of the liver-derived clone may be due to the existence of polymorphism or some kind of RNA editing.

```
                                          ┌►α
human: MWVTKLLPALLLQHVLLHLLLLPIAIPYAEGHKKRRNTIHEFKKSAKTTL   50
hu-2:  -------------------------------QR-----------------   50
rat:  M--G-----V--------------VT------Q------L-----------   51

human: IKIDPALKIKTKKVNTADQCANRCTRNNGLPFTCKAFVFDKARKQCLWFP  100
hu-2:  --------------------------K-----------------------  100
rat:   T-E--LV--------S--E-----I--K-F-----------S--R-Y-Y-  101

human: FNSMSSGVKKEFGHEFDLYENKDYIRNCIIGKGRSYKGTVSITKSGIKCQ  150
hu-2:  --------------------------------------------------  150
rat:   ----------G-----------------------G---------------  151

human: PWSSMIPHEHSFLPSSYRGKDLQENYCRNPRGEEGGPWCFTSNPEVRYEV  200
hu-2:  --------------------------------------------------  200
rat:   --------------------------------------------------  201

human: CDIPQCSEVECMTCNGESYRGLMDHTESGKICQRWDHQTPHRHKFLPERY  250
hu-2:  --------------------------------------------------  250
rat:   ----------------------P--------T-----Q------------  251

human: PDKGFDDNYCRNPDGQPRPWCYTLDPHTRWEYCAIKTCADNTVNDTDVPM  300
hu-2:  ------------------------------------------M------L  300
rat:   ---------------K----------D---------M--HSA--E-----  301

human: ETTECIQGQGEGYRGTANTIWNGIPCQRWDSQYPHKHDMTPENFKCKDLR  350
hu-2:  ----------------V------------------E--------------  350
rat:   ------K---------T----------------------I----------  351

human: ENYCRNPDGSESPWCFTTDPNIRVGYCSQIPNCDMSNGQDCYRGNGKNYM  400
hu-2:  ------------------------------------H-------------  400
rat:   ---------A-----------------------K--V-S-----------  401

human: GNLSQTRSGLTCSMWNKNMEDLHRHIFWEPDASKLNENYCRNPDDDAHGP  450
hu-2:  ---------------D----------------------------------  450
rat:   ----K----------D------------------TK--------------  451
                                                   ┌►β
human: WCYTGNPLIPWDYCPISRCEGDTTPTIVNLDHPVISCAKTKQLRVVNGIP  500
hu-2:  --------I-----------------------------------------  500
rat:   --------V-----------------------------------------  501

human: TRTNVGWMISLRYRNKHICGGSLIKESWVLTARQCFPSP   DLKDYEAWL  548
hu-2:  ----I---V------------------------------   ---------  548
rat:   -Q-T----V--K--------------------------A-NK---------  551

human: GIHDVHGRGEEKRKQVLNVSQLVYGPEGSDLVLMKLARPAVLDDFVNTID  598
hu-2:  ---------D--C-------------------------------------  598
rat:   ------E--------I--I--------------L------I--N--S---  601

human: LPNYGCTIPEKTSCSVYGWGYTGLINYDGLLRVAHLYIMGNEKCSQHHRG  648
hu-2:  ---------------------------Y--------------------R-  648
rat:   --S---------T--I----------A---------------------Q-  651

human: KVTLNESEICAGAEKIGSGPCEGDYGGPLVCEQHKMRMVLGVIVPGRGCA  698
hu-2:  --------I--------------------V--------------------  698
rat:   --------L--------------------I--------------------  701

human: IPNRPGIFVRVAYYAKWIHKIILTYKVPQS                      728
hu-2:  ------------------------------                      728
rat:   --------------------V-----L                         728
```

Fig. 1. Alignment of amino acid sequences of rat and human HGF. Amino acid numbers are given on the right. Identical amino acids are indicated by dashes in the sequence of human HGF. Amino acid sequences of human HGF deduced from cDNAs derived from human liver and leukocytes are indicated as "human" and "hu-2", respectively.

We recently identified the N-terminus of recombinant human HGF and rat HGF purified from CCl_4-treated rat liver as histidine at position 32 and glutamine at position 32 modified to pyroglutamic acid, and the N-terminus of recombinant human HGF obtained from a cDNA library of leukocytes (see below) as glutamine at position 32 modified to pyroglutamic acid (our unpublished results).

A schematic representation of the processing of pre-proHGF is shown in Fig. 2. Most of the first 31 amino acids are hydrophobic, a feature that is typical of a signal sequence. The α-chain extents from amino acid 32 to 494, and the β-chain from 495 to 728. After the biosynthesis, N-terminal signal peptide is proteolytically cleaved, and one chain

HGF is separated by a trypsin-like protease at an Arg-Val site. Thus, the α-chain consists of 463 amino acids, and the β-chain of 234 amino acids. HGF contains four putative aspargine-linked glycosylation sites, which are located at positions 294 and 402 of the α-chain and at positions 566 and 653 of the β-chain. A diagram of the structure of the predicted mature human HGF is shown in Fig. 3. One prominent structural feature is four homologous triple looped, kringle domains in the α-chain. An interchain S-S bridge may be formed between Cys 487 in the α-chain and Cys 604 in the β-chain. We found that a biologically active HGF could be expressed from HGF cDNA in COS-1 cells (Nakamura et al., 1989; Seki et al., 1990).

HGF has considerable homology (20-40%) with several proteins involved in the fibrinolytic process or blood coagulation, such as plasmin, prothrombin, tissue plasminogen activator, urokinase-type plasminogen activator, and coagulation factor XII. All the above proteins also contain kringle domains. Plasminogen and plasmin contain five kringle domains, but neither plasminogen nor plasmin have HGF activity. On the other hand, HGF has no protease activity, since the His and Ser residues of the protease active site in plasminogen are replaced by Gln and Tyr, respectively, in the HGF β-chain.

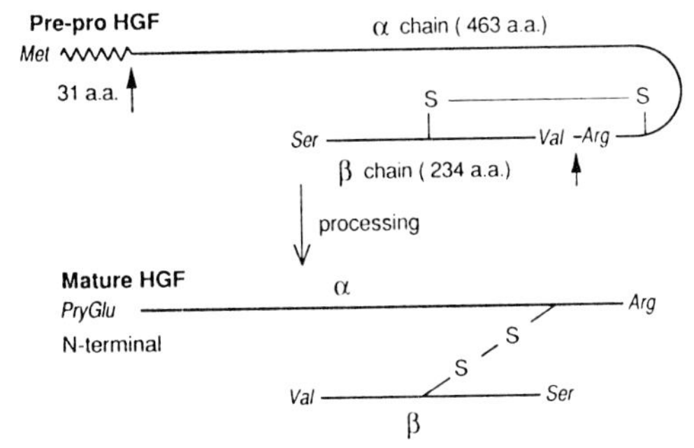

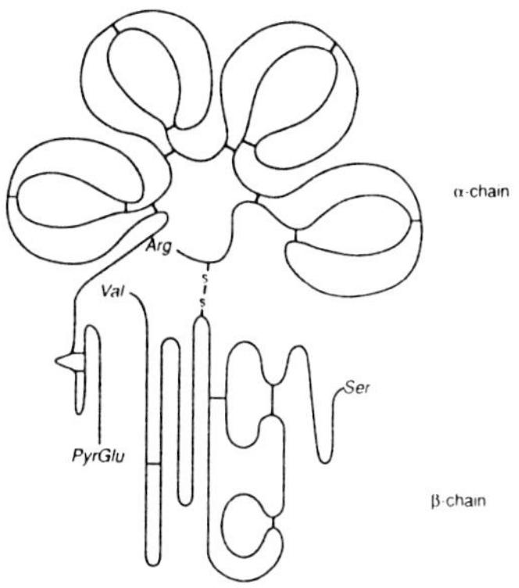

Fig. 2 (Left). Schematic representative of the processing of pre-proHGF. The wavy line open box represent the signal peptide, respectively. The solid arrows indicate processing sites.

Fig. 3 (Right). Schematic structure of predicted mature human HGF. The S-S bridge connecting the α- and β-chains is formed between Cys487 in the α-chain and Cys604 in the β-chain.

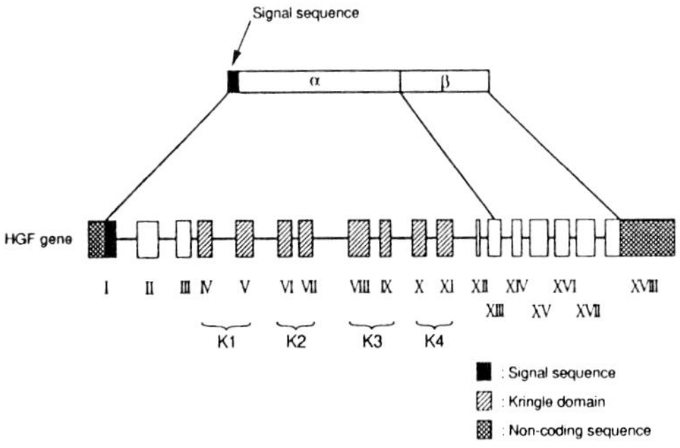

Fig. 4. Exon-intron structure of the gene encoding human HGF.

The HGF gene is composed of 18 exons and 17 introns and spans about 70 kb (Seki et al., 1991). The exon-intron structure of the HGF gene is shown in Fig. 4. The first exon contains the 5'-untranslated region and the signal peptide. The next ten exons encode the α-chain, which contains four kringle domains. Each kringle domain is encoded by two exons, as in other proteins containing kringle domains. The twelfth exon contains the short spacer region between the α- and β-chains. The overall organization of the HGF gene is highly homologous to that of plasminogen. Therefore, the HGF gene is probably evolutionary related to plasminogen.

BIOLOGICAL ACTIVITIES OF HGF

HGF is the most potent mitogen for adult rat hepatocytes in primary culture: it is 2-3 times as effective as EGF and transforming growth factor-α (TGF-α) in stimulating DNA synthesis in the cells. Moreover its maximal dose is 60 pM to 90 pM, which is 1/20 of those of EGF and TGF-α, and its effect is additive to EGF or TGF-α. In the presence of EGF, HGF, and insulin, over 80% of adult rat hepatocytes enter the S phase. The biological activity of HGF is lost by treatment with heat, acid, or trypsin digestion. HGF has no species-specificity: rat HGF strongly stimulates DNA synthesis of human, dog, pig and mouse hepatocytes as well as rat cells, and reversely human HGF stimulates DNA synthesis in rat hepatocytes, as effectively as in human hepatocytes.

The original purification of HGF was based on the stimulation of DNA synthesis of adult rat hepatocytes in primary culture, so that the peptide was named hepatocyte growth factor (HGF) based on this biological activity. However, the effect of HGF is not restricted to hepatocyte growth. HGF has no effect on DNA synthesis of non-parenchymal hepatocytes or fibroblast cell lines such as NIH 3T3 and Balb/c 3T3 cells, but it stimulates DNA synthesis of normal rabbit renal tubular epithelial cells (Igawa et al., 1991), normal human epidermal melanocytes (Matsumoto et al., 1991) and keratinocytes (Matsumoto et al., 1991), and non-transformed epithelial cell lines such as Mv1Lu cells derived from mink lung epithelium. In addition to stimulating cell growth, HGF markedly enhanced the motility of human keratinocytes (Matsumoto et al., 1991) and canine kidney epithelial cells (MDCK cells). Moreover, HGF remarkably inhibited the growth of several tumor cells such as B6/F1 melanoma and HepG2 hepatoma cells (our unpublished data). Indeed, hepatocellular carcinoma cells stably transfected with an albumin-HGF expression vector exhibited growth inhibition *in vitro*, and these cells produced tumors that averaged only 10% of the size of controls when transplanted into nude mice (Shiota et al., 1991). The physiological significances of these activities are unknown, but as increases in of cell growth and cell motility would enhance tissue repair and organogenesis during embryogenesis, HGF may be involved in these processes. The biological activities and typical target cells of HGF are summarized in Table 1.

Recently, other biologically active factors with HGF-like activity have been purified to homogeneity, using other assay systems to monitor their purification. Stoker and his colleagues identified a factor that they called "scatter factor", which was secreted by MRC-5 fibroblasts derived from human embryonic lung. Scatter factor enhanced the motility and scattering of the epithelial cell line MDCK (Stoker et al., 1987). The amino-terminal sequence of the purified scatter factor was found to be very similar to that of rat HGF (Gherardi & Stoker, 1990). Moreover, the purified scatter factor stimulated the DNA synthesis of cultured rat hepatocytes dose-dependently (Bhargava et al., 1991; Furlong et al., 1991). Similarly, a fibroblast-derived tumor cytotoxic factor (F-TCF), recently purified from conditioned medium of human embryonic lung fibroblasts and sequenced, was also found to be the same as HGF (Higashio et al., 1990).

Table 1. Biological activities and typical target cells of HGF.

Biological activity	Target cells
Growth promotion	Mature hepatocytes Renal tubular epithelial cells Epidermal keratinocytes Epidermal melanocytes Mv1Lu (mink lung epithelial cells) Balb/MK (mouse keratinocytes)
Stimulation of migration	Epidermal keratinocytes MDCK (canine kidney epithelial cells) A431 (human epidermoid carcinoma) HepG2 (human hepatoma) Lu99 (human lung carcinoma)
Growth inhibition	B6/F1 (mouse melanoma) KB (human squamous cell carcinoma) HepG2

HGF RECEPTOR

We recently identified a single-class of high affinity receptors for HGF on rat hepatocytes and plasma membranes from rat liver (Higuchi & Nakamura, 1991). Rat hepatocytes express about 500-600 binding sites/cell with a Kd of 20-30 pM. The binding of ^{125}I-HGF to the plasma membranes is not competitive with those of other growth factors or plasmin. Affinity cross-linking of ^{125}I-HGF to plasma membranes from rat liver revealed that the apparent Mr of the HGF receptor is approximately 220kD, as determined SDS-PAGE under non-reducing conditions. Therefore, a low number of binding sites and high affinity to HGF seem to be characteristics of the HGF receptor. We detected the HGF receptor in various tissues, such as the liver, lung, kidney, adrenal, and pituitary, and found that it was expressed by various epithelial cells, including rabbit renal tubular epithelial cells, normal human epidermal keratinocytes and melanocytes, and A431 (human squamous cell carcinoma), B6F1 (mouse melanoma), and HepG2 (human hepatoma) cells (unpublished data).

HGF AND LIVER REGENERATION

1) Growth regulation of hepatocytes by cell-cell contact

Cell growth, differentiation and tissue organization are regulated not only by humoral factors, but also by cell-cell contact from the cytosocial environment. The regulations of growth and differentiated functions of mature hepatocytes through cell-cell contact were elucidated in *in vitro* studies using adult rat hepatocytes in primary culture (Nakamura et al., 1983b; Yoshimoto et al., 1983; Nakamura et al., 1984c; Nakamura et al., 1984d). Although rat hepatocytes in primary culture can proliferate in response to growth factors, their growth response to these factors largely depends on cell density. In cultures at high cell density, the hepatocytes form tight cell-cell contact, and remain in the quiescent G0 phase (differentiated state): they do not proliferate in the presence of excess amounts of growth factors, but fully express liver specific differentiated phenotypes, such as tyrosine aminotransferase, serine dehydratase, tryptophan oxygenase, and triglyceride synthesis. In cultures at lower cell density, the cells do not form tight cell-cell contact, and their liver specific functions are suppressed: these cells in the G1 phase (proliferative) can respond to growth factors and their cell cycle progresses from the G1 to the S phase. The regulation of G0-G1 cell cycle transition in mature hepatocytes through cell-cell contact is regulated by a plasma membrane protein named "Cell Surface Modulator (CSM)" (Nakamura et al., 1983b; Nakamura et al., 1984c; Nakamura et al., 1984d). When CSM is added to adult rat hepatocytes cultured at low cell density, the cells do not respond to mitogens. After treatments with heat or trypsin, CSM activity was lost completely. CSM was extracted from liver plasma membranes with 4% octylglucoside in 4 M guanidine-HCl and found to have an apparent molecular mass of 670kD, as determined by molecular sieve chromatography (Nakamura et al., 1984c).

This cell surface mechanism may also operate *in vivo* : In intact lobules, CSM on the hepatocyte cell membrane will signal suppression of growth and expression of differentiated functions of neighboring cells. However, if this cell surface mechanism is impaired as the result of some insult such as partial hepatectomy or hepatitis, the suppression of growth of hepatocytes may be released and the cells may progress from the G0 to the G1 phase. The existence of this mechanism is supported by the finding that cell-cell contact between hepatocytes is loosened in regenerating liver *in vivo* (Meyer et al., 1981). Thus, after liver injury, loss of tight cell-cell contact may induce G0-G1 cell cycle transition and provide the conditions for hepatocytes to respond to HGF.

2) HGF and liver regeneration after hepatitis

The blood GPT and GOT activities increase markedly after CCl_4 administration reaching maxima in 24 h. The HGF activities in the sera correlated well with the severity of hepatitis. HGF activity in the livers of rats also increases markedly 12 h after CCl_4 administration and were 20 times higher than normal after 30 h. Moreover, HGF was purified from the livers of rats treated with CCl_4 (Asami et al., 1991). This increase in the HGF may represent increased net synthesis of HGF in the injured liver, as suggested by northern hybridization studies (Fig. 5) (Kinoshita et al., 1989): the HGF mRNA increased markedly 5 h after CCl_4 administration and reached a maximum after 10 h.

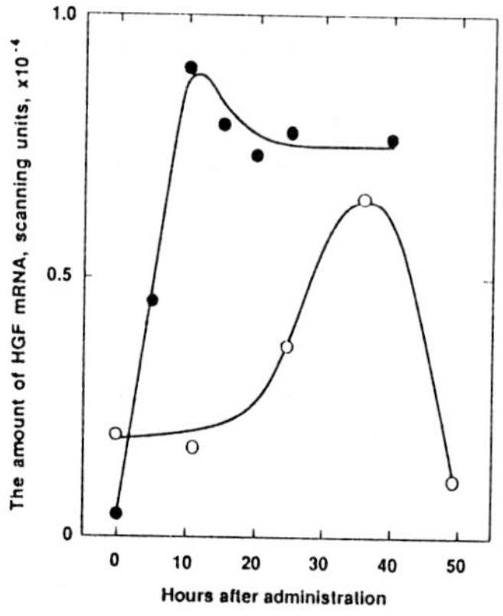

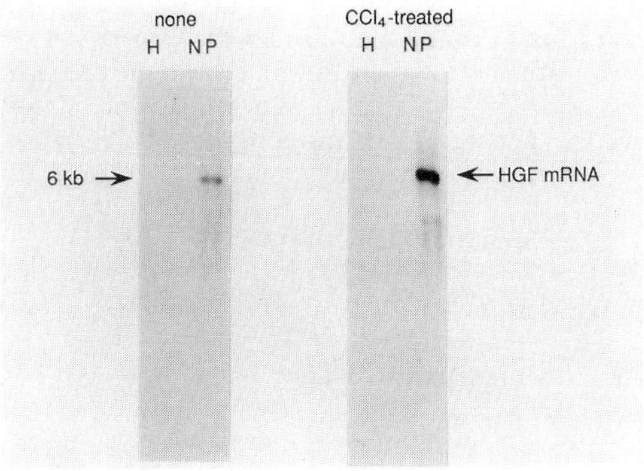

Fig. 5 (Left). Time courses of changes in HGF mRNA level in the liver of rats treated with CCl_4 or D-galactosamine. Poly(A)$^+$ RNAs were extracted from the livers at the indicated times after treatment with CCl_4 (●) or D-galactosamine (○) and analyzed by northern hybridization.

Fig. 6 (Right). HGF mRNA levels in parenchymal and non-parenchymal liver cells of rats with or without CCl_4-treatment. Liver cells were isolated by *in situ* perfusion with collagenase, and parenchymal hepatocytes and non-parenchymal liver cells were then separated by differential centrifugation. H, parenchymal hepatocytes; NP, non-parenchymal liver cells.

Increase of HGF mRNA in the liver of rats was also observed after administration of another potent hepatotoxin, D-galactosamine. The HGF mRNA level increased 24 h after D-galactosamine-administration, reaching a peak after 36 h. Induction of HGF mRNA by D-galactosamine is significantly slower than that after CCl_4 treatment, the difference perhaps being related to differences in the mechanisms by which these compounds elicit hepatocellular injury. D-galactosamine-induced hepatitis occurs over a longer period than CCl_4-induced hepatitis. Therefore, there is a good correlation between the increases in HGF mRNA levels in the liver and the degrees of liver damage.

As described above, the liver is one of the main organs producing HGF, and HGF production increases after liver injury. Therefore, we next examined which liver cells produce HGF after liver injury. Northern blot hybridization analysis showed that HGF mRNA was present in only non-parenchymal liver cells and that their HGF mRNA level increased markedly after CCl_4-administration, as seen in Fig. 6 (Kinoshita et al., 1989). To identify the non-parenchymal liver cells that produced HGF, HGF mRNA was detected by *in situ* hybridization of liver sections (Noji et al., 1990). Results showed that Kupffer cells and sinusoidal endothelial cells were the main cells that produced HGF in the liver. Therefore, the growth of parenchymal hepatocytes during liver regeneration after hepatitis may be mainly regulated by HGF synthesized by the non-parenchymal liver cells, presumably Kupffer cells and sinusoidal endothelial cells, that is, by a paracrine system. The induction of HGF is not restricted to hepatitis: We found that HGF mRNA also increased markedly in the liver of rats after partial ligation of the portal vein (ischemic damage to the liver) and after physical pressure (crushed liver) (manuscript in preparation).

3) Liver regeneration after partial hepatectomy

After 70% hepatectomy of the liver of rats, the HGF activity in the liver remnant begins to increase within 24 hours. The HGF mRNA level in the liver remnant also increases after 12 hours reaching a maximum after 24 hours, whereas the increases in the HGF activity and mRNA level were much less and occurred later than after CCl_4 administration (Kinoshita et al., 1991). Because the initial peak of DNA synthesis in the liver remnant was observed about 24 hours after the hepatectomy, the initial mitogenic signal should act within 10 hours. Strikingly, the increase of HGF activity in the plasma of hepatectomized rats was observed as early as 3 hours after partial hepatectomy. Therefore, newly synthesized HGF in the liver is unlikely to trigger the initial DNA , but may function to sustain subsequent hepatocyte growth and functional maturation. In contrast, HGF derived from extrahepatic organs or cells *via* the blood circulation is probably the actual trigger for liver regeneration. Supportive evidence for this conclusion is the finding that the number of HGF receptors on the plasma membranes of the liver remnant decreased markedly within 3 hours after partial hepatectomy. Fig. 7 shows the change in [^{125}I]-HGF binding to plasma membranes of livers obtained at various times after CCl_4 administration and partial hepatectomy (Higuchi & Nakamura, 1991). Probably, the decrease of HGF binding results from occupation and/or internalization of receptors of HGF. Therefore, Fig. 7 indicates that HGF should act as a mitogen for hepatocytes *in vivo* after liver injury by either CCl_4-administration or partial hepatectomy.

As described above, HGF mRNA was detected in various rat tissues, such as the lung, kidney, and spleen as well as liver, and rat platelets were also found to contain relatively large amounts of HGF. If HGF in these organs or cells is produced and secreted in response to liver injuries, HGF should act as a hepatotrophic factor through an endocrine mechanism. Therefore, there may be two pathways for the action of HGF in liver regeneration: a paracrine pathway, and an endocrine pathway. In hepatitis induced by CCl_4 administration, HGF produced by non-parenchymal liver cells may be predominant, whereas after partial hepatectomy, HGF supplied through the endocrine pathway may have a predominant effect on liver regeneration.

3) Possible mechanism of liver regeneration

Fig. 8 summarizes the putative mechanisms involved in liver regeneration. In normal intact liver, mature hepatocytes are in the G0 state and are in tight cell-cell contact to organize liver lobules, because CSM on the cell membrane gives a signal to suppress growth and stimulate liver-specific functions. When the liver is injured such as by hepatitis or partial hepatectomy, cell-cell contact of the hepatocytes is loosened. The hepatocytes are then released from growth suppression by CSM and tend to move to the G1 state, in which they can response to mitogenic signals for movement to the S phase. HGF, produced and secreted by Kupffer cells and sinusoidal endothelial in the liver and HGF produced in other organs such as lung, kidney and spleen acts in paracrine and endocrine fashions to stimulate liver regeneration.

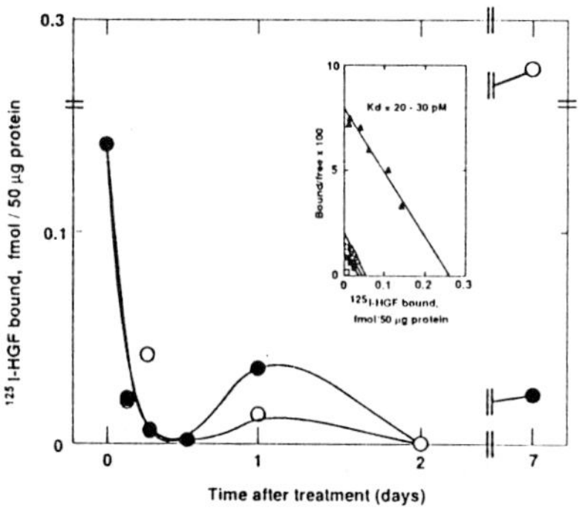

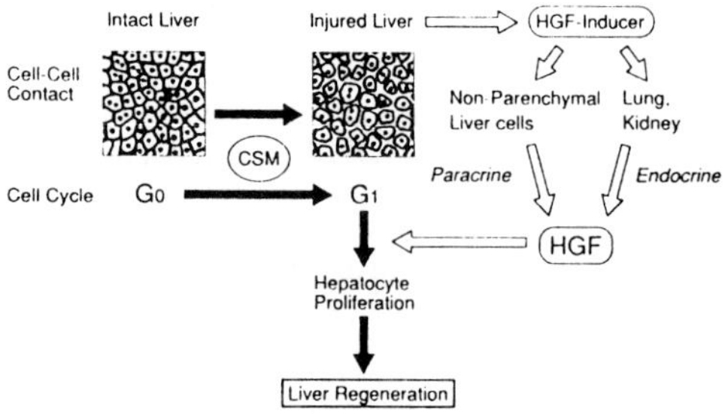

Fig. 7 (Left). Changes in specific binding of ^{125}I-HGF to liver plasma membranes after partial hepatectomy or hepatitis induced by CCl_4 treatment. Plasma membranes were purified from the residual liver of hepatectomized rats (○) or liver from CCl_4-treated rats (●) at the indicated time. Specific binding of ^{125}I-HGF to the membranes is shown. The inset shows a Scatchard plot: ▲, normal liver; 3 hours (■) and 12 hours (□) after partial hepatectomy; 3 hours (○) and 24 hours (△) after CCl_4 treatment.

Fig. 8 (Right). Possible mechanisms involved in liver regeneration.

Acknowledgement: This work was supported by a Research Grant for Science and Cancer from the Ministry of Education, Science and Culture of Japan and by research grants from the Princess Takamatsu Cancer Research Fund, the Cell Science Research Foundation, the Terumo Life Science Foundation, and the Kurata Foundation.

REFERENCES

Asami, O., Ihara, I., Shimidzu, N., Shimizu, S., Tomita, Y., Ichihara, A., & Nakamura, T. (1991) Purification and characterization of hepatocyte growth factor from injured liver of carbon tetrachloride-treated rats. J. Biochem. 109, 8-13.

Bhargava, M., Joseph, A., Li, Y., Pang, S., Goldberg, I., Setter, E., Donovan, M.A., Zarneger, R., Michalopoulos, G.A., Nakamura, T., & Rosen, E.M. (1991): Scatter factor and hepatocyte growth factor: comparison of biologic and immunologic reactivity, submitted to publication.

Bucher, N.L.R. (1963): Regeneration of mammalian liver. Int. Rev. Cytol. 15, 245-300.

Furlong, R.A., Takehara, T., Taylor, W.G., Nakamura, T., & Rubin, J.S.,(1991): Comparison of biological and immunochemical properties indicates that scatter factor and hepatocyte growth factor are the same protein. J. Cell Science., submitted to publication.

Gherardi, E. & Stoker, M. (1990): Hepatocytes and scatter factor. Nature 346, 228.

Higashio, K., Shima, N., Goto, M., Itagaki, Y., Nagao, M., Yasuda, H., & Morinaga, T. (1990): Identity of a tumor cytotoxic factor from human fibroblasts and hepatocyte growth factor, Biochem. Biophys. Res. Commun. 170, 397-404.

Higuchi, O. & Nakamura, T.(1991): Identification and change in the receptor for hepatocyte growth factor in rat liver after partial hepatectomy or induced hepatitis. Biochem. Biophys. Res. Commun. 176, 599-607.

Igawa, T., Kanda, S., Kanetake, H., Saitoh, Y., Ichihara, A., Tomita, Y., & Nakamura, T. (1991): Hepatocyte growth factor is a potent mitogen for cultured rabbit tubular epithelial cells, Biochem. Biophys. Res. Commun. 174, 831-838.

Kinoshita, Y., Tashiro, K., & Nakamura, T. (1989): Marked increase of HGF mRNA in non-parenchymal liver cells of rats treated with hepatotoxins, Biochem. Biophys. Res. Commun. 165, 1229-1234.

Kinoshita, T., Hirao, S., Matsumoto, K., & Nakamura, T. (1991): Possible endocrine control by hepatocyte growth factor of liver regeneration after partial hepatectomy, Biochem. Biophys. Res. Commun., in press.

Matsumoto, K., Tajima, H., & Nakamura, T. (1991): Hepatocyte growth factor is a potent stimulator of human melanocyte DNA synthesis and growth, Biochem. Biophys. Res. Commun. 176, 45-51.

Matsumoto, K., Hashimoto, K., Yoshikawa, K., & Nakamura, T. (1991): Marked stimulation of growth and motility of human keratinocytes by hepatocyte growth factor, Exp. Cell. Res. submitted to publication.

Meyer, D.J., Yancy, M., & Revel, J.-P. (1981): Intercellular communication in normal and regenerating rat liver: a quantitative analysis. J. Cell Biol. 91, 505-523.

Nakamura, T., Tomita, Y., & Ichihara, A. (1983a): Density-dependent growth control of adult rat hepatocytes in primary culture. J. Biochem. 94, 1029-1035.

Nakamura, T., Yoshimoto, K., Nakayama, Y., Tomita, Y., & Ichihara, A. (1983b): Reciprocal modulation of growth and differentiated functions of mature rat hepatocytes in primary culture by cell-cell contact and cell membranes. Proc. Natl. Acad. Sci. USA 80, 7229-7233.

Nakamura, T., Teramoto, H., Tomita, Y., & Ichihara, A. (1984a): L-Proline is an essential amino acid for hepatocyte growth in culture. Biochem. Biophys. Res. Commun. 122, 884-891.

Nakamura, T., Nawa, K. & Ichihara, A. (1984b): Partial purification and characterization of hepatocyte growth factor from serum of hepatectomized rats. Biochem. Biophys. Res. Commun. 122, 1450-1459.

Nakamura, T., Nakayama, Y., & Ichihara, A. (1984c): Reciprocal modulation of growth and liver functions of mature rat hepatocytes in primary culture by an extract of hepatic plasma membranes. J. Biol. Chem. 259, 8056-8058.

Nakamura, T., Nakayama, Y., Teramoto, H., Nawa, K., & Ichihara, A. (1984d): Loss of reciprocal modulations of growth and liver function of hepatoma cells in culture by contact with cells and cell membranes, Proc. Natl. Acad. Sci. USA 81, 6398-6402.

Nakamura, T., Teramoto, H., & Ichihara, A. (1986): Purification and characterization of a growth factor from rat platelets for mature parenchymal hepatocytes in primary cultures. Proc. Natl. Acad. Sci. USA 83, 6489-6493.

Nakamura, T., Nawa, K., Ichihara, A., Kaise, A., & Nishino, T. (1987): Subunit structure of hepatocyte growth factor from rat platelets. FEBS Lett. 224, 311-318.

Nakamura, T., Nishizawa, T., Hagiya, M., Seki, T., Shimonishi, M., Sugiura, A., Tashiro, K. & Shimizu, S. (1989): Molecular cloning and expression of human hepatocyte growth factor. Nature 342, 440-443.

Noji, S., Tashiro, K., Koyama, E., Nohno, T., Ohyama, K., Taniguchi, S., & Nakamura, T. (1990) Expression of hepatocyte growth factor gene in endothelial and Kupffer cells of damaged rat livers, as revealed by *in situ* hybridization. Biochem. Biophys. Res. Commun. 173, 42-47.

Seki, T., Ihara, I., Sugimura, A., Shimonishi, M., Nishizawa, T., Asami, O., Hagiya, M., Nakamura, T., & Shimizu, S. (1990): Isolation and expression of cDNA for different form of hepatocyte growth factor from human leukocytes, Biochem. Biophys. Res. Commun., 172, 321-327.

Seki, T., Hagiya, M., Shimonishi, M., Nakamura, T., & Shimizu, S. (1991): Organization of the human hepatocyte growth factor-encoding gene. Gene, in press.

Shiota, G., Rhoads, D.B., Nakamura, T., & Schmidt, E.V. (1991): Hepatocyte growth factor inhibits growth of hepatocellular carcinoma cells. Proc. Natl. Acad. Sci. USA, submitted to publication.

Stoker, M., Gherardi, E., Perryman, M., & Gray, J. (1987): Scatter factor is a fibroblast-derived modulator of epithelial cell mobility. Nature 327, 239-242.

Tashiro, K., Hagiya, M., Nishizawa, T., Seki, T., Shimonishi, M., Shimizu, S., & Nakamura T. (1990): Deduced primary structure of rat hepatocyte growth factor and expression of the mRNA in rat tissues. Proc. Natl. Acad. Sci. USA 87, 3200-3204.

Tomita, Y., Nakamura, T., & Ichihara, A. (1981): Control of DNA synthesis and ornithine decarboxylase activity by hormones and amino acids in primary cultures of adult rat hepatocytes. Exp. Cell. Res. 135, 361-371.

Yoshimoto, K., Nakamura, T., & Ichihara, A. (1983): Reciprocal effects of epidermal growth factor on key lipogenic enzymes in primary cultures of adult rat hepatocytes: Induction of glucose-6-phosphate dehydrogenase and suppression of malic enzyme and lipogenesis. J. Biol. Chem. 258, 12355-12360.

Cellular and Molecular Aspects of Cirrhosis. Eds B. Clément, A. Guillouzo. Colloque INSERM/John Libbey Eurotext Ltd. © 1992, Vol. 216, pp. 265-276

Cyclin A and liver cell proliferation

Frédérique Zindy [1], Jian Wang [1], Eugénia Lamas [1], Xavier Chenivesse [1], Berthold Henglein [1], Christian Bréchot [1,2]

[1] *INSERM U 75, CHU Necker, 156, rue de Vaugirard, 75742 Paris Cedex 15;* [2] *Unité d'Hépatologie, Hôpital Laënnec, rue de Sèvres, 75007, Paris, France*

ABSTRACT :
We have previously reported the identification of hepatitis B virus (HBV) integration in an intron of cyclin A gene in an early hepatocellular carcinoma and hence the isolation of human cyclin A cDNA.
We have constructed a cDNA library of the original tumor (tumor HEN) and isolated several hybrid HBV-cyclin A cDNAs. These cDNAs have the coding capacity for a HBV-cyclin A fusion protein. In the chimeric protein, the N-terminal of cyclin A, including the signals for signals for cyclin degradation, was deleted and replaced by viral preS2/S sequences while the rest of cyclin A remained intact. HBV integration in the cyclin A gene resulted in the overexpression of hybrid HBV-cyclin A transcripts that code for a stabilized cyclin A. In addition, we have investigated cyclin A expression in a primary culture of normal rat hepatocytes and during rat liver regeneration after partial hepatectomy. In both cases, cyclin A mRNA and protein accumulate as the cells enter S phase. Moreover we microinjected anti-sense DNA constructs for cyclin A, resulting in effective inhibition of S phase entry.

In conclusion, we showed in this paper an analysis of the expression pattern of cyclin A gene in the original tumor which supports the hypothesis of insertional mutagenesis of HBV, and a study of the role of cyclin A in a normal cell cycle which indicates its involvement in G1/S transition. That cyclin A is involved in S phase may provide new clues as to its potential role in carcinogenesis.

INTRODUCTION :
Cyclins play a major role in the cell cycle regulation. Two classes of cyclins, G1 and M cyclins, have been identified in fission (Booher and Beach, 1988 ; Forsburg and Nurse, 1991) and budding yeast (Hadwiger et al., 1989 ; Nash et al., 1988 ; Ghiara et al., 1991). They cooperate with the gene products of cdc2/cdc28 kinases in driving the cell through G1/S and G2/M boundaries. In higher eukaryotes, several cyclins (cyclins A, B, C, D and E) have been isolated. The cyclin B is a mitotic cyclin, which associates to the $p34^{cdc2}$ protein kinase to initiate mitosis and meiosis (Draetta et

al., 1989 ; Labbé et al., 1989 ; Meijer et al., 1989 ; Gautier et al., 1990). The C, D and E type cyclins seem to act in G1/S boundary since they can rescue G1 cyclin deficient mutants in S. Cerevisiae (Xiong et al., 1991 ; Matsushime et al., 1991 ; Motokura et al., 1991 ; Koff et al., 1991).
Cyclin A can also associate with $p34^{cdc2}$, but this complex is formed and active in advance of the $p34^{cdc2}$/cyclin B complex (Swenson et al., 1986 ; Draetta et al., 1989 ; Minshull et al., 1990 ; Pines and Hunter, 1990). However, several lines of evidence suggest that cyclin A may also have a role in the S phase. First, addition of cyclin A to a G1 phase extract was sufficient to initiate SV40 DNA replication in vitro (D'urso et al., 1990) ; second, microinjection of anti-sense cyclin A DNA into cultured cell blocked the initiation of DNA synthesis (see section 2 of this paper) and third, cyclin A associates to a $p34^{cdc2}$ related protein ($p33^{cdc2}$ or CDK2) that functions in S phase (Pines and Hunter, 1990 ; Fang & Newport, 1991 ; Tsai et al., 1991).
We have previously reported the identification of hepatitis B virus (HBV) DNA integration in human cyclin A gene in an early hepatocellular carcinoma (HCC) (Wang et al., 1990). Chronic HBV infection has been associated with the development of HCC by extensive epidemiological studies (Beasley, 1988). There are several mechanisms which account for the role played by HBV in hepatocarcinogenesis. HBV induces cirrhosis, a premalignant state (Chisari et al, 1990). In addition, HBV likely exerts a direct effect on cell transformation by transactivation of the x and truncated PréS2/S viral proteins (Kim et al, 1991) as well by insertional mutagenesis. This latter mechanism has been well illustrated in woodchucks infected with the woodchuck hepatitis virus (WHV) where WHV DNA was found integrated in the C-myc or N-myc gene in 30% of the tumor studied, most of them with an elevated expression of these oncogenes (Fourel et al., 1990). In human, however, there is only one report in which HBV DNA was found to integrate in the gene coding for a retinoic acid receptor β in HCC (Dejean et al., 1986 ; de The et al., 1987).
In the present manuscript we will focus on two implications of our results :
1) a detailed analysis of the expression pattern of cyclin A gene in the original tumor (tumor HEN) which supports the hypothesis of insertional mutagenesis.
2) An analysis of the role of cyclin A in a normal cell cycle which indicates its involvement in G1/S transition.

RESULTS :

1) HBV and cyclin A expression in tumor HEN

In Northern blots of the original tumor HEN, both cyclin A and HBV probes detected the same two polyadenylated transcripts of 2.7 and 1.7 kb, which were nearly the same size as the normal cyclin A transcripts but quite different from that of HBV. These bands were undetectable in the non-tumorous liver of the same patient. A cDNA library was constructed in lambda gt10 with mRNAs from the tumor and hybrid HBV cyclin A transcripts were caracterised.
The genomic structure of the human cyclin A gene has been established in our laboratory (Henglein et al., in preparation). A comparaison with the HBV integration site indicated that the HBV sequences integrated in the first intron of cyclin A gene (Fig. 1). Two representative cDNAs, 1.7 and 2.7 kb respectively, have been completely sequenced. The results indicated that hybrid transcripts

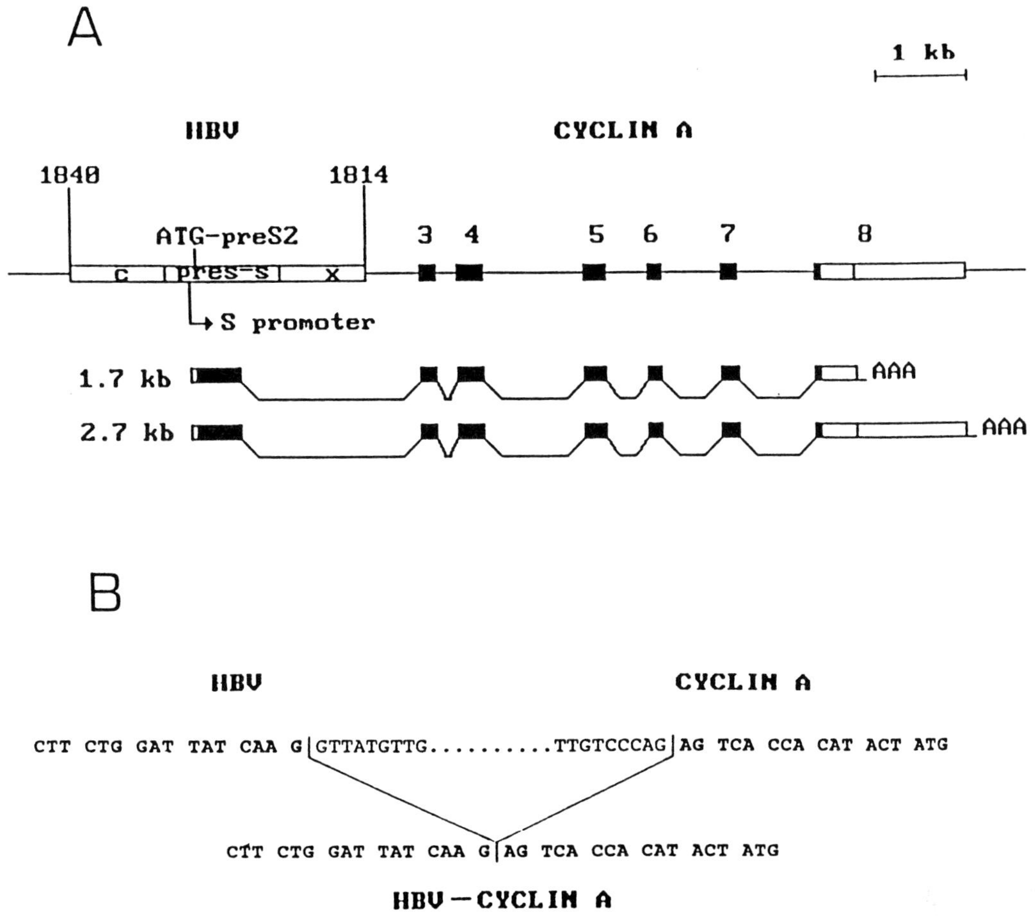

Fig. 1 A : Genomic structure of human cyclin A gene in the HBV integration site (upper) and structure of the hybrid cDNAs (lower). The cyclin A exons are numbered, the black boxs represent the coding sequences and the blanked boxs represent non coding exons, arrow indicate the initiation site of transcription from viral S promoter. The poly (A) tails in the two cDNAs mark the two commonly used polyadenylation sites for normal cyclin A transcription. **B : Sequence of HBV-cyclin A junction in the hybrid cDNAs.** The splicing manner is indicated.

were produced by splicing between HBV and cyclin A sequences, using a cryptic splice donnor site in the middle of viral S gene and the normal splice acceptor site of the third exon of cyclin A gene. A primer extension assay, confirmed that the hybrid transcripts were initiated from the viral Pre S2/S promoter (data not shown).
Sequence analysis showed that the HBV open reading frame was fused to that of the cyclin A in the hybrid cDNAs which code for an HBV-cyclin A fusion protein of 430 amino acids. In the chimeric protein, the N-terminal 152 amino acids of cyclin A were reimplaced by 150 amino acids from the viral PreS2 and a part of S regions whereas the

C-terminal two third of cyclin A, including the cyclin box, remained intact (Fig. 1). In vitro translation of the hybrid cDNA produced a 54 KD protein (slightly smaller than normal cyclin A). The N-terminal domain of cyclin A contains the signals for its degradation by the ubiquitin pathway, (Glotzer et al., 1991). An in vitro degradation assay recently indicated that the deletion of the N-terminal of cyclin A has indeed stabilized cyclin A (data not shown).

2) Cyclin A is required in S phase in normal epithelial cells.

Until now, the investigations on cyclins have been performed either in invertebrates or in transformed mammalian cells. Therefore, we chose to investigate cyclin A expression in normal epithelial cells. With this purpose, we have studied cyclin A mRNA and protein in primary culture of rat hepatocytes and in rat liver regeneration. This approach was associated to experiments based on microinjecting an anti-sense cyclin A cDNA.

In vitro cultured hepatocytes can be maintained for 8 days in serum-free medium supplemented with dexamethasone and insulin (referred to as untreated hepatocytes). Alternatively, culturing cells in serum-free medium supplemented with insulin, pyruvate and epidermal growth factor (EGF) (referred to as treated hepatocytes), stimulates DNA synthesis in most hepatocytes (around 80%), with a maximum at day 3 of culture (Mc Gowan, 1986). Using these experimental conditions, we established primary rat hepatocytes culture confirming that maximum DNA synthesis, shown by ^{3}H-thymidine incorporation, occured on day 3 in treated hepatocytes (fig. 2A). When the hepatocytes were untreated, DNA synthesis was barely detectable. Initial experiments used Northern analysis of cyclin A mRNAs. Cyclin A mRNA was not detected in untreated hepatocytes (fig. 2B). In contrast, in treated hepatocytes, the accumulation of cyclin A mRNA increased to a maximum at day 2-4 and then decreased (fig. 2B). This accumulation of transcripts coincided with maximal ^{3}H-thymidine incorporation. To determine if these transcripts were effectively related to protein expression, we also analyzed total cellular protein from cultured hepatocytes by means of immunoblotting with affinity purified polyclonal antibodies raised against human cyclin A. In primary culture, cyclin A protein was detectable from day 2 to day 5 with a maximum at day 3 in treated hepatocytes (i.e. at the time of DNA synthesis) (fig. 2C). Furthermore, we analyzed the localization of cyclin A in cultured hepatocytes. The staining of cyclin A was preferentially localized into the nucleus. At day 3 of culture, high amount of cells were labelled for cyclin A whereas at day 1 of culture, only few cells were stained (data not shown).

To determine if this observation also true in-vivo, the expression of cyclin A was analysed in regenerating liver at various times after partial hepatectomy (PH). Indeed, PH partially synchronizes the hepatocytes proliferative phase (30-40%) during the first mitosis. The growth process includes a distinct prereplicative phase of hypertrophy which lasts for 12-16 hrs after PH and a replicative phase in which hepatocytes undergo DNA replication (peak et 24 hrs) and then division (peak at 30 hrs) (Bucher and Malt, 1971 ; Grisham, 1962).

Therefore, we analyzed liver samples obtained at 16 to 32 hrs after PH. After 32 hrs, further points were not analyzed due to the loss of cellular synchronisation. ^{3}H-thymidine incorporation was detected with a maximum at 24 hrs after PH (fig. 3A). Northern blot analysis revealed cyclin A mRNA at a very low level before and 16 hrs after

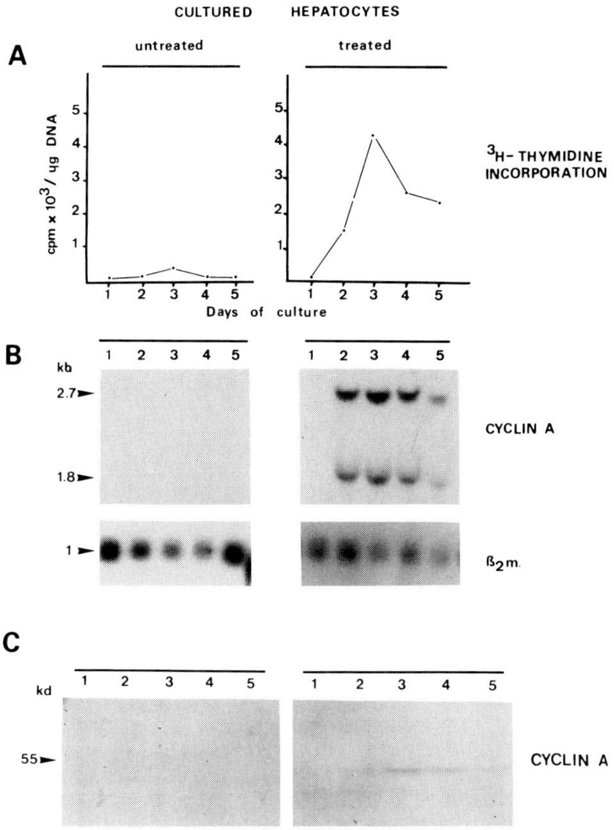

Fig. 2 : Cyclin A expression and ^{3}H-Thymidine incorporation in cultured hepatocytes. Hepatocytes were isolated from 2-month-old male Wistar rats and cultured in serum-free medium supplemented with dexamethasone (1μM) and insulin (200nUI/ml) (untreated hepatocytes) or in serum-free medium supplemented with insulin (20 m UI/ml), pyruvate (20 mM) and epidermal growth factor (50ng/ml) (treated hepatocytes). Hepatocytes untreated or treated by growth factors were harversted at the indicated times. ^{3}H-thymidine incorporation was measured (A), cyclin A mRNAs were analyzed by Northern blot normalized relative to B2 microglobulin mRNAs (B2m.) (B), and cyclin A protein was analyzed by Western blot (C).

PH (fig. 3B). Cyclin A mRNA accumulation increased at 20 hrs with a maximum level from 24 hrs to 32 hrs after PH corresponding respectively to the period in which maximal DNA synthesis and mitosis take place. Cyclin A protein was not detected before or 16 hrs after PH (fig. 3C) ; its level was maintained from 24-26 hrs (time of DNA synthesis) to 32 hrs (time of mitosis).

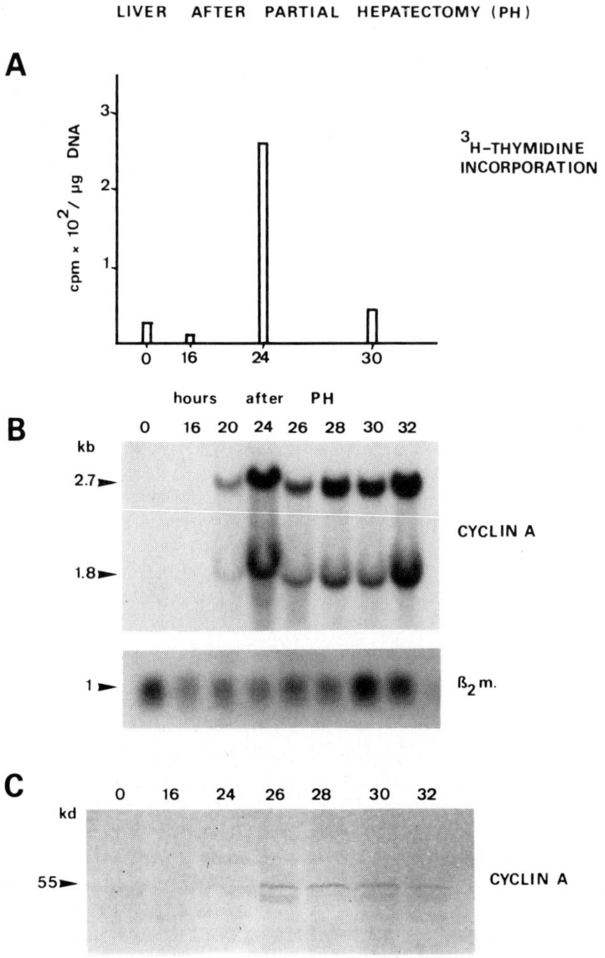

Fig. 3 : cyclin A expression and ^{3}H-thymidine incorporation in regenerating liver after partial hepatectomy. Male Wistar rats were subjected to 70% partial hepatectomy and liver was removed at the indicated times after hepatectomy. ^{3}H-thymidine incorporation was measured (A), cyclin A mRNAs were analyzed by Northern blot normalized relative to B2 microglobulin (B2m.) (B), and cyclin A protein was analyzed by Western blot.

To examine further the effects of changes in cyclin A mRNA and protein levels, we investigated the consequences on S phase transit of artificially inhibiting cyclin A synthesis. We inhibited cyclin A synthesis through microinjection of plasmid constructs encoding anti-sense human cyclin A cDNA under the control of SV40 promoter-enhancer element. At various times after plating, cultured rat hepatocytes stimulated by growth factors were microinjected with the anti-sense cyclin A construct, a sense cyclin A construct or an anti-sense human cyclin B cDNA under the control of an SV40 promotor-enhancer element. The effects of injection were assessed by following the incorporation of 5-bromo-deoxyuridine (5-Br-DU) (i.e. S-phase transit). Injected cells were relocated by inclusion of a non-specific antibody in the injection solutions which was subsequently stained after immunofluorescence with anti-5-Br-DU. Cells were injected 2-3 days after plating and labelled from injection until the end of day 4. Each microinjection experiment was performed three times, involving the injection of 30 to 40 cells every time. Under normal conditions, treated hepatocytes synthetized DNA between the end of day 2 and day 5 (as controlled by ^{3}H-thymidine and 5-Br-DU incorporation). The pattern of 5-Br-DU staining was similar in cells injected with the sense cyclin A construct (data not shown) and in cells injected with the anti-sense cyclin B construct (fig. 4 pannels A and B) which showed between 50 to 85% of DNA synthesis, a level similar to that achieved in the surrounding non injected cells. In contrast, cells injected with the anti-sense cyclin A construct (fig. 4 pannels C-F, and table 1), showed no evidence of DNA synthesis if injected during day 2 (C and D) or day 3 (E and F) ; we detected no evidence of nuclear staining for cyclin A in injected cells (data not shown). Surrounding uninjected cells proceeded normally to transit S-phase. This effect was observed in all the cells injected with the anti-sense constructs from the end of day 2 until day 3.

DISCUSSION :

In this paper, we have both analyzed the HBV and cyclin A expression in the tumor HEN and further caracterized the role of cyclin A in a normal cell cycle.

Concerning the tumor HEN, we have provided strong evidence for a role of HBV in a step of liver cell transformation by insertional mutagenesis. Indeed we showed an increased level of hybrid transcripts HBV-cyclin A, potentially coding for a stabilized chimeric protein. There are several possibilities to account for its effect on the cell phenotype. Loss of the degradation signals in the N-terminal part of the cyclin A, together with initiation from the Pre S2/S viral promoter, may lead to an increased and constitutive synthesis of cyclin A. In addition it is also plausible that the membranous PreS2/S protein may markedly change the localization in the cell of the protein. Finally the viral sequences at the N-terminal part include a truncated form of PreS/S which may have retained a transactivating effect on cellular oncogenes (Kekule et al., 1990 ; Caselman et al., 1990). These different possibilities are being explored through in vitro transfection of cell cultures and in vivo experiments on transgenic mice.

In order to clarify the involvement of cyclin A in carcinogenesis, we have also adressed the issue of its potential role in the G1/S phase of the cell cycle. The present study provides two lines of evidence for the requirement of cyclin A for the cell to proceed to S phase. First, cyclin A mRNA and protein are accumulated as the cells enter S phase in hepatocytes in-vitro and in-vivo. Secondly, the microinjection of an anti-sense cyclin A cDNA inhibited DNA synthesis in cultured normal epithelial cells. The involvememt of cyclin A in the S phase was further supported by the specific inhibition of DNA synthesis following the microinjection of an anti-sense cyclin A while an anti-sense cyclin B cDNA did not inhibit DNA synthesis. Therefore, our observation, based on normal epithelial cells analyzed in-vitro and in-vivo, does imply that cyclin A is not only a mitotic cyclin but also acts at S phase. This finding is also

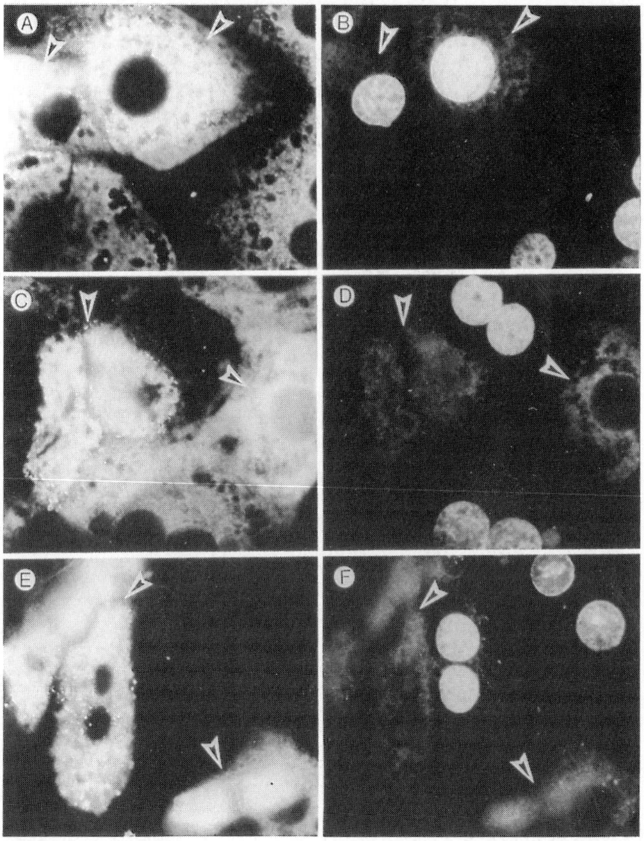

Fig. 4 : effect on DNA synthesis in cultured hepatocytes of overexpression of anti-sense cyclin constructs. To examine the involvement of cyclin A in S phase transit in cultured hepatocytes, cells stimulated by growth factors (day 0) were microinjected with either anti-sense human cyclin A or B cDNA under transcriptional regulation of a SV40 enhancer element. Immediately afterwards, cells were incubated in the presence of 5-Br-DU.
Cells were stained for the distribution of 5-Br-DU (panels B, D, F) and subsequently for the non-specific anti-serum co-injected with the DNA (panels A, C, E). Shown are cells injected on the second day of culture (panels A-D) and cells injected on the third day of culture (panels E and F). Cells were microinjected with either an anti-sense cyclin B (panels A-B), or anti-sense cyclin A (panels C-F) cDNA constructs. Arrowed are the injected cells.

consistent with recent in-vitro reports based on cell-free replication of simian virus 40 DNA (D'Urso et al, 1990). In view of our present observation on the role of cyclin A in S phase, it is interesting to note that cyclin A has been recently shown to associate to E_2F transcription factor in S phase (Mudryj et al,

1991), and to be included in a complex containing the retinoblastinoma protein and the DRTF1 transcription factor (related to E2F) (Bandara et al, 1991). It is therefore possible that cyclin A plays a role in regulation of transcription. Our result also raises the question as to the nature of cdc2 protein kinase which associates to cyclin A. Cyclin A has been shown to complex both to $p34^{cdc2}$ as well as to a $p33^{cdc2}$ (Pines and Hunter, 1990), recently referred to as CDCK2 (Tsai et al., 1991).
Therefore, this study might be important with regard to the potential involvement of cyclin A in cell transformation. Indeed, cyclin A has been shown to associate with the E1A protein of adenovirus in infected cells (Giordano et al 1983). In addition, hepatitis B virus DNA has integrated into the cyclin A gene in a human primary liver cancer. That cyclin A is involved in S phase may provide new clues as to its potential role in carcinogenesis.

REFERENCES

Bandara, L.R. & La Thangue, N.B. (1991) : Cyclin A and the retinoblastoma gene product complex with a common transcription factor. Nature 351, 494-497.

Beasley, R.P. (1988) : Hepatitis B virus : the major etiology of hepatocellular carcinoma. Cancer Res. 61, 1942-1956.

Booher, R., and Beach, D. (1988) : Involvement of cdc13+ in mitotic control in Schizosacchromyces pombe : possible interaction of the gene product with microtubules. EMBO J. 7, 2321-2327.

Bucher, N.L.R. & Malt, R.A. (1971) : Regeneration of liver and kidney. Little, Brown & Co, New-York, 1-278.

Caselman, W.H., Meyer, M., Kekule, A.S., Lauer, U., Hofscheneider, P.H. & Koshy, R. (1990) : A trans-activator function is generated by integration of hepatitis B virus preS/S sequences in human hepatocellular carcinoma DNA. Proc. Natl. Acad. Sci. USA 87, 2970-2974.

Chisari, F.V., Klopchin, K., Moriyama, T., Pasquinelli, C., Dunsford, H.A., Sell, S. Pinkert, C.A., Brinster, R.L. & Palmer, R.D. 1990 : Molecular pathogenesis of hepatocellular carcinoma in hepatitis B virus transgenic mice. Cell 59, 1145-1156.

Dejean, A., Bougueleret, L., Grzeschik, K.H., & Tiollais, P. (1986) : Hepatitis B virus DNA integration in a sequence homologous to v-erb-A and steroid receptor gene in a hepatocellular carcinoma. Nature 322, 70-72.

Draetta, G. Luca, F., Westendorf, J., Brizuela, L., Ruderman, J. & Beach, D. (1989) : cdc2 protein kinase is complexed with both cyclin A and B : evidence for proteolytic inactivation of MPF. Cell 56, 829-838.

Fang, F. & Newport, J.W. (1991) : Evidence that the G1-S and G2-M transitions are controlled by differnt cdc2 proteins in higher eukaryotes. Cell, 66, 731-742.

Forsburg, S.L., and Nurse, P. (1991) : Identification of a G1-type cyclin puc1+ in the fission yeast Schizosaccharomyces pombe. Nature 351, 245-248.

Fourel, G., Trepo, C., Bougueleret, L., Henglein, B., Ponzetto, A., Tiollais, P. & Buendia, M.A. (1990) : Frequent activation of N-myc genes by hepadnavirus insertion in woodchuck liver tumours. Nature 347, 294-298.

Gautier, J., Minshull, J. Lohka, M., Glotzer, M., Hunt, & Maller, J.L. (1990) : Cyclin is a compoment of maturing-promoting -factor from Xenopus. Cell 60, 487-494.

Ghiara, J.B., Richardson, H.E., Sugimoto, K., Henze, M., Lew, D.J., Wittenberg, C. & Reed, S.I. (1991) : A cyclin B homolog in S. cerevisiae : chronic activation of the cdc28 protein kinase prevents exit from mitosis. Cell 65, 163-174.

Giordanno, A., Whyte, P., Harlow, Ed., Franza, B.R., Beach, D., Draetta, G. (1989) : A 60 kd cdc2-associated polypeptide complexes with the E1A proteins in adenovirus-infected cells. Cell 58, 981-990.

Glotzer, M., Murray, A.W. & Kirschner, M.W. (1991) : Cyclin is degraded by the ubiquitin pathway. Nature 349, 132-137.

Grisham, J.W., (1962) : A morphologic study of deoxyribonucleic acid synthesis and cell proliferation in regenerating rat liver ; autoradiography with Thymidine-^{3}H. Cancer Res. 22, 842-849.

Hadwiger, J.A., Wittenberg, C., Richardson, H.E., de Barros Lopes, M. & Reed, S.I. (1989) :A family of cyclin homologs that control the G1 phase in yeast. Proc. Natl. Acad. Sci. USA 86, 6255-6259.

Kekulé, A.S., Lauer, U., Meyer, M., Caselman, W.H., Hofschneider, P.H. & Koshy, R. (1990) : The preS2/S region of integrated hepatitis B virus encodes a transcriptionnal transactivator. Nature 343, 457-460.

Kim, C.M., Koike, K., Saito, I., Miyamura, T. & Jay, G. (1991) : HBx gene of hepatitis B virus induces liver cancer in transgenic mice. Nature 351, 317-320.

Koff, A., Cross, A., Fisher, A., Schuma, J., Le Guellec, K., Philippe, M. & Roberts, J.M. (1991) : Human cyclin E, a new cyclin that interacts with two members of the cdc2 gene family. Cell 66, 1217-1228.

Labbé, J.C., Capony, J.P., Caput, D., Cavadore, J.C., Derancourt, J., Kaghad, M., Lelias, J.M., Picard, A. & Dorée, M. (1989) : MPF from starfish oocytes at first meiotic metaphase is a heterodimer containing one molecule of cdc2 and one molecule of cyclin B. EMBO J. 8, 3053-3058.

Matsushime, H., Roussel, M.F., Ashum, R.A. & Sherr, C.J. (1991) : Colony-stimulating factor 1 regulates novel cyclins during the G1 phase of the cell cycle. Cell 65, 701-713.

Meijer, L., Arion, D., Golsteyn, R., Pines, J., Brizuela, L., Hunt, T. & Beach, D. (1989) :Cyclin is a compoment of the sea urchin egg M-phase specific histone H1 kinase. EMBO J. 8, 2275-2282.

Mc Gowan, J.A. (1986) : prolifération des hépatocytes en culture Research in... Isolated and cultured hepatocytes. INSERM/John Libbey Eurotext, 13-40.

Minshull, J., Golsteyn, R., Hill, C.S. & Hunt T. (1990) :The A- and B-type cyclin associated cdc2 kinase in Xenopus turn on and off at different times in the cell cycle. Embo J. 9, 2865-2875.

Motokura, T., Bloom, T., Kim, H.G., Juppner, H., Ruderman, J.V., Kronenberg, H.M. & Arnold, A. (1991) : A novel cyclin encoded by a bcl1-linked candidate oncogene. Nature 350, 512-515.

Nash, R., Tokiwa, G., Anand, S., Erickson, K. & Futcher, A.B. (1988) : The WHI1+ gene of Saccharomyces cerevisiae tethers

cell division to cell size and is a cyclin homolog. EMBO J. 7, 4335-4346.
Pines, J., & Hunter, T. (1990) : Human cyclin A is adenovirus E1A -associated protein p60 and behaves differently from cyclin B. Nature 346, 760-763.
Swenson, K.I., Farell, K.M. & Ruderman, J.V. (1986) : The clam embryo protein cyclin A induces entry into M phase and resumption of meiosis in Xenopus oocytes. Cell 47, 861-870.
de Thé, H., Marchio, A., Tiollais, P. & Dejean, A. (1987) : A novel steroid thyroid hormone receptor-related gene inappropriately expressed in human hepatocellular carcinoma. Nature 330, 667-670.
Tsai, L.H., Harlow, E. & Meyerson, M. (1991) : Isolation of the cdk2 gene that encodes the cyclin A- and adenovirus E1A -associated p33 kinase. Nature 353, 174-177.
D'Urso, G., Marraciano, R.L., Marchak, D.K., & Roberts, J.M. (1990) : Cell cycle control of DNA replication by a homologue from human cells of the $p34^{cdc2}$ protein kinase. Science 250, 786-791.
Wang, J., Chenivesse, X., Henglein, B., Bréchot, C. (1990) : Hepatitis B virus integration in a cyclin A gene in a hepatocellular carcinoma. Nature 343, 555-557.
Xiong, Y., Connolly, T., Futcher, B. & Beach, D. (1991) : Human D -type cyclin. Cell 65, 691-699.

Résumé

Nous avons décrit précédemment l'intégration de l'ADN du virus de l'hépatite B (VHB) dans un intron du gène de la cycline A dans un cancer du foie. Ce travail nous a permis d'isoler l'ADNc de la cycline A humaine.
Nous avons construit une banque d'ADNc à partir de la tumeur originale (tumeur HEN) et isolé plusieurs ADNc hybrides VHB-cycline A. Ces ADNc hybrides présentent une phase ouverte de lecture codant pour une protéine de fusion qui comprend la partie N-terminale de la protéine préS2/S suivie de la cycline A. Cependant la partie N-terminale de la cycline A, impliquée dans sa dégradation, est délétée. L'intégration du VHB dans le gène de la cycline A rend compte de la surexpression des transcripts hybrides VHB-cycline A codant pour une protéine stabilisée.
De plus, nous avons étudié l'expression du gène de la cycline A dans les hépatocytes de rat en culture primaire et dans le foie de rat en régénération après hépatectomie partielle. Dans les deux cas, les ARNm et la protéine cycline A s'accumulent au moment où les cellules rentrent en phase S. La microinjection de plasmides contenant l'ADNc antisens de la cycline A inhibe la synthèse de l'ADN.
En conclusion, nous avons analysé le profil d'expression de la cycline A dans la tumeur HEN. Les résultats obtenus renforcent l'hypothèse d'une mutagénèse insertionnelle du VHB. Par ailleurs, nous avons montré, dans les hépatocytes, que la cycline A est impliquée dans la transition G1/S du cycle cellulaire. L'ensemble de ces résultats apportent de nouvelles données quant au rôle de la cycline A dans la carcinogénèse.

Cellular and Molecular Aspects of Cirrhosis. Eds B. Clément, A. Guillouzo. Colloque INSERM/John Libbey Eurotext Ltd. © 1992, Vol. 216, pp. 277-285

Oncogenes and cell cycle in adult hepatocytes

Pascal Loyer, Denis Glaise, Laurent Meijer * and Christiane Guguen-Guillouzo

*INSERM U 49, Hôpital Pontchaillou, 35033 Rennes and * CNRS, Station Biologique, Roscoff, France*

ABSTRACT

A sequential activation of proto-oncogenes, including c-fos, c-myc,p53 the jun and the ras families, has been reported to parallel hepatocyte growth activity during liver regeneration after two-third hepatectomy. However, the mechanism(s) by which these proto-oncogenes may participate to the control of hepatocyte cell cycle progression remain(s) unclear. Particularly, their relation with the cdc2protein kinase activity is unknown. The aim of this work was 1) to analyze the different phases of the cell cycle of growing hepatocytes exposed to Epidermal Growth Factor (EGF) + pyruvate in primary culture ; 2) to characterize in parallel the cdc2 protein and its Histone H1 activity (H1k) ; 3) to determine the sequence of proto-oncogene activation in this model of normal proliferating cells. Isolated adult rat hepatocytes were cultured in a medium containing EGF, insulin and pyruvate. The S phase started 48 hours (hrs) after cell seeding and maximal DNA synthesis occurred at 84 hrs, the maximum of mitosis being around 96 hrs. When extracts were made throughout the cell cycle, cdc2 protein was detected only after 54 hrs and increased in amount thereafter, reaching a maximum at 84 hrs. Unexpectedly, no protein was detected during G1 and early S phases. In addition, quantification of the tyrosine 15 phosphorylated form of cdc2 protein showed an accumulation during the S phase followed by a gradual disappearance, indicative of the progression through the G2 and M phases. This finding was confirmed by activation of H1k. Transient increased amounts of c-fos and c-jun transcripts were observed during liver tissue disruption, and in isolated cells. Then, c-myc and jun B were expressed at a high levels up to the cell entrance in S phase (48 hrs), while p53 and jun D occurred during the G1 phase and remained overexpressed all along the cell cycle. C-Ki-ras slightly was expressed during the G1 phase and strongly increased at the G1/S transition. These results show that cdc2 plays a major role on the G2/M transition, but not on the G1/S transition, in rat hepatocytes. They strongly suggest that the G1/S-associated proto-oncogene activation is not directly induced by this mitosis-promoting factor.

INTRODUCTION

In normal liver, cells divide at a very low rate (<< 1% daily) and at the adult stage this tissue keeps the possibility to regenerate after partial mass loss (Higgins and Anderson, 1931). Partial hepatectomy (PHT) triggers the proliferation of liver cells which undergo DNA synthesis and division up to mass tissue recovery in a few days. (Grisham, 1962 ; Fabrikant, 1968). This regenerative process can be mimicked *in vitro* and advantageously

used to futher analyze the mechanisms that control the cell cycle progression. Different *in vitro* models have been described to allow hepatocyte DNA synthesis (Table 1). Among them, addition of insulin + Epidermal Growth Factor (EGF) + pyruvate was found as the most efficient supplied medium (EGFpyr) to induce an intense DNA replicative phase. However, unexpectedly only few mitotic figures were reported(Richman and al., 1976 ; Hasegawa and al, 1980 ; Friedman and al., 1981 ; McGowan et al., 1981; Hasegawa et al., 1982 ; St Hilaire and Jones, 1982 ; Strain et al., 1982 ; Russell et al., 1984 ; McGowan, 1986).
P34Cdc2 gene has been described to encode a cell cycle kinase protein, considered as a master effector which could control the restriction points (G1/S and G2/M transitions) in fission yeast Saccharomyces pombe cell cycle (Nurse and Bissett, 1981 ; Piggott, et al., 1982). More recently, p34cdc2 has been also shown to play a crucial role in G2/M transition in a large range of proliferating eukaryotic cells (Arion et al., 1988 ; Draetta and Beach, 1988 ; Draetta et al., 1988 ; Lee et al., 1988). However, in mammalians, its role in G1/S transition is still yet discussed. Indeed, data from different transformed cell lines seemed to confirm a p34cdc2 control of G1/S transition in contrast with others which suggested that G1/S and G2/M transitions may be controlled by distinct cell cycle kinases (Elledge and Spottswood, 1991 ; Fang and Newport, 1991 ; Paris et al.,1991).We have devised experiments on hepatocytes using the EGFpyr model to define the role of p34cdc2 in normal proliferating cells.
Numerous studies have described a sequential proto-oncogene activation after PHT (Corral et al., 1985 ; Thompson et al., 1986 ; Sobczack et al., 1989 ; Morello et al., 1990), underlying for each of them distinct role(s) on the cell cycle progression (Fig. 1). However, this activation sequence of proto-oncogenes remained largely controversed when compared to other proliferating cell systems. Thus, in regenerating liver, c-fos, c-myc and jun expression occurred during the G0/G1 transition and/or early G1 phase, and are so called immediate-early proto-oncogenes. In contrast, in several synchronized *in vitro* cell lines, the specific induction of c-myc related to the G1 phase was not evidenced (Thompson et al., 1985 ; Waitz and Loidl, 1991), and in a recent report of Carter et al. (1991) on synchronized WI-38 human fibroblasts, a late overexpression of c-jun at the G1/S boundary was clearly shown. Only few reports described proto-oncogene expression in hepatocyte primary cultures. We previously demonstrated a transient overexpression of c-fos after tissue disruption of rat liver, and a maintenance of c-myc in long-term culture of normal adult rat hepatocytes (Etienne et al., 1988). Sawada et al. (1989) also showed activation of c-myc in short-term cultured hepatocytes treated or not with EGF and suggested that hepatocytes might progress from G0 to the G1 phase even in absence of DNA synthesis. This hypothesis was confirmed by Ikeda et al. (1989).
Here, we have established the sequence of proto-oncogene activation in dividing hepatocytes in relation with the cell cycle progression and p34cdc2 expression.

TABLE 1 : MAJOR HUMORAL GROWTH STIMULATING FACTORS OF ADULT HEPATOCYTES.

Mitogenic factors	Co-mitogenic factors
EGF(McGowan, 1986)	Norepinephrin
TGF α	Vasopressin
HBGF-I or FGF	Oestrogens
Hepatopoietin A or HGF (Nakamura & al, 1988)	Angiotensin I and II
	Insulin
PDGF(Strain & al, 1982)	Glucagon

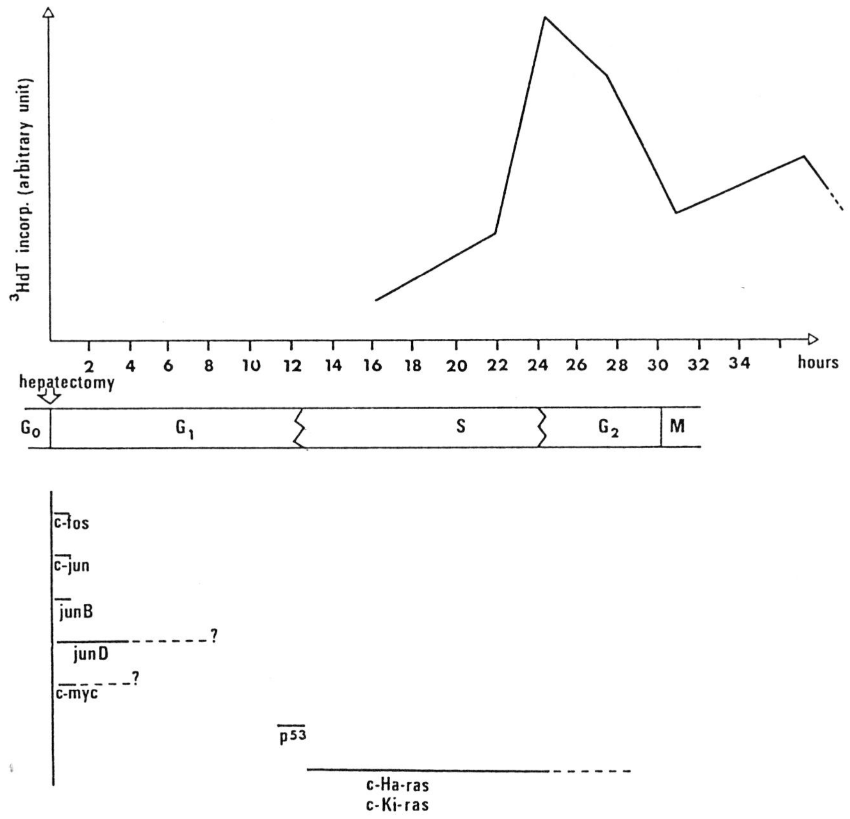

Figure 1: Schematic representation of the sequential proto-oncogene activation during rat liver regeneration.

RESULTS

Cell cycle of normal adult hepatocytes stimulated to proliferate in vitro.

When the basal medium (MEM/199; 2V/1V), containing insulin (5 ug/ml) and glucocorticoids (0.1 uM, hydrocortisone) was used, no (H^3)thymidine incorporation was detectable during the first 36 hours of culture, and only very low DNA synthesis could be observed from 2 to 6 days of culture. In contrast, when both EGF (50ng/ml) and pyruvate (20mM) were added to the basal medium, we found DNA synthesis, at least 10-fold increased (Fig. 2). Interestingly, no DNA synthesis occurred before 36 hrs of culture whatever the culture medium used, indicating a G1 phase time-lapse of 36 hrs. The S phase started 36 hrs after seeding and maximum of DNA synthesis was found at around 84hrs. Futhermore, numerous typical mitotic figures could be seen, indicating the high rate of divisions (Fig. 3). To confirm this point, mitotic index was established by counting the cells blocked in M phase by colcemid treatment. It was low (< 1/1000) during the first 48 hrs after plating, increased up to 10% at 72hrs and reached a maximum (50%) at around 96hrs. Thereafter DNA synthesis and mitotic rate decreased abruptly,

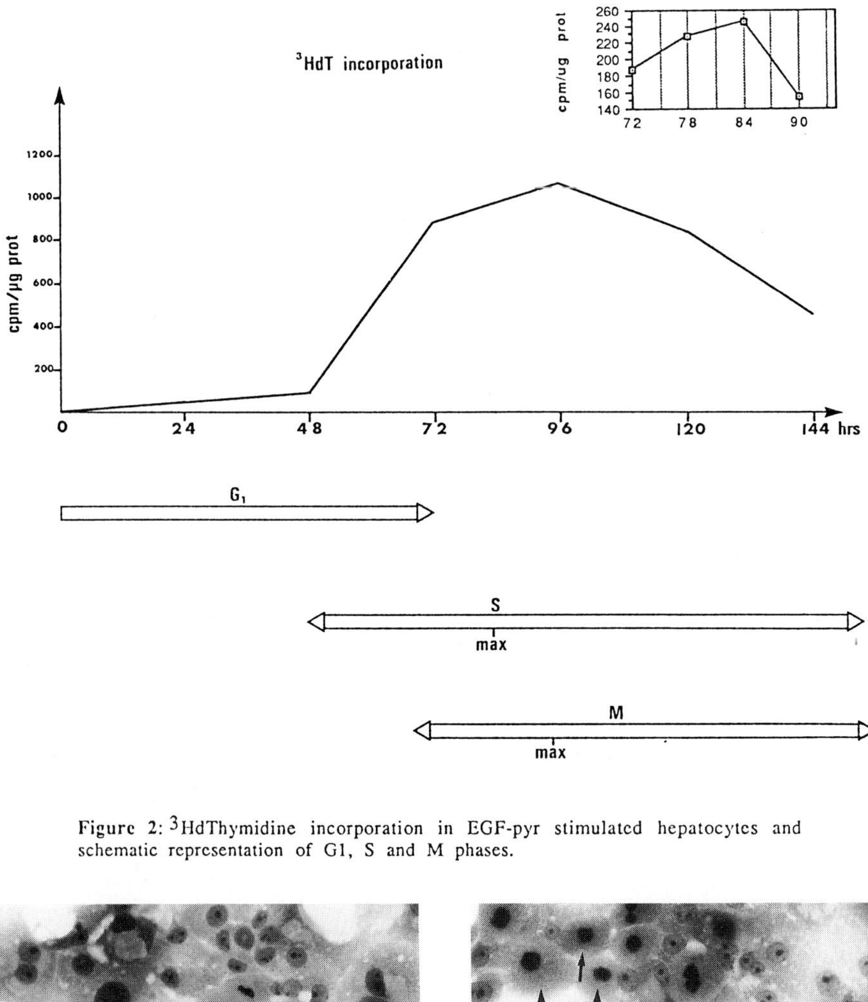

Figure 2: ^{3}HdThymidine incorporation in EGF-pyr stimulated hepatocytes and schematic representation of G1, S and M phases.

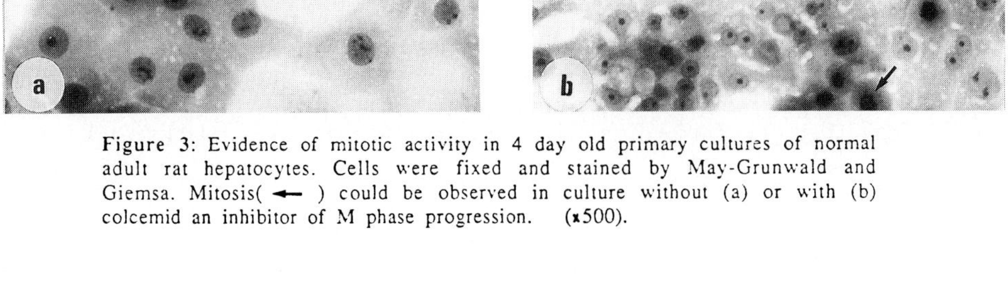

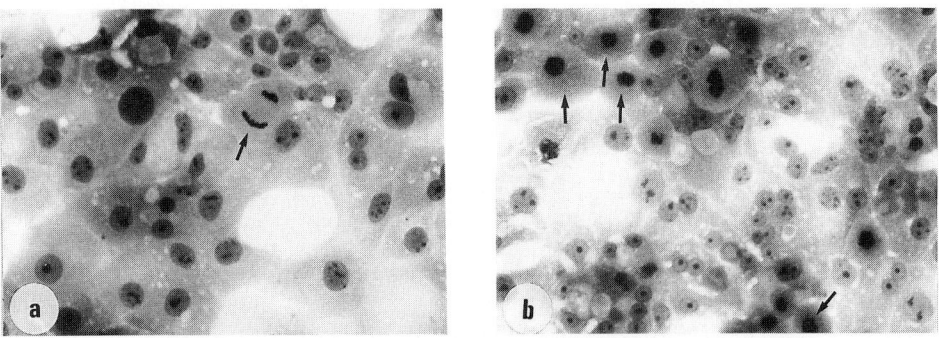

Figure 3: Evidence of mitotic activity in 4 day old primary cultures of normal adult rat hepatocytes. Cells were fixed and stained by May-Grunwald and Giemsa. Mitosis(←) could be observed in culture without (a) or with (b) colcemid an inhibitor of M phase progression. (x500).

corresponding to less than 5% of mitotic cells per day. Taken together these results show that EGFpyr induced most hepatocytes to enter the G1 and S phases in a synchronized manner and to progress through one complete cell cycle. This makes stimulated hepatocyte culture a very appropriate model for analyzing the different events which control progression through the different phases.

P34Cdc2 protein kinase expression along the cell cycle of normal hepatocytes in culture.

We have used the EGFpyr model of normal dividing hepatocytes to define the p34cdc2 expression through the cell cycle and to determine its role in G1/S and G2/M transitions (Fig. 4).
By northern blot analysis, we failed to detect the p34cdc2 mRNA during the first 36 hrs after plating. A faint band was detected after 48 hrs of culture. Its expression gradually increased up to a maximum between 72-84 hrs, and decreased thereafter. P34cdc2 protein was detected by western-blotting. It appeared as a faint band only 54 hrs after plating, and increased with time until 84 hrs, remained stable, and drastically decreased after 120 hrs of culture. These results indicated that DNA synthesis takes place several hours

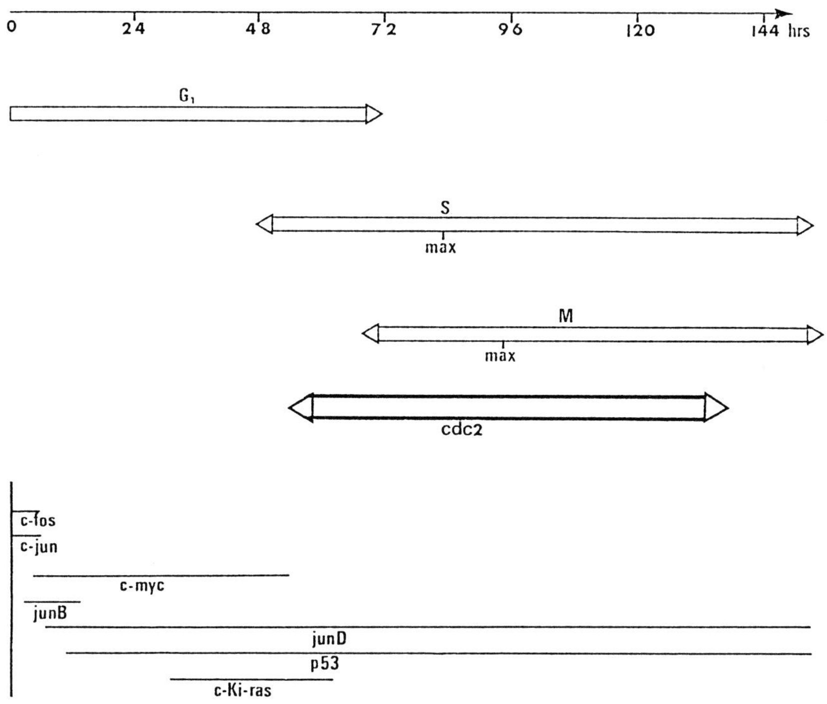

Figure 4: Schematic representation of the sequential cdc2 and proto-oncogene activation during cell cycle of normal adult rat hepatocytes cultured in EGFpyr medium.

before p34cdc2 synthesis. In addition, the cascade of phosphorylation/dephosphorylation and kinase activity of this protein was followed along the cell cycle. Quantitation of tyrosine15 phosphorylated form of cdc2, which is an inactive form of this protein kinase, showed no expression during G1 phase, an accumulation during S phase and as expected, a decrease after the peak of DNA synthesis in parallel to the cell progression towards the G2 and M phases. Moreover, the cdc2 kinase activity (using histone H1 as substrat) was found very high at 84 hrs of culture just before the peak of mitosis.
From these data, we may conclude that p34cdc2 could not be implicated in G1/S transition whereas it might control the G2/M transition.

Proto-oncogene activation during the cell cycle of dividing hepatocytes.

In order to progress in the understanding of the role of different proto-oncogenes in the mitotic cycle we have analyzed the level expression of 5 of them well-known to be overexpressed in liver after partial hepatectomy: c-fos, c-myc, p53, c-Ki-ras and jun family (Corral et al., 1985 ; Thompson et al., 1986 ; Sobczack et al., 1989; Morello et al., 1990).All these proto-oncogenes were also induced in EGFpyr stimulated hepatocyte model (Fig. 4). C-fos and c-jun overexpression took place very early during cell isolation indicating that hepatocytes entered in G1 phase, following tissue disruption. In contrast, jun D, jun B, c-myc expression increased in isolated cells and reached a maximum 6 hrs after plating. P53 was weakly expressed in freshly isolated cells, slightly increased 6 hrs after plating and highly expressed at 2 hrs. Thereafter, jun B and c-myc decreased whereas jun D and p53 were maintained all along the cell cycle, including the S and M phases. We have confirmed the G1-related expression of c-myc by using sodium butyrate which blocks the cells in early G1 phase. Treated hepatocytes exhibited a high level of c-myc mRNA all along the culture time. For c-Ki-ras, a faint band was detected in whole liver and in freshly isolated hepatocytes. It was slightly enhanced at 6 and 24 hrs, reached a maximum at 48 hrs and declined thereafter.

CONCLUSION

During the past decade, cell cycle regulation has been extensively studied. Thus, a great number of genes have been identified to play role in the cell cycle progression. Among them proto-oncogenes and cell cycle kinases were the most studied and numerous data were reported about their(s) cell cycle regulation(s) and function(s). These genes are studied in a large range of species, *in vivo* and *in vitro*. This heterogeneity of models was probably one of the reasons of conflicting data about functions of this group of genes. Moreover, in cultured mammalian cells, proto-oncogene expression is dependant on the transformation state of the cell lines. For these reasons, we have used primary cultures of normal rat hepatocytes and we have stimulated their growth activity in order to study cdc2 and proto-oncogene expression through the cell cycle. We showed a sequential proto-oncogene activation including c-fos, c-jun and c-myc, jun B,jun D and p53, c-Ki-ras which correspond to early enter in G1, progression in G1 and G1/S transition phases respectively. Cdc2 kinase protein appeared transiently expressed and capable to actively phosphorylate histone H1 in normal proliferating hepatocytes. Our data strongly evidence that cdc2 plays a major role on the G2/M transition, but not on the G1/S transition. Further experiments should be devised to define the cell cycle protein(s) implicated in the G1/S transition.

REFERENCES

Arion, D., Meijer L., Brizuela, L. & Beach, D. (1988): Cdc2 is a component of the M phase-specific Histone H1 kinase : Evidence for identity with MPF. *Cell* 55, 371-378.

Carter, R., Cosenza, S.C., Pena, A., Lipson, K., Soprano, D.R. & Soprano, K.J. (1991): A potential role for c-jun in cell cycle progression through late G1 and S.*Oncogene* 6, 229-235.

Corral, M., Tichoniky, L., Guguen-guillouzo, C.,Corcos, D., Raymonjean, M., Paris, B., Kruh, J. & Defer, N. (1985): Expression of c-fos oncogene during hepatocarcinogenesis, liver regeneration and synchronized HTC cells. *Exp. cell Res.* 160, 427-434.
Draetta, G. & Beach, D. (1988): Activation of cdc2 protein kinase during mitosis in human cells: cell cycle-dependent phosphorylation and subunit rearrangement. *Cell* 54, 17-26.
Draetta, G., Piwnica-Worms, H., Morrison, D., Druker, B., Roberts, T. & Beach, D. (1988): Human cdc2 protein kinase is a major cell-cycle regulated tyrosine kinase substrate. *Nature* 336, 738-744.
Elledge, S.J. & Spottswood, M.R.(1991): A new human p34 protein kinase, CDK2, identified by complementation of a cdc28 mutation in Saccharomyces cerevisiae, is a homolog of Xenopus Egl. *EMBO J.* 10, 2653-2659.
Etienne, P. L., Baffet, G., Desvergne, B., Boisnard-Rissel, M., Glaise, D. & Guguen-Guillouzo, C. (1988): Transient expression of c-fos and constant expression of c-myc in freshly isolated and cultured normal adult rat hepatocytes. *Oncogene Res.* 3, 255-262.
Fang, F. Newport, J.W. (1991): Evidence that the G1-S and G2-M transitions are controlled by different cdc2 proteins in higher eukaryotes. *Cell* 66, 731-742.
Fabrikant, J. I.(1968): The kinetic of cellular proliferation in regenerating liver. *J. Cell. Biol.* 36, 551-565.
Friedman, D., Claus, T., Pilkis, S. & Pine, G. (1981): Hormonal regulation of DNA synthesis in primary cultures of adult rat hepatocytes- Action of glucagon. *Exp. Cell. Res.* 135, 283-290.
Grisham, J.W. (1962): A morphologic study of deoxyribonucleic acid synthesis and cell proliferation in regenerating rat liver. Autoradiography with Thymidine-H^3. *Cancer Res.* 22, 842-849.
Hasegawa, K., Namai, K. & Koga, M. (1980): Induction of DNA synthesis in adult rat hepatocytes cultured in a serum free medium. *Biochem. Biophys. Res. Commun.* 95, 243-249.
Hasegawa, K., Watanabe, K. & Koga, M. (1982): Induction of mitosis in primary cultures of adult rat hepatocytes under serum free conditions. *Biochem. Biophys. Res. Commun.* 104, 259-265.
Higgins, G.M. & Anderson, R.M. (1931): Exprimental pathology of liver; Restoration of the liver of the white rat following partial surgical removal. *Arch. Pathol.* 12,186-202.
Ikeda T., Sawada N., Fujiniga K., Minase, T. & Mori, M. (1989): C-H-ras gene is expressed at the G1 phase in primary cultures of hepatocytes. *Exp. Cell. Res.* 185, 292-296.
Lee, M. G., Norbury, C.J., Spurr, N.K. & Nurse, P. (1988): Regulated expression and phosphorylation of a possible mammalian cell-cycle control protein. *Nature* 333, 676-679.
Mc.Gowan, J.A. (1986). Prolifération des hépatocytes en culture. Recherche en : *Hépatocytes en culture.* A. Guillouzo and C. Guguen-Guillouzo (eds.), pp. 13-40. INSERM, Paris and John Libbey Eurotext, London.
McGowan, J.A., Strain, A.J., Bucher, N. L. (1981): DNA synthesis in primary cultures of adult rat hepatocytes in adefined medium: effects of epidermal growth factor, insulin, glucagon, and cyclic-AMP. *J. Cell. Physiol.* 108, 353-363.
Morello, D., Lavenu, A. & Babinet, (1990): Differential regulation and expression of jun, c-fos and c-myc proto-oncogenes during mouse liver regeneration and after inhibition of protein synthesis. *Oncogene* 5, 1511-1519.
Nakamura, T., Nishizawa, T., Hagiya, M., Seki, T., Shimonishi, M., Sugimura, A., Tashiro, K. & Shimizu, S. (1988): Molecular cloning and expression of human hepatocyte growth factor. *Nature* 342, 440-443.
Nurse, P. & Bissett, Y. (1981): Gene required in G1 for commitment to cell cycle and in G2 for control of mitosis in fission yeast. *Nature* 292, 558-560.
Paris, J., Le Guellec, R., Couturier, A., Le Guellec, K., Omilli, F., Camonis, J., MacNeill, S. & Philippe, M. (1991): Cloning by differential screening of a xenopus cDNA coding for a protein highly homologous to cdc2. *Proc. Natl. Acad. Sci. USA* 88, 1039-1043.
Piggott, J., Rai, R. & Carter, B.(1982): A bifonctional gene product involved in two phases of the yeast cell cycle. *Nature* 298, 391-393.

Richman, R.A., Claus, T.H., Pilkis, S. & Friedman, D.L.(1976): Hormonal stimulation of DNA synthesis in primary cultures of adult rat hepatocytes. *Proc. Natl. Acad. Sci.* 73, 3589-3593.

Russell, W.E., McGowan, J.A. & Bucher, N.L.R. (1984): Partial characteriza-tion of a hepatocytes growth factor from rat platelets. *J. Cell. Physiol.* 119, 183-192.

Sawada, N.(1989): Hepatocytes from old rats retain responsiveness of c-myc expression to EGF in primary culture but do not enter S phase. *Exp. Cell Res.* 5, 584-588.

St Hilaire, R.J. & Jones, A. L.(1982): Epidermal growth factor: Its biological and metabolic effects with emphasis on the hepatocytes. *Hepatology* 2, 601-613.

Sobczack, J., Mechti, N., Tournier, M.F., Blanchard, J.M. & Duguet, M.(1989): C-myc and c-fos gene regulation during mouse liver regeneration. *Oncogene* 4, 1503-1508.

Strain, A.J., McGowan, J.A. & Bucher, N.L.(1982): Stimulation of DNA synthesis in primary culture of adult rat hepatocytes by rat platelet-associated substance(s). *In Vitro* 18, 108-116.

Thompson, N.L., Mead, J.E., Braun, L., Goyette, M., Shank, P.R.& Fausto, N. (1986): Sequential proto-oncogene expression during rat liver regeneration. *Cancer Res.* 46, 3111-3117.

Thompson, C. B., Challoner, P. B., Neiman, P. E. & Groudine, M. (1985): Levels of c-myc oncogene mRNA are invariant throughout the cell cycle.*Nature* 314, 363-366.

Waitz, W. & Loidl, P.(1991): Cell cycle dependent association of c-myc protein with the nuclear matrix. *Oncogene* 6, 29-35.

Résumé

Une activation séquentielle de proto-oncogenes dont c-fos, c-myc, p53, les familles jun et ras, est corrélée à la croissance des hépatocytes au cours du processus régénératif qui suit l'hépatectomie (HTP) expérimentale. Cependant, le(s) mécanisme(s) par le(s)quel(s) ces proto-oncogenes participent au contrôle de la progression des hépatocytes dans le cycle cellulaire reste(nt) obscur(s). En particulier, leur relation avec la protéine kinase cdc2 considérée comme une kinase clef du cycle cellulaire, demeure inconnue. Dans ce travail, nous nous sommes proposés 1) d'analyser les différentes phases du cycle cellulaire des hépatocytes normaux induits à proliférer sous l'effet combiné de l'Epidermal Growth Factor (EGF) et du pyruvate ; 2) de caractériser l'expression de cdc2 et de déterminer son activité kinase au cours des differentes phases du cycle cellulaire ; 3) de déterminer la séquence d'activation de divers proto-oncogenes dans ce modèle de cellules normales prolifératives. Les hépatocytes isolés de rat sont cultivés dans un milieu supplémenté en insuline, EGF et pyruvate. La phase S débute environ 48 heures (hrs) après l'ensemencement et le maximum de synthèse d' ADN se produit à 84 hrs et l'indice mitotique maximal se situe à 96 hrs. Dans les cultures récoltées à différents moments du cycle cellulaire, la protéine cdc2 n'était détectable que 54 hrs après l'ensemencement et son expression augmentait progressivement jusqu'à 84 hrs. D'une façon surprenante cette protéine était indétectable en phase G1 et en phase S précoce. De plus, la forme phosphorylée sur la tyrosine 15 de cdc2 était accumulée durant la phase S, puis disparaissait progressivement, indiquant une progression vers les phases G2 et M. Ce résultat était confirmé par l'activité histone H1 kinase. Une augmentation transitoire des messagers codant pour c-fos et c-jun était observée pendant la dissociation du foie et dans les hépatocytes isolés. C-myc et jun B étaient fortement surexprimés jusqu'à l'entrée en phase S alors que jun D et p53 étaient difficilement détectés en phase G1 et surexprimés tout au long du cycle cellulaire. Le taux du messager c-Ki-ras était faiblement exprimé durant la phase G1 et très augmenté à la transition G1/S. Ces résultats montrent que cdc2 joue un rôle majeur dans la transition G2/M, mais pas G1/S, dans les hépatocytes de rat. Ils suggèrent fortement que l'activation des proto-oncogènes associés à la transition G1/S n'est pas directement induite par ce factor mitotique.

Cellular and Molecular Aspects of Cirrhosis. Eds B. Clément, A. Guillouzo. Colloque INSERM/John Libbey Eurotext Ltd. © 1992, Vol. 216, pp. 287-298

Phenotypic characteristics and neoplastic transformation of primitive epithelial cells derived from rat liver and pancreas

Snorri S. Thorgeirsson, Anthony C. Huggett and Hanne Cathrine Bisgaard

Laboratory of Experimental Carcinogenesis, National Cancer Institute, Bethesda, Maryland 20892, USA

SUMMARY

Epithelial cell lines having extended capacity to proliferate in vitro were established from adult rat liver and pancreas. The cell lines exhibited almost identical phenotypes as judged by both morphological appearance and biochemical characterization. The cytokeratin expression in the hepatic and pancreatic epithelial cell lines revealed a unique coexpression and filament formation of the "simple" epithelial type II cytokeratins 7 and 8 with type I cytokeratin 14. These data indicate a common cell of origin for primitive epithelial cells isolated from rat liver and pancreas. Transformation of rat liver derived epithelial cells by both chemical carcinogens and oncogenes results in the generation of a wide range of tumors including hepatocellular carcinoma, cholangiocarcinoma, and hepatoblastoma as well as sarcoma and mixed epithelial-mesenchymal tumors (Tsao & Grisham, 1987; Garfield *et al.*, 1988). Transplantation of rat liver epithelial cells spontaneously transformed in vitro resulted in formation of hepatocellular carcinomas. The appearance of morphologically aberrant transformants correlated directly with an increased resistance of the population to the growth inhibitory effects of TGF-ß1.

Taken together these data indicate that rat liver epithelial cells represent a progeny from a progenitor cell compartment in the liver that may be a "target" for chemical and biological agents involved in hepatocarcinogenesis, and suggest that acquisition of resistance to the effects of growth inhibitors such as TGF-ß1 is an important and possibly essential stage in the spontaneous transformation of these cells. Furthermore, we hypothesized that a similar progenitor cell compartment exists in rat pancreas and that these cells may also be involved in pancreatic carcinogenesis.

INTRODUCTION

The rat liver and pancreas have a common embryonic origin, both being derived from almost identical regions of the primitive gut endoderm. These organs are comprised of predominantly epithelial cells, which based on their expression of cytokeratins, have been characterized as simple epithelia (Moll *et al.*, 1982). In the early fetal period, hepatic cells express predominantly cytokeratins 8, 14, and 18 (Germain *et al.*, 1988a,b; Marceau, 1990). However, as cell differentiation proceeds in the liver along the hepatocytic or biliary epithelial lineages a more complex pattern of cytokeratin expression arises. While hepatocytes express primarily cytokeratins 8 and 18, biliary epithelial cells express cytokeratins 7, 8, 18, and 19 (Marceau, 1990). Interestingly, the cytokeratin expression in adult pancreas parallels that seen in the liver, specifically, pancreatic acinar cells express cytokeratins 8 and 18 while pancreatic ductal cells express cytokeratins 7, 8, 18, and 19 (Marceau, 1990).

Recently it has been reported that hepatocytes appear in the pancreas of rats during aging (Chiu, 1987) or after feeding a diet deficient in copper (Reddy *et al.*, 1984; Rao *et al.*, 1989). The pancreatic hepatocytes in $Cu2^{+}$-deficient animals seem to arise from periductular or ductular cells in a manner very similar, if not identical, to the oval cell derived hepatocytes in livers of animals exposed to chemical hepatocarcinogens (Farber, 1984; Evarts *et al.*, 1987; Rao *et al.*, 1989). Thus, we and others have hypothesized that a "stem" cell compartment of common embryonic origin is present in both the liver and pancreas (Sell, 1990; Thorgeirsson & Evarts, 1991; Bisgaard & Thorgeirsson, 1991; Fig. 1).

Extensive research in hepatocarcinogenesis has revealed that one of the earliest cellular responses to chemical hepatocarcinogens in the rat involves the proliferation of cells located around the terminal bile ductules followed by the appearance of a rapidly growing population of small distinct epithelial cells characterized by oval nuclei and dense cytoplasm (Farber, 1984; Sell, 1990). These cells, commonly referred to as "oval cells," have been shown to be multipotent cells which can differentiate into hepatocytes as well as other cell lineages (Inaoka, 1967; Grisham *et al.*, 1974; Evarts *et al.*, 1987; Evarts *et al.*, 1989; Evarts *et al.*, 1990). Additionally, oval cells can undergo intestinal metaplasia (Tatematsu *et al.*, 1985) and may also differentiate into pancreatic tissue in rat liver (Kimbrough *et al.*, 1972; Rao *et al.*, 1986). Presence of both "oval" cells and exocrine pancreatic tissue similar to that seen in human liver has recently been observed (Wolf *et al.*, 1990; Hsia, C.-H. & Thorgeirsson S.S., unpublished data). During the early stages of oval cell proliferation, a majority of the small epithelial cells seem to express cytokeratins similar to that of biliary ductular cells (Germain *et al.*, 1985; Dunsford *et al.*, 1989; Dunsford & Sell, 1989; Evarts *et al.*, 1990).

Recent studies have indicated that the development of hepatocarcinogenesis following hepatitis B virus infection is the result of the increased proliferation and associated spontaneous transformation of liver cells consequent to the induction of a chronic inflammatory response, rather than due to insertion of a viral transforming gene or protooncogene activation following virus integration (Chisari *et al.*, 1989). It is likely that this process involves spontaneous mutations of key regulatory genes or epigenetic events altering gene expression within the target cell populations in the liver. Similar mechanisms are likely to be involved in the progression of hepatocarcinogenesis following initiation with chemical carcinogens. An increased rate of spontaneous transformation within the preneoplastic cell population may result from the increased rate of cell turnover that is commonly observed in the hepatic lesions derived following the exposure of animals to carcinogens (Rotstein *et al.*, 1986; Takematsu *et al.*, 1987). Thus it is proposed that liver stem cells, which are capable of multiple cell divisions, are likely targets for spontaneous transformation following either hepatitis virus or carcinogen insult.

Spontaneous transformation in vitro may represent a better model for the study of the stepwise process of carcinogenesis than the direct transformation of cells with potent transforming agents. Using such a system it may be possible to dissect out distinct cell types representing phenotypes at different stages of the neoplastic process. We have derived spontaneous transformants of normal

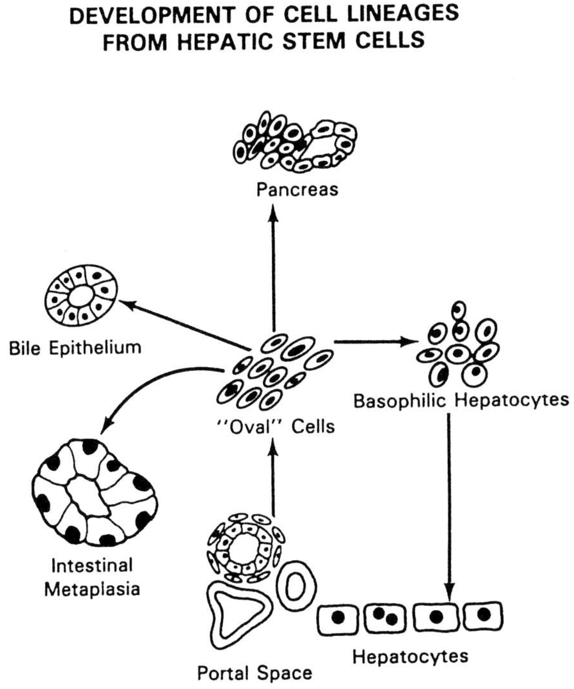

Fig. 1. Hypothetical scheme for development of cell lineages in rat liver.

diploid rat liver epithelial cells and used this model system to investigate whether spontaneous transformation in vitro is associated with the development of a TGF-ß1 resistant phenotype.

RESULTS AND DISCUSSION

Epithelial cell lines having extended capacity to proliferate in vitro were established from adult rat liver and pancreas. The clonal lines RLEAM7 and RLEAM12 (Rat Liver Epithelial Adult Male clones #7 and #12) were established from a 9 week old male Fischer rat (Bisgaard & Thorgeirsson, 1991). The clonal line RLESF13 (Rat Liver Epithelial Suckling Female clone #13) was established from a 10 day old female Fischer rat as previously described (McMahon *et al.*, 1986).

The clonal lines RPEAM3 and RPEAM4 (Rat Pancreas Epithelial Adult Male clones #3 and #4) were established from pancreas of a 9 week old male Fischer rat (Bisgaard & Thorgeirsson, 1991). The cell line FR (Epidermis, Germ-free fetal rat) was obtained from the American Type Culture Collection (Rockville, MD).

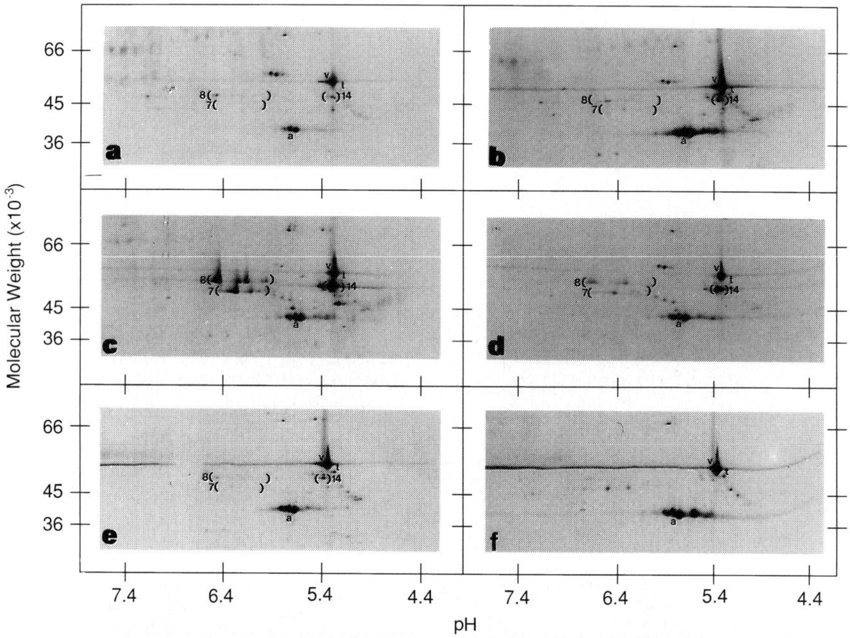

Fig. 2. Two-dimensional electrophoretic patterns of [^{35}S]-methionine labelled cytoskeletal proteins extracted (a) RLEAM7 passage 13, (b) RLEAM12 passage 11, (c) RPEAM3 passage 9 and (d) RPEAM4 passage 9, (e) RLESF13 passage 18, (f) FR. Abscissa, pH range; ordinate, molecular weight x 103. The abbreviations used are: 7, cytokeratin 7; 8, cytokeratin 8; 14, cytokeratin 14; a, actin; v, vimentin; t, ß-tubulin (From Bisgaard & Thorgeirsson 1991, with permission).

The two-dimensional gel patterns of ^{35}S-methionine labelled intermediate filaments extracted from RLEAM7, RLEAM12, RPEAM3, RPEAM4, RLESF13 and FR are shown in Fig. 2. Relatively few intermediate filament proteins were present in the cell lines. For identification, the polypeptides were transferred to nitrocellulose and their location visualized by immunostaining with specific antibodies (data not shown). The two-dimensional gel analysis performed on our established cell lines showed that cytokeratins 7, 8 and 14 were synthesized in several of the cell lines. Immunofluorescent localization of cytokeratins 8 and 14 revealed formation of filament bundles expanding from the nucleus to the membrane. Filament formation of cytokeratins normally requires expression of distinct pairs of type I and type II cytokeratins, the normal counterpart for cytokeratin 8 being cytokeratin 18 (Hatzfeld & Franke, 1985). However, we were unable to detect an equivalent of cytokeratin 18 as well as 19 in the cell lines at early as well as late passage number in vitro. Cytokeratin 8 has been shown to be indiscriminate when forming filaments in reconstituted systems in vitro (Hatzfeld & Franke, 1985). In addition, it has been suggested to act as an indiscriminate type II cytokeratin in filament formation with other type I cytokeratins such as 19 in intestinal epithelia and MCF-7 cells (Moll *et al*., 1982). In view of the coexpression of cytokeratins 8 and 14 observed in the RLEAM12 after prolonged passage in vitro and our inability to detect cytokeratins 18, 19 and 5, it seems reasonable to suggest that cytokeratin 8 acts as the type II partner in filament formation with cytokeratin 14 in all our epithelial cell lines. Whether cytokeratin 7 can act as an indiscriminate cytokeratin in filament formation in the epithelial cell lines is presently under investigation.

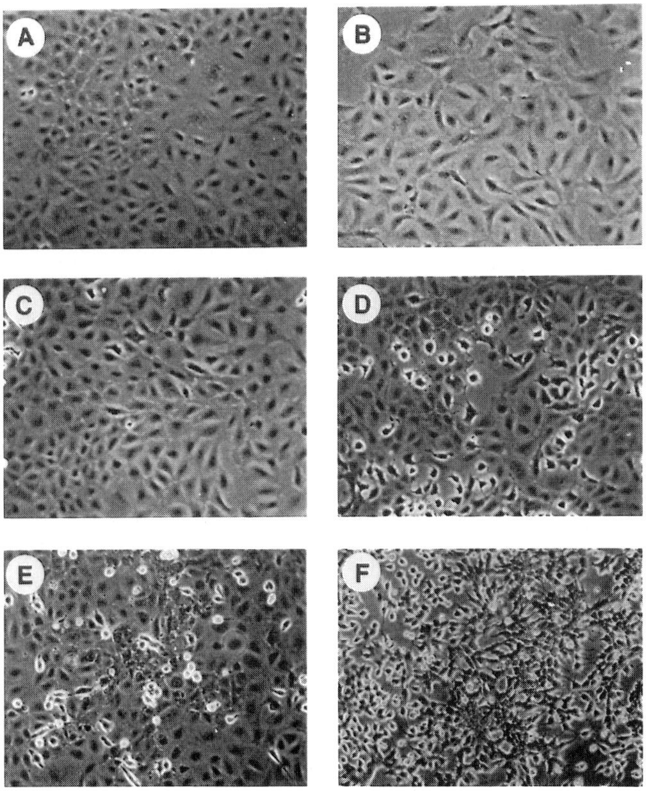

Fig. 3. Morphology of RLESF13 cells during spontaneous transformation. A: passage 32. B: passage 34. C: passage 36. D passage 37. E: passage 38. F: passage 39 (From Huggett *et al*., 1991, with permission).

A few cells showing an aberrant morphology were observed in the RLESF13 cell cultures at passage 36 (about 108 population doublings following original cloning of RLESF13 cells) and by passage 39 about 95% of the cell population was comprised of morphologically transformed cells as shown in Fig. 3 (Huggett *et al.*, in press 1991).

The majority of the cell lines cloned out from the passage 36 population showed a similar transformed morphology, consisting of small cells with little cytoplasm and an enlarged nucleus compared to the original early passage RLESF13 cells. Seven of these cell lines (A2T, A5T, B1T, B3T, B5T, C3T, C4T) were selected for further analysis. Only a few apparently normal clones were obtained and these were further single-cell cloned to ensure that there was no contamination with individual transformed cells. During this second cloning procedure one of the apparently normal cell lines, B4N, underwent a morphological transformation to the transformed phenotype described above. The remaining cell lines continued to exhibit a similar normal epithelial morphology to the early passage RLE«13 cells although they tended to be more irregular and less cuboidal.

There was no clear relationship between morphological transformation and doubling time in monolayer culture (Table 1). In contrast, the anchorage-independent growth of the cells was related to transformation in that all of the morphologically transformed cell lines formed colonies in soft agar while no colonies were obtained for any of the normal clones (Table 1). EGF (5 ng/ml) produced a marked stimulation of colony formation by A2T and B3T cells but had little effect on the other cell lines.

The effects of TGF-ß1 on DNA synthesis in RLESF13 cells during serial passaging are illustrated in Fig. 4. TGF-ß1 had potent inhibitory activity on DNA synthesis in early passage (passages 18-35) RLESF13 cells, with greater than 90% inhibition produced with a TGF-ß1 concentration of 300 pg/ml, and about a 40% inhibition with 30 pg/ml TGF-ß1. However at later passages the cells became resistant to the antiproliferative effect of TGF-ß1, such that by passage 43 the cell population showed little inhibition of DNA synthesis in the presence of TGF-ß1 at a concentration of 30 pg/ml, and only about 20% inhibition at 300 pg/ml. These findings correlated with the appearance of morphologically aberrant cells in the RLESF13 populations at the later passages.

In order to assess whether the development of resistance to TGF-ß1 growth inhibition was merely a function of passaging, general to the whole population, or associated with the development of individual spontaneously transformed cells, the effect of TGF-ß1 on DNA synthesis in the clonal cell lines was examined (Fig. 5). Each of these cell lines was investigated at the fourth passage following their cloning. The clones with a near-normal morphology [B4T, B7(96), E5(96-2)] showed a similar inhibition of DNA synthesis with TGF-ß1 (300 pg/ml) as observed in RLESF13 cells at passage 13. DNA synthesis in these normal cell lines was also inhibited by TGF-ß1 at a concentration of 30 pg/ml although they appeared to be slightly more resistant to this TGF-ß1 concentration than the early passage RLESF13 cells. In contrast, all of the morphologically aberrant clones were completely resistant to 30 pg/ml TGF-ß1 and they exhibited a much reduced inhibition of DNA synthesis with 300 pg/ml TGF-ß1 than was observed for the more normal-looking cell lines. A wide range of inhibitory responses to 300 pg/ml TGF-ß1 were obtained and four of the clones (A2T, A5T, B3T, B4N) were as resistant to TGF-ß1 as the rat liver tumor-derived RC-3 cell line, which was used as a control (Chapekar *et al.*, 1989).

TABLE 1 *Phenotypic properties of spontaneously-transformed RLE cells*

Cell Line	Doubling Time (h)	Soft Agar Growth[a] -EGF	Soft Agar Growth[a] +EGF	γGT Activity[b]	Tumorigenicity Incidence	Tumorigenicity Latency[c] (days)	Tumorigenicity Growth Rate[d] (mm^2/day)
RLEØ13	24.6 ± 1.7	0.0	0.0	--	0/5	-	0/0
B4T	14.9 ± 0.2	0.0	0.0	--	0/5	-	0/0
B7(96)	19.8 ± 1.7	0.0	0.0	--	0/5	-	0/0
E5(96-2)	29.7 ± 3.5	0.0	0.0	--	0/5	-	0/0
A2T	20.6 ± 0.8	3.5 ± 0.3	29.2 ± 4.8	++	5/5	6 ± 0.7	38.8 ± 6.0
A5T	20.9 ± 1.4	8.8 ± 0.6	11.3 ± 2.5	++	5/5	6 ± 0.8	36.1 ± 3.4
B1T	23.2 ± 1.0	2.3 ± 0.5	2.7 ± 0.7	+	5/5	7 ± 0.8	21.5 ± 3.1
B3T	18.1 ± 0.3	3.1 ± 0.1	33.1 ± 3.5	++	5/5	9 ± 1.2	10.8 ± 1.0
B4N	14.6 ± 1.0	17.4 ± 1.7	21.3 ± 0.6	--	5/5	9 ± 0.5	21.7 ± 1.9
B5T	18.5 ± 0.8	2.8 ± 0.6	3.6 ± 0.9	+	5/5	6 ± 0.1	13.1 ± 0.3
C3T	20.3 ± 0.6	6.9 ± 1.4	8.6 ± 0.5	++	5/5	7 ± 0.9	26.6 ± 3.8
C4T	15.0 ± 1.3	33.7 ± 2.7	33.6 ± 1.0	+	5/5	8 ± 0.8	13.8 ± 0.9

[a] Colony forming efficiency (%), EGF (5 ng/ml)

[b] Histochemical staining for γGT activity: -- no detectable staining; ++ all cells show intense staining

[c] Within one month

[d] Diameter x depth

From Huggett *et al.*, 1991

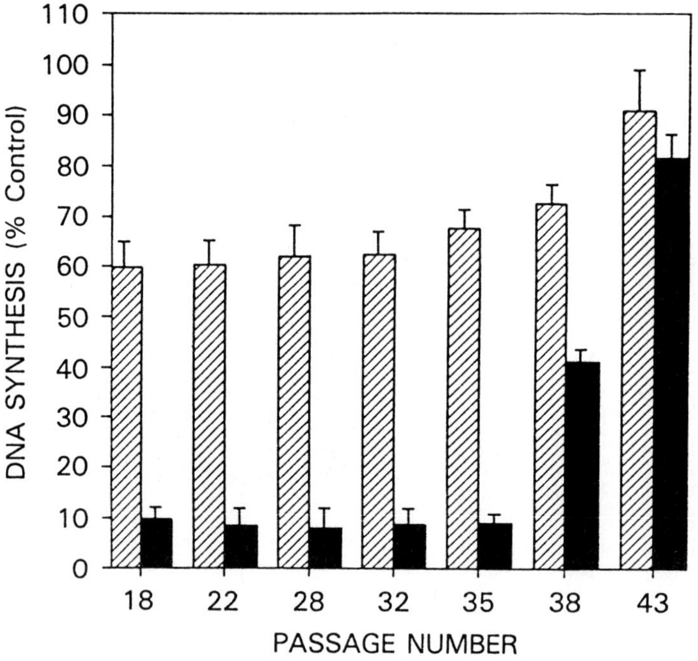

Fig. 4. Effect of TGF-ß1 on DNA synthesis in RLESF13 cells at different passages during spontaneous transformation. (mean ± SD, n=8). Hatched bar: 30 pg/ml; Solid bar: 300 pg/ml (From Huggett *et al.*, 1991 with permission).

In this study we have confirmed that temporary maintenance of hepatic epithelial cell populations at confluence before passaging can result in the generation of spontaneous transformants after about 100 population doublings (Lee *et al.*, 1989). The appearance of morphologically aberrant transformants in the rat liver epithelial cell population correlated directly with an increased resistance of the population to the growth inhibitory effects of TGF-ß1. Clonal cell lines derived from the transformants were resistant to TGF-ß1 dependent inhibition of DNA synthesis. These cell lines were also highly tumorigenic, aneuploid with characteristic gross chromosomal abnormalities and expressed a number of phenotypic markers common to RLE cells transformed by oncogenes or chemicals. In contrast, apparently normal-looking cell lines cloned from the same population were non-tumorigenic, near-diploid and were as sensitive to TGF-ß1 as early passage normal rat liver epithelial cells. These findings suggest that acquisition of resistance to the effects of growth inhibitors such as TGF-ß1 is an important and possibly essential step in the spontaneous transformation of rat liver epithelial cells.

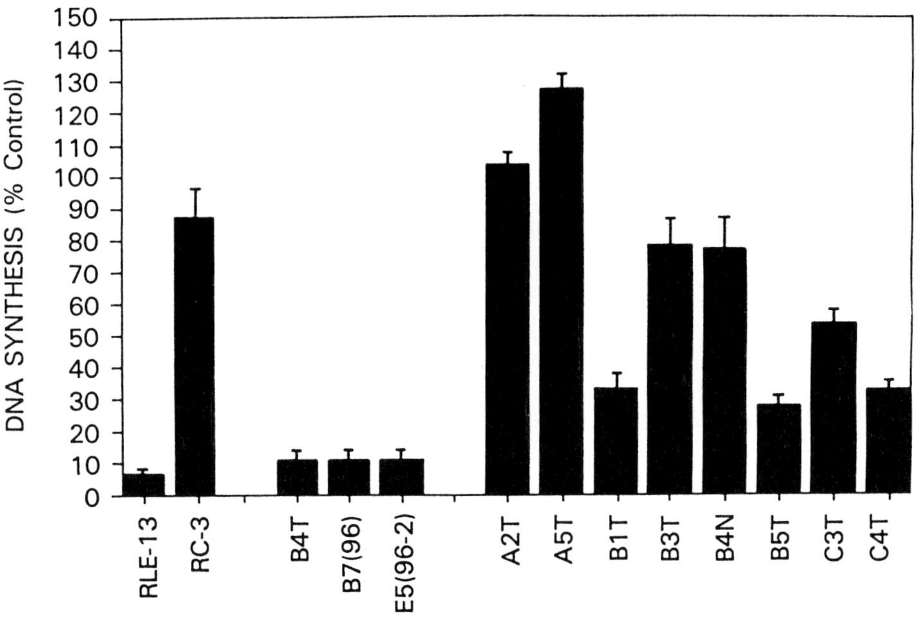

Fig. 5. Effect of TGF-ß1 (300 pg/ml) on DNA synthesis on the clonal cell lines derived from the mixed RLESF13 cell population at passage 6. (mean ± SD, n=8). RC-3 is a rat hepatocellular carcinoma cell line previously shown to be resistant to TGF-ß1 (From Huggett *et al.*, 1991 with permission).

REFERENCES

Bisgaard, H.C. & Thorgeirsson, S.S. (1991): Evidence for a common cell of origin for primitive epithelial cells isolated from rat liver and pancreas. *J. Cell. Physiol.* 147, 333-343.

Chapekar, M.S., Huggett, A.C., & Thorgeirsson, S.S. (1989): Growth modulatory effects of a liver-derived growth inhibitor, transforming growth factor beta 1, and recombinant tumor necrosis factor alpha, in normal and neoplastic cells. *Exp. Cell Res.* 185, 247-257.

Chisari, F.V., Klopchin, K., Moriyama, T., Pasquinellic, C., Dunsford, H.A., Sell, S., Pinkert, C.A., Brinster, R.L., & Palmiter, R.D. (1989). Molecular pathogenesis of hepatocellular carcinoma in hepatitis B virus transgenic mice. *Cell* 59, 1145-1156.

Chiu, T. (1987): Focal eosinophilic hypertrophic cells in the rat pancreas. *Toxicol. Pathol.* 15, 331-333.

Dunsford, H.A., Karnasuta, C., Hunt, J.M., & Sell, S. (1989): Different lineages of chemically induced hepatocellular carcinoma in rats defined by monoclonal antibodies. *Cancer Res.* 49, 4894-4900.

Dunsford, H.A. & Sell, S. (1989): Production of monoclonal antibodies to pre-neoplastic liver cell populations induced by chemical carcinogens in rats and to transplantable Morris hepatomas. *Cancer Res.* 49, 4887-4893.

Evarts, R.P., Nagy, P., Marsden, E. & Thorgeirsson, S.S. (1987): A precursor-product relationship exists between oval cells and hepatocytes in rat liver. *Carcinogenesis* 8, 1737-1740.

Evarts, R.P., Nagy, P., Nakatsukasa, H., Marsden, E. & Thorgeirsson, S.S. (1989): In vivo differentiation of rat liver oval cells into hepatocytes. *Cancer Res.* 49, 1541-1547.

Evarts, R.P., Nakatsukasa, H., Marsden, E., Hsia, C-C., Dunsford, H.A., & Thorgeirsson, S.S. (1990): Cellular and molecular changes in the early stages of chemical hepatocarcinogenesis in the rat. *Cancer Res.* 50, 3439-3444.

Farber, E. (1984): The multistep nature of cancer development. *Cancer Res.* 44, 4217-4223.

Garfield, S., Huber, B.E., Nagy, P., Cordingley, M.G., & Thorgeirsson, S.S. (1988): Neoplastic transformation and lineage switching of rat liver epithelial cells by retrovirus-associated oncogenes. *Mol. Carcinog.* 1, 189-195.

Germain, L., Blouin, M-J., & Marceau, N. (19881): Biliary epithelial and hepatocytic cell lineage relationships in embryonic rat liver as determined by the differential expression of cytokeratins, α-fetoprotein, albumin, and cell surface-exposed components. *Cancer Res.* 48, 4909-4918.

Germain, L., Goyette, R., & Marceau, N. (1985): Differential cytokeratin and α-fetoprotein expression in morphologically distinct cells emerging at early stages of rat hepatocarcinogenesis. *Cancer Res.* 45, 673-681.

Germain, L., Noel, M., Gourdeau, H., & Marceau, N. (1988b): Promotion of growth and differentiation of ductular oval cells in primary culture. *Cancer Res.* 48, 368-378.

Grisham, J.W., Thal, S.B., & Nagel, A. (1974): Cellular derivation of continuously cultured epithelial cells from normal rat liver. In *Gene expression and carcinogenesis in cultured liver*, ed. L.E. Gerschenson & E. Thompson, New York: Academic Press.

Hatzfeld, M. & Franke, W.W. (1985): Pair formation and promiscuity of cytokeratins: Formation in vitro of heterotypic complexes and intermediate-sized filaments by homologous and heterologous recombinations of purified polypeptides. *J. Cell. Biol.* 101, 1826-1842.

Huggett, A.C., Ellis, P.A., Ford, C.P., Hampton, L.L., Rimoldi, D., & Thorgeirsson, S.S. (1991): Development of resistance to the growth inhibitory effect of transforming growth factor beta-1 during the spontaneous transformation of rat liver epithelial cells. *Cancer Res.*, In press.

Inaoka, Y. (1967): Significance of the so-called oval cell proliferation during azo-dye hepatocarcinogenesis. *GANN* 58, 355-366.

Kimbrough, R.D., Linder, R.E., & Gaines, T.B. (1972): Morphological changes in liver of rats fed polychlorinated biphenyls. *Arch. Environ. Health* 25, 354.

Lee, L.W., Tsao, M-S., Grisham, J.W., & Smith, G.J. (1989): Emergence of neoplastic transformants spontaneously or after exposure to N-methyl-N'-nitro-N-nitrosoguanidine in populations of rat liver epithelial cells cultured under selective and nonselective conditions. *Am. J. Pathol.* 135, 63-71.

Marceau, N. (1990): Biology of diseases: cell lineages and differentiation programs in epidermal, urothelial and hepatic tissues and their neoplasms. *Lab. Invest.* 63, 4-20.

McMahon, J.B., Richards, D.W., del Campo, A.A., Song, M.-K.H., & Thorgeirsson, S.S. (1986): Differential effects of transforming growth factor-β on proliferation of normal and malignant rat liver epithelial cells in culture. *Cancer Res.* 46, 4667-4671.

Moll, R., Franke, W.W., Schiller, D.C., Geiger, B., & Krepler, R. (1982): The catalog of human cytokeratin: patterns of expression in normal epithelia, tumors and cultured cell. *Cell* 31, 11-24.

Rao, M.S., Bendayan, R.D., Kimbrough, R.D., & Reddy, J.K. (1986): Characterization of pancreatic-type tissue in the liver of rat induced by polychlorinated biphenyls. *J. Histochem. Cytochem.* 34, 197-201.

Rao, M.S., Dwiwedi, R.S., Yeldandi, A.V., Subbarao, V., Tan, X., Usman, M.I., Thangada, S., Nemali, M.R., Kumar, S., Scarpelli, D.G., & Reddy, J.K. (1989): Role of periductal and ductular epithelial cells of the adult rat pancreas in pancreatic hepatocyte lineage: A change in the differentiation commitment. *Am. J. Pathol.* 134, 1069-1086.

Reddy, J.K., Rao, M.S., Qureshai, S.A., Reddy, M.K., Scarpelli, D.G., & Lalwani, N.D. (1984): Induction and origin of hepatocytes in pancreas. *J. Cell. Biol.* 98, 2082-2090.

Rotstein, J., Sarma, D.S.R., & Farber, E. (1986): Sequential alterations in growth control and cell dynamics of rat hepatocytes in early precancerous steps in hepatocarcinogenesis. *Cancer Res.* 46, 2377-2385.

Sell, S. (1990): Is there a liver stem cell? *Cancer Res.*, 50, 3811-3815.

Takematsu, M., Lee, G., Hayes, A., & Farber, E. (1987): Progression of hepatocarcinogenesis: Differences in growth and behavior of transplants of early and late hepatocyte nodules in the rat spleen. *Cancer Res.* 47, 4699-4705.

Tatematsu, M., Thohru, K., Medline, A., & Farber, E. (1985): Intestinal metaplasia as a common option of oval cells in relation to cholangiofibrosis in the livers of rats exposed to 2-acetylaminofluorene. *Lab. Invest.* 52, 354.

Thorgeirsson, S.S. & Evarts, R.P. (1991): Experimental hepatocarcinogenesis: Relationship between oval cells and hepatocytes in rat liver. In *Advances in Applied Biotechnology Series, Vol. 13. Etiology, Pathology, and Treatment of Hepatocellular Carcinoma in North America*, ed. E. Tabor, A.M. Di Bisceglie, Y & R.H. Purcell, pp. 171-175. Houston, Texas: Gulf Publishing Co.

Tsao, M.-S. & Grisham, J.W. (1987): Hepatocarcinomas, cholangiocarcinomas and hepatoblastomas produced by chemically transformed cultured rat liver epithelial cells: a light and electron microscopic analysis. *Am. J. Pathol.* 127, 168-181.

Wolf, H.K., Burchette, J.L., Garcia, J.A., & Michalopoulos, G. (1990): Exocrine pancreatic tissues in human liver: a metaplastic process? *Am. J. Surg. Pathol.* 14, 590-595.

Résumé

Des lignées de cellules épithéliales ayant une forte capacité à proliférer *in vitro* ont été obtenues à partir du foie et du pancréas de rat adulte. Ces lignées possédaient des phénotypes très comparables si l'on en juge par leur aspect morphologique et des critères biochimiques. L'analyse des cytokératines dans les lignées d'origine hépatique et pancréatique a révélé une co-expression et une formation de filaments tout à fait uniques qui associaient les cytokératines 7 et 8 de type épithelial II et la cytokératine 14 de type épithélial I. Les résultats indiquent que les cellules épithéliales primitives provenant du foie et du pancréas de rat ont une origine cellulaire commune. La transformation des cellules épithéliales d'origine hépatique par des carcinogènes chimiques et des oncogènes conduit à la formation de tumeurs diverses notamment des carcinomes hépatocellulaires, des cholangiocarcinomes, des hépatoblastomes ainsi que des sarcomes et des tumeurs mixtes épithélio-mésenchymateuses. La transplantation de cellules épithéliales de foie de rat spontanément transformées *in vitro* donne naissance à des carcinomes hépatocellulaires. L'apparition de cellules transformées morphologiquement aberrantes est corrélée à une résistance accrue de ces cellules à l'inhibition de croissance induite par le TGF-β1.

Les résultats dans leur ensemble, indiquent que les cellules épithéliales de foie de rat constituent une source pour un compartiment de cellules souches dans le foie, qui pourraient être la cible des agents chimiques et biologiques impliqués dans l'hépatocarcinogénèse et suggèrent que l'acquisition d'une résistance aux effets des inhibiteurs de croissance tels que le $TGF\beta_1$, est une étape importante voire essentielle dans la transformation spontanée de ces cellules. De plus, nous avons émis l'hypothèse qu'un compartiment identique de cellules souches existe dans le pancréas et que ces cellules peuvent également être impliquées dans la carcinogénèse pancréatique.

Cellular and Molecular Aspects of Cirrhosis. Eds B. Clément, A. Guillouzo. Colloque INSERM/John Libbey Eurotext Ltd. © 1992, Vol. 216, pp. 299-306

Tissue specific expression of multiple gamma glutamyl transpeptidase mRNAs

Yannick Laperche and Georges Guellaen

INSERM U 99, Hôpital Henri Mondor, 94010 Créteil, France

ABSTRACT : Gamma-glutamyl transpeptidase is an heterodimeric glycoprotein located on the outer surface of the plasma membrane. It catalyzes the degradation of glutathione and allows the recovery of cysteine from extracellular GSH by the cell. The two GGT subunits are synthetized as a single precursor which is glycosylated and then cleaved into two subunits. In rat and human, GGT is mainly expressed in tissues very active in detoxication reactions (kidney, intestine) or in protein synthesis (pancreas, intestine). In the liver the activity is low but inducible in several hepato-biliary diseases. We demonstrated that the rat GGT precursor is encoded by four different mRNAs with alternate 5' ends. The four mRNAs are encoded on the single copy GGT gene from multiple promoters which exhibit a strong tissue specificity. In human, several genes have been identified and mapped at the locus q111-q112 on the chromosome 22. Among these genes, one produces multiple transcripts, a situation which is similar to that found in the rat. In conclusion, in rat, and posssibly in human, the tissue specificity of the GGT expression is based on the use of multiple promoters which are expressed and controlled independently.

Gamma-glutamyl transpeptidase (GGT) is a heterodimeric enzyme involved in the catabolism of extra-cellular glutathione (GSH). This ubiquitous tripeptide found in a millimolar range concentrations in many cells, serves as a substrate for GSH peroxidase and GSH transferase ; therefore, it plays a critical role in the cell protection against peroxides, electrophilic drugs and carcinogen metabolites (Meister and Anderson, 1983). The liver is the major source of circulating glutahione (Lauterburgh *et al.*, 1984). The hepatocytes, which are the only cells able to synthetize cysteine, produce a large amount of GSH which is released into the blood stream or into the bile as free GSH or GSH conjugated to electrophilic compounds. Reduced glutathione is cleared from the plasma compartment and from the gastro-intestinal tract by organs like kidney or intestine (Lauterburgh *et al.*, 1984). These organs rely largely on an extracellular supply of cysteine for intracellular GSH and protein synthesis, and also to maintain the thiol redox status. The use extracellular GSH involves first its degradation which is initiated on the outer surface of the epithelial cell membranes by gamma-glutamyl transpeptidase (Meister and Anderson, 1983).

Gamma-glutamyl transpeptidase biosynthesis has been investigated by pulse chase experiments in kidney slices (Nash and Tate, 1982), in hepatoma tissue culture cells (Barouki *et al.*, 1984)), as well as in a cell-free translation system (Finidori *et al.*, 1984). These studies demonstrated that the two glycosylated subunits are synthetized as a single precursor (Mr : 63, 000) which then is glycosylated (Mr : 79, 000) and cleaved into two mature subunits (Mr : 58, 000 and 28, 000). The anchorage to the membrane occurs through an uncleaved amino terminal signal sequence located on the heavy subunit ; the slight subunit bears the catalytical site (Meister and Anderson, 1983) and is linked to the heavy subunit by electrostatic interactions. The sequence of the precursor deduced from the cDNA (Laperche *et al*, 1986) confirmed the GGT insertion into the membrane through its uncleaved signal sequence and the orientation of the NH_2 terminus of the heavy chain in the cytoplasm (type II orientation). This type of protein orientation, although uncommon, has been described for several brush border hydrolases (Semenza, 1986).

Tissues very active in detoxication reactions (kidney, intestine) or in protein synthesis (pancreas, intestine, seminal vesicles, epididymis) exhibit the highest GGT activities (Meister and Anderson, 1983). However, in the adult liver, an organ also involved in detoxication reactions, the GGT activity is low and is located mainly in the bile duct cells. The GGT activity increases during chronic alcoholism in humans (Rosalki and Rau, 1972) and in the early stages of chemical hepatocarcinogenesis in the rat (Hanigan and Pitot, 1985), two situations in which there is an increase in glutathione consumption. The GGT expression has an opposite developmental pattern in tissues like the kidney and the intestine which use circulating glutathione, as compared to the liver which produces it. In the kidney, the activity increases from the fetal to the adult stage (Jacquemin *et al.*,1990) and a high GGT activity is considered as a part of the differentiation program of the proximal tubule. In the liver, the high GGT activity at the fetal stage decreases sharply at birth. The high GGT activity found in hepatomas and preneoplastic liver cells has been viewed as a marker of cellular dedifferentiation which indicates a reversion to the fetal phenotype (Hanigan and Pitot, 1985).

The elucidation of the biochemical processes involved in the regulation of GGT activity as well as in its tissue specificity clearly requires a detailed analysis at the gene level. We demonstrated that the rat GGT precursor can be encoded by four different GGT mRNAs (mRNAs $_{I, II, III}$ and $_{IV}$) which are expressed in a tissue specific manner (Darbouy *et al.*, 1991). We cloned two full length cDNA sequences which hybridize to 2.2 kb GGT mRNAs. These two mRNAs (I and II) share the same sequence up to the nucleotide 144 upstream of the initiation codon but have alternate sequences (154 and 138 bases) at their 5' ends. (Fig. 1).

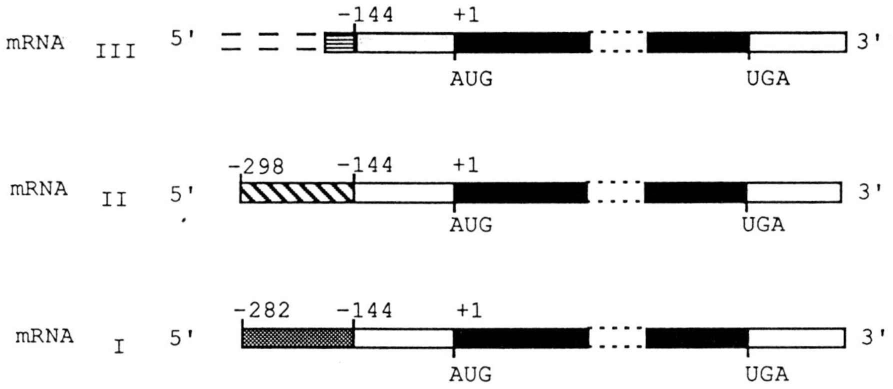

Fig. 1 Schematic representation of the rat GGT mRNAs. Coding (black area) and non coding (open area) region common to the three mRNAs. Sequences specific for $mRNA_I$ (stippled area), $mRNA_{II}$ (hatched area) and $mRNA_{III}$ (stripped area).

By using the two alternate sequences of $mRNA_I$ and $_{II}$ as specific probes we observed that the $mRNA_I$ and $mRNA_{II}$ are specifically expressed in the kidney and accumulate in the distal part of the proximal convoluted tubule (pars recta) (Chobert *et al.*, 1991). By Northern blot analysis, neither of these two transcripts can be detected in the other tissues, or cell investigated (liver, intestine, lactating mammary gland, HTC hepatoma cells). In these tissues two other GGT transcripts with a larger size (2.4 kb and 2.5 kb) were clearly observed on the Northern blot (Darbouy *et al.*, 1991). Analysis of the GGT mRNAs by ribonuclease H mapping shows that the four mRNA species have heterogeneous 5' ends that fully account for the size heterogeneity observed on a Northern blot. This is in agreement with the sequence of a cDNA isolated from a library prepared from an ethoxyquin treated liver. This sequence, which corresponds to the $mRNA_{III}$ (Griffiths and Manson, 1989 ; Darbouy *et al.*, 1991), differs in its 5' untranslated region from the sequences reported for the two rat kidney GGT cDNAs (Fig. 1). The GGT mRNA heterogeneity, limited to the length and the structure of the 5' untranslated region, excludes the synthesis of GGT isoforms with different primary structures.

In the rat, the four GGT mRNAs are encoded from a single copy gene (Pawlak *et al.*, 1988). The organization of the cDNA sequences on the 5' end of this gene reveals that the multiple GGT mRNAs are transcribed from at least three independent promoters as reported on Fig. 2. The promoter activity of the GGT genomic sequences immediately upstream the leader exons for $mRNA_I$ (P_1) and $mRNA_{II}$ (P_2), was demonstrated by transient transfections of sequences, coupled to the chloramphenicol acetyltransferase gene, into a pig kidney epithelial cell line (LLCPK) (Kurauchi *et al.*, 1991). Together with the human aldolase A (Maire *et al.*, 1987)) and the rat IGF_{II} genes (Ueno *et al.*, 1988) the rat GGT gene appears to be another example of a gene transcribed from at least three promoters.

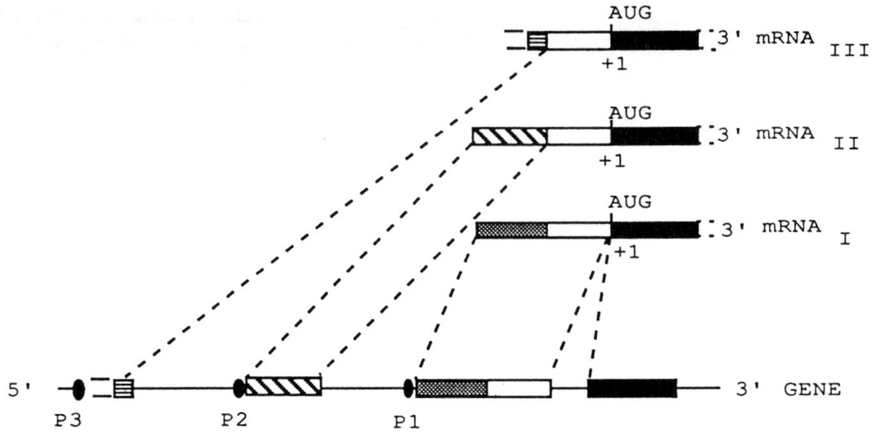

Fig. 2 Schematic representation of the structure of the 5' end of the rat GGT gene and of three GGT primary transcripts. Exons are represented by boxes and intron are shown by lines connecting the exons. The black boxes correspond to the first translated exon.

The use of multiple promoters affords a flexibility in the control of gene expression. Each promoter can be regulated independently in response to a particular stimulus (Carlson and Botstein, 1982) a tissue-specific factor (Young *et al.*, 1981), or at a particular developmental stage (Benyajati *et al.*, 1983). Northern blot analysis revealed a strong tissue specificity in the expression of the multiple GGT mRNA transcripts. This tissue and cell specificity, in the GGT mRNA accumulation, gives a physiological significance to the synthesis of multiple GGT transcripts which are coding for the same protein. The GGT promoters I and II appear to be active only in the kidney whereas the accumulation of $mRNA_{IV}$ is restricted to the small intestine and some hepatoma cells. The synthesis of multiple mRNAs with alternate leader sequences also allows a regulation at the post-transcriptional level. However the effects of the 5' non-coding regions on the stability and the translational efficiency of the different GGT mRNA species have not been investigated yet.

In human tissues, the levels of GGT activity are comparable to those found in rat tissues and no difference has been reported in the GGT regulation between these two species. In human, however, several GGT genomic sequences have been characterized which correspond to four different genes located on the chromosome 22 at the locus q111-q112 (Pawlak *et al.*, 1988 ; Bulle *et al.*, 1987). These different genes arise most probably by recent duplications of a unique gene after the evolutionary divergence of rat from that of human. Integration of processed GGT sequences into the human genome can be excluded since all the GGT genes have an intron-exon structure.

Three human cDNAs which cover the entire GGT precursor open reading frame and extend in the 5' non coding region of the mRNA, have been cloned from placenta (De Meyts *et al.*, 1988)), fetal liver (Sakamuro *et al.*, 1988) and the HepG2 hepatoma (Goodspeed *et al.*, 1989) . All these sequences are 100% homologous in their coding regions and differ only from the nucleotide 88 upstream the AUG (Fig.3).

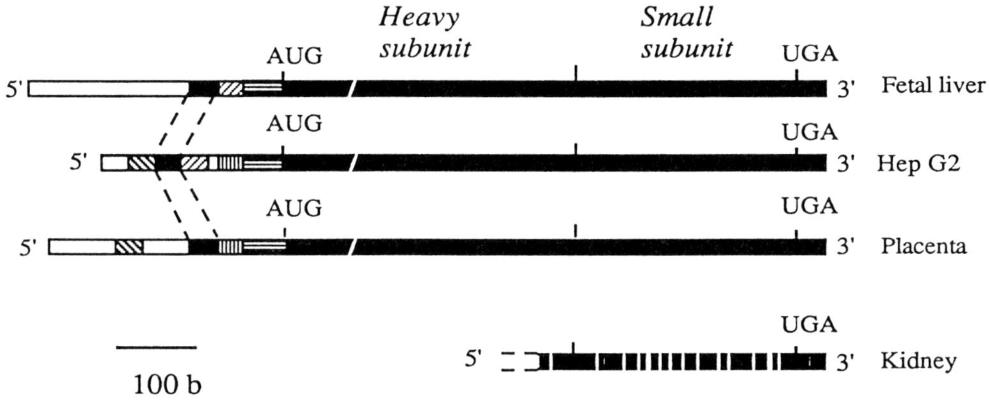

Fig. 3 Schematic representation of the human GGT mRNAs. Sequences common to three mRNAs (black area). Sequences homologous between two mRNAs (hatched and stripped area). Specific sequences for each mRNA (open area).

These data show that these three mRNAs are encoded by the same gene, otherwise point mutations scattered all over the coding sequence would have been observed. In the 5' non coding sequences, 100% homologous boxes are detected among the different cDNAs but at varying positions with respect to the AUG ; such an organization is also compatible with the expression from a single gene. It is not known whether these three human GGT cDNAs are full length ; therefore, there is no sufficient information to conclude whether all these mRNAs arise from the alternate splicing of one or multiple primary transcripts initiated on one or several promoters on the gene.

According to these results, the human GGT multigene family does not give rise to the production of GGT isoforms. Among the duplicated genes, one of them seems to be functional and produces multiple transcripts, a situation which is similar to that found in the rat . Recently, another cDNA was obtained from a human kidney library. Its sequence, which displays point mutations and a deletion as compared to the other cDNAs, reveals the transcription from another GGT gene (Pawlak *et al.*, 1989). However this cDNA sequence covers only the 3' half of the reading frame and it cannot be concluded if it could correspond to a functional mRNA.

In conclusion in the rat, and possibly in human, the tissue specificity of the GGT expression is based on the use of multiple promoters which are expressed and controlled independently. The multiple GGT isoforms reported in several rat and human tissues would not differ in their protein backbone but only in terms of glycosylation or other post-translational modifications. The study of the expression of the different GGT promoters will be valuable in the identification of the proteins that contribute to the GGT gene regulation.

REFERENCES :

Barouki, R., Finidori, J., Chobert, M.N., Aggerbeck, M., Laperche, Y. and Hanoune, J. (1984) Biosynthesis and processing of γ-glutamyl transpeptidase in hepatoma tissue culture cells. *J. Biol. Chem.*, 259, 7970-7974.

Benyajati, C., Spoerel, N., Haymerle, H. and Ashburner, M. (1983) : The messenger RNA for alcohol deshydrogenase in *Drosophila melanogaster* differs in its 5' end in different developmental stages. *Cell*, 33, 125-133.

Bulle, F., Mattei, M.G., Siegrist, S., Pawlak, A., Passage, E., Chobert, M.N., Laperche, Y. and Guellaën, G. (1987) Assignment of the human γ-glutamyl transferase gene to the long arm of chromosome 22. *Human Genet.*,76, 283-286.

Carlson, M. and Botstein, D. (1982) : Two differentially regulated mRNAs with different 5' ends encode secreted and intracellular forms of yeast invertase. *Cell*, 28, 145-154.

Chobert, M.N., Lahuna, O., Lebargy, F., Kurauchi, O., Darbouy, M., Bernaudin J.F., Guellaën, G., Barouki, R. and Laperche, Y. (1991) : Tissue-specific expression of two-γ-glutamyl transpeptidase mRNAs with alternative 5' ends encoded by a single copy gene in the rat. *J. Biol. Chem.*, 265, 2352-2357.

Darbouy, M., Chobert, M.N., Lahuna, O., Okamoto, T., Bonvalet, J.P., Farman, N. and Laperche, Y. (1991) : Tissue-specific expression of multiple γ-glutamyl transpeptidase mRNAs in rat epithelia. *Am. J. Physiol.* (in press).

De Meyts, E.R., Heisterkamp, N. and Groffen, J. (1988) : Cloning and nucleotide sequence of human γ-glutamyl transpeptidase. *Proc. Natl. Acad. Sci. USA*, 85, 8840-8844.

Finidori, J., Laperche, Y., Haguenauer-Tsapis, R., Barouki, R., Guellaën, G. and Hanoune, J. (1984) : In vivo biosynthesis and membrane insertion of γ-glutamyl transpeptidase. *J. Biol. Chem.*, 259, 4687-4690.

Goodspeed, D.C., Dunn, T.J., Miller, C.D. and Pitot, H. (1989) : Human γ-glutamyl transpeptidase cDNA : comparison of hepatoma and kidney mRNA in the human and rat. *Gene*, 76, 1-9.

Griffiths, S.A. and Manson, M. (1989) : Multiple mRNA species for rat γ-glutamyl transpeptidase appears to be transcribed from a single gene. *Cancer Lett.* 46, 69-74.

Hanigan, M.H. and Pitot, H.C. (1985) γ-glutamyl transpeptidase, its role in hepatocarcinogenesis. *Carcinogenesis,* 6, 165-172.

Jacquemin, E.F., Bulle, F., Bernaudin, J.F., Wellman, M., Hugon, R.N., Guellaën, G. and Hadchouel, M. (1990) : Pattern of expression of γ-glutamyl transpeptidase in rat liver and kidney during development : study by immunochemistry and *in situ* hybridization. *J. Pediatr. Gastroenterol. Nutr.,* 11, 89-95.

Kurauchi, O., Lahuna, O., Darbouy, M., Aggerbeck, M., Chobert, M.N., and Laperche, Y. (1991) : Organization of the 5' end of the rat γ-glutamyl transpeptidase gene : structure of a promoter active in the kidney. *Biochemistry,* 30, 1618-1623.

Laperche, Y., Bulle, F., Aissani, T., Chobert, M.N., Aggerbeck, M., Hanoune, J. and Guellaën, G. (1986) : Molecular cloning and nucleotide sequence of the rat kidney γ-glutamyl transpeptidase. *Proc. Natl. Acad. Sci. USA.* 83, 937-941.

Lauterburg, B.H., Adams, J.D. and Mitchell, J.R. (1984) : Hepatic glutathione homeostasis in the rat : efflux accounts for glutathione turnover. *Hepatology,* 4, 586-590.

Maire, P.S., Gautron, M., Hakim, V., Gregori, C., Mennecier, F. and Kahn, A. (1987) : Characterization of three optional promoters in the 5' region of the human aldolase A gene. *J. Mol. Biol.,* 197, 425-438.

Meister, A. and Anderson, M.E. (1983) : Glutathione. *Ann. Rev. Biochem.* 52, 711-760.

Nash, B. and Tate, S.S. (1982) : Biosynthesis of rat renal γ-glutamyl transpeptidase. *J. Biol. Chem.,* 257, 585-588.

Pawlak, A., Lahuna, O., Bulle, F., Suzuki, A., Ferry, N., Siegrist, S., Chikhi, N., Chobert, M.N., Guellaën, G. and Laperche, Y. (1988) : γ-glutamyl transpeptidase gene : a single copy gene in the rat and a multigene family in the human genome. *J. Biol. Chem.,* 268, 9913-9916.

Pawlak, A., Wu, S.J., Bulle, F., Suzuki, A., Chikhi, N., Ferry, N., Baik, J.H., Siegrist, S., and Guellaën, G. (1989) : Different γ-glutamyl transpeptidase mRNAs are expressed in human liver and kidney. *Biochem. Biophys. Res. Comm.,* 164, 912-918.

Reynolds, G.A., Basu, S.K., Osborne, T.F., Chin, D.J., Gil, G., Brown, M.S., Goldstein, J.L. and Luskey, K.L. (1984) : HMG CoA reductase : A negatively regulated gene with unusual promoter and 5' untranslated regions, *Cell,* 38, 275-285.

Rosalki, S.B. and Rau, D. (1972) : Serum γ-glutamyl transpeptidase activity in alcoholism. *Clin. Chim. Acta.,* 39, 41-47.

Sakamuro, D., Yamazoe, M., Matsuda, Y., Kangawa, K., Taniguchi, N., Matsuo, H., Yoshikawa, H. and Ogasawara, N. (1988) : The primary structure of human γ-glutamyl transpeptidase. *Gene*, 73, 1-9.

Semenza, G. (1986) : Anchoring and biosynthesis of stalked brush border membrane proteins : glycosidases and peptidases of enterocytes and renal tubuli. *Ann. Rev. Cell. Biol.* 2, 255-313.

Ueno, T.I., Takahashi, K., Matsuguchi, T., Endo, H. and Yamamoto, M. (1988) : Transcritpional deviation of the rat insulin-like growth factor II gene initiated at three alternative leader-exons, between neonatal tissues and ascites hepatomas. *Biochem. Biophys. Acta*, 950, 411-419.

Young, R.A., Hagenbuchle, O. and Schibler, U. (1981) : A single mouse α amylase gene specifies two different tissue-specific mRNAs. *Cell*, 23, 451-458.

Résumé : La gamma-glutamyl transpeptidase est une glycoprotéine composée de deux sous-unités localisées à la face externe de la membrane plasmique. Elle catalyse la dégradation du glutathion et permet la réabsorption de la cystéine à partir du glutathion extracellulaire. Les deux sous-unités de la GGT sont synthétisées à partir d'un précurseur commun glycosylé. Chez le rat et chez l'homme, la GGT est surtout exprimée dans le rein, l'intestin et le pancréas. Dans le foie l'activité de la GGT est faible mais elle est induite lors de nombreuses maladies hépatiques. Chez le rat, nous avons montré que le précurseur de la GGT est codé par quatre ARN messagers qui ne diffèrent que par leur extrémité 5'. Ces ARNm sont transcrits à partir d'un seul gène comprenant plusieurs promoteurs dont l'expression varie suivant les tissus. Chez l'homme plusieurs gènes de la GGT ont été localisés sur le chromosome 22 dans le locus q111-q112 ; l'un de ces gènes code pour plusieurs mRNAs. En résumé, chez le rat et probablement chez l'homme, la spécificité tissulaire de l'expression de la GGT est liée à l'expression indépendante de plusieurs promoteurs sur un même gène.

Cellular and Molecular Aspects of Cirrhosis. Eds B. Clément, A. Guillouzo. Colloque INSERM/John Libbey Eurotext Ltd. © 1992, Vol. 216, pp. 307-310

Kupffer cells release a 95kD gelatinase

P.J. Winwood, P. Kowalski-Saunders, I. Green, G. Murphy *, R. Hembry * and M.J.P. Arthur

Medicine II, Southampton General Hospital, Tremona Road, Southampton, Hampshire SO9 AXY, UK;
** Cell and Molecular Biology Department, Strangeways Research Laboratory, Cambridge, UK*

INTRODUCTION

In liver fibrosis an important early event is the replacement of the normal basement membrane-like matrix, in the subendothelial space of Disse, by interstitial (types I and III) collagens (Bissell, 1990). Lipocytes (fat storing or Ito cells) are the main cellular source of interstitial collagens (Friedman et al, 1985) and are activated by degradation of the normal subendothelial matrix (Friedman 1989). In normal basement membrane, type IV collagen is arranged in a lattice framework and provides structural integrity (Yurchenco and Schittny, 1990). Monocytes secrete a 95-97kD type IV collagenase/gelatinase (Welgus et al, 1990) which degrades subendothelial matrix. In this study we have demonstrated that Kupffer cells, which are activated in liver injury (Arthur et al, 1988) release an identical enzyme and may therefore promote liver fibrosis.

METHODS

Cells and cell culture conditions Kupffer cells (KC) were isolated from normal rat livers by pronase/collagenase perfusion and purified by arabinogalactan density gradient centrifugation followed by centrifugal elutriation, as previously described (Arthur et al, 1989). KC cultures were 94% pure up to 7 days as assessed by morphology, endogenous peroxidase staining and immunostaining for ED1 and ED2 (Hardonk et al, 1989). After 7 days lipocyte outgrowth occurred (10% at 9 days).

Analysis of gelatinase activity Gelatin degrading activity in serum-free Kupffer cell conditioned media (KCCM) was detected by gelatin-substrate SDS-PAGE (Herron et al, 1986). Quantitative analysis of gelatinase activity was measured by degradation of ^{14}C-gelatin (Arthur et al, 1989).

Immunostaining for 95kD gelatinase Kupffer cells were immunostained using sheep anti-pig 95kD gelatinase (Murphy et al, 1989).

RESULTS

Substrate gel analysis of Kupffer cell conditioned media By gelatin-substrate SDS-PAGE, KCCM from 4 day cultures contained gelatinase activity, Mr95kD (Fig. 1), extending to 75kD, consistent with the presence of cleaved activated forms (88kD and 75kD) as described for the monocyte derived enzyme (Murphy et al, 1989). KCCM from 9 day cultures contained 95kD and 66kD gelatinase activity (Fig. 1). In contrast KCCM had no degradative activity against casein, (Fig. 2) indicating substrate specificity. In the presence of 10mM EDTA, gelatinase activity in KCCM was completely inhibited but 1mM phenylmethylsulfonylfluoride (PMSF) and 2mM N-ethyl-malemide (NEM) had no effect (Fig. 3) indicating that KC gelatinase is a metalloproteinase.

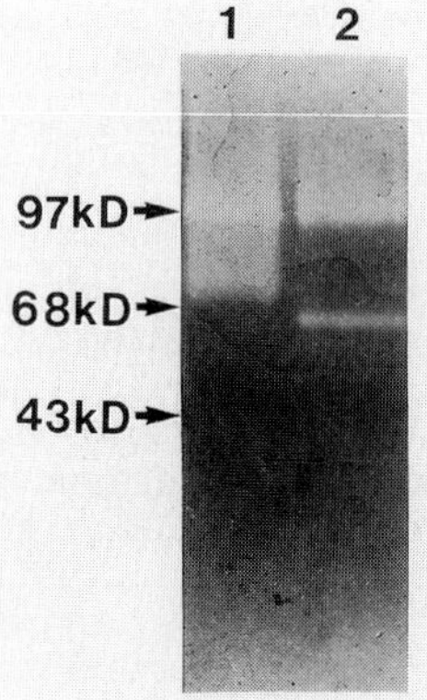

Fig. 1. Gelatin substrate SDS-PAGE. Lane 1; KCCM (4 day old cultures) demonstrating gelatinase activity of Mr 95 and 75kD. Lane 2; KCCM (9 day old cultures) with gelatinase activity of Mr 95kD and 66kD.

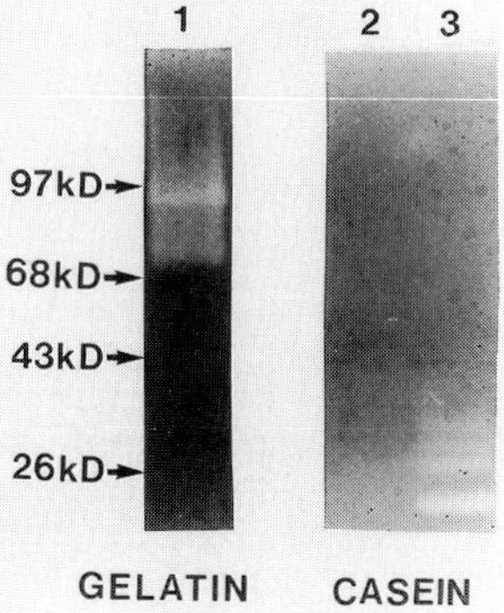

Fig. 2. Substrate SDS-PAGE. Lane 1; KCCM with 95kD gelatinase activity. Lane 2; KCCM run on a gel with casein incorporated as substrate has no degradative activity. Lane 3; trypsin (positive control).

Quantitative analysis of gelatin degrading activity The addition of 1mM aminophenyl mercuric acetate (APMA), an organomercurial, to KCCM caused an increase in measurable activity from a mean of 2.8 to 5.23 mU gelatinase/μg DNA/24 hours (Fig. 5a; $p<0.05$, n=20), indicating that KC-derived 95kD gelatinase is released partially in latent form.

Kupffer cell activation Culture of KC in the presence of 50ng/ml phorbol myristate acetate (PMA) caused an increase in release of total gelatinase activity (Fig. 5b) (following APMA activation) from 3.59 to 9.49 mU/μg DNA/24 hours ($p<0.05$, n=5).

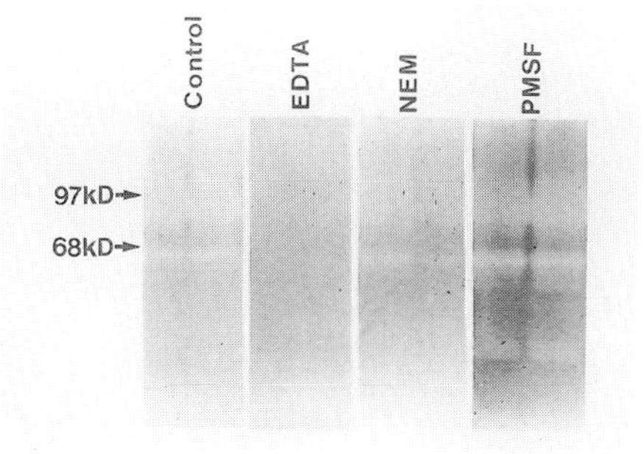

Fig. 3. Gelatin substrate SDS -PAGE. EDTA inhibits gelatinase activity whereas NEM and PMSF have no effect.

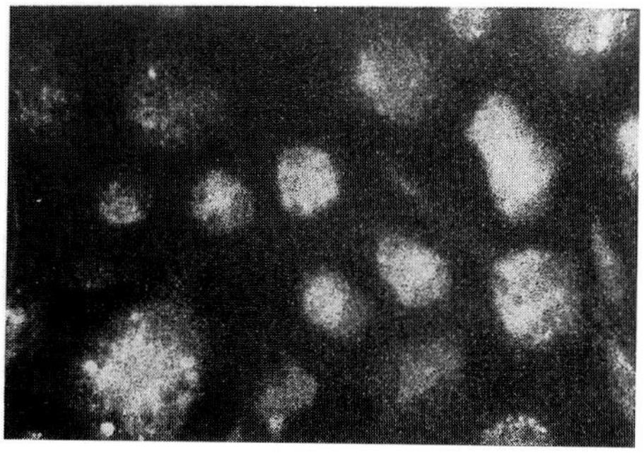

Fig. 4. Perinuclear staining of 95kD type IV collagenase/ gelatinase by immunofluorescence in Kupffer cells.

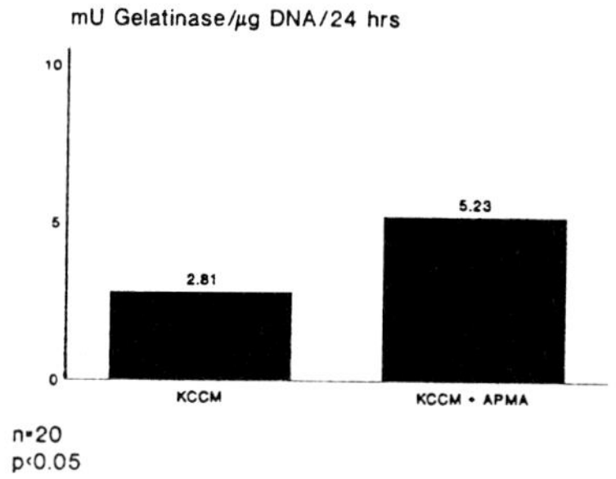

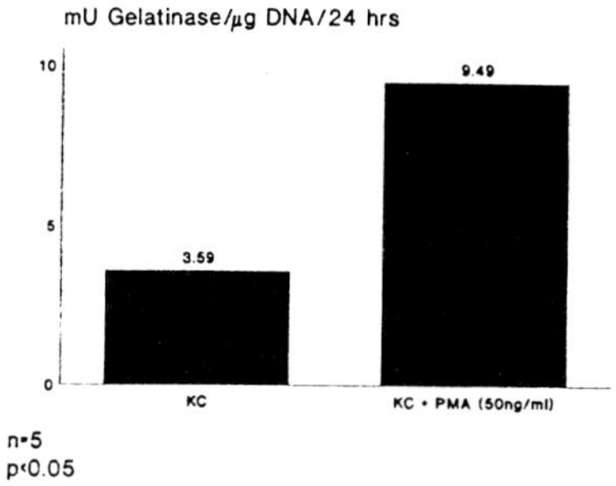

Fig. 5. Gelatinase activity in KCCM (<7 day old cultures). 5a) APMA activates latent activity in KCCM; 5b) PMA (50ng/ml) increases release of total (APMA-activated) gelatinase activity.

DISCUSSION

The normal hepatic subendothelial matrix plays an important role in maintaining cell specific functions. It's degradation results in promotion of liver fibrosis via lipocyte activation (Friedman et al, 1989) and impaired hepatocellular function (Bissell et al, 1990). This study demonstrates that Kupffer cells (hepatic macrophages) release a 95kD gelatinase which has matrix-degrading activity. The evidence presented here suggests that it is identical to monocyte-derived 95-97kD type IV collagenase/ gelatinase (Murphy et al, 1989). It is a metalloproteinase, with no activity against casein and is released in a latent form. Also, immunostaining with an antibody raised to neutrophil-derived type IV collagenase/gelatinase stained KC positively (Fig. 6). The 66kD gelatinase activity at 9 days in primary culture (Fig. 1) probably derived from the 10% lipocytes contaminating the KC at this stage (Arthur et al, 1989), however it may also represent a switch in gene products by dedifferentiating KC.

The function of KC 95kD gelatinase is yet to be clearly defined but it is likely that it facilitates migration across the space of Disse particularly during the inflammatory response. This is supported by our observation that activated KC (subjected to PMA), as occur in liver injury (Arthur et al, 1988), secrete large quantities of gelatinase (Fig. 5b). We suggest that KC-derived 95kD gelatinase is also an important factor in the initiation of liver fibrosis.

REFERENCES

Arthur, M.J.P., Kowalski-Saunders, P. & Wright, R. (1988): Effect of endotoxin on release of reactive oxygen intermediates by rat hepatic macrophages. Gastroenterology 95, 1588-1594.

Arthur, M.J.P., Friedman, S.L., Roll, F.J. & Bissell, D.M. (1989): Lipocytes from normal rat liver release a neutral metalloproteinase that degrdes basement membrane (type IV) collagen. J. Clin. Invest. 84, 1076-85.

Bissell, D.M., Friedman, S.L., Maher, J.J. & Roll, F.J. (1990): Connective tissue biology and hepatic fibrosis: Report of a conference. Hepatology 11, 488-498.

Friedman, S.L., Roll, F.J., Boyles, J. & Bissell, D.M. (1985): Hepatic lipocytes: the principal collagen-producing cells of normal rat liver. Proc. Natl. Acad. Sci. USA 82, 8681-8685.

Friedman, S.L., Roll, F.J., Boyles, J., Arenson, D.M. & Bissell, D.M. (1989): Maintenance of differentiated phenotype of cultured rat hepatic lipocytes by basement membrane matrix. J. Biol. Chem. 264, 10756-10762.

Hardonk, M.J., Huitema, S. & Kondstool, J. (1989): Immuno-histochemical methods in the study of liver sinusoidal cells. In Cells of the Hepatic Sinusoid, Vol 2, ed. E. Wisse, D.L. Knook & K. Decker, pp. 482-487. Rijswick: The Kupffer Cell Foundation.

Herron, G.S., Banda, M.J., Clark, E.J., Gavrillovic, J. & Werb, Z. (1986): Secretion of metalloproteinases by stimulated capillary endothelial cells. J. Biol. Chem. 261, 2814-2818.

Murphy, G., Ward, R., Hembry, R.M., Reynolds, J.J., Kuhn, K. & Trygvasson, K. (1989): Characterisation of a gelatinase from pig polymorphonuclear leukocytes. Biochem. J. 258, 465-472.

Welgus, H.G., Campbell, E.J., Curry, J.D., Eisen, A.Z., Senior, R.M., Wilhelm, S.M. & Goldberg, G.I. (1990): Neutral metalloproteinases produced by human mononuclear phagocytes. J. Clin. Invest. 86, 1496-1502.

Yurchenco, P.D. & Schittny, J.C. (1990): Molecular architecture of basement membranes. FASEB J. 4, 1577-1590.

Cellular and Molecular Aspects of Cirrhosis. Eds B. Clément, A. Guillouzo. Colloque INSERM/John Libbey Eurotext Ltd. © 1992, Vol. 216, pp. 311-314

A model of paracrine regulation of hepatocellular proliferation

Dieter H. Meyer, Max G. Bachem and Axel M. Gressner *

Department of Clinical Chemistry and Central Laboratory, Philipps University, Baldingerstrasse, 3550 Marburg, Germany

* *Corresponding author*

Abstract: The paracrine regulation of hepatocyte proliferation by Kupffer cells and myofibroblast-like cells was studied. Conditioned media from Kupffer cells and Myofibroblast-like cells inhibit the replicative (hydroxyurea-sensitive) DNA synthesis dose-dependently in primary culture of hepatocytes. The cytokine responsible for the inhibition was identified as TGFβ. After neutralization of active TGFβ in these media, DNA synthesis is stimulated in quiescent hepatocytes via TGFα. Hybridization experiments confirm the expression of both TGFβ and TGFα in Kupffer cells and myofibroblast-like cells. Our data support the finding that Kupffer cells and myofibroblast-like cells might regulate liver regeneration in both directions depending on the proportion of secreted TGFα and TGFβ and on the activation status of TGFβ which is secreted mostly in the latent form.

Introduction: In healthy liver the proliferative turnover is at a relatively low level, but after acute and chronic liver injury a highly increased cell proliferation is observed (Michalopoulos 1990). The mechanisms for the regulation of hepatocellular proliferation are still poorly understood, although there are evidences for metabolic cooperation of Kuffer cells (KC) and hepatocytes. KC have also been implicated in the regulation of hepatocyte proliferation in vitro but contradictory results were communicated (Mayanskii et al. 1977; Katsumoto et al. 1989). Fat storing cells (FSC), which are the main site of retinoid storage in liver (Hendriks et al. 1987) proliferate in the area of tissue injury (Enzan 1985), transform into myofibroblast-like cells (MFblC), and synthesize a broad spectrum of extracellular matrix components (Friedman 1990; Gressner and Bachem 1990). Thus, these cells play a prominent role in tissue repair after wounding and in the development of fibrosis. The interaction of FSC and MFblC with endothelial cells (Braun et al. 1988) and KC by paracrine mechanisms (Bachem et al. 1988) and even autocrine regulatory loops (Mead J.E. and Fausto N. 1989) have been identified, which involve the opposite effects of transforming growth factors (TGF) type α and β. We have shown recently that Kupffer cells modulate the mitotic activity of cultured fat storing cells in both ways depending on the activity of TGFα and β (Meyer et al. 1990). TGFα and TGFβ are important activators and inhibitors, respectively, of hepatocyte proliferation and are thought to play central roles in the regulation of liver cell regeneration (Braun et al. 1988). In the present study we present evidence that KC and MFblC stimulate and inhibit hepatocyte DNA synthesis in vitro determined by the ratio of active TGFβ to TGFα.

Methods: *Chemicals:* Rat TGFα, TGFβ and rat TGFα decapeptide (aminoacid residues 34-43) (Nestor et al 1985) were obtained from Bachem Biochemica (Heidelberg, FRG). Neutralizing antibodies against TGFβ were from British Biotechnology Ltd. (Oxford, UK). The 44 base long TGFα oligonucleotide probe was purchased from Dianova (Hamburg, FRG). The porcine TGFβ c-DNA probe (pTGFβ33) was kindly provided by Dr. P. Kondaiah (NIH, Bethesda, USA).

Isolation and culture of hepatocytes, fat storing cells and Kupffer cells: All cells were prepared from male Sprague-Dawley rats following previously described procedures (Meyer et al. 1990).

Viability of isolated *hepatocytes* checked by trypan blue exclusion was > 90 % and contamination with vimentin/desmin-positive cells was below 0.4 %. The cells were seeded with a density of 5 $\times 10^4/cm^2$ and cultured in Hanks F-12 medium (0.2 % BSA, 0.02 U/ml insulin, 1 % penicillin/streptomycin). Medium was changed 2 h and 20 h after seeding. Additions of factors (TGF alpha, beta) and of conditioned media were made at the same times. *Fat storing cells* (FSC) were seeded with a density of 3.8×10^6 and maintained as monolayers in DMEM (10 % (v/v) fetal calf serum (FCS)). Medium changes were made every second day beginning 16 h after seeding. After reaching confluency primary cultured cells were subcultured by trypsinization and reseeding. Cells were passaged for a 2nd time after a further incubation period of 14 days. The purity of freshly isolated FSC was at least 90 %, cell viability was more than 80 % and the yield ranged from 2×10^7 to 5×10^7 cells/liver. With the first medium change most of the contaminating cells were removed and the monolayers were essentially free of impurities.

Kupffer cells were seeded with a density of 0.4 x 10^6cells/cm^2 and incubated for 2 h in 15 ml DMEM containing 10 % FCS. After 2 h FCS in the medium was changed to 0.2 % BSA. Viability was greater than 90 %, purity was greater than 95 %.

Conditioned medium was harvested after a 24 h incubation period in absence of fetal calf serum. Half of the conditioned medium was acidified (pH 2.0) with HCl for 30 min. and reneutralized. Native and transiently acidified media were dialyzed (MW cut off 3500) against 100 vol Hanks F-12 medium at 4°C.

[3H]thymidine incorporation: The incorporation of [^{3}H]thymidine (1 µCi/ml medium) into the DNA of hepatocytes was measured over a 24 h incubation period beginning 20 h after seeding following a previously described protocol (Zerbe and Gressner 1988).

Competitive radioligand binding assay: TGFβ and TGFα in Kupffer cell conditioned media were quantitated using competitive radioligand binding assays as described in Meyer et al. 1990.

Northern and dot blotting: Total RNA from KC was isolated as described by Chomczynski and Sacchi (1987), separated by gel electrophoresis and blotted on Hybond N membranes. The measurement of ribosomal S6-protein gene expression was used as internal standard. Hybridization was carried out under high stringency conditions.

<u>Results:</u> *Effect of Kupffer cell conditioned medium on the proliferation of EGF-stimulated hepatocytes.* Conditioned medium from Kupffer cells caused a dose-dependent inhibition of [^{3}H]-thymidine incorporation into the DNA of hepatocytes stimulated in vitro by addition of 25 ng/ml EGF (fig. 1). Medium, which had been transiently acidified before addition to hepatocyte cultures, was constantly more potent than native conditioned medium. The inhibitory effect of KC-conditioned medium could be reduced and even completely abolished by preincubation of the medium with increasing concentrations of neutralizing polyclonal antibodies against TGFβ (fig. 2).

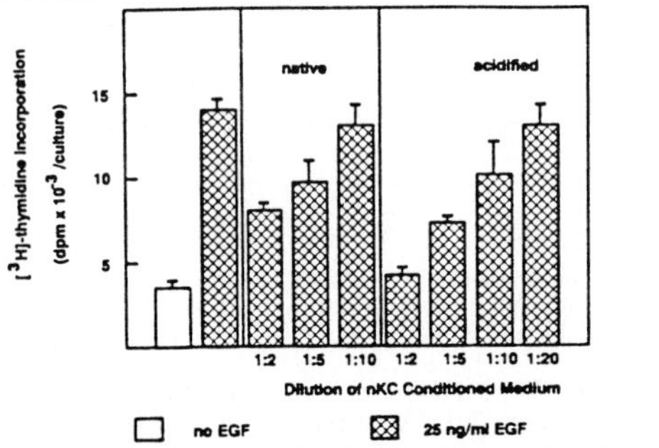

Fig. 1: ***Inhibition of EGF stimulated DNA synthesis in hepatocytes by native and transiently acidified conditioned medium from cultured Kupffer cells.*** *Epidermal growth factor (EGF) was added 2 h and 20 h after plating simultaneously with conditioned medium. Control represents DNA synthesis of parenchymal cells in the absence of EGF. Mean values ± S.D. of four experiments are shown.*

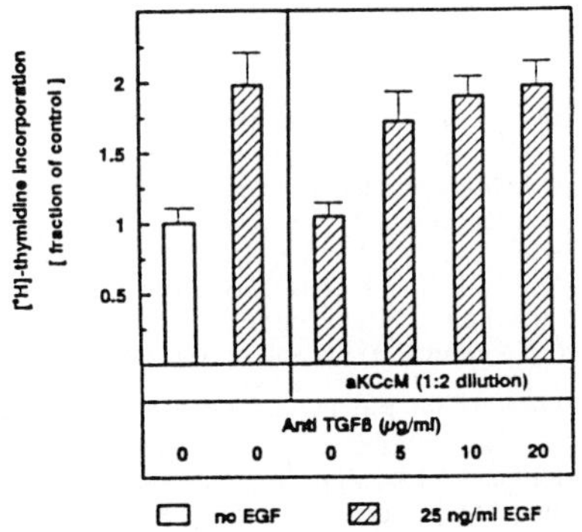

Fig. 2: ***Effect of anti-TGFβ antibodies on the inhibitory action of conditioned medium from Kupffer cell cultures on hepatocellular [³H]-thymidine incorporation.*** *Transiently acidified KC medium (aKCcM) at a 1:2 dilution was incubated for 2 h with increasing amounts of neutralizing anti-TGFβ prior to the addition to hepatocytes stimulated by EGF. Mean values ± S.D. of four experiments are shown.*

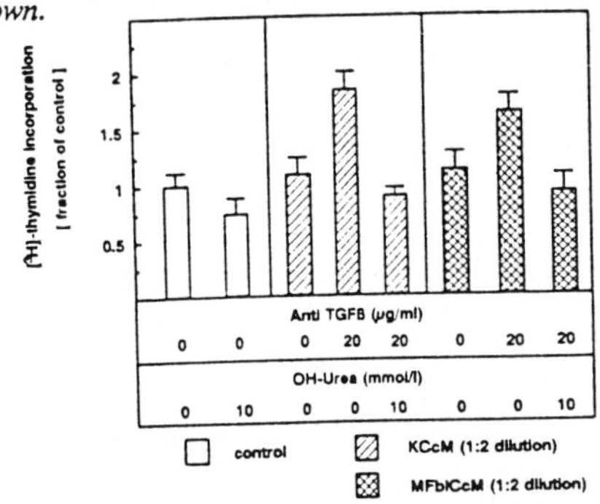

Fig. 3: ***Effect of conditioned medium from Kupffer cells and transformed FSC (Myofibroblast like cells)*** *on unstimulated hepatocellular DNA synthesis in absence and presence of hydroxyurea (10 mM). Conditioned media and OH-Urea were added 2 h and 20 h after plating. In one portion of the conditioned medium TGFβ was neutralized by preincubation at 37°C for 2 h with 20 ug/ml anti-TGFβ before addition to hepatocyte cultures. Mean values ± S.D. of four experiments are shown.*

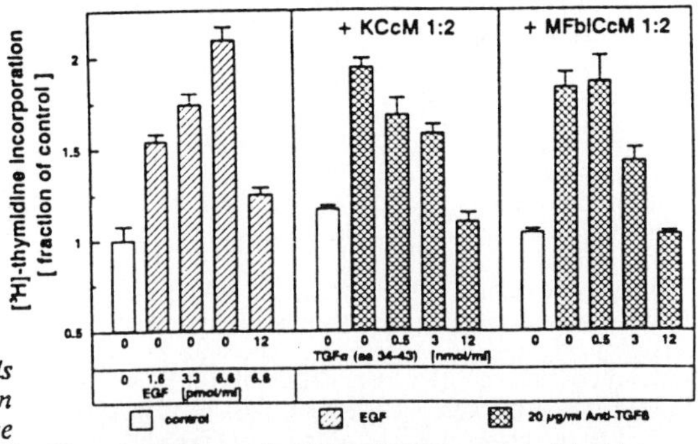

Fig. 4: ***Effect of TGFα/EGF-receptor blocking on stimulated hepatocyte proliferation*** *by competing TGFα peptide. Conditioned medium was pretreated for 2 h with anti-TGFβ and added 2 h and 20 h after plating simultanously with increasing amounts of competing TGFα peptide (aminoacid residues 34-43).*

Effects of Kupffer cell conditioned medium (KCcM) on the proliferation of quiescent hepatocytes. Native and transiently acidified Kupffer cell media had no effect on the [^{3}H]-thymidine incorporation into the DNA of hepatocytes, cultured in Hanks F-12 medium in the absence of growth factors. When preincubated with 20 ug/ml neutralizing anti-TGFβ antibodies a dose dependent, hydroxyurea-sensitve growth stimulatory effect of KCcM was observed (fig. 3). Competitive inhibition of the binding of TGFα-receptors on hepatocytes by addition of the 10 aminoacid long TGFα-(aa 34-43)-polypeptide (Nestor et al. 1985), the proliferation stimulatory effect of KCcM was reduced and even completely abolished at a peptide concentration of 12 pmol/ml (fig. 4).

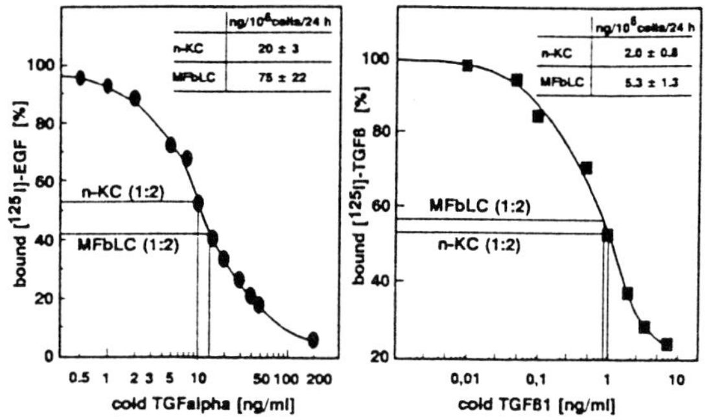

Fig 5: Binding of(^{125}I)TGFβ and (^{125}I)TGFα, resp. to hepatocytes at the first day of primary culture in the presence of increasing concentrations of unlabeled TGFβ and TGFα, resp. Competitions of conditioned media from Kupffer cells and Myofibroblast-like cells are indicated.

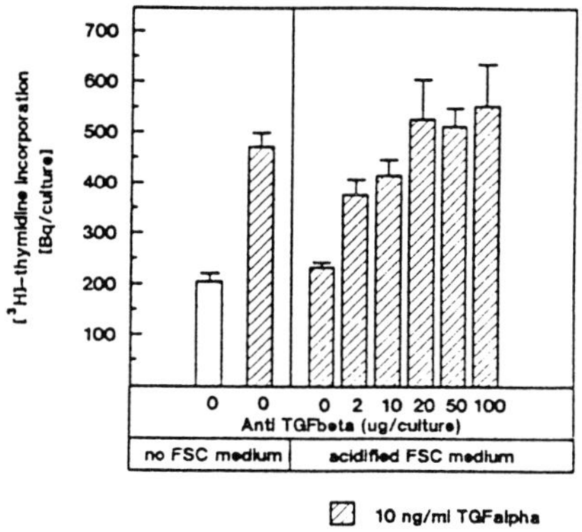

Fig. 7: Effect of anti-TGF beta antibodies on the inhibitory action of MFblCcM on hepatocellular [^{3}H]-thymidine incorporation. Transiently acidified FSC medium at 1 : 4 dilution was incubated for 2 h with increasing amounts of antibody prior to the addition to hepatocyte cultures stimulated by TGF alpha.

Effects of conditioned medium from transformed FSC (myofibroblast-like cells) on hepatocyte proliferation. Like KCcM MFblC conditioned medium inhibited the EGF-stimulated proliferation of hepatocytes (fig. 7). Preincubation of the media with anti-TGFβ antiserum resulted in a complete neutralization of the inhibitory effect (fig. 7). Conditioned medium from primary cultured FSC did not show this inhibitory effect. (data not shown).
To substantiate the hypothesis, that conditioned media of MFbLC might also stimulate hepatocyte proliferation, we studied the effects of MFbLCcM on the proliferation of quiescent hepatocytes.
Similar to KCcM MFblCcM stimulated dose dependently [^{3}H]-thymidine incorporation into the DNA of hepatocytes, if TGFβ in the media was neutralized by anti-TGFβ antibodies (fig. 4). Again, the proliferation stimulatory effect was abolished by competition with TGFα receptor using the TGFα receptor blocking TGFα-(aa34-43)-peptide (fig. 4). The concentration of TGFα/β was found to be 24 ± 7 ng/ml and 1.8 ± 0.4 ng/ml, resp. in the conditioned media added to hepatocyte cultures. The production rates of the factors by MFblC are given in fig. 5. Autoradiographs, which demonstrate the expression of TGFα and β in MFBLC are shown in fig. 6B.

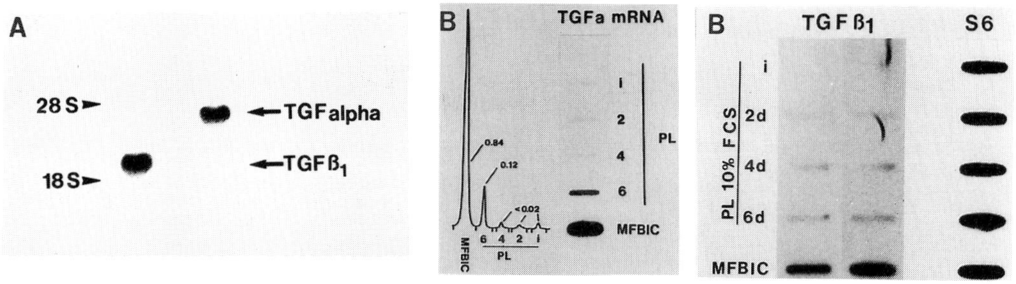

Fig. 6: Hybridization of total RNA from cultured KC and FSC for TGFβ and TGFα.
A) 20 ug RNA from 24 h cultured KC was separated by agarose gel electrophoresis under denaturating conditions and hybridized with ^{32}P-labeled probes for TGFβ and TGFα resp. The positions of the 28S and 18S RNA are indicated.
B) 20 ug RNA from FSC in culture isolated 2, 4, 6 days times after seeding and from MFblC was slot blotted on hybond N membranes and hybridized for TGFα and TGFβ. The relative amount of RNA-DNA hybrides was measured by laser densitomety of the autoradiographs.

Discussion: KC produce a large variety of cytokines and cell growth modulation factors (for review see Decker 1990). The cooperative action of these soluble mediators in conditioned media has not been clearly defined. In the present study we identified in KC conditioned media TGFα and TGFβ as the most important mediators influencing hepatocellular proliferation. Results similar to those with KC were obtained with myofibroblast-like cell conditioned medium, showing that transformed FSC, which accumulate in areas of tissue damage, produce both transforming growth factors. As shown by radioligand binding assays, conditioned media from KC and MFblC contained TGFβ mostly in the latent, biologically inactive form. The proliferation of EGF/TGFα stimulated hepatocytes was inhibited by conditioned media from KC amd MFblC and this effect was pronounced using medium in which TGFβ was activated. These results together with the finding that the growth inhibiting activity can be neutralized by anti-TGFβ antibodies suggest that the growth inhibitory activity is due to TGFβ. Hybridization of total RNA from KC and MFblC with a cDNA probe for TGFβ1 showed the expression of mRNA encoding for TGFβ. The previous finding that KCcM will generally stimulate hepatocyte proliferation (Katsumoto et al. 1989) could not be confirmed. Only after neutralization of TGFβ in KCcM and MFblCcM the replicative, hydroxyurea-sensitive fraction of DNA synthesis (Cleaver 1969) of quiescent hepatocytes was stimulated. This effect was abolished by addition of a TGFα specific decapeptide (amino acid residues 34 - 43), which competes with EGF and TGFα for receptor binding, but does not affect itself cell proliferation (Nestor et al. 1985). The data indicate, that TGFα or EGF might be stimulatory mediators for hepatocyte proliferation. In fact, we measured biologically significant amounts of TGFα/EGF in the conditioned media. Hybridization with a TGFα specific oligonucleotide probe showed TGFα mRNA expression in KC and MFblC. These results together with the observation, that the effects of EGF and TGFα, which are known to induce hepatocellular proliferation (for review see Michalopoulos 1990) are similar to the effect of KCcM and MFblCcM in which TGFβ was blocked suggest that TGFα is the effector in KCcM and in MFblCcM which stimulates hepatocyte DNA synthesis under culture conditions reported here.

Conclusion: The above mentioned data and the observation that TGFα and TGFβ are sequentially expressed in regenerating liver (Fausto and Mead 1989 ; Nakatsukasa et al. 1990) support strongly the assumption that both TGFs play a central role in the up and down regulation of liver regeneration. Cellular sources in the liver of TGFα are hepatocytes (Fausto 1990) and nonparenchymal cell as shown here. The close contacts between FSC. MFblC, KC and hepatocytes in situ and the observation that in regenerating liver TGFα and TGFβ are expressed in nonparenchymal cells in the perisinusoidal area (Fausto 1990; Nakatsukasa 1990; Armendariz-Borunda et al. 1990) suggest that Kupffer cells and transformed fat storing cells might play a central role in the paracrine control of hepatocyte regeneration in situ.

References:

Armendariz-Borunda J., Seyer J.M., Kang A.H., Raghow R. (1990): Regulation of TGFβ gene expression in rat liver intoxicated with carbon tetrachloride. *FASEB J.* 4, 215 - 221.

Bachem M.G., Meyer D., Schäfer W. Gressner A.M. (1989): Evaluation of fibrogenic polypeptide mediators stimulating fat storing cell proliferation and/or proteoglycan synthesis *In: The liver, metabolism and ageing, Topics in aging research in Europe, Vol 12,* ed. Woodhouse K.W., Yelland C. and James O.F.W., pp169 - 177. EURAGE Rijswijk,.

Braun L., Mead J.E., Panzica M., Mikumo R., Bell G.I., Fausto N. (1988): Transforming growth factor beta mRNA increases during liver regeneration. A possible paracrine mechanism of growth regulation, *Proc. Natl. Acad.Sci. USA* 85, 1539-1543.

Chomcynski P. and Sacchi N. (1987): Single-step method of RNA isolation by acid guanidinium thiocynat-phenol-chloroform extraction. *Anal. Biochem.* 162, 156 - 159.

Cleaver J.E. (1969): Repair replication of mammalian cell DNA: effects of compounds that inhibit DNA synthesis of dark repair. *Radiat. Res.* 37, 334 - 349.

Decker K. (1990): Biologically active products of stimulated liver macrophages (Kupffer cells) *Eur. J. Biochem.* 192: 245 - 261.

Enzan H. (1985) Proliferation of ITO cells (fat storing cells) in acute carbon tetrachloride liver injury. *Acta Pathol. Jpn.* 35, 1301 - 1308.

Fausto N. (1990): Hepatic regeneration. *In: Hepatology. A textbook of liver disease.* ed. Zakim D., Boyer T.D., pp 49 - 65. W.B. Saunders Co.

Fausto N., Mead E. (1989): Regulation of liver growth: protooncogenes and transforming growth factors. *Lab. Invest.* 60, 4 - 13.

Friedman S.L. (1990): Cellular sources of collagen and regulation of collagen production in liver. *Seminars in liver disease* 10, 20-29.

Gressner A.M. and Bachem M.G. (1990): Cellular sources of noncollagenous matrix proteins: role of fat-storing cells in fibrogenesis. *Seminars in liver disease* 10,; 30 - 46.

Hendriks H.F.J., Brouwer A., Knook D.L. (1987): The role of hepatic fat storing (Stellate) cells in retinoid metabolism. *Hepatology* 7, 1368 - 1371.

Katsumoto F. Miyazaki K., Nakayama F. (1989): Stimulation od DNA synthesis in hepatocytes by Kupffer cells after partial hepatectomy. *Hepatology* 9, 405 - 410.

Mayanskii D.N., Shcherbakov,V.I., Mirokhanov (1977): Effect of Kupffer cell block at different times after partial hepatectomy on hepatocyte regeneration. *Biul. Eksp. Biol. Med.* 84, 616 - 618.

Mead J.E. Fausto N. (1989): Transforming growth factor alpha may be a physiological regulator of liver regeneration by means of an autocrine mechanism. *Proc. Natl. Acad. Sci. USA* 86, 1558 - 1562.

Meyer D.H. Bachem M.G. and Gressner A.M. (1990): Modulation of hepatic lipocyte proteoglycan synthesis and proliferation by Kupffer cell-derived transforming growth factors type β1 and type α. *Biochem. Biophys. Res. Commun.* 171, 1122 - 1129.

Michalopoulos G.K. (1990): Liver regeneration: molecular mechanisms of growth control. *FASEB J.* 4, 176 - 187.

Nakatsukasa H., Evarts R.P., Hsia C.-C. and Thorgeirsson S.S. (1990): Transforming growth factor-β1 and type I procollagen transcripts during regeneration and early fibrosis of rat liver. *Lab. Invest.* 63, 171 -180.

Nestor, Jr. J.J., Mewman S.R., DeLustro B., Torado G.J., and Schreiber A.B. (1985): A synthetic fragment of rat transforming growth factor α with receptor binding and antigenic properties. *Biochem Biophys. Res. Commun.* 129, 226-232.

Zerbe O. and Gressner A.M. (1988): Proliferation of fat storing cells is stimulated by secretions of Kupffer cells from normal and injured liver. *Exp. Mol. Pathol.* 49, 87 - 101.

Cellular and Molecular Aspects of Cirrhosis. Eds B. Clément, A. Guillouzo. Colloque INSERM/John Libbey Eurotext Ltd. © 1992, Vol. 216, pp. 315-318

Hepatocyte growth factor (HGF) expression in rat liver cells

Peter Schirmacher, Albert Geerts [(1)], Antonello Pietrangelo [(2)], Hans P. Dienes and Charles E. Rogler [(2)]

Institute of Pathology, University of Mainz, Langenbeckstrasse 1, D-6500 Mainz, Germany, [(1)] Laboratory for Cell Biology and Histology, Free University Brussel, Laarbeeklaan 103, B-1090 Brussel-Jette Belgium, and [(2)] Liver Research Center, Albert Einstein College of Medicine, 1300 Morris Park Avenue, Bronx, NY 10461 USA

It has long been known that liver tissue efficiently reacts to acute damage with increased replication of parenchymal cells. A serum-derived and liver-expressed growth factor, which seems to be the major stimulus has recently been purified from various species, cloned, and termed Hepatocyte Growth Factor (HGF) (Nakamura et al., 1989; Zarnegar and Michalopoulos, 1989). HGF-expression has also been detected in several non-hepatic tissues, but recent results indicate that HGF may additionally and predominantly act by paracrine mechanisms (Kinoshita et al., 1989). Therefore it is important to exactly determine the HGF-expressing liver cell population, especially because the results concerning hepatic HGF-production have been conflicting. Zarnegar et al. (1990) have not detected HGF in liver tissue by immunohistochemistry and sequential purification, while HGF-transcripts have been identified in poly A(+) RNA from rat and human liver and attributed to non-parenchymal liver cells (Kinoshita et al., 1989).
Using a rat HGF-cDNA we have performed in situ hybridization with ^{35}S-labeled riboprobes to localize HGF-expressing cells in normal liver tissue from adult male Sprague-Dawley rats. Specific signals were distributed in a single cell pattern and preferentially located in acinar zone 1 and 2 (Fig. 1A). Bright field observations clearly demonstrated that only sinusoidal cells expressed HGF (Fig. 1C), while parenchymal cells (PC) and cells in the portal tracts including bile duct epithelium (Fig. 1D) were negative. Moreover, it was obvious that only a subpopulation of sinusoidal cells expressed HGF, because a significant number of sinusoidal cells did not contain HGF-transcripts (Fig. 1C, arrows). To exactly determine the HGF-expressing subpopulation of sinusoidal liver cells we have analyzed RNA extracted from isolated and purified liver cells for HGF steady state transcript levels by Northern blot hybridization. The relevant liver cell populations were isolated and purified as described recently (Rogiers et al., 1987; Van Bossuyt et al., 1988; De Bleser et al., 1991; Schirmacher et al., 1991) and representative aliquots of the different fractions were characterized and quantitated for their composition by transmission electron microscopy (data not shown). Only the fat-storing cell (FSC) fraction contained the specific 6kb HGF-transcripts, while PC and Kupffer cells (KC) were negative (Fig. 2A). A faint specific

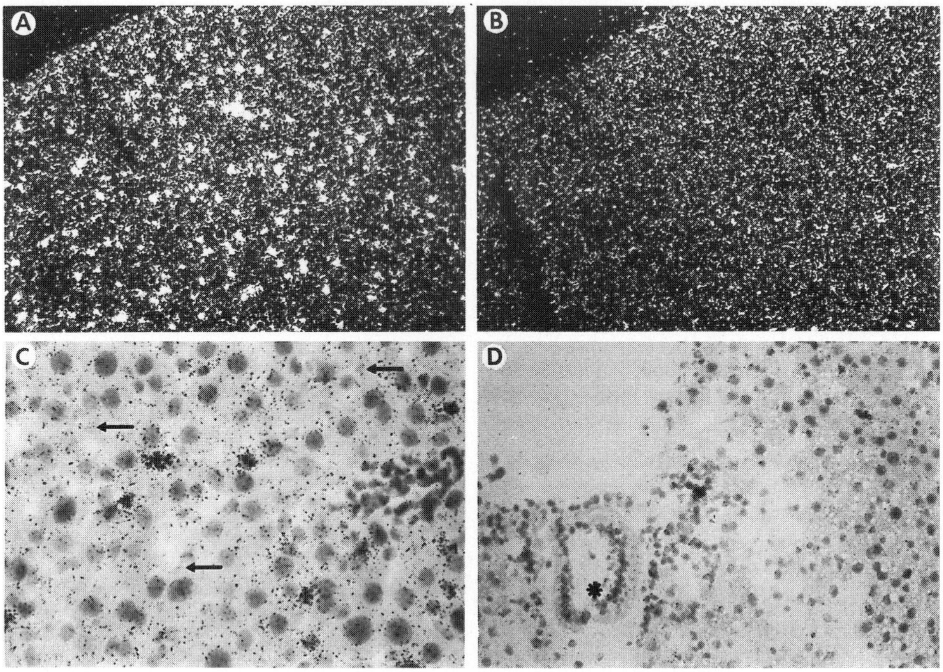

Fig. 1

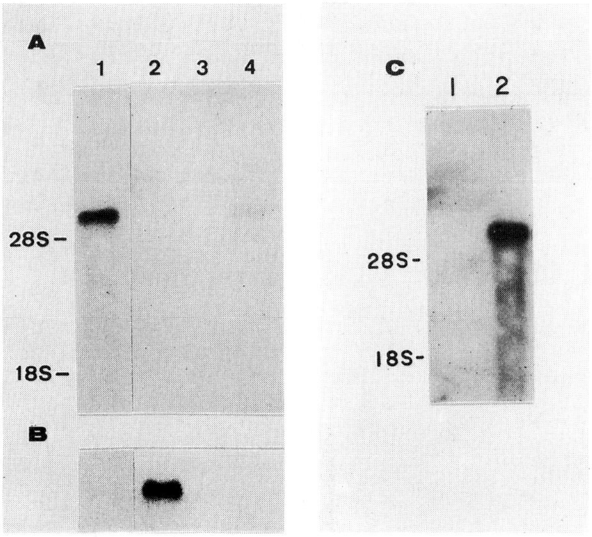

Fig. 2

band present in the endothelial cell (EC) fraction was due to a minor contamination of the EC-fraction with FSC as calculated by comparing the densitometry scanning of the hybridization signals with the quantitative composition of the different cell fractions.
Chronic inflammation of the liver or culturing of isolated FSC on a plastic substrate leads to activation of FSC, which is morphologically characterized by their transition into a myofibroblast-like phenotype. By Northern hybridization of total RNA (Fig 2B) and poly A(+) RNA (data not shown) extracted from myofibroblast-like cells derived from FSC, it was determined that this cell population completely lacked HGF-expression.
The in vivo significance of this observation is indicated by the observation that the number of HGF-expressing sinusoidal cells, which rises significantly during acute CCl_4 induced liver damage, is lower in cirrhotic rat liver tissue then even in normal liver tissue. Especially in the vicinity of fibrous septa HGF-expressing cells are missing (data not shown).
The in situ and Northern hybridization data demonstrate that among normal rat liver cells only FSC express HGF transcripts in significant amounts. This is in disagreement with results published by Noji et al. (1990), who have described HGF-expression in EC and KC. In our hands the data solely derived from in situ hybridization experiments do not allow the specific assignment of the observed signal to EC and KC, nor do they exclude HGF-expression in FSC.
HGF-expression in FSC, which are situated in a strategic position of the hepatic microenvironment, raises several considerations: (i) expression of a growth factor constitutes a new function of FSC, which is fundamentally different from their known ability to store vitamin A and synthesize connective tissue molecules. (ii) It strengthens the idea of a preferentially paracrine interaction of FSC and PC in regeneration following liver damage, although further expression studies involving the recently identified HGF-receptor (Bottaro et al. 1991) are required. (iii) As HGF is most likely identical to the so-called Scatter Factor (Gherardi & Stoker, 1990),

---

Fig. 1: In situ hybridization for HGF-transcripts in normal rat liver: (A) Specific hybridization with HGF-antisense riboprobe demonstrates single cells positive for HGF mRNA in the liver parenchyma (dark field). (B) Control hybridization with HGF-sense riboprobe (dark field). (C) Specific hybridization with HGF-antisense riboprobe (bright field). Positive signal in sinusoidal cells (smaller, oval nuclei). Parenchymal cells (large cells with large, round nuclei) and a small portal tract (right side) are negative for HGF mRNA. Some sinusoidal lining cells (arrows) are also negative for HGF mRNA. (D) Specific hybridization with HGF-antisense riboprobe (bright field). Large intrahepatic bile duct negative for HGF mRNA.

Fig. 2: Analysis for HGF gene expression in different rat liver cell populations by Northern hybridization of total cellular RNA: (A) Freshly isolated liver cells: (1) fat-storing cells, (2) parenchymal cells, (3) Kupffer cells, (4) Endothelial cells. (B) Rehybridization of (A) with a rat albumin cDNA-probe (C) Loss of HGF gene expression in myofibroblast-like cells derived from fat-storing cells after 30 days culturing (1), compared to freshly isolated fat-storing cells (2).

a differential auto-/paracrine regulatory function of HGF on (other) sinusoidal cells seems likely.
The loss of HGF-expression during myofibroblast-like transition of FSC is of possible significance for chronic liver disease. In fibrotic and cirrhotic liver tissue failure of the activated FSC-population to express sufficient HGF may contribute to an impairment of parenchymal cell regeneration and finally to liver insufficiency.

REFERENCES

Bottaro, D.P., Rubin, J.S., Faletto, D.L., Chan, A.M.-L., Kmiecik, T.E., Vande Woude G.F., and Aaronson S.A. (1991): Identification of the hepatocyte growth factor receptor as the c-met proto-oncogene product. Science 251, 802-804.

De Bleser, P., Geerts, A., Van Eyken, P., Vrijsen, R., Lazou, J.M., Desmet, V., and Wisse, E. (1991): Tenascin synthesis in cultured rat liver fat-storing cells. In Cells of the hepatic sinusoid, Vol 3, eds. E. Wisse, D.L. Knook, R. McCuskey, Kupffer Cell Foundation (in press).

Gherardi, E., and Stoker, M. (1990): Hepatocytes and scatter factor. Nature 346, 228.

Kinoshita, T., Tashiro, K., and Nakamura, T. (1989): Marked increase of HGF mRNA in non-parenchymal liver cells of rats treated with hepatotoxins. Biochem. Biophys. Res. Comm. 165, 1229-1234.

Nakamura, T., Nishizawa, T., Hagiya, M., Seki, T., Shimonishi, M., Sugimura, A., Tashiro, K., and Shimizu, S. (1989): Molecular cloning and expression of human hepatocyte growth factor. Nature 342, 440-443.

Noji, S., Tashiro, K., Koyama, E., Nohno, T., Ohyama, K., Taniguchi, S., and Nakamura, T. (1990): Expression of hepatocyte growth factor gene in endothelial and Kupffer cells of damaged rat livers, as revealed by in situ hybridization. Biochem. Biophys. Res. Comm. 173, 42-47.

Rogiers, V., Paeme, G., Sonck, W., and Vercruysse, A. (1987): Metabolism of procyclidine in isolated rat hepatocytes. Xenobiotica 17, 849-857.

Schirmacher, P., Geerts, A., Pietrangelo, A., Dienes, H.P., and Rogler, C.E. (1991): Hepatocyte growth factor/hepatopoietin A is expressed in fat-storing cells from rat liver, but not myofibroblast-like cells derived from fat-storing cells. Hepatology (in press).

Van Bossuyt, H., Bouwens, L., and Wisse, E. (1988): Isolation, purification and culture of sinusoidal liver cells. In Sinusoids in human liver: health and disease, eds. P. Bioulac-Sage and C. Balabaud, pp. 1-16, Kupffer Cell Foundation.

Zarnegar, R. & Michalopoulos G. (1989): Purification and biological characterization of human hepatopoietin A, a polypeptide growth factor for hepatocytes. Cancer Res. 49, 3314-3320.

Zarnegar, R., Muga, S., Rahija, R., Michalopoulos, G. (1990): Tissue distribution of hepatopoietin-A: A heparin-binding polypeptide growth factor for hepatocytes. Proc. Natl. Acad. Sci. USA 87, 3200-3204.

Cellular and Molecular Aspects of Cirrhosis. Eds B. Clément, A. Guillouzo. Colloque INSERM/John Libbey Eurotext Ltd. © 1992, Vol. 216, pp. 319-322

CCAAT/enhancer binding protein (C/EBP) : role in physiologial regulation of liver regeneration ?

David Mischoulon, Basabi Rana, Gregory S. Robinson, Nancy L.R. Bucher and Stephen R. Farmer *

Departments of Biochemistry and Pathology, Boston University School of Medicine, Boston, MA 02118, USA

* *Corresponding author*

In adult liver, the hepatocytes, which are normally quiescent, are induced to proliferate by an excessive workload, which is imposed experimentally in the rat by partial hepatectomy or by somewhat less effective but non-surgical means. The growth process appears to be signalled by hormones and growth factors circulating in the blood. Partial hepatectomy is followed by an initial, major outburst of proliferative activity which peaks at about 24 hours and is tightly regulated, diminishing proportionately as the cell population is restored. Such regulation has suggested an interplay between growth stimulatory and growth inhibitory factors that balance growth rate against metabolic demands.

Hepatocytes, freshly isolated and cultured, respond in a similar way to most of the soluble growth effectors proposed as regulators within the animal. None of these is liver specific, however, and the physiological mechanisms through which they translate a metabolic workload into a growth response, that is limited to liver, remain obscure. We are investigating how a soluble growth effector, Epidermal Growth Factor (EGF), influences the activities of a particular gene, C/EBP. C/EBP, whose product is a transcription factor, controls a number of genes that regulate energy metabolism (stearoyl acyl-CoA desaturase, PEP carboxykinase) as well as other liver functions such as production of albumin, transthyretin, alpha and beta-fibrinogen, alpha-1-antitrypsin, alcohol dehydrogenase, carbamyl phosphate synthetase, Apolipoprotein B-100 and others (McKnight et al, 1989). Overall, it is thought to function as a growth-suppressor/differentiation promoter gene. Our studies are directed towards finding how fully C/EBP is implicated in the hepatic regenerative scheme, and the mechanisms through which metabolic processes, hormones, and growth factors implement its various functions. Other liver specific and growth related genes (especially several immediate early genes) are examined as liver function and cell-cycle markers. To the extent feasible, parallel studies are carried out in livers regenerating within the animal and in normal hepatocytes exposed to growth effectors in vitro.

Expression of C/EBP mRNA during liver regeneration

To determine the relative abundance of C/EBP mRNA during liver regeneration, we isolated total RNA from livers (Chomczynski & Sacchi, 1987) at various times following a 2/3 partial hepatectomy (Higgins & Anderson, 1931) and analyzed the expression of mRNAs by Northern blot hybridization (Bond & Farmer, 1983). Figure 1A reveals an abrupt drop in C/EBP mRNA levels within the first 3 hours of regeneration as the hepatocytes move from G_0 into G_1. This low level of expression remains quite constant until 19 hours post-hepatectomy, when there is a second drop that corresponds with passage of cells into S phase, indicated by induction of histone 3.2 mRNA (Delisle et al, 1983). Soon after this phase, there is a gradual increase in C/EBP mRNA which returns to near-normal values by 72 hours (Fig.1B), a time when hepatic regeneration is beginning to shut down. Partial hepatectomy induces a slight acute phase response, presumably due to surgical stress, but stress alone appears to have little or no effect on C/EBP mRNA expression, as indicated by the control samples taken at corresponding intervals following sham operation (see Fig.1B, 4S vs 4R).

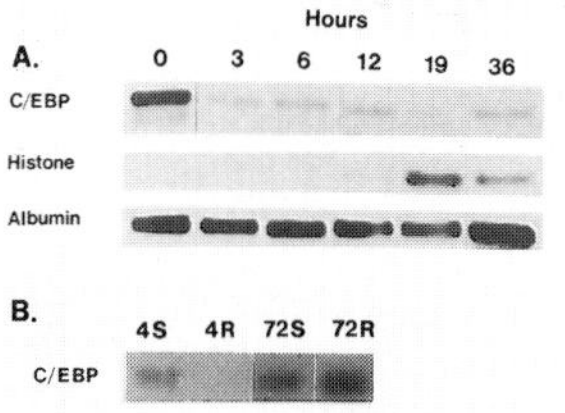

Fig. 1: Abundance of C/EBP mRNA during liver regeneration.
A. Northern blot analysis of total RNA isolated from livers at the indicated times following a 2/3 partial hepatectomy. An albumin probe was used to control for equal loading. *B*. Northern blot of total RNA from 4hr (4R) and 72hr (72R) regenerating liver and corresponding sham controls (4S, 72S).

Transcriptional activity of the C/EBP gene during liver regeneration

Many hepatic genes, both liver specific and growth-associated, are regulated at a transcriptional level. We therefore performed a series of nuclear run on assays (Greenberg & Ziff,1984; Bellas & Farmer,1991) to assess whether C/EBP expression was similarly regulated. Figure 2 shows that transcription of the rat liver C/EBP gene decreases at least 2 fold within an hour following hepatectomy, reaching a 5 fold reduced level of transcription by 2 hours and remaining at this low level of expression through S phase (25 hours posthepatectomy). As observed for C/EBP mRNA levels, there is a similar increase in the transcription of C/EBP gene after this phase of the cell cycle, returning to control liver levels by 72 hours. The increased transcription of the actin gene at 15 mins, the c-myc gene at 60 mins and the fibronectin gene at 120 mins likely corresponds to the activation of a program of immediate early genes accompanying the G_0/G_1 transition (Lau & Nathans,1987; Carpenter & Wahl,1990), and the increased transcription of histone 3.2 gene corresponds to the entry of hepatocytes into S phase at 24 hours (Delisle et al,1983; Bucher et al,1990). The assay performed on sham hepatectomized animals at 1 hour indicates that the decrease in C/EBP transcription results exclusively from liver growth, and not the stress of the operation.

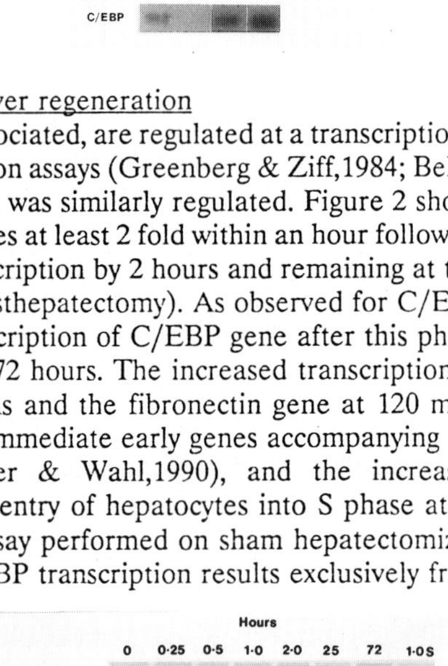

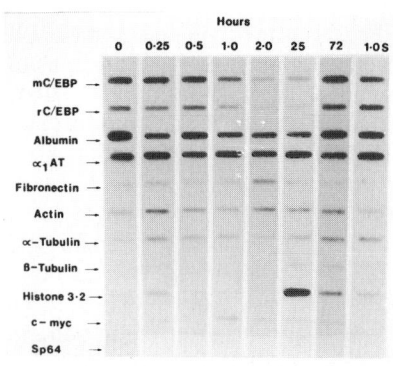

Fig. 2: Transcriptional activity of the C/EBP gene relative to other abundant liver genes during liver regeneration.
Run-on assays were performed on equal numbers of nuclei isolated from total liver at the indicated times following a partial hepatectomy (7.5 X 10^7 nuclei per set). 1S corresponds to a sham operation taken at 1 hr. The genes assayed correspond to the various cDNA probes used: mC/EBP = a mouse cDNA probe; rC/EBP = a rat cDNA probe; α_1(I)AT = alpha1-antitrypsin; Sp64 = control plasmid.

The effect of EGF on the expression of C/EBP mRNA in short term cultures of hepatocytes

The kinetics of inhibition of C/EBP gene expression during liver regeneration shown in Figs. 1 and 2 suggested that this process may be regulated by effectors that control the activation of quiescent hepatocytes into the cell cycle. Epidermal Growth Factor (EGF) has been shown to be a potent hepatic mitogen both in the animal and in culture (Bucher et al, 1978; Richman et al, 1976). We therefore assessed whether the expression of C/EBP in cultured hepatocytes was influenced by EGF. Figure 3 shows a Northern blot analysis of total RNA isolated from hepatocytes cultured on rat tail collagen (Seglen, 1976; Ben-Ze'ev et al, 1988) in the presence or absence of EGF (10ng/ml). EGF causes a significant decrease in expression of C/EBP mRNA by 3 hours, and this effect is most pronounced by 4 hours.

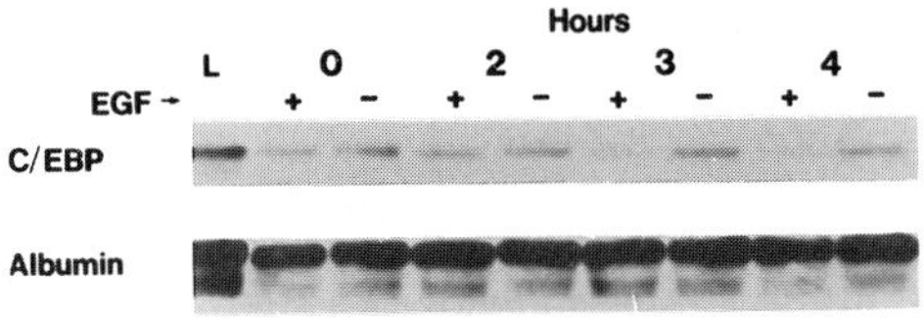

Fig. 3: The effect of EGF on the expression of C/EBP mRNA in hepatocytes cultured under conventional conditions with or without EGF.
Hepatocytes were plated at a concentration of 350X10^3 cells/1.5ml onto Lux 100mm tissue culture dishes coated with rat tail dry collagen (RTd). Cells were maintained at 37°C, in air + 5% CO_2, and harvested at the indicated times. Total RNA (25ug) isolated from hepatocytes was subjected to Northern blot analysis as in Fig. 1A. An albumin probe was used to control for equal loading.

Down-regulation of C/EBP mRNA during liver regeneration and in cultured hepatocytes is dependent on protein synthesis, and has multiple levels of regulation.

Activation of the early growth response in hepatocytes involves the so-called immediate early genes which do not require prior protein synthesis, but rather seem to depend on transduction of second messenger signals directly to the regulatory elements within these growth-related genes. Since the down-regulation of C/EBP occurs early, and is transcriptionally regulated, we examined the possible relation to the immediate early gene family. We found, however, that inhibition of protein synthesis by injection of cycloheximide 15 minutes prior to partial hepatectomy prevents the usual post-hepatectomy down-regulation of C/EBP (Fig.4). As controls we included c-myc, c-jun, and jun B mRNAs, which Fig.4 shows were superinduced in response to cycloheximide treatment (Mohn et al, 1990), indicating that the drug dosage was sufficient to alter immediate early gene responses. As within the animal, cycloheximide similarly blocked the down-regulation of C/EBP in growth factor stimulated hepatocyte cultures (Fig.5).

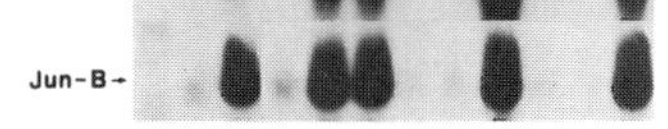

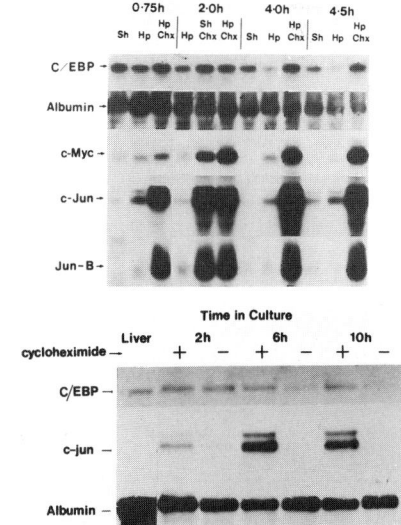

Fig. 4: Effect of cycloheximide on the down-regulation of C/EBP expression in regenerating liver.
Rats were partially hepatectomized and, where indicated, injected with cycloheximide (50mg/200g rat) 15 mins. prior to surgery. RNA was isolated at the indicated times, and subjected to Northern blot analysis. Sh = sham; Hp = hepatectomy; Chx = cycloheximide.

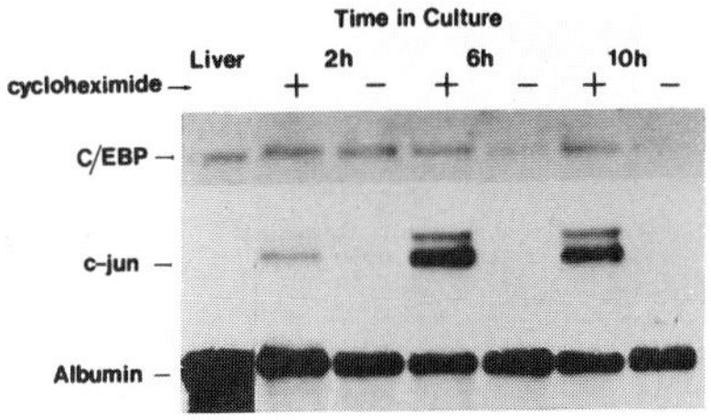

Fig. 5: Effect of cycloheximide on the down-regulation of C/EBP expression in hepatocyte cultures.
Hepatocytes were cultured on RTd as in Fig.3, and treated with cycloheximide (10ug/ml) or carrier buffer (saline). Cells were harvested at the indicated times and RNA was subjected to Northern blot analysis.

The effect of cycloheximide on C/EBP gene expression may involve regulation at a transcriptional or posttranscriptional level. To gain insight into the possible mechanisms involved, we assessed whether cycloheximide had an effect on the rate of turnover of the C/EBP mRNA. We therefore measured C/EBP mRNA by Northern blots following the inhibition of transcription with actinomycin D in hepatocytes cultured in the presence or absence of cycloheximide. Figure 6 (filled bars) shows the extensive decrease in C/EBP mRNA in response to culture of hepatocytes in growth medium alone; addition of act D results in an even greater decrease in mRNA levels during the 8 hr culture period indicating that the normal turnover rate of C/EBP mRNA is extremely rapid. Cycloheximide, as in Fig.5, again inhibits C/EBP mRNA down-regulation, and this occurs also even when mRNA synthesis is blocked by act D, suggesting that the effect of cycloheximide is to stabilize the C/EBP mRNA rather than increase the rate of C/EBP transcription.

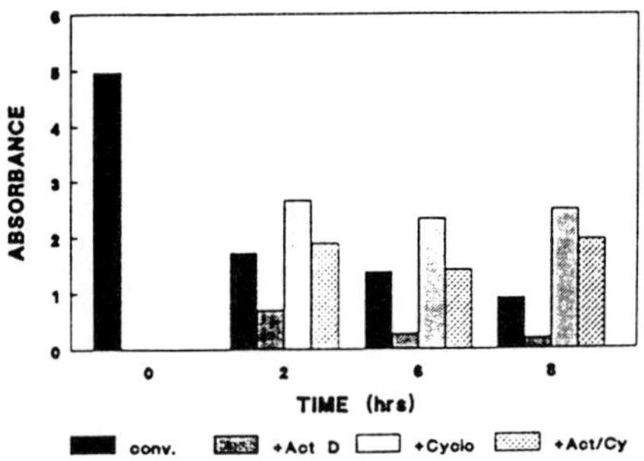

Fig. 6: Effects of cycloheximide and actinomycin D on C/EBP down-regulation in hepatocyte cultures. Hepatocytes were cultured as in Fig.5, with or without cycloheximide (10ug/ml) and actinomycin D (5ug/ml). Cells were harvested at the indicated times, and RNA was subjected to Northern blot analysis. conv. = conventional cultures, i.e. cells on RTd with EGF and insulin. The intensity of the autoradiograph was quantified by laser densitometry, and plotted as a bar graph.

Our data suggest that C/EBP expression undergoes cell cycle-related changes that are similar in vitro and in vivo. Expression of C/EBP appears to be transcriptionally regulated in regenerating liver, and decreases during early regeneration, suggesting that C/EBP may have an anti-proliferative role in normal liver. Activation of quiescent hepatocytes into the cell cycle may require that C/EBP expression be depressed, perhaps by EGF or other known hepatocyte mitogens. On the basis of inhibition of protein and mRNA synthesis with cycloheximide and actinomycin D respectively, **a)** C/EBP expression seems to be dependent on prior protein synthesis, **b)** C/EBP mRNA has a rapid rate of turnover, **c)** C/EBP expression is controlled both at transcriptional and post-transcriptional levels. Further studies are underway to assess the role C/EBP may play in the physiological regulation of liver regeneration.

We are grateful to Drs. S.L. McKnight and J.E. Darnell for providing the rat and mouse C/EBP cDNAs, respectively. We also thank our Research Associates Y.H. Xie, F. Lin, and B. Radner for valuable assistance. D.M. acknowledges the support of the C.E. Culpeper Foundation, and the K. Grunebaum Cancer Research Foundation. This work was supported by grants #CA39049 from the N.I.H. and #2237 from the Council for Tobacco Research.

Bellas, R.E. & Farmer, S.R.(1991): *J. Biol. Chem.* **266**:12008-12014

Ben-Ze'ev, A., Robinson, G.S., Bucher, N.L.R. & Farmer, S.R.(1988): *Proc. Natl. Acad. Sci. USA* **85**:2161-2165

Bond, J.F. & Farmer, S.R. (1983): *Molec. Cell. Biol.* **3**: 1333-1342

Bucher, N.L.R., Patel, U. & Cohen, S. (1978): *Adv. Enzyme Reg.* **16**:205-213

Bucher, N.L.R., Robinson, G.S. & Farmer, S.R. (1990): *Seminars in Liver Disease* **10**:11-19

Carpenter, G. & Wahl, M.I. (1990): *Handb. Exp. Pharmacol.* **951**:69-171

Chomczynski, P. & Sacchi, N. (1987): *Anal. Biochem.* **162**:156-159

Delisle, A.J., Graves, R.A., Marzluff, W.F. & Johnson, L.F. (1983): *Mol. Cell Biol.* **3**:1920-1929

Greenberg, M.E. & Ziff, E.B. (1984): *Nature* **311**:433-37

Higgins, G.M. & Anderson, R.M. (1931): *Arch. Pathol.* **12**:186

Lau, L.F. & Nathans, D. (1987): *Proc. Natl. Acad. Sci. USA* **84**:1182-1186

McKnight, S.L., Lane, M.D. & Gluecksohn-Walsh, S. (1989): *Genes and Dev.* **3**:2021-2024

Mohn, K.L., Laz, T., Melby, A.E. & Taub, R. (1990): *J. Biol. Chem.* **265**:21916-21921

Richman, R.A., Claus, T.H., Pilkis, S.J. & Friedman, D.L. (1976): *Proc. Natl. Acad. Sci. USA* **73**:3589-3593

Seglen. P.O. (1976): *Meth. Cell Biol.* **13**: 29-83

Cellular and Molecular Aspects of Cirrhosis. Eds B. Clément, A. Guillouzo. Colloque INSERM/John Libbey Eurotext Ltd. © 1992, Vol. 216, pp. 323-326

Cirrhosis, liver cell dysplasia, hepatocarcinoma : histological evidence for this sequence ?

Brigitte Le Bail, Paulette Bioulac-Sage and Charles Balabaud

Laboratoire des Interactions Cellulaires Université de Bordeaux II, 146, rue Léo Saignat, 33076 Bordeaux Cedex, France

SUMMARY

It has been suggested that macroregenerative nodule are preferential sites of degenerescence in cirrhotic livers.We studied 14 macronodules (8 - 15mm) selected during gross examination of the cirrhotic livers of 5 patients undergoing liver transplantation. Histology indicated for all 14 adenomatous hyperplasia; 4 nodules had areas of large liver cell dysplasia; 12 presented foci of small liver cell dysplasia of varying degrees of severity according to the intensity of nuclear crowding, cytoplasmic basophilia and architectural disarray. One of these foci could be considered a very well differentiated (grade I) "in situ" hepatocellular carcinoma. Like hepatoma cells, the small dysplastic hepatocytes had an increased nucleo-cytoplasmic ratio; they were often depleted in glycogen and iron; they expressed more p 21- *ras* oncoprotein and Ki 67 proliferative index was increased in these foci. In conclusion, small liver cell dysplasia is frequent in cirrhotic macronodules of adenomatous hyperplasia. As it shares many morphological and functional similarities with hepatoma cells, we think that its preneoplastic potentiality must be taken into account.

INTRODUCTION

It has been shown in experimental hepatocarcinogenesis in the rat that hyperplastic nodules are intermediary premalignant lesions preceeding the development of hepatocellular carcinoma (Farber &Sarma, 1987). In human cirrhosis, two kinds of liver cell dysplasia have been described but there is still controversy regarding their preneoplastic potential (Crawford, 1990). On the other hand, cirrhotic macronodules consisting of adenomatoid hyperplasia are suspected to be the preferential sites for the malignant transformation (Arakawa **et al.,** 1986; Furuya **et al.** , 1988; Wada **et al.** , 1988; Takayama **et al.** , 1990). The aim of this study was to document the histology of cirrhotic macronodules and to look for possible morphological, morphometric, histochemical or immunohistochemical arguments for a transition from benign to malignant lesions.

MATERIAL AND METHODS

Fourteen macronodules (8 to 15 mm in diameter) were taken from 5 cirrhotic livers from patients undergoing liver transplantation for end stage cirrhosis of alcoholic and/or viral origin; a hepatocellular carcinoma was associated in two of them.

Macronodules were defined at gross examination as sizable nodules bulging on their cut surface; the minimal diameter chosen was 8 mm for micro-macronodular cirrhosis.

For histology, haematoxylin-eosin-safran, PAS, perls and reticulin stains were used. ***Large liver cell dysplasia (LLCD)*** was defined as cellular and nuclear enlargement with a normal nuclear-cytoplasmic ratio, nuclear pleomorphism, hyperchromasia and possible multiple nuclei and nucleoli (Anthony ***et al.***, 1973). ***Small liver cell dysplasia (SLCD)*** was characterized by a decreased volume of cytoplasm associated with a moderate increase in nuclear size, resulting in an increased nucleo-cytoplasmic ratio, in the absence of patent nuclear atypia (Watanabe ***et al.***, 1983). ***Adenomatoid hyperplasia*** was diagnosed for macronodules surrounded by a condensed rim of fibrous tissue, and composed of one large or several confluent regenerating nodules, containing occasional portal tracts (Edmonson, 1976). Immunohistochemistry was performed on paraffin sections to detect the following antigens: HBs, HBc , AFP, ACE, α-1 AT (Dako), p 21- *ras* (Oncogene Science); Ki 67 (Dako) proliferative index was determined on frozen sections. Morphometric analysis (IBAS I, Kontron computer, software version 5.42, 1984) was carried out on one typical nodule; groups of 100 cells were tested for cellular (C) and nuclear (N) areas, N/C, and a nuclear form factor PE= 4 π x area / perimeter.

RESULTS

Histology : all 14 macronodules presented the characteristics of adenomatoid hyperplasia.They were composed of hepatocytes of normal or reduced size, with normal or enhanced cytoplasmic eosinophilia, arranged in one- or two-thick plates, with occasional areas of moderate hypercellularity (cobblestoning). Siderosis or fatty change was possible. In addition, 4/14 contained areas of LLCD, situated at the periphery of the nodule, often associated with inflammatory cells. Most interestingly, 12/14 of the macronodules presented foci of SLCD of varying degree. SLCD was considered mild , moderate or severe after appreciation of the severity of the following three criteria: nuclear crowding, cytoplasmic basophilia, and architectural disarray (pseudoglandular, glandular or trabecular arrangements). In one nodule, a foci presenting as a "nodule-in-nodule" was considered a very well differentiated (grade I) "in situ" hepatocellular carcinoma; it was associated with foci of severe and moderate SLCD and with LLCD. In LLCD areas, special stains indicated no modification of the reticulin network, variable amounts of glycogen, and occasional iron overload in hemosiderotic livers. In SLCD, the reticulin network was often decreased and disorganized; cells were generally poor in glycogen and resistant to iron accumulation. Ag HBs was sometimes found in LLCD; in SLCD foci, the amount of Ag HBs and HBc was very low, clearly inferior to that of the rest of the liver. AFP and α-1AT were not detectable in the macronodules. Ki 67 proliferative index was increased, particularly in dysplastic areas of SLCD type, reaching the level of 5% of the hepatocytes, which is superposable to the level in low grade hepatocellular carcinoma and superior to the level in a classic cirrhotic nodule. Expression of p21- *ras* oncoprotein was increased and detectable both in LLCD at the periphery of the macronodules (as in the rest of the cirrhotic liver) and in SLCD, particularly close to portal tracts. Morphometric analysis clearly demonstrated two types of dysplastic cells: SLCD and LLCD. (C) and (N/C) of SLCD (125± 40 μm^2 and 17,7% respectively) was intermediary between normal hepatocyte (151±44 μm^2 and 10,3%) and grade 1 hepatocellular carcinoma (107± 32 μm^2 and 22%). Cells of LLCD type were 6 times larger than normal (C: 1070± 410 μm^2) , but had a normal N/C ratio (11,5%). Nuclear form (Pe) of SLCD was identical to normal hepatocytes, while (Pe) of LLCD was close to those of grade 1 hepatocellular carcinoma.

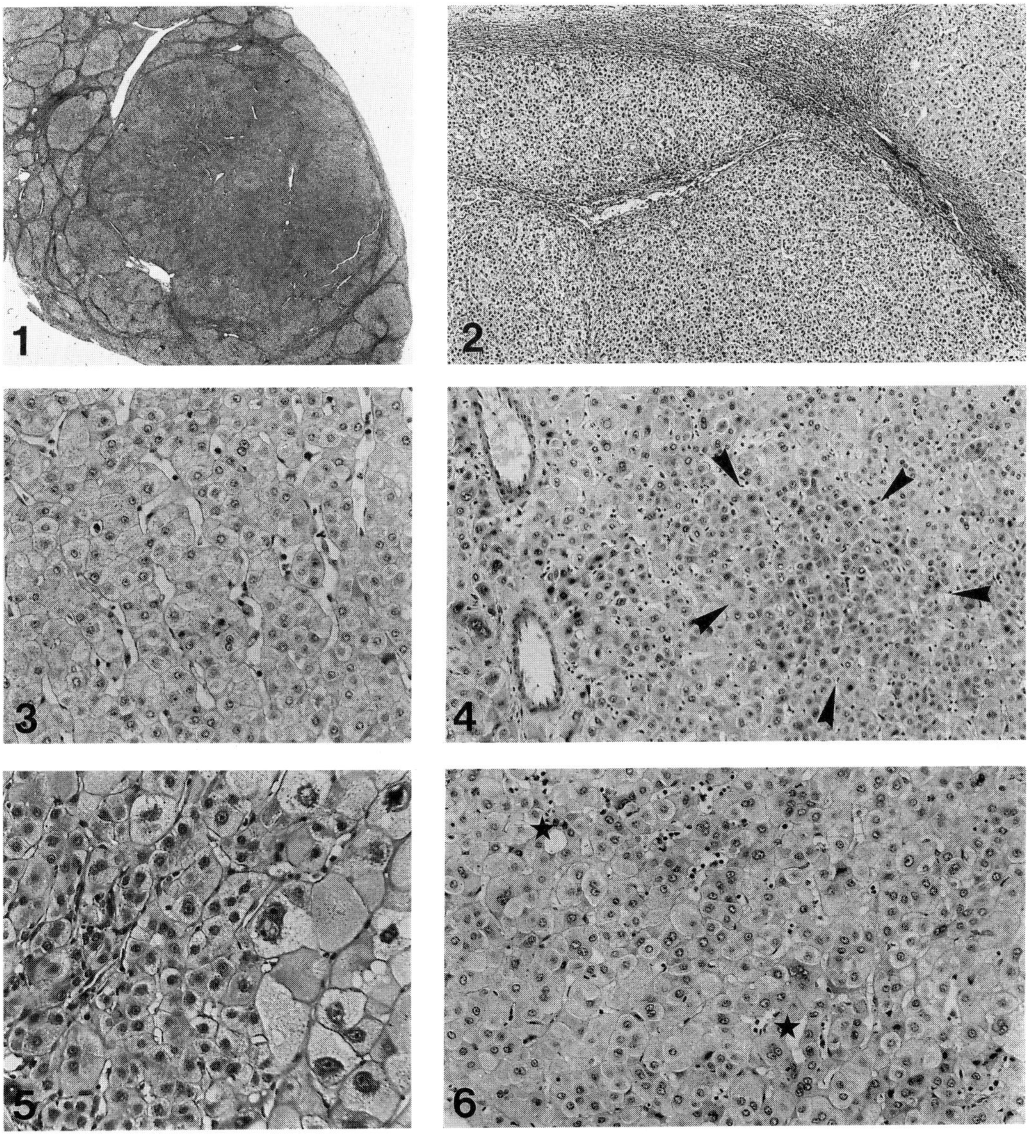

LEGENDS. (1) Histological section of a 17 mm diameter macronodule (micro-macronodular viral cirrhosis). (2) General view of a nodule of adenomatoid hyperplasia, surrounded by a condensed rim of collagen, containing a portal tract, with slight hypercellularity, near a normal cirrhotic nodule (top right), G x 55. (3) Adenomatoid hyperplasia: one- or two- cell thick plates of normal hepatocytes, G x 175 . (4) Hypercellular foci of small and basophilic dysplastic cells in an adenomatous hyperplastic nodule, G x 110 . (5) Association of small liver cell dysplasia (left) and large liver cell dysplasia (right) in viral cirrhosis, G x 190 . (6) Mild to severe small liver cell dysplasia, characterized by nuclear crowding, basophilic cell foci, thickened plates and glandular arrangements (stars), Gx 145 .

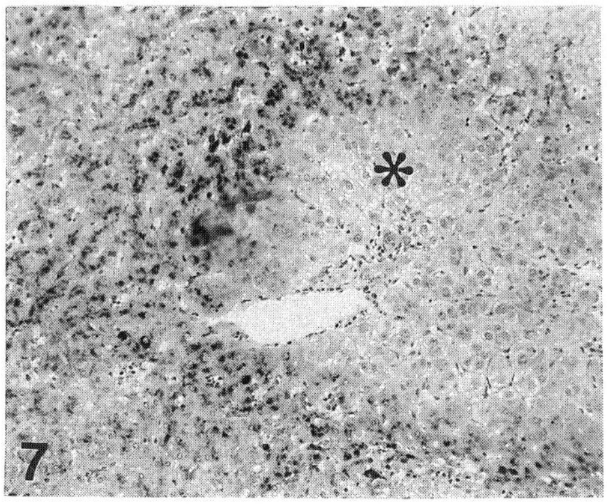

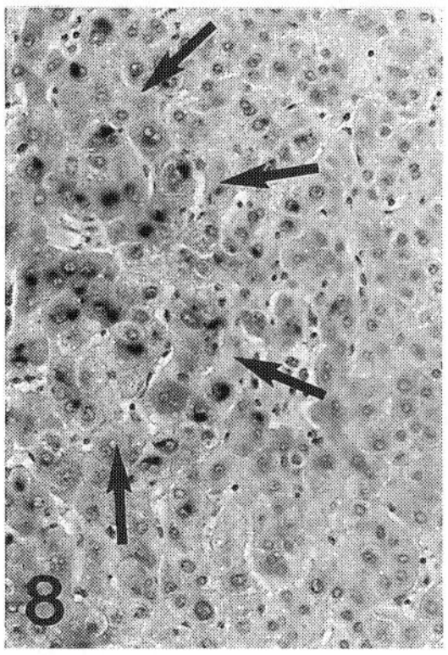

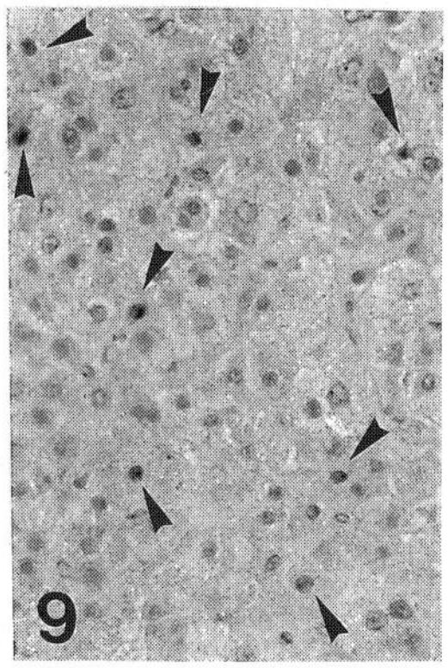

LEGENDS. (7) Focus of small dysplastic hepatocytes (asterisk) resistant to iron accumulation in an alcoholic liver with hemosiderosis (Perls stain), G x 110. (8) Marked expression of p 21-*ras* oncoprotein, appearing as cytoplasmic globular inclusions, in a focus of small cells in a macronodule (immunoperoxydase, paraffin section), G x 145 . (9) Increased antigen Ki 67 expression in a focus of small liver cell dysplasia, appearing as small nuclear dots (immunoperoxydase, frozen section) , G x 175 .

CONCLUSION

In our study, macroregenerative nodules histologically correspond to adenomatoid hyperplasia. They frequently display areas of liver cell dysplasia of both small and large cell type; foci of well differenciated hepatocellular carcinoma, appearing as a " nodule-in -nodule" may be associated. LLCD may be the morphological evidence of hepatocellular dystrophic regeneration, closely linked to the presence of hepatitis B or C virus ; there are no clear morphological, architectural, immuno/histochemical arguments to indicate that this is a preneoplastic condition. On the contrary, SLCD cells share many similarities with cells of well differentiated hepatocellular carcinoma: small size, increased nucleo-cytoplasmic ratio, architectural disarray, enhanced Ki 67 proliferative index and p 21- *ras* oncoprotein expression, a tendency towards a reduction in glycogen content and a resistance to iron accumulation.The exact nature and origin of SLCD (dedifferenciated hepatocytes ?or cells derived from "stem cells"?) is still unknown, but it would seem that the preneoplastic potentiality of this lesion should be taken into account.

REFERENCES

Anthony, P.P.et al. (1973): Liver cell dysplasia: a premalignant condition. *J. Clin. Pathol.* 26, 217-223.

Arakawa, M. et al. (1986): Emergence of malignant lesions within an adenomatous hyperplastic nodule in a cirrhotic liver. *Gastroenterology* 91, 198- 208.

Crawford, J.M. (1990): Pathologic assessment of liver cell dysplasia and benign liver tumors: differenciation from malignant tumors. *Sem. Diag. Pathol.* 7, 115-128.

Edmonson, H.A. (1976): Benign epithelial tumors and tumor-like lesions of the liver. In *Hepatocellular carcinoma* , ed. K. Okuda & R.L. Peters, pp.309-330. New York:Wiley.

Farber, E. & Sarma, D.S.R. (1987): Biology of disease. Hepatocarcinogenesis: a dynamic cellular perspective. *Lab. Invest*. 56, 4-22.

Furuya, K. et al. (1988): Macroregenerative nodule of the liver: a clinicopathologic study of 345 autopsy cases of chronic liver diseases. *Cancer* 61, 99-105.

Takayama, T. et al. (1990): Malignant transformation of adenomatous hyperplasia to hepatocellular carcinoma. *Lancet* 33, 1150-1153.

Wada, K. et al. Large regenerative nodules and dysplastic nodules in cirrhotic livers: a histopathological study. *Hepatology* 8, 1684-1688.

Watanabe, S. et al. (1983): Morphologic studies of liver cell dysplasia. *Cancer* 51, 2197-2205.

Cellular and Molecular Aspects of Cirrhosis. Eds B. Clément, A. Guillouzo. Colloque INSERM/John Libbey Eurotext Ltd. © 1992, Vol. 216, pp. 327-330

Expression of drug metabolizing enzymes in human $HepG_2$ hepatoma cells

Olivier Fardel, Fabrice Morel, Damrong Ratanasavanh, Alain Fautrel, Philippe Beaune * and André Guillouzo

*INSERM U 49, Hôpital Pontchaillou, Rennes and * INSERM U 75, Laboratoire d'Enzymologie Médicale, CHU Necker, Paris, France*

INTRODUCTION

Cultured hepatocytes are now widely used as a model system in pharmacotoxicological research (Guillouzo et al., 1990). Since various functions, including drug metabolic capacity, often differ between laboratory animals and humans, the use of human hepatocytes is of a great interest for studying drug metabolism and toxicity. Human hepatocytes in primary culture have moreover been shown to express cytochrome P-450 enzymes and respond to inducers (Diaz et al., 1990 ; Morel et al., 1990) ; they have been used to analyse metabolism of many drugs, including caffeine (Ratanasavanh et al., 1990) and mitoxantrone (Cano et al., 1988), and toxicity of various hepatotoxins, e.g. aflatoxin B_1 (Bégué et al., 1988). However the erratic availability and individual functional variations of human hepatocytes make their extensive use difficult. Consequently human hepatoma cell lines could represent an interesting and convenient alternative model for pharmacological and toxicological studies, provided that they express at a sufficient level drug metabolizing enzymes. Several hepatoma cell lines have been reported to express some phase I and phase II drug reactions. However discrepancies exist from one study to another. This led us to measure various phase I and phase II drug metabolizing enzymes in the human $HepG_2$ hepatoma cell line. $HepG_2$ cells have been derived from a human hepatocarcinoma (Aden et al., 1979) and are known to express various liver functions (Knowles et al., 1980), including synthesis of the major plasma proteins, receptors for insulin, transferrin and epidermal growth factor, and low density lipoproteins.

MATERIALS AND METHODS

Cell culture

$HepG_2$ cells were cultured in a mixture of 75 % minimal essential medium and 25 % medium 199, supplemented with 10 % fetal calf serum and were analysed at confluency. Some drug metabolizing enzyme inducers such as rifampicin (RIF, 50 µM), 3-methylcholanthrene (3-MC, 5 µM), dexamethasone (DEX, 100 µM) and sodium phenobarbital (PB, 3.2 mM) were added daily to cultures during 3 days.
Human hepatocytes were prepared by the two step collagenase perfusion method and cultured as previously described (Guguen-Guillouzo et al., 1982).

This work was supported by INSERM and ARC (Contract number 6604).

Preparation of microsomes and immunoblot analysis

Preparation of microsomes from $HepG_2$ cells and human hepatocytes was performed by differential centrifugation (Morel et al., 1990). Microsomal proteins were separated by sodium dodecyl sulfate/polyacrylamide-gel electrophoresis (Laemmli, 1970) and then electrophoretically transferred to nitrocellulose sheets as previously described (Towbin et al., 1979). Nitrocellulose sheets were blocked for 1 hr with phosphate buffer saline containing 0.15 M NaCl, 3 % bovine serum albumin, 10 % fetal calf serum and 0.5 % Tween 20. Antisera against cytochromes P-450 IA, IIC and IIIA and glutathione S-transferases (GST) alpha and mu (Bioprep laboratory, Dublin) were used as the primary antibody at appropriate dilutions. Biotinylated anti-immunoglobulins were used as the secondary antibody. Blots were developed using the Vectastain ABC kit (Vector laboratory, Burlingame, CA) and 4-chloro-1-naphthol (Sigma) as the substrate.

Drug metabolic assays

Metabolism of acetanilide, phenacetin, paracetamol and procainamide were studied by high pressure liquid chromatography. Metabolites of phenacetin, acetanilide and paracetamol were separated on a C_{18} nucleosil column and were detected at 250 nm. Procainamide metabolites were analysed on a spherisorb C_{18} column and were detected at 280 nm. Results were expressed as amount of metabolites formed per 24 hr culture per µg DNA and were mean ± SD of 4 experiments. Cellular DNA content was determined according to Labarca and Paigen (1980).

RESULTS

Expression of phase I drug metabolizing enzymes

Analysis by western blotting showed that cytochromes P450 IA, IIC and IIIA were present if any at very low levels in $HepG_2$ cells, while these drug metabolizing enzymes were clearly detectable in normal human hepatocytes.Treatment by DEX or RIF increased markedly cytochrome P450 IIIA (Fig. 1). Exposure to 3-MC enhanced cytochrome P450 IA protein level (Fig. 2) as well as acetanilide and phenacetin metabolism (Fig. 3) which is mediated by cytochrome P450 IA.

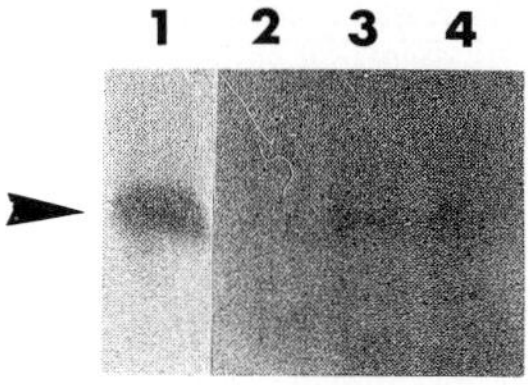

Figure 1 : Expression of cytochrome P450 IIIA in $HepG_2$ cells either untreated (2) or after exposure to DEX (3) and RIF (4) and in normal untreated human hepatocytes (1). Arrow indicates the position of cytochrome P450 IIIA.

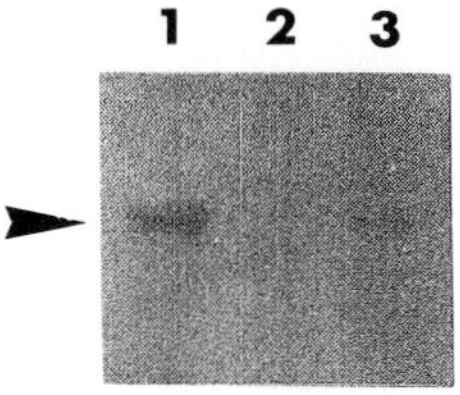

Figure 2 : Expression of cytochrome P450 IA in $HepG_2$ cells either untreated (2) or after exposure to 3-MC (3) and in normal untreated human hepatocytes (1). Arrow indicates the position of cytochrome P450 IA.

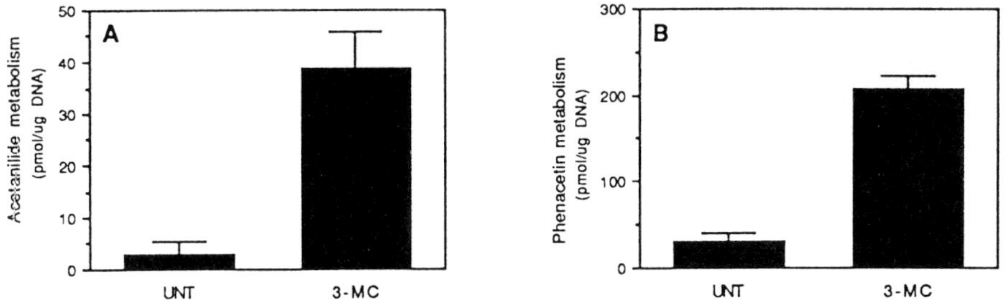

Figure 3 : Induction of acetanilide (A) and phenacetin (B) metabolism in $HepG_2$ cells after exposure to 3-MC (UNT: untreated cells).

Expression of phase II drug metabolizing enzymes

By western blotting GST alpha or mu classes were not detected while they were clearly evidenced in human hepatocytes. Sulfotransferase activity assayed by determination of the formation of paracetamol sulfoconjugated products was low in $HepG_2$ cells (Fig. 4), as well as N-acetyl transferase activity estimated by determination of N-acetyl procainamide metabolites (Fig. 4). UDP-glucuronosyl conjugates of paracetamol were not detected, thus suggesting that UDP-glucuronosyl transferase activity was absent or very low in $HepG_2$ cells. None of the inducers tested had a marked effect on sulfotransferase or N-acetyl transferase activity.

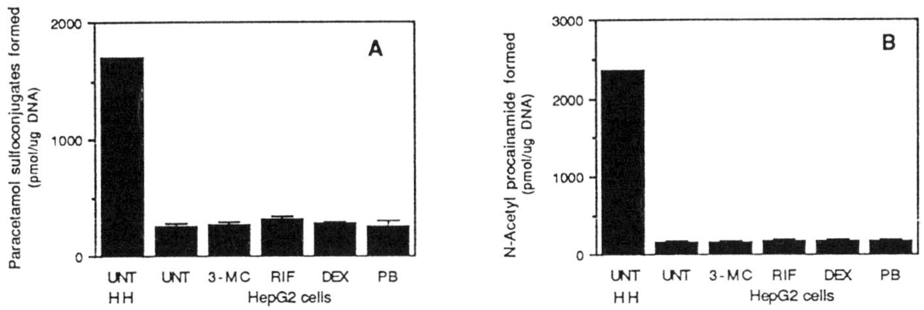

Figure 4 : Sulfotransferase (A) and N-acetyl transferase (B) activity in $HepG_2$ cells after exposure to various inducers and in normal human hepatocytes (HH) (UNT: untreated cells).

DISCUSSION

Our results showed that various drug metabolizing enzymes, including phase I and phase II enzymes, were undetected or present only in low amount in $HepG_2$ cells. These findings are in agreement with previous studies which showed low mixed function oxidase activity (Grant et al., 1988) and failed to evidence cytochromes P450 IIC and IIIA (Cresteil et al., 1988) or UDP-glucuronosyl transferase activity (Le Bot et al., 1991) in $HepG_2$ cells.

Compared to human hepatocytes HepG2 cells poorly metabolized acetanilide, phenacetin and procainamide in our culture conditions. Similarly all drug metabolizing enzymes analysed were expressed at much more lower levels. However, some drug metabolizing enzymes which were induced in human hepatocytes (Morel et al., 1990), were also enhanced in $HepG_2$ cells after xenobiotic exposure. Exposure of $HepG_2$ cells to 3-MC resulted in an increase in cytochrome P450 IA content and in metabolic rate of acetanilide and phenacetin while treatment by RIF and DEX increased cytochrome P450 IIIA. These results support the idea that some regulatory mechanisms of drug metabolizing enzymes are preserved in human hepatoma cells. Recent studies have also shown that drug metabolizing enzymes could be modulated by drug inducers (Dawson et al., 1985), exposure to aryl hydrocarbons (Cresteil et Eisen, 1988) or culture conditions (Doodstar et al., 1988). This suggests that although they cannot replace human hepatocytes for analysis of drug metabolism in vitro, $HepG_2$ cells could represent an interesting model for studying the regulation of some human drug metabolizing enzymes.

REFERENCES

Aden, D.P., Fogel, A., Plotkin, S., Danjanov, I. & Knowles, B.B. (1979): Controlled synthesis of HBsAg in a differentiated human liver carcinoma-derived cell line. *Nature* 282, 615-616.

Bégué, J.M., Baffet, G., Campion, J.P. & Guillouzo, A. (1988): Differential response of primary cultures of human and rat hepatocytes to aflatoxin B_1-induced cytotoxicity and protection by the hepatoprotective agent (+)-cyanidanol-3. *Biol. Cell* 63, 327-333.

Cano, J.P., Rahmani, R., Fabre, G., Richard, B., Lacarelle, B., Bertault-Peres, P., De Sousa, G., Fabre, I., Placidi, M., Coulange, C., Ducros, M. & Rampal, M. (1988): Human hepatocytes as an alternative model to the use of animals in experiments. In *Liver Cells and Drugs*, ed. A. Guillouzo, vol. 164, pp. 301-307. Paris: INSERM and London: John Libbey.

Cresteil, T & Eisen, H.J. (1988): Regulation of human cytochrome P1-450 gene. In *Liver Cells and Drugs*, ed. A. Guillouzo, Vol. 164, pp. 301-307. Paris: INSERM and London: John Libbey.

Dawson, J.R., Adams, D.J. & Wolf, C.R. (1985): Induction of drug metabolizing enzymes in human liver cell line $HepG_2$. *FEBS Lett.* 183, 219-222.

Diaz, D., Fabre, I., Daujat, M., Saint Aubert, B., Bories, P., Michel, H. & Maurel, P. (1990): Omeprazole is an aryl hydrocarbon-like inducer of human hepatic cytochrome P-450. *Gastroenterology* 99, 737-747.

Doodstar, H., Duthie, S.J., Burke, M.D., Melvin, W.T. & Grant, M.H. (1988): The influence of culture medium composition on drug metabolizing activities of the human liver-derived $HepG_2$ cell line. *FEBS Lett.* 241, 15-18.

Grant, M.H., Duthie, S.J., Gray, A.G. & Burki, M.D.(1988): Mixed function oxidase and UDP-glucuronyltransferase activities in the human Hep G_2 hepatoma cell line. *Biochem. Pharmacol.* 37, 4111-4116.

Guguen-Guillouzo, C., Campion, J.P., Brissot, P., Glaise, D., Launois, B., Bourel, M. & Guillouzo, A. (1980): High yield preparation of isolated human adult hepatocytes by enzymatic perfusion of the liver. *Cell Biol. Int. Rep.* 6, 625-628.

Guillouzo, A., Morel, F., Ratanasavanh, D., Chesne, C. & Guguen-Guillouzo, C. (1990): Long-term culture of functional hepatocytes. *Toxicol. in Vitro* 4, 415-427.

Knowles, B.B., Howe, C.C. & Aden, D.P. (1980):Human hepatocellular carcinoma cell lines secrete the major plasma proteins and hepatitis B surface antigen. *Science* 209, 497-499.

Labarca, C. & Paigen P. (1980): A simple , rapid and sensitive DNA assay procedure. *Anal. Biochem.* 102, 344-352.

Laemmli, U.K. (1970): Cleavage of structural proteins during the assembly of the head of the bacteriophage T4. *Nature* 227, 680-685.

Le Bot, M.A., Glaise, D., Kernaleguen, D., Ratanasavanh, D., Carlhant, D., Riche, C. & Guillouzo, A. (1991): Metabolism of doxorubicin, daunorubicin and epirubicin in human and rat hepatoma cells. *Pharmacol. Res.* 24, 243-252.

Morel, F., Beaune, P.H., Ratanasavanh, D., Flinois, J.P., Yang, C., Guengerich, F.P. & Guillouzo, A. (1990): Expression of cytochrome P-450 enzymes in cultured human hepatocytes. *Eur. J. Biochem.* 191, 437-444.

Ratanasavanh, D., Berthou, F., Dreano, Y., Mondine, P., Guillouzo, A. & Riché, C. (1990): Methylcholanthrene but not phenobarbital enhances caffeine and theophylline metabolism in cultured adult human hepatocytes. *Biochem. Pharmacol.* 266, 683-688.

Towbin, H., Staehelin T. & Gordon J. (1979): Electrophoretic transfer of proteins from polyacrylamide gels to nitrocellulose sheets : procedures and some applications. *Proc. Natl. Acad. Sci. USA* 76, 4350-4354.

Clinical aspects

Aspects cliniques

Cellular and Molecular Aspects of Cirrhosis. Eds B. Clément, A. Guillouzo. Colloque INSERM/John Libbey Eurotext Ltd. © 1992, Vol. 216, pp. 333-343

Significance of serum matrix proteins in the diagnosis of cirrhosis

P. Frank and E.G. Hahn

Medizinische Klinik I mit Poliklinik der Friedrich-Alexander-Universität Erlangen-Nürnberg Krankenhausstrasse 12, D-8520 Erlangen, Germany

I)SUMMARY

During the last ten years, based on the growing knowledge about structure, function and metabolism of extracellular matrix and the need for a non-invasive diagnostic tool, several tests have been developped to measure different circulating connective tissue-related components. The number of published methods and their application to different clinical situations is increasing rapidly. There is still controversy about many findings, the following, however, is most widely accepted:

An increase of the **aminoterminal propeptide of type III procollagen** appears to correlate with the activity of hepatic fibrogenesis and thus to predict the development of chronic active fibrogenic liver disease, to differentiate alcoholic fatty liver from alcoholic hepatitis, chronic active from persistent viral hepatitis and to predict survival in primary biliary cirrhosis.

The **propeptides of type IV collagen** reflect the turnover of basement membrane collagen and can help distinguish between chronic persistent and active hepatitis. Furthermore they are helpful in the assessment of fibrogenic liver disease in small children where PIIINP has failed to be of any use.

Laminin P_1, too, mirrors the turnover of basement membrane collagen and displays a good correlation to elevated portal pressure in fibrosis/cirrhosis.

Collagen type VI and **undulin** mainly reflect fibrolysis and remodelling of the interstitial connective tissue.

Some essays have been commercially available for several years now, there are more to come.

High hopes of finding a means to diagnose liver fibrosis/ cirrhosis by serum markers have not been fulfilled (yet) and histology is still required to establish the diagnosis. But for the first time firm conclusions can be drawn about the activity of fibrogenesis, fibrolysis or both by monitoring one or a combination of these extracellular matrix components.

II) INTRODUCTION

Liver fibrosis is one of the most important factors of disturbed liver function. The development of fibrosis is usually a slow process that cannot be diagnosed or predicted by conventional blood tests, which are tailored to detect or quantitate hepatobiliary function or to reflect cell injury of the parenchymal organ. Therefore histopathology is, and will be, the mainstay for the diagnosis of liver fibrosis and cirrhosis. The prognosis, however, is closely linked to the development of excess connective tissue and the clinician needs information about the activity and the reversability of fibrosis.
In this context it is necessary to clearly define what we are talking about: **fibrosis** is a histomorphological term for the presence of excess connective tissue at a certain point in time; **cirrhosis** is characterized by fibrosis plus the conversion of normal liver architecture into structurally abnormal nodules. **Fibrogenesis** and **fibrolysis** are defined as net accumulation and net loss, respectively, of connective tissue between two given points in time (e.g. between two biopsies), caused by an imbalance between synthesis and degradation of connective tissue. The histological assessment of the extent of fibrosis/cirrhosis shows a certain state of the tissue at the time of biopsy. Since specific methods of estimating the fibrogenic activity like measurement of mRNA for a certain collagen are not yet feasible for routine use, we are restricted to indirect methods like counting the number of inflammatory cells. Thus at present histological evaluation cannot reflect the fibrogenic activity and furthermore as an invasive method has obvious drawbacks which limit its repeated use for follow-up purposes.

During the last ten years, with growing knowledge about structure, function and metabolism of extracellular matrix and the need for a non-invasive diagnostic tool, new methods based on immunological detection of well defined chemical components of connective tissue have been introduced. But different contributions of various tissues to the blood pools of extracellular matrix components make matters more complicated than initially expected, when radioimmunological methods for procollagen propeptides were first described and a direct relationship between collagen deposition and serum levels of propeptides was assumed.
By now several tests have been developed to measure different circulating connective tissue-related components; some of them are commercially available, and the number of published methods and their application to different clinical situations is increasing rapidly.

The composition of the hepatic connective tissue in health and disease is well-known (Hahn et al,1980), structure and localisation of its components have been reviewed recently (Schuppan,1990). Enzymes and metabolic products of collagen and extracellular glycoproteins have been widely used for some time to quantitate altered connective tissue metabolism as summarized in Table 1.
Today, we know that for future clinical use, only the measurement of the specific proteins (see Table 1) is promising.

Table 1. Enzymes and metabolic products that have been used (+) to quantitate altered connective tissue metabolism in liver disease

	Biopsy	Serum/Plasma	Urine
General			
Proline	+	+	+
Hydroxyproline	+[a]	+[b]	+
(^{14}C)/(^{3}H)proline transformation into hydroxyproline	+	-	-
Prolyl hydroxylase			
-activity	+	+	-
-immunoreactive	+	+	-
Galactosylhydroxylysyl glycosyl transferase	+	+	-
Lysyl oxidase	+	+	-
Collagenase	+[b]	-	-
β-N-acetylglucosaminidase	+	+	+
Specific proteins			
Procollagen peptides			
-type I	-	+	-
-type III	+	+	+
7-s collagen	+	+	+
NC1 peptide	+	+	+
Type IV collagen	+	+	+
Type VI collagen	+	+	-
Laminin	+	+	+
Undulin	+	+	-

[a] Measures collagen content
[b] Measures collagen degradation

III) COLLAGEN DERIVED ANTIGENS

1) The aminoterminal propeptide of procollagen type III (PIIINP)

Type III collagen is a major component of interstitial connective tissue synthesized in the the early phase of fibroproliferative response as a larger precursor molecule. During fibril formation the additional peptide sequences (propeptides) at both the aminoterminal and the carboxyterminal end are cleaved off stoichiometrically by specific endoproteinases, but, since a significant proportion of PIIINP is retained on the surface and set free during degradation of collagen fibrils, the initial assumption that PIIINP levels only reflect fibrogenesis have been proven wrong.
Two more things make interpretations rather difficult:
- Circulating PIIINP is heterogenous, consisting of at least 4 fractions, 2 of higher molecular weight, that may represent intact or only partly processed procollagen type III molecules, a minor fraction of intact propeptide (Col 1-3, M_r 45000) and a quantitatively predominant degradation product of PIIINP (Col 1, M_r 10000) (Niemelä et al,1982). Furthermore, the proportions of

the fractions can vary in one patient's serum during different phases of a disease (Niemelä et al,1983).
- Lately more information is available about the metabolism of circulating PIIINP, which is of major importance for the interpretation of the serum levels. Up to 70% of radiolabelled PIIINP, injected intravenously, can be recovered from rat liver, indicating that the liver is strongly involved in its metabolism. PIIINP is specifically bound to and internalized by sinusoidal endothelial cells (Smedsrod,1988) and elevated serum levels may be at least partly due to reduced endothelial function in diseased liver (Bentsen et al,1989). There is evidence that larger propeptide antigen forms are mainly metabolized in the liver (Bentsen et al,1988) whereas smaller degradation products (Col1) are mainly degraded and cleared by the kidneys; Col1 appears to be excreted via bile and urine (Smedsrod,1988).

The many radioimmunoassays, that have been used in different laboratories, show different avidity for the different fractions of PIIINP (see above) which makes it difficult to compare the published studies.
Three methods are available commercially:

a) <u>RIAgnost PIIIP</u> (Behringwerke, Marburg, Germany) is a non-equilibrium inhibition RIA based on the bovine antigen-antibody system with crossreactivity for human PIIINP. The avidity of the rabbit antibodies for the intact PIIINP is about 10-fold higher than for the fragment Col1. In normal adult serum however, there is a predominance of Col1 which causes a flat slope of inhibition when plotted against the standard. Therefore, three serum dilutions and calculations by a "50% intercept method" have to be performed, which has been criticized in the past (Risteli & Risteli,1986). This kit was used in most of the clinical studies to date.

b) <u>Fab-PIIIP</u> (Behringwerke, Marburg, Germany) uses antibody Fab fragments. The almost equal sensitivity for intact PIIINP and fragment Col 1 leads to parallel inhibition curves for serum; only one single dilution is necessary.

c) <u>PIIIP</u> (Farmos Diagnostica, Oulunsalo, Finland), the newest of the three, is based on highly purified human PIIINP and primarily detects the intact propeptide. It needs only one dilution of serum sample. Similarly an easy to perform coated tube RIA using two different monoclonal antibodies against PIIINP, developed by Behringwerke, is thought to be specific for intact PIIINP.

A lot of studies - more cross-sectional than follow-up - have been done, the findings and conclusions are sometimes very controversal. Yet, it seems clear, that very high PIIINP concentrations are found, when there is marked inflammation (e.g. acute viral hepatitis, alcoholic hepatitis) or in malignancy (Hatahara et al,1984); silent, subclinical accumulation of connective tissue (e.g. hemochromatosis) has little impact. These findings could lead to the conclusion that in acute situations de novo synthesis and a concomitant breakdown of procollagen type III may contribute to the elevation of PIIINP, whereas in slower processes the inhibition of normal fibrolysis may play a role (Colombo et al,1985). For clinical use, there is not sufficient correlation between PIIINP levels and the extent of fibrosis or

cirrhosis in any of the examined liver diseases except for PBC (Eriksson & Zettervall,1986; Niemelä et al,1988), where it allows to even predict survival. In inactive cirrhosis there is little or no increase, but it may predict the development of hepatoma (Hatahara et al, 1984). Undoutably, persistent elevations of PIIINP correlate with the activity of hepatic fibrogenesis and predict the development of chronic active fibrogenic liver disease. It is possible to differentiate between alcoholic fatty liver and alcoholic hepatitis and between chronic active and persistent viral hepatitis, the RIAgnost obviously being more distinctive than the Fab assay (Rohde et al,1983; Schneider et al,1989). PIIINP is not a useful marker of fibrogenesis in small children, because growth related procollagen turnover exceeds that of the diseased liver with one exception - Indian childhood cirrhosis (Trivedi et al,1987). Other serum assays are more suitable for this age group (see below).
What might be promising for the future is the finding, that in rat models of chronic CCl_4-intoxication and of choline/vitamin deficiency the area under the curve of elevated serum PIIINP, measured individually as follow-up, can predict the extent of fibrosis at a chosen point in time. A combination of the RIAgnost and the Fab assay may allow a more exact assessment of the (im)balance between synthesis and degradation of connective tissue in different liver diseases; the Fab assay picking up the smaller degradation fragment Col 1.

2) The carboxyterminal propeptide of procollagen type I (PICP)

To our present knowledge PICP, unlike PIIINP, is completely cleaved off during collagen fibril formation and therefore should provide a means to directly measure fibrogenesis. However, since type I collagen is present in mature bone and tendon, the basic serum level of PICP is comparably high and changes in the liver connective tissue contribute too little to the overall pool to matter much.
Little is known about the metabolism and elimination of this serum antigen.
The radioimmunoassay for PICP was already developed in 1974 (Taubman et al,1974). The theoretical drawbacks have been confirmed by studies in alcoholic liver disease where PICP showed less pronounced differentiation between hepatitis and fatty liver than PIIINP. It is not known, how much of the PICP increase is due to impaired clearance in the liver. The same difficulties apply to assays for PINP that have been used in PBC (Taubman et al,1976), where in contrast to PIIINP no increases in serum PINP were seen.

3) Collagen type VI (CVI)

The structure of collagen type VI is different from the fibril forming types I,II and V. Its triple helical part, for which a specific RIA has been developed (Schuppan et al,1985) is shorter, the amino- and carboxyterminal propeptides contributing about 2/3 to the molecule. Collagen type VI is not processed during microfibril formation and its content in human liver is far lower than that of type I or III collagen (Hahn & Schuppan,1985). Almost nothing is known about its origin and metabolism.

The serum antigen is heterogenous, probably due to degradation.

Circulating CVI in liver diseased patients does not correlate with PIIINP or propeptides of type IV collagen (Schuppan et al,1985).
No clinical studies have been published so far. The diagnostic value is altogether very much debatable, but a combination of PIIINP and CVI, which are essentially codistributed in most tissues, including the liver, could give some information about the equilibrium between fibrogenesis and fibrolysis by indicating a shift towards the first when CVI relative to PIIINP goes down.

IV) BASEMENT MEMBRANE DERIVED ANTIGENS

Metabolism of basement membrane components and that of the connective tissue are interrelated. In hepatic fibrosis new formation of basement membranes in the space of Disse, leading to sinusoidal capillarisation and proliferation of bile ducts and blood vessels, increases the amount of type IV collagen and laminin.

1) The **propeptide of basement membrane (type IV) collagen**

No propeptides are released prior to or during the deposition of type IV collagen. Metabolism and elimination routes are currently unknown.

The aminoterminal part, known as 7s collagen domain (or PIVNP) and the carboxyterminal part, known as NC1 domain (or PIVCP) have been isolated and used to establish several radioimmunoassays (Risteli et al,1981; Schuppan et al,1986). The antigenic material in serum is homogenous, it is thought to result from degradation and thus mirror fibrolysis, which, again, may induce a higher rate of fibrogenesis as shown on mRNA level in a rat model (Savolainen et al,1988), especially when bile ductular and vascular proliferation are involved (Milani et al,1989). Therefore PIVNP and PIVCP probably reflect the turnover of basement membrane collagen.
Several clinical studies have been performed, in which PIVNP and PIVCP parallel the results of PIIINP with marked elevations in alcoholic hepatitis (Niemelä et al,1985) and chronic active hepatitis and normal levels in chronic persistent hepatitis (Misaki et al,1990). In liver cirrhosis, however, contrarily to PIIINP, PIVCP exhibits the highest elevations (Hayasaka et al,1990). According to new studies PIVNP levels significantly differentiate between acute and subfulminant hepatitis B (Sotaniemi et al,submitted) and asymptomatic and symptomatic PBC (Fukutomi et al,submitted). In small children PIVNP/PIVCP serum levels are only moderately raised (Trivedi et al,1987; Danne et al,1988) which makes them a helpful marker in fibrogenic liver diseases like Indian childhood cirrhosis or biliary atresia, where they reach up to 12-fold levels above normal and where PIIINP fails to be of any use.

2) **Laminin P_1** ($LamP_1$)

In the liver laminin (M_r 900000) - a major non-collagenous glycoprotein of basement membranes, important for cellular adhesion, differentiation, gene expression and metastasis - is codistributed with type IV collagen. Its most antigenic parts are located in two relatively protease-resistent areas of the molecule, called fragments 1 and 2.

RIAs for both have been developed, however, only for fragment 1 (termed $LamP_1$ - P standing for pepsin; M_r 300000) two human antigen assays are available: one based on complete antibodies, the other on antibody Fab-fragments. The first requires the "50% intercept method", the latter - commercially available (Behringwerke, Marburg, Germany) - needs only one dilution of the sample. Both tests have been criticized in the past: the complete antibody kit because of the need for the intercept method, the Fab modification because its units were artificial and did not indicate any defined biological activity.
The antigenic material is heterogenous and like PIVNP/PIVCP reflects basement membrane turnover.
The clinical value of $LamP_1$ in adults must be questioned, because apart from statistically significant (but only 1,5- to 2-fold) elevations in alcoholic hepatitis combined with compromised liver function (Annoni et al,1989) and the differentiation of subfulminant from acute hepatitis B in one publication (Sotaniemi et al,submitted) the changes in serum concentration in any other condition are neglectable. There seems to be a correlation with raised portal pressure (Gressner et al,1986); however, the question arises how useful this parameter can possibly be for monitoring a single patient. In children, like PIVNP, $LamP_1$ could be useful: in Indian childhood cirrhosis $LamP_1$ is highly elevated and shows a good correlation with PIVNP and the histological degree of necrosis, inflammation and fibrosis (Trivedi et al,1987).

V) OTHER EXTRACELLULAR MATRIX GLYCOPROTEINS

1) Undulin (Un)

Undulin, an extracellular glycoprotein, that has been characterized only recently (M_r 700000) and named so because of its association with uniform undulating fibers of collagen, is suggested to play a role in the supramolecular organisation of fibril bundles (Schuppan,1990). In liver fibrosis its normally regular pattern appears disrupted and diminished.
An inhibition ELISA, for determination in the serum, has been developed (Schuppan D:personal communication) and the first studies in patients are under way. From preliminary data it can be suspected that it mainly reflects fibrolysis and remodelling of the interstitial connective tissue.

2) Fibronectin

Fibronectin, an ubiquitous glycoprotein (M_r 500000), is associated with basement membranes as well as interstitial collagens; it mediates cellular adhesion to collagens, fibrin and heparin via specific domains (Hynes,1985). It is mainly produced by hepatocytes and in the liver has a similar distribution to that of type I and type III collagen (Hahn et al,1980). Synthesis and distribution of fibronectin vary in physiological and pathological states; however, in liver fibrosis a marked accumulation precedes the deposition of the other extracellular matrix components.

Quantitative measurements of fibronectin are based on immunochemical assays, but, perhaps depending on the method used, different investigators have reported widely differing values. Known factors that influence plasma levels include age, sex, renal function, nutritional status, hormones and cytokines. Plasma fibronectin levels have been measured in patients with various liver diseases. The only finding generally accepted is a decrease in acute fulminant hepatitis (Almasio et al,1986). In any other condition this parameter failed to be of much value.

Table 2. Extracellular matrix protein levels in different liver diseases

	PIIINP	PICP	PIVP	LamP1
alcoholic liver disease :				
fatty liver	(+)	(+)		(+)
hepatitis	++	+	+	++
cirrhosis	(+)[a]	(+)	++	+
viral hepatitis :				
acute	++		+	normal
chron.active	+	normal	+	(+)
chron.persist.	(+)	normal	normal	normal
cirrhosis	(+)	(+)	++	+/++
primary biliary cirrhosis :				
asymptomatic	+		(+)	(+)
symptomatic	+		+	+
hemochromatosis :	(+)			
Indian childhood cirrhosis:	++[b]		+	+
liver carcinoma :	++		+	+

[a] depending on fibrogenic activity
[b] elevation mainly due to growth related procollagen turnover

REFERENCES

Almasio PL, Hughes RD, Williams R (1986): Characterization of the molecular forms of fibronectin in fulminant hepatic failure. Hepatology 6:1340-1352

Annoni G, Colombo M, Cantaluppi MC, Khlat B, Lampertico P, Rojkind M (1989): Serum type III procollagen peptide and laminin (Lam-P1) detect alcoholic hepatitis in chronic

alcohol abusers.Hepatology 9(5):693-697
Bentsen KD, Boesby S, Kirkegaard P, Hansen CP, Jensen SL, Horslev-Petersen K, Lorenzen I (1988): Is the aminoterminal propeptide of type III procollagen degraded in the liver? A study of type III procollagen peptide in serum during liver transplantation in pigs. J Hepatol 6:144-150
Bentsen KD, Henriksen JH, Boesby S, Horslev-Peterson K and Lorenzen I (1989): Hepatic and renal extraction of circulating type III procollagen amino-terminal propeptide and hyaluronan in pig. J hepatol 9:177-183
Colombo M, Annoni G, Donato MF, Conte D, Martines D, Zaramella MG, Bianchi PA, Piperno A, Tiribelli C (1985): Serum type III procollagen peptide in alcoholic liver disease and idiopathic hemochromatosis:its relationship to hepatic fibrosis, activity of the disease and iron overload. Hepatology 5:475-479
Danne T, Decker J, Schuppan D, Burger W, Enders I, Hahn EG, Charissis G, Weber B (1988): Serum levels of laminin P1 and type IV collagen in healthy children and children with insulin-dependent diabetes mellitus. In: Gubler MC, Sternberg M, eds. Progress in basement membrane research, renal and related aspects in health and disease. John Libbey:315-322
Eriksson S, Zettervall O (1986): The N-terminal propeptide of collagen type III in serum as a prognostic indicator in primary biliary cirrhosis. J Hepatol 2:370-378
Fukutomi T, Sakamoto S, Isobe H, Nawata H (submitted): Clinical significance of the serum levels of type IV collagen 7s domain in the patients with primary biliary cirrhosis. Hepatology
Gressner AM, Tittor W, Negwer A, Pick-Kober KH (1986): Serum concentrations of laminin and aminoterminal propeptide of type III procollagen in relation to the portal venous pressure of fibrotic liver disease. Clin Chim Acta 161:249-258
Hahn EG, Schuppan D (1985): Ethanol and fibrogenesis in the liver. In: Seitz HK, Kommerell B, eds. Alcohol related diseases in gastroenterology. Berlin: Springer, 124-153
Hahn EG, Wick G, Pencev D, Timpl R (1980): Distribution of basement membrane proteins in normal and fibrotic human liver: collagen type IV, laminin and fibronectin. Gut 21:63-71
Hatahara T, Igarashi S, Funaki N (1984): High concentrations of N-terminal peptide of type III procollagen in the sera of patients with various cancers, with special reference to liver cancer. Gann 75:130-137
Hayasaka A, Schuppan D, Ohnishi K, Okuda K, Hahn EG (1990): Serum concentrations of the carboxyterminal cross-linking domain of procollagen type IV (NC1) and the aminoterminal propeptide of procollagen type III (PIIIP) in chronic liver disease. J Hepatol 10:17-22
Hynes RO (1985): Molecular biology of fibronectin. Annu Rev Cell 1:67-90
Milani S, Herbst H, Schuppan D, Kim KY, Hahn EG, Stein H (1989): In situ hybridization for procollagen types I,III, and IV mRNA: evidence for predominant expression in non-parenchymal liver cells. Hepatology 10:84-92
Misaki M, Shima T, Yano Y, Sumita Y, Kano U, Murata T, Watanabe S, Suzuki S (1990): Basement membrane-related and type III procollagen-related antigens in serum of patients with

chronic viral liver disease. Clin Chem 36/3:522-524
Niemelä O, Risteli L, Sotaniemi EA, Risteli J (1982): Heterogeneity of the antigens related to the aminoterminal propeptide of type III procollagen. Clin Chim Acta 124:39-44
Niemelä O, Risteli L, Sotaniemi EA, Risteli J (1985): Type IV collagen and laminin-related antigens in human serum in alcoholic liver disease. Eur J Clin Invest 15:132-137
Niemelä O, Risteli L, Sotaniemi EA, Risteli J (1983): Aminoterminal propeptide of type III procollagen in serum in alcoholic liver disease. Gastroenterology 85:254-259
Niemelä O, Risteli L, Sotaniemi EA, Stenbäck F, Risteli J (1988): Serum basement membrane and type III procollagen related antigens in primary biliary cirrhosis. J Hepatol 6:307-314
Risteli L, Risteli J (1986): Radioimmunoassays for monitoring connective tissue metabolism. Rheumatology 10:216-245
Risteli J, Rohde H, Timpl R (1981): Sensitive radioimmunoassays for 7s collagen and laminin. Anal Biochem 113:372-378
Rohde H, Langer I, Krieg T, Timpl R (1983): Serum and urine analysis of the aminoterminal procollagen peptide type III by radioimmunoassay with antibody Fab fragments. Coll Rel Res 3:371-379
Savolainen ER, Brocks D, Ala-Kokko L, Kivirikko KI (1988): Serum concentration of the N-terminal propeptide of type III procollagen and two type IV collagen fragments and gene expression of the respective collagen types in liver in rats with dimethylnitrosamine-induced hepatic fibrosis. Biochem J 249:753-759
Schneider M, Voss B, Högemann B, Eberhardt G, Gerlach U (1989): Evaluation of serum laminin P1, procollagen-III peptides, and N-acetyl-β-glucosaminidase for monitoring the activity of liver fibrosis. Hepato-gastroenterol 36: 506-510
Schuppan D, Besser M, Schwarting R, Hahn EG (1986): Radioimmunoassay for the carboxyterminal cross-linking domain of type IV (basement membrane) procollagen in body fluids. J Clin Invest 78:241-248
Schuppan D (1990): Structure of the extracellular matrix in normal and fibrotic liver: collagens and glycoproteins. Sem Liv Dis 10:1-10
Schuppan D, Rühlmann T, Hahn EG (1985): Radioimmunoassay for human type VI collagen and its application to tissue and body fluids. Analyt Biochem 149:238-247
Smedsrod B (1988): Aminoterminal propeptide of type III procollagen is cleared from the circulation by receptor-mediated endocytosis in liver endothelial cells. Coll Rel Res 8:375-388
Sotaniemi EA, Mungan Z, Risteli L, Stenbäck FG, Ökten A, Yalcin S, Risteli J (submitted): Serum and hepatic type III procollagen and basement membrane antigens in hepatitis B virus liver disease. J Hepatol
Taubmann MB, Kammerman S, Goldberg B (1976): Radioimmunoassay of procollagen in serum of patients with Paget's disease of bone. Proc Soc Exp Biol Med 152:284-286
Taubmann MB, Goldberg B,Sherr CJ (1974): Radioimmunoassay for human procollagen. Science 186:1115-1119
Trivedi P, Risteli J, Risteli L, Tanner Ms, Bhave S, Pandit AN, Mowat AP (1987): Serum type III procollagen and basement membrane proteins as noninvasive markers of hepatic pathology in Indian childhood cirrhosis. Hepatology 7:1249-1253

Résumé

Au cours des dix dernières années, grâce aux connaissances accrues sur la structure, les fonctions et le métabolisme de la matrice extracellulaire, afin de développer des outils diagnostics non-invasifs, plusieurs tests ont été mis au point pour mesurer différents composants de la matrice extracellulaire circulants. Le nombre de méthodes publiées et leur application à différentes situations cliniques augmentent rapidement. Bien qu'il y ait encore des controverses sur beaucoup de données, les résultats suivants sont le plus généralement admis :

- Une augmentation du propeptide aminoterminal du procollagène de type III montre une corrélation avec l'activité de fibrogénèse hépatique et donc prédit le développement d'une maladie chronique active fibrogène du foie, différencie la stéatose de l'hépatite alcoolique et l'hépatite virale chronique active de celle qui est persistante, et enfin permet une prédiction de la survie dans les cirrhoses biliaires primitives.
- Les propeptides du collagène de type IV sont le reflet du turnover du collagène des lames basales et peuvent aider à distinguer entre les hépatites chroniques persistantes et actives. De plus, ils servent à l'évaluation des maladies fibrosantes du jeune enfant chez qui le PIIINP n'a donné aucun résultat.
- De même, la laminine P1 reflète le turnover du collagène des lames basales et montre une bonne corrélation avec l'hypertension portale dans la fibrose et la cirrhose.
- Le collagène de type VI et l'onduline sont principalement associés à la fibrolyse et au remodelage du tissu conjonctif interstitiel.

Des tests sont disponibles commercialement depuis plusieurs années et d'autres sont en préparation. Le besoin important de moyens diagnostics de la fibrose et de la cirrhose du foie par des marqueurs sériques n'est pas encore satisfait et l'histologie est encore indispensable. Mais pour la première fois, des conclusions claires peuvent être établies quant à l'activité de la fibrogénèse et/ou la fibrolyse en contrôlant l'un ou une combinaison des composants de la matrice extracellulaire.

Cellular and Molecular Aspects of Cirrhosis. Eds B. Clément, A. Guillouzo. Colloque INSERM/John Libbey Eurotext Ltd. © 1992, Vol. 216, pp. 345-349

Ursodeoxycholic acid for primary biliary cirrhosis : effects and mechanisms of action

Raoul Poupon [(1)], Yvon Calmus [(1)] and Renée E. Poupon [(2)]

[(1)] *Service d'Hépatologie and INSERM U 181, Hôpital Saint-Antoine, 184, rue du Faubourg Saint-Antoine, 75571 Paris Cedex, France and* [(2)] *INSERM U 221, Villejuif, France*

Primary biliary cirrhosis (PBC) is a chronic cholestatic disease, characterized by portal inflammation and focal and segmental necrosis of interlobular bile ducts (1). As in other forms of long-term obstructive cholestasis, lobular lesions, fibrosis and eventually cirrhosis may occur. The terminal phase is characterized by hyperbilirubinemia, a major decrease in the number of intrahepatic bile ducts and extensive fibrosis or cirrhosis. Orthotopic liver transplantation is currently the treatment of choice for end-stage patients (2). Although the etiology of PBC is unknown, many clinical, serological and histological features suggest that immunological factors are of primary importance in the pathogenesis and progression of the disease (1). Numerous drugs have been evaluated in controlled trials for the medical therapy of PBC : corticosteroids, azathioprine, chlorambucil, cyclosporine, D-penicillamine, colchicine. Most of them have been chosen for their immunosuppressive properties, to decrease portal inflammation and thus to limit bile duct destruction. These drugs, particularly cyclosporine, show a degree of efficacy, but also have major side effects which make their long-term use hazardous (3).

In 1987, we proposed UDCA as a novel therapeutic approach in PBC (4). The rationale for its use is the following : In chronic biliary obstruction, bile acids accumulate in the liver. Endogenous bile acids are hepatotoxic. At high concentrations, they induce cholestasis, cytotoxicity and, when administered chronically, they can induce ductular proliferation, fibrosis and cirrhosis in certain species. In contrast, UDCA is a hydrophilic non-hepatotoxic bile acid both in vitro and in man. In some models, UDCA can prevent both cholestasis and cell damage induced by biliary obstruction or bile acid administration (5-7). We therefore postulated that changes in the composition of the endogenous bile acid pool induced by long-term ingestion of UDCA might be beneficial to patients with PBC (8).

To test this hypothesis, we carried out an uncontrolled pilot study which effectiveley indicated that major improvement occurred (4). Other studies have suggested that UDCA treatment could also have beneficial effects in other chronic cholestatic diseases. To confirm and extend these preliminary results, we designed a controlled trial comparing the efficacy and tolerance of UDCA and a placebo (9,10). In this review article, the results of the trial will be summarized and some aspects of the mechanisms of action of UDCA will be discussed.

UDCA for the treatment of PBC.

Our double-blind, multicenter controlled trial comparing the efficacy of UDCA to that of placebo in PBC was conducted for two years. The end-point chosen to assess efficacy was a treatment failure, defined by one of the three following criteria : (a) a doubling of the bilirubin level to more than 70 μM; (b) the occurrence of a severe complication of cirrhosis, i.e. ascites, variceal bleeding or encephalopathy; and (c) the occurrence of a side-effect requiring interruption of therapy. According to these criteria, we estimated the treatment failure rate at 30 % in the placebo group and 5 % in the

UDCA group. The calculated number of patients required to show a difference between the two groups with an a risk of 5 % and a ß risk of 10 % was at least 100. Following randomization, 73 patients received UDCA (13-15 mg/kg/day) and 73 the placebo. The two groups were well matched with respect to age and sex. In the UDCA group, there were more stages 3 and 4 patients than in the placebo group (51 % vs 42 %), although the difference was not significant.

Treatment failure was analyzed by the Kaplan-Meier method. Treatment failed in 6 patients on UDCA and in 13 on placebo. The difference is statistically significant in the logrank test at the level of 5 %. There was one side effect requiring interruption of therapy in each group. To take into account the patients' condition at entry, we used a Cox regression model. After adjusting for imbalance in prognostic variables, i.e. bilirubin, age, albumin and cirrhosis, UDCA was more effective than placebo with a p value of less than 0.01, and the relative risk of failure was 3 times higher in the placebo group. Pruritus resolved partially or completely in 40 % of the patients assigned to UDCA but in only 19 % of those receiving placebo. With regard to biochemical and immune parameters, there was a strong improvement under UDCA therapy. The time courses of bilirubin, cholesterol, alkaline phosphatase, gGT and transaminase activities were radically improved. A risk score, combining five prognostic variables (bilirubin, albumin, prothrombin time, age and edema) has been proposed for PBC by the group of the Mayo clinic (11). At one and two years, the difference of this score between the two groups was very clear-cut. This suggests that UDCA would prolong survival in PBC. Unexpectedly, there was also marked improvement in the immune parameters, including IgG levels, IgM levels and to a lesser extent anti-mitochondrial antibody titers. The histologic study showed that bile duct paucity, portal inflammation, bile duct proliferation, piece-meal necrosis and cholestasis significantly improved in the patients receiving UDCA. There was no difference in terms of fibrosis. The overall score reflecting histological severity markedly improved in UDCA treated patients.

Effect of bile acids on the Major histocompatibility complex (MHC) expression.

The beneficial effect of UDCA in PBC was initially thought to result only from a reduction of the toxic effect of endogenous bile acids (6,7). Indeed, endogenous bile acids of the pool are largely replaced by non-toxic UDCA during long-term administration of UDCA (8). However, the effect of UDCA on the immunological abnormalities observed during the trial (improvement of IgM and antimitochondrial antibodies levels) suggested that UDCA could also have immunoregulating properties (9,10). We report here the results of recent works showing that bile acids are able to modulate hepatic MHC expression.

The hepatic expression of MHC molecules is normally limited : class I expression is restricted to sinusoidal and biliary cells while class II expression is mostly restricted to sinusoidal cells (12-14). However, hepatic MHC expression is enhanced in immune-mediated diseases such as autoimmune diseases, viral hepatitis and allograft rejection (15-17). MHC antigens play a major role in the immune response (18). It is well established that the immunogenicity of a cell or a tissue is proportional to its MHC class II expression, while the presence of MHC class I molecules is required for an efficient cytolysis of a target cell by cytotoxic T cells. Therefore, the abnormal expression of MHC could play a role in the induction and/or the evolution of immune-mediated liver diseases. It is generally assumed that MHC expression is modulated by immune mediators. The most potent of them are interferon and TNF, which strongly increase both MHC class I and MHC class II expression. In contrast, corticosteroids and cyclosporine suppress MHC expression (19).

Aberrant hepatic expression of MHC molecules has been documented in PBC (16,17). A first study was undertaken to evaluate the effects of UDCA therapy on this expression (16). Twelve untreated patients with PBC were compared to 8 patients treated for at least a year by 13 to 15 mg/kg/d of UDCA and to 8 control patients without hepatobiliary disease. MHC expression was studied by an immunofluorescence technique. No class I molecules were expressed on hepatocytes of control subjects. In contrast, there was a strong expression on hepatocytes of untreated PBC patients. UDCA treatment induced a dramatic reduction of HLA class I expression. No class II molecules were expressed in bile ducts of controls. In contrast, there was a strong class II expression of bile ducts of PBC patients, without significant difference of expression between treated and untreated patients. These results suggest that cholestasis itself can induce aberrant expression of MHC class I molecules on hepatocytes. The beneficial effect of UDCA on this expression could result from an improvement in cholestasis or a direct effect of UDCA on hepatocytes.

In a subsequent work, effect of cholestasis itself (20) on MHC expression was evaluated (21-22). We first assessed hepatic expression during extrahepatic cholestasis in man (21). Six patients with extrahepatic cholestasis and 8 control patients without hepatobiliary disease were studied. Hepatocyte MHC class I expression was present in 6/6 cholestatic patients and in 0/8 control subjects. Hepatocytes did not express MHC class II in either group. Class II expression was observed on a few bile ducts in 3/6 cholestatic patients. We then evaluated experimentally the effect of cholestasis on MHC expression of hepatocytes and determined if cyclosporine and corticosteroids, used in the treatment of autoimmune diseases and in the prevention of allograft rejection, might modulate this expression (22). Cholestasis was induced in rats by ligation-section of the common bile duct. Hepatocytes, obtained by liver perfusion with EDTA, were labelled with either a mouse anti-rat MHC class I or a mouse anti-rat MHC class II monoclonal antibody and counted by cytofluorimetry. Five groups of rats were studied : controls, 3-day cholestasis, 5-day cholestasis, 5-day cholestasis associated with cyclosporin treatment, and finally, 5-day cholestasis plus steroid treatment. About 10 % of the control hepatocytes were positive for MHC class I antigens; hepatocytes were class II negative. After three days of cholestasis, 50 % of the hepatocytes were positive for MHC class I antigens. After five days of cholestasis, 84 % of the hepatocytes were positive for MHC class I antigens. After five days of cholestasis and treatment by cyclosporin or corticosteroids, about 80 % of the hepatocytes remained positive for MHC class I antigens. MHC class II expression was not modified either by cholestasis or by cyclosporine or steroid treatments. These results show that extrahepatic cholestasis induces MHC class I expression by hepatocytes. High doses of corticosteroids or cyclosporine, which are known to prevent cytokine release, had no effect on the abnormal MHC expression of hepatocytes, suggesting that an immune mechanism is not involved in this abnormal expression. The previously shown beneficial effect of UDCA during PBC is an indirect evidence to suggest that bile acids may directly enhance hepatocyte MHC expression.

Therefore, we decided to study the effect of individual bile acids on isolated hepatocytes. Normal human hepatocytes were isolated from five patients who underwent surgical liver resection by two step collagenase liver perfusion. Hepatocytes were placed in medium containing one of the following bile acids : (a) Chenodeoxycholic acid (CDCA), (a model of endogenous bile acid), 100-500 µM; (b) UDCA 100-500 µM; (c) Tauroursodeoxycholic acid (TUDCA) 100-500 µM; (d) CDCA 100 µM and UDCA 100 µM; (e) CDCA 100 µM and TUDCA 100 µM. After 4 days of culture in the presence of bile acids, the monolayer of flattened hepatocytes was incubated in EDTA to detach the hepatocytes. Cytofluorimetric analysis was performed using monoclonal anti-class I or anti-class II antibodies. MHC class I expression was found on 25 % of control hepatocytes. CDCA induced an hyperexpression of class I MHC molecules, which was dose-dependent for concentrations ranging from 100 to 500 µM. In contrast, UDCA or his tauroconjugate had no significant effect. CDCA, UDCA, TUDCA had no effect on hepatocyte MHC class II expression, which did not exceed 10 % of the cells. Furthermore, the addition of UDCA (100 µM) or TUDCA (100 µM) to CDCA (100 µM) suppressed the hyperexpression of HLA class I on the human hepatocytes (Hillaire S et al., Submitted).

Conclusion.

Administration of UDCA in patients with PBC (a) improves clinical, biochemical, immune and histological parameters of the disease; (b) slows the progression of the disease and reduces the incidence of complications which can require liver transplantation; (c) is not associated with adverse effects.

UDCA could be effective by replacing hepatotoxic endogenous bile acids which accumulate in the liver during cholestasis. However, recent data suggest that UDCA could also have immunomodulating properties. Indeed, endogenous bile acids are able to enhance MHC class I expression in hepatocytes. Overexpression of these molecules in PBC could result from the accumulation of endogenous bile acids in the liver and could play a role in the progression of the disease by rendering hepatocytes more susceptible to immune destruction. UDCA has little or no effects on MHC expression and could even reverse the effects of endogenous bile acids.

UDCA could have also beneficial effects in other liver diseases where MHC expression plays a role, such as viral hepatitis, allograft rejection, autoimmune diseases, graft-versus-host disease.

References.

1. Kaplan MM (1987) : Primary biliary cirrhosis. *N Engl J Med* 316, 521-528.

2. Markus BH, Dickson ER, Grambsch PM (1989) : Efficacy of liver transplantation in patients with primary biliary cirrhosis. *N Engl J Med* 320, 1709-1713.

3. Kaplan MM (1989) : Medical treatment of primary biliary cirrhosis. *Semin Liv Dis* 9, 138-143.

4. Poupon R, Chrétien Y, Poupon RE, Ballet F, Calmus Y, Darnis F (1987) : Is ursodeoxycholic acid an effective treatment for primary biliary cirrhosis ? *Lancet* i, 834-836.

5. Schmucker D, Otha M, Kanai S, Sata Y, Kitani K (1990) : Hepatic injury induced by bile salts : correlation between biochemical and morphological events. *Hepatology* 12, 1216-1221.

6. Galle PR, Theilmann L, Raedsch R, Otto G, Stiehl A (1990) : Ursodeoxycholate reduces hepatotoxicity of bile salts in parimary human hepatocytes. *Hepatology* 12, 486-491.

7. Heuman DM, Mills AS, McCall J, Hymelon PB, Pandak WM, Vlahcevic ZR (1991) : Conjugates of ursodeoxycholate protect against cholestasis and hepatocellular necrosis caused by more hydrophobic bile salt. *Gastroenterology* 100, 203-211.

8. Marteau P, Chazouillères O, Myara A, Jian R, Rambaud JC, Poupon R (1990) : Effect of chronic administration of ursodeoxycholic acid on the ileal absorption of endogenous bile acids in man. *Hepatology* 12, 1206-1208.

9. Poupon RE, Eschwege E, Poupon R and the UDCA-PBC study group (1990) : Ursodeoxycholic acid for the treatment of primary biliary cirrhosis. *J Hepatol* 11, 16-21.

10. Poupon RE, Balkau B, Eschwege E, Poupon R and the UDCA-PBC study group (1991) : A multicenter double blind trial of ursodiol for the treatment of primary biliary cirrhosis. *N Engl J Med* 324, 1548-54.

11. Dickson ER, Grambsch PM, Fleming TR, Fisher LD, Langworthy A (1989) : Prognosis in primary biliary cirrhosis : Model for decision making. *Hepatology* 10, 1-7.

12. Franco A, Barnaba V, Balsano C, Musca C, Balsano F (1988) : Expression of class I and class II Major Histocompatibility Complex Antigens on human hepatocytes. *Hepatology* 8, 449-454.

13. Lautenschlager I, Taskinen E, Inkinen K, Lehto VP, Virtanen I, Hayry P 1984) : Distribution of the major histocompatibility complex antigens on different cellular components of human liver. *Cell Immunol* 85: 191-200.

14. Rouger P, Poupon R, Gane P, Mallissen B, Darnis F, Salmon C (1986) : Expression of blood group antigens including HLA markers in human adult liver. *Tissue Antigens* 27, 78-86.

15. Ballardini G, Bianchi FB, Mirakian R, Fallani M, Pisi E, Bottazo GF (1987) : HLA-A,B,C, HLA-D/DR and HLA-D/DQ expression on unfixed liver biopsy sections from patients with chronic liver disease. *Clin Exp Immunol* 70, 35-46.

16. Calmus Y, Gane P, Rouger P, Poupon R (1990) : Hepatic expression of class I and class II major histocompatibility complex molecules in primary biliary cirrhosis : Effect of ursodeoxycholic acid. *Hepatology* 11, 12-15.

17. Nagafuchi Y, Scheuer PJ (1986) : Hepatic ß2-microglobulin distribution in primary biliary cirrhosis. *J Hepatol* 2, 73-80.

18. Schwartz RH (1984) : The role of gene products of the major histocompatibility complex in T cell activation and cellular interactions. *In: Fundamental Immunology* (Paul WE) Raven Press, New York, 379-438.

19. Calmus Y, Weill B, Poupon R (1991) : Expression hépatique des molécules du complexe majeur d'histocompatibilité. *Gastroenterol Clin Biol* 15, 110-119.

20. Innes GK, Nagafuchi Y, Fuller BJ, Hobbs KEF (1988) : Increased expression of major histocompatibility antigens in the liver as a result of cholestasis. *Transplantation* 45, 749-752.

21. Calmus Y, Gane P, Boucher E, Arvieux C, Poupon RY (1990) : Cholestasis induces abnormal and aberrant HLA expression in the human liver. *J Hepatol* 11, S14.

22. Arvieux C, Calmus Y, Gane P, Rouger P, Nordlinger B, Poupon R (1990) : Quantitation and modulation of major histocompatibility complex (MHC) expression : The effect of cholestasis and immunosuppressive drugs. *J Hepatol* 11, S2.

Résumé

La cirrhose biliaire primitive est une maladie chronique cholestatique de cause indéterminée caractérisée par une inflammation portale et une nécrose des cellules biliaires des canaux de petit et de moyen calibre. Ces lésions ont pour conséquences la destruction des canaux biliaires, une cholestase généralement progressivement croissante. Comme dans les autres formes de cholestase extrahépatique prolongée, des lésions lobulaires, une fibrose, voire une cirrhose, peuvent survenir. La transplantation hépatique est le traitement de choix des patients ayant une maladie évoluée. Nous avons proposé l'acide ursodésoxycholique (UDCA) comme nouvelle approche thérapeutique de la maladie. En effet, les lésions hépatiques observées dans les maladies chroniques cholestatiques pourraient être dues au moins en partie à l'accumulation d'acides biliaires endogènes dans le foie. L'UDCA est un acide biliaire dénué de toute cytotoxicité chez l'homme et in vitro. Aussi, il a été postulé que l'administration continue d'UDCA, en modifiant la composition du pool des acides biliaires endogènes, pourrait avoir un effet bénéfique chez les patients ayant une maladie biliaire chronique cholestatique et plus précisément une cirrhose biliaire primitive. Cette hypothèse est maintenant confirmée par les résultats de l'essai contrôlé en double aveugle ayant inclus 146 patients, suivis pendant deux ans. Cet essai montre que l'UDCA diminue l'incidence des complications de la maladie considérée comme des indices d'entrée dans la phase terminale de la maladie, et fournit par ailleurs une amélioration clinique, biochimique et histologique. Les mécanismes par lesquels l'UDCA modifie l'évolution de cette maladie pourraient être les suivants : (a) l'UDCA modifie la composition des acides biliaires circulants en inhibant l'absorption iléale active des acides biliaires endogènes, (b) l'UDCA a aussi un effet direct cytoprotecteur sur les hépatocytes ; (c) finalement, nous avons maintenant des preuves que les acides biliaires et l'UDCA interfèrent également avec le système immunitaire ; en particulier l'UDCA inhibe l'expression anormale des molécules du complexe majeur d'histocompatibilité induite par les acides biliaires endogènes.

Cellular and Molecular Aspects of Cirrhosis. Eds B. Clément, A. Guillouzo. Colloque INSERM/John Libbey Eurotext Ltd. © 1992, Vol. 216, pp. 351-355

Protective effect of ursodeoxycholic acid on secondary biliary cirrhosis and ethinyl estradiol induced cholestasis in the rat

Serge Erlinger, Jorge-Luis Poo, Emmanuel Jacquemin, Gérard Feldmann [1], Alain Braillon and Didier Lebrec

Unité de Recherches de Physiopathologie Hépatique, INSERM U 24, Hôpital Beaujon, 92118 Clichy and [1] Unité de Recherches Structure et Fonction des Cellules Hépatiques, INSERM U 327, Faculté Xavier Bichat, 75018 Paris, France

SUMMARY

The authors have examined the influence of ursodeoxycholic acid (UDCA) on biliary cirrhosis induced by bile duct ligation and on cholestasis induced by ethinyl estradiol (EE) in the rat. The bile acid was given to 19 rats with bile duct ligation and 7 rats with EE-induced cholestasis. In rats with bile duct ligation, as compared to controls, UDCA-treated rats developed cirrhosis less frequently, had less fibrosis and less ductular proliferation.In rats receiving EE, cholestasis was less severe in UDCA-treated rats than in controls. It is concluded that UDCA limits fibrosis induced by bile duct ligation and protects against EE-induced cholestasis.

Ursodeoxycholic acid (UDCA) has recently been proposed as a potential treatment of cholestatic liver diseases, mainly primary biliary cirrhosis and primary sclerosing cholangitis. There are several experimental studies showing a "protective" effect of UDCA in acute cholestasis induced by bile acids (Kitani & Kanai, 1982). However, with the exception of a preliminary study (Krol et al., 1983), experimental studies on chronic cholestasis are lacking. In this study, we have examined the influence of chronic administration of UDCA in bile duct-ligated rats and in rats receiving ethinyl estradiol.

The purpose of the study was two-fold : 1) to examine the effect of UDCA on liver histology and portal hypertension in bile duct-ligated rats ; 2) to examine the effect of UDCA on bile flow and bile salt secretion in rats with ethinyl estradiol induced cholestasis.

METHODS

1) Bile duct ligation.

Thirty-five male Sprage-Dawley rats had bile duct ligation-section on day 0, using a technique previously described (Lee et al., 1986). Three days after this operation, the animals were randomly allocated to two-groups : in one group (n=19), the animals received UDCA by gavage at the dose 5 mg/kg ; in the other group (n=16), the animals received a placebo. Twenty-eight days after operation, the animals were operated again, portal pressure was measured, a complete hemodynamic study (which will not be described here) was performed. Then, the liver was removed, weighed, and coded specimens were taken, fixed, and examined by light microscopy with morphometric analysis.

2) Ethinyl estradiol-induced cholestasis.
Twenty-six female Sprague-Dawley rats were used. In group 1 (controls, n=7) the animals received only the solvents of ethinyl estradiol (propylene glycol) and of UDCA (Na_2CO_3 0.15 M, NaCl 0.15 M, 1:1, vol/vol, pH 7.8). In group 2 (ethinyl estradiol, n=7), the animals received ethinyl estradiol at the dose of 5 $mg.kg^{-1}.d^{-1}$ intraperitoneally for 10 days, and the solvent of UDCA. In group 3 (n=6), the animals received ethinyl estradiol at the same dose, for 10 days, and UDCA (gavage) at the dose of 25 $mg.kg^{-1}.d^{-1}$ for the same duration. In group 4 (n=6), the animals received ethinyl estradiol at the same dose, and UDCA at the dose of 500 $mg.kg^{-1}.d^{-1}$ for the same duration. On day eleven, a catheter was placed in the common bile duct under general anesthesia, and bile flow and bile salt secretion were measured by standard methods. Biliary bile acids were separated and quantitated by HPLC.

RESULTS

1) Bile duct ligation
Liver weight was significantly lower in UDCA-treated animals (5.1 ± 0.3 g/100 g b. wt.) than in rats receiving placebo (6.6 ± 0.3 g/100 g ; $p<0.005$). In rats receiving placebo, 13 rats (out of 16) developped cirrhosis, while in rats treated with UDCA, only 7 out of 19 rats had cirrhosis. The difference was significant ($p<0.01$). Portal pressure (Fig. 1) was significantly lower in UDCA-treated rats (12.7 ± 0.5 mmHg) than in rats receiving placebo (17.1 ± 0.5 mmHg ; ($p<0.05$)

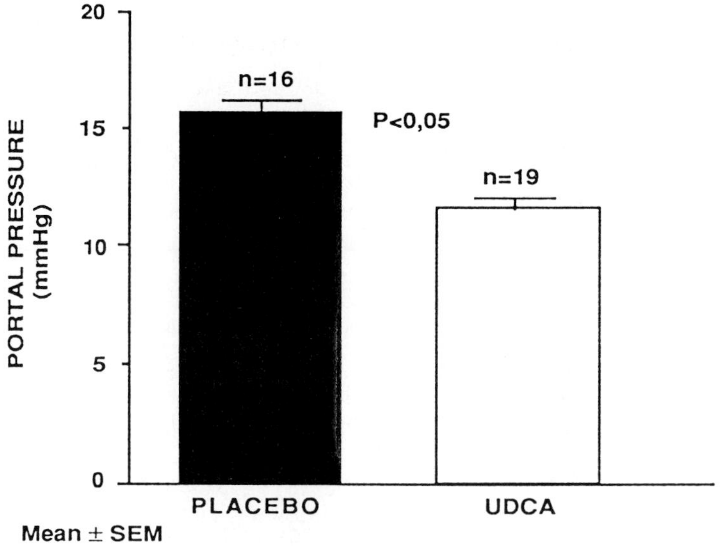

Fig. 1. Influence of ursodeoxycholic acid (UDCA) on the development of chirrhosis in bile duct-ligated rats. In placebo-treated rats, 13 out of 16 rats had cirrhosis. In UDCA-treated rats, 7 out of 19 had cirrhosis.

Morphometric analysis showed that bile duct volume fraction and connective tissue fraction (Fig. 2) were significantly lower in UDCA-treated animals than in those receiving placebo. Similarly, hepatocyte volume fraction and sinusoidal space volume fraction were significantly higher in UDCA-treated rats than in those receiving placebo (data no shown).

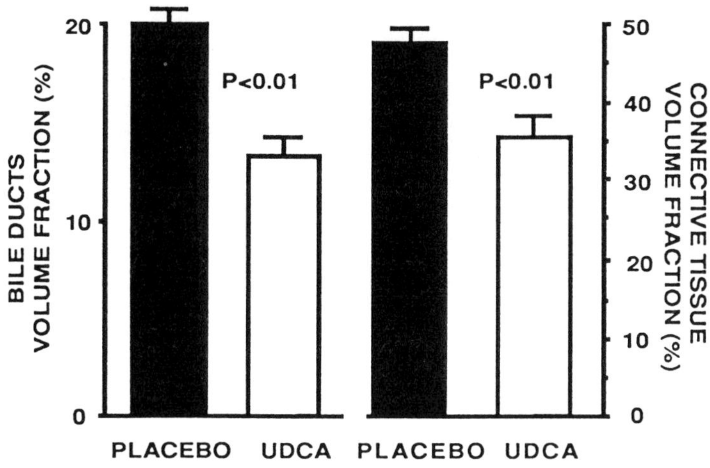

Fig. 2. Morphometric analysis of liver sections (light microscopy) in placebo and UDCA-reated rats. Left : bile ductular volume. Right : connective tissue volume. Bile ductular volume and connective tissue volume were significantly lower in UDCA-treated animals than in controls.

2) Ethinyl estradiol-induced cholestasis

In rats treated with ethinyl estradiol alone for 10 days, bile flow (Fig. 3) and bile salt secretion (not shown) were significantly lower than in controls (receiving only the solvents). In rats treated with ethinyl estradiol and UDCA at both doses (25 and 500 $mg.kg^{-1}.d^{-1}$), bile flow (Fig. 3) and bile salt secretion (not shown) were significantly higher than in rats receiving ethinyl estradiol alone. Bile salt secretion was not different from that of controls. HPLC analysis showed a significant enrichment of biliary bile acids with UDCA in the animals receiving the bile acid.

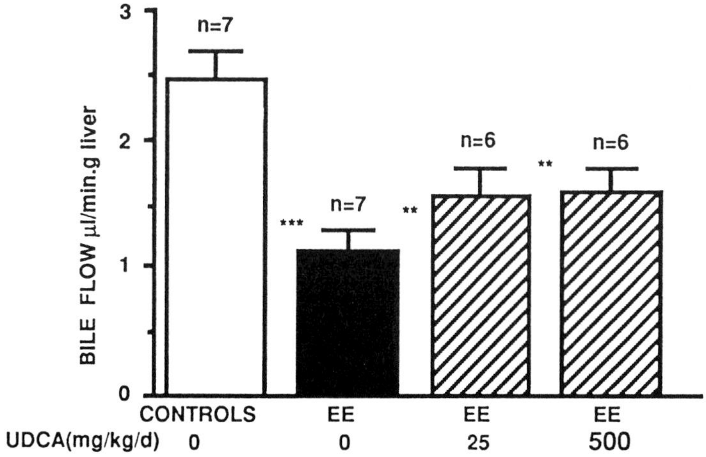

Fig. 3. Influence of UDCA on bile flow in rats treated with ethinyl estradiol. Bile flow was significantly higher in rats treated with ethinyl estradiol (25 and 500 $mg.kg^{-1}.d^{-1}$) than in those receiving ethinyl estradiol alone.

DISCUSSION

We have used two experimental models of cholestasis to test the possibility that UDCA may be beneficial. One is biliary cirrhosis induced bile duct ligation. In this model, the animals develop bile ductular proliferation, fibrosis and, after 1 month, cirrhosis is found in most of the rats (Kountouras et al., 1984). In parallel, portal hypertension and the hemodynamic alterations associated with cirrhosis are found (Lee et al., 1986). In 1983, Hardison and his colleagues showed that chronic administration of tauro-UDCA (two weeks before and two weeks after bile duct ligation) reduced ductular proliferation and portal inflammation in bile duct-ligated hamsters (Krol et al., 1983). We tried to determine wether a one-month oral administration of UDCA in bile duct-ligated rats could prevent cirrhosis and improve portal hypertension. We found than the incidence of cirrhosis defined macroscopically and histologically was significantly lower among the animals with bile duct ligation receiving UDCA (5 $mg.kg^{-1}.d^{-1}$) than in those receiving a placebo under the same conditions. In parallel, portal pressure was significantly lower in UDCA-treated animals than in controls.

In the animals which did not have cirrhosis, there were histological abnormalities. We thought it was important to perform a quantitative analysis of these abnormalities in order to have a valid comparison between UDCA and placebo-treated animals. For this, we used morphometry and analyzed four variables : bile ductular volume, connective tissue volume, hepatocyte volume and sinusoidal volume. These variables were expressed as fraction of total volume. Again, we found significant differences between UDCA-treated animals and animals receiving a placebo. Bile ductular volume and connective tissue volume were significantly lower in UDCA-treated animals than in placebo-treated controls (indicating less ductular proliferation and less fibrosis in the treated animals). Hepatocyte volume and sinusoidal volume were significantly higher in UDCA-treated animals than in controls (indicating a higher hepatic mass and sinusoidal space in the treated animals).

The second experimental model used in this study was estrogen-induced cholestasis. Estrogen administration has been known for a long time to induce cholestasis in several animal species, including the rat (see Kreek, 1987). The mechanism of cholestasis is not fully understood : it may involve inhibition of plasma membrane Na^{+},K^{+}-ATPase, increased permeability of the paracellular pathway with "back-leakage" of bile constituents into plasma, and alterations of plasma membrane composition and fluidity (Kreek, 1987).

This study confirmed that ethinyl estradiol administration for 10 days resulted in a significant decrease in bile flow and bile salt secretion. The animals treated with UDCA at the doses used (25 and 500 $mg.kg^{-1}.d^{-1}$) had a significant improvement in bile flow and bile salt secretion, which were not significantly different from those of normal animals. In parallel, the percentage of UDCA in bile increased. We chose these doses because it has been established that, in normal rats, a dose of 500 $mg.kg.^{-1}.d^{-1}$ was necessary to produce an enrichment of the pool of bile acids with UDCA similar to that obtained by therapeutic doses in man (Parquet et al., 1981 ; Raicht et al., 1978), i.e. approximately 70% of total bile acids. Actually, we foundd a similar effect at the lowest dose of 25 $mg.kg^{-1}.d^{-1}$.

The mechanism of "protection" (or reversal of cholestasis) by UDCA cannot be inferred from these studies. Further experiments are in progress, in particular to measure sucrose biliary clearance and examine the influence of UDCA on biliary permeability to sucrose. Information would also be needed on Na^{+},K^{+}-ATPase activity and lipid composition of the plasma membrane.

REFERENCES

1. Kitani, K. & Kanai, S. (1982) : Tauroursodeoxycholate prevents taurocholate induced cholestasis. *Life Sci.* 30, 515-523.
2. Kountouras, J. et al. (1984) : Prolonged bile duct obstruction : a new experimental model for cirrhosis in the rat. *Br. J. Exp. Path.* 65, 305-311.
3. Kreek, M.J. (1987) : Female sex steroids and cholestasis. *Semin. Liver Dis.* 7, 8-23.
4. Krol, T. et al. (1983) : Tauroursodeoxycholate (TUDC) reduces ductular proliferation and portal inflammation in bile-duct-ligated hamsters. *Hepatology.* 3, 881 (Abstract).
5. Lee, S.S. et al. (1986) : Hemodynamic characterization of chronic bile duct-ligated rats : effets of pentobarbital sodium. *Am. J. Physiol.* 251, G176-180.
6. Parquet, M. et al. (1981) : Pharmacokinetics and metabolism of $[^{14}C]$ursodeoxycholic acid in the rat. *Biochim. Biophys. Acta* 665, 299-305.
7. Raicht, R.F. et al. (1978) : Ursodeoxycholic acid. Effects on sterol metabolism in rats. *Biochim. Biophys. Acta* 531, 1-8.

Résumé

Les auteurs ont examiné l'influence de l'acide ursodésoxycholique (AUDC) sur la cirhose biliaire induite par la ligature du cholédoque et la cholestase induite par l'éthinyl estradiol (EE) chez le rat. L'acide biliaire a été donné à 19 rats ayant une ligature du cholédoque et à 7 rats ayant une cholestase induite par l'EE.Chez les rats ayant une ligature du cholédoque, les animaux traités par l'AUDC, comparés aux témoins, avaient moins fréquemment une cirrhose, moins de fibrose et moins de prolifération ductulaire. Chez les rats recevant de l'EE, la cholestase était moins marquée chez les animaux traités par l'AUDC que chez les témoins. Il est conclu que l'AUDC limite la fibrose induite par la ligature du cholédoque et protège contre la cholestase induite par l'EE chez le rat.

Cellular and Molecular Aspects of Cirrhosis. Eds B. Clément, A. Guillouzo. Colloque INSERM/John Libbey Eurotext Ltd. © 1992, Vol. 216, pp. 357-367

New perspectives in the therapy of chronic viral hepatitis

Isabelle Fourel [(1)], Thierry Bizollon [(2)] and Christian Trépo [(1)]

[(1)] INSERM U 271, Lyon and [(2)] Service d'Hépatologie, Hôtel Dieu, Paris, France

SUMMARY : *Hepatitis B virus (HBV) causes both acute and chronic infections. The latter represents a major risk of developing hepatocellular carcinoma (HCC). The goal of antiviral therapy for chronic HBV infection is to prevent progression to HCC. The available antiviral protocols lack efficacy. The problems for the development of anti-HBV drugs were the very limited host range of HBV and the lack of any tissue culture system in which to propagate HBV. Discovery of HBV-like viruses in animals and the advent of molecular cloning techniques led to rapid advances. Several tools are presently available to evaluate both in vitro and in vivo the inhibitory effects of potential antiviral compounds. They include: a) hepatocyte culture supporting the complete viral cycle ; b) hepatoma cell lines transfected with viral DNA supporting continuously viral replication ; c) animal models including the duck and the woodchuck. In this review, we have summarized the recent studies on evaluation of antiviral compounds (inhibitors of the viral DNA polymerase) both in vitro and in vivo and the clinical trials. More work in this area is also needed but new approaches may soon begin to shed light in this area.*

Chronic HCV hepatitis has only been studied in the clinical setting sofar.

I. INTRODUCTION

In 10 per cent of exposed subjects, the hepatitis B virus (HBV) induces chronic hepatitis which is often associated with liver cirrhosis and hepatocellular carcinoma (HCC) (Popper et al. 1987). The aim of antiviral therapy is to interrupt the progression of chronic hepatitis to HCC. The first studies were based on an empirical approach through clinical trials. They have been since then revisited using the new tools, presently available, presented below. The current treatments of chronic hepatitis B infection using vidarabine monophosphate or alpha interferon are far from satisfactory since therapy is effective in only one-third of patients (Jacyna et al., 1990). The major problems met for the development of anti-HBV drugs were the absence of an *in vitro* system as well as an available animal model. HBV does not readily replicate in culture cells and does not infect common animal models. The discovery of other naturally occuring animal viruses with similar properties and the development of molecular biology techniques allowed to better understand the potential targets of antiviral compounds. With the progress in the culture of hepatocytes and in the transfection techniques of viral DNA in different cell lines, a number of assay systems have been developed. These systems have allowed the first *in vitro* evaluations of the inhibitory effects of potential antiviral compounds against hepadnaviruses. The development is still at an early stage, but several important findings have already been made.

In the following, we will briefly describe the physiopathological basis of the antiviral therapy, the HBV-family, and its virus replication cycle as well as the present antiviral compounds. Furthermore, we will summarize the different studies on evaluation of antiviral compounds *in vivo* in the HBV animal models and *in vitro* in the available cellular models as well as the different approaches for the development of new antiviral strategies. In the last part of this review, progress in clinical trials will be also presented.

Physiopathological basis of antiviral therapy. During HBV infections, the hepatic lesions observed are not mediated by HBV but by the immune response against the viral antigens, probably the capsid antigens expressed on hepatocyte membrane (Thomas et al., 1984). Both hepatocyte necrosis and inflammation lead to the development of cirrhosis and HCC. The inhibition of the viral replication is aimed at suppressing the immunological target of the immune response which is responsible for hepatic lesions and stopping the progession of cirrhosis to HCC. It is noteworthy that during chronic HBV infection, the deficient immune response leads to partial elimination of infected hepatocytes. One can postulate that for this reason, current treatments are not sufficiently effective. Therefore, a second type of treatment improving the immune response against HBV, eventually associated with the inhibitors of the viral replication, must be taken into account.

Hepadnaviruses. HBV is the prototype member of the Hepadnaviruses which include the hepatitis viruses of woodchuck (woodchuck hepatitis virus, WHV), Pekin duck (duck hepatitis B virus, DHBV) and ground squirrel (ground squirrel hepatitis virus, GHSV) (Ganem & Varmus, 1987). More recently, other virus (not well characterized) were described in heron and in tree squirrel (Mason & taylor, 1989).

These hepatotropic DNA viruses share unique ultrastructure, molecular and biological features. The replication of Hepadnavirus is strikingly different from all other DNA viruses in that it involves the reverse transcription of an RNA intermediate by a virus-encoded reverse transcriptase (Summer & Mason, 1982). All hepadnaviruses have the capacity to produce either acute or chronic infections in their host. Among the animal models of human hepatitis B, the woodchuck seems to be the most relevant model for the study of HBV. In addition, the natural history of the chronic infection progressing to HCC is similar in man and in woodchucks. In ground squirrel, the percentage of carrier developping HCC is lower and in ducks, the oncogenic potential of the viral infection is controversial (Ganem & Varmus, 1987 ; Mason & Taylor 1989).

Hepadnavirus replication : potential targets of anti-viral compounds. Virus attachment to the hepatocyte membrane and penetration in the cell appear to be mediated through a specific cellular receptor, recognizing the pre-S proteins of HBV envelope (Neurath et al., 1986). After the uncoating of the virus, the relaxed circular genome is converted to a supercoiled DNA that probably serves as the template for synthesis of viral RNAs. Among these, viral pregenomic is reverse transcripted in viral DNA by the endogenous viral DNA polymerase which works as a retroviral reverse transcriptase. Following the synthesis of the first DNA strand, second strand synthesis is initiated by the viral DNA polymerase (Summers & Mason, 1982). Reverse transcription step is not a common cellular process, therefore one can expect to inhibit specifically the viral replication by using inhibitors of reverse transcriptase. Circumstantial evidence suggests that supercoiled viral DNA form is maintained, in the nucleus, through an intracellular pathway prior to virus release rather than through reinfection of cells by progeny virus particles (Wu et al, 1990). Furthermore, the amount of this supercoiled DNA is modulated by the expression of pre-S antigens (Summers et al, 1990). As a consequence, this nuclear viral DNA seems to play an important part in hepadnavirus replication.

Present antiviral compounds. In theory, each of the essential steps of viral replication cycle can be regarded as a target for inhibition of viral replication. Nevertheless, no step is really specific for the virus and it is not easy to interfere with viral replication without damaging host cells. In most of the cases, the viral targets are viral enzymes such as polymerases and kinases. The present antiviral compounds are nucleoside analogues mainly effective against herpes virus and retrovirus like the arabinosyl derivatives, acyclovir and their related compounds and the 2'3' dideoxynucleoside analogues (De Clercq, 1988). Moreover, interferons with both antiviral activity and complex immunomodulatory properties, are also used to treat some viral infections.

II. STUDY OF THE INHIBITORS OF HBV REPLICATION IN BOTH CELLULAR AND ANIMAL MODELS

Evaluation of anti-HBV compounds *in vivo* in animal models.

In duck. *In vivo* evaluation of anti-HBV compounds was mainly carried out in adult ducks. The antiviral compounds used in these studies were inhibitors of the DNA polymerase DNA dependant (vidarabine, acyclovir, foscarnet) or RNA dependant (suramin, dideoxynucleoside analogues). Vidarabine administered at higher doses than those used in human, induced a transient inhibitory effect on DHBV replication (Hirota et al., 1986). The same phenomenon was observed with acyclovir (Zuckerman 1987; Freiman et al., 1990) and with foscarnet (Sherker et al., 1987). During the course of treatment, viral replication decreased considerably. Nevertheless, after the cessation of treatment, viral replication returned to pretreatment levels. The analysis of liver biopsies obtained during treatment showed that the supercoiled DNA form was the less affected by therapy. Among the nucleoside analogues, known as anti-reverse transcriptase, the purine 2'3' dideoxyribonucleoside analogues were the most potent inhibitors. Thus an 2'3' dideoxyadenosine analogue induced a swift disappearance of serum DHBV in treated animals (Lee et al., 1990). Nevertheless, the pyrimidine 2'3'dideoxycytidine showed antiviral activity on DHBV replication (Kassianides et al., 1989). By contrast, azidothymidine had no inhibitory effect on viral replication (Haritani et al., 1989). Suramin, a drug used in the treatment of sleeping-sickness, was reported to also induce a transient inhibition of viral replication (Zuckerman, 1987).

In ground squirrel and woodchuck. In ground squirrel, vidarabine monophosphate (ara-AMP) and ganciclovir induced a weak suppression of the viral replication (Smee et al., 1985). By contrast, in woodchuck, ara-AMP at dosage used in human therapy, caused a significant depression of viral DNA synthesis from the first day of treatment. However, the inhibitory effect was transient and viral replication rebounced immediatly after discontinuation of therapy as observed in human. Among the 2'fluorinated arabinosyl-pyrimidine nucleosides, potent inhibitors of the DNA polymerase of the Hepadnavirus, fluoroethyl*ara*uracil induced a significant inhibition of the viral replication. After stopping therapy, viral replication returned slowly to pretreatment level. The antiviral effect was immediate but not permanent. This compound was also effective by oral route. By contrast, fluoroiodo*ara*cytosine and fluoromethyl*ara*uracil abolished completely the viral replication in all treated animals. Unfortunately, these compounds were associated with toxicity (Fourel et al., 1990). Although further studies are needed to better document the optimal regimen, these compounds offer new hopes for human therapy. Plants, used in India including a traditionnal treatment of jaundice, were studied in animal models. A first experiment has shown that when a crude extract from the plant *Phyllanthus* was given to chronically infected woodchuck, the majority of the animals responded with a decrease in surface viral antigen titer and fall of DNA polymerase in serum (Venkateswaran et al., 1987). The chemical compounds responsible for the potential antiviral activity are still unknown. Moreover, these results were not confirmed in chronically infected ducks (Niu et al., 1990).

Evaluation of anti-HBV compounds in cellular models. The important progress made in both liver perfusion and hepatocyte culture, have allowed the development of hepatocyte culture systems supporting viral replication (Tuttleman et al., 1986 ; Uchida et al., 1988). Some conditions of culture (dimethylsulfoxide in primary culture, coculture with epithelial cells), have allowed to maintain hepatocytes in a fully differentiated state for a long time (Gripon et al., 1988 ; Pugh et al., 1989 ; Fourel et al., 1989). An alternative to this cell system, technically more simple, is the use of cell lines transfected with HBV DNA and supporting continuously viral replication. Several cell lines have been yet described using highly differentiated hepatoma cell lines (Hep G2, Huh6, Huh7) (Mason & Taylor, 1989). These systems have provided new tools to evaluate the efficacy of antiviral compounds on the different steps of viral replication.

Duck hepatocyte culture. Cultured duck hepatocytes have mainly been used for the evaluation of anti-HBV compounds. These studies are still at an early stage and only nucleoside analogues, known as antihepadnaviruses, antiherpetic drugs or antiretrovirus compounds, were assessed.

Antiviral compounds known as potent inhibitors of the DHBV DNA polymerase (foscarnet, ara-AMP, fluoromethyl*ara*uracil, fluoroiodo*ara*-cytosine), were found effective also on viral replication in this duck hepatocyte culture system (Fourel et al., 1989). Nevertheless, the inhibitory effect was transient. The 2'3'dideoxynucleoside analogues have been reported to inhibit DHBV replication (Lee et al., 1989 ; Yokoda et al., 1990). Recently, it was shown that the new class of phosphonylmethoxypropyl purine and -pyrimidine derivatives exhibited inhibitory effects on DHBV replication (Yokoda et al., 1990). Finally, several compounds acting at the level of viral supercoiled form have been identified *ie* novobiocin and nalidixic acid (Civitico et al., 1990). Recent *in vitro* experiences suggested that suramin inhibits infection of duck hepatocytes by DHBV, probably by blocking virus uptake without affecting viral DNA synthesis once cells are infected (Petcu et al., 1990).

Transfected cell lines. Thanks to these experimental systems, a number of antiviral compounds specially nucleoside analogues and interferons have already been assessed. New potent antiviral compounds were selected such as a carboxyclic analogue of 2'-deoxyguanosine (Price et al., 1989 ; Lampertico et al., 1991), the 3'fluoro dideoxyribonucleoside derivatives (Matthes et., 1990) as well as phosphonylmethoxypropyl purines (Yokota et al., 1991) and derivatives of oxetanicin (a novel nucleoside isolated from bacteria) (Nagahata et al., 1989). The selective index of these compounds was found to be good and they were efficient at low concentration. Among interferons studied, the interferon β specially inhibited HBV DNA synthesis (Ueda et al., 1989).

Conclusion. The recently described cell culture systems suitable for *in vitro* infection or transfection and replication of hepadnavirus have allowed to select new potent anti-HBV agents. To evaluate the new antiviral agents, it seems that the most adequate system will be a primary hepatocyte culture system rather than transfected cancerous cell lines. These cells have lost several hepatocyte functions as well as cellular receptors which are involved in the recognition of chemical species. Furthermore, the intracellular viral DNA forms which were found were relaxed circular form and single stranded form but not always the supercoiled form. It seems, therefore, that in these artificial systems the viral replication could initiate from viral integrated sequences, by contrast to the physiological replication cycle.

III. OUTLOOK FOR EXPERIMENTAL INVESTIGATIONS

Over the past ten years, significant progress for the study of HBV and research of anti-HBV compounds have been done. Two main approaches have been developped in the chemotherapy of HBV infections *ie* the search for new models of HBV infection and to the evaluation of antihepadnavirus therapies.

New models. Some investigators began to consider transgenic mice for model studies and have generated and described several transgenic mouse lines expressing HBV sequences. It was shown that viral replication could occur in these transgenic mice (Chisari et al., 1989). This model should allow to study both the different aspects and the therapy of chronic HBV infection. In an other field, the inoculation of hepatoma cell lines supporting HBV replication in nude mice does offer new possibilities for *in vivo* screening of potential anti-HBV compounds (Zhai et al., 1990). At last, new cell systems were recently described *ie* both the infection of the hepatoma cell line HepG2 (Bichini et al.,1990) and of the hematopoïetic cell line named K562 (Steinberg et al., 1989). These systems could be used to evaluate inhibitors of viral infection.

New antiviral strategies. Antiviral compounds are only partly effective. To improve their activity, the targeting of antiviral compounds to the liver could be considered. It is possible to target drugs by coupling antiviral compounds with substrate of known hepatocyte receptors. Recently, studies in human have been carried out with ara-AMP coupled with lactosaminated albumin (Fiume et al., 1987). The preliminary results were very promising and further studies are conducted in woodchucks. An other possibility to target the antiviral compounds is the use of liposomes again promising results have been obtained (Ishihara et al. 1991).

One can also expect to improve the activity of antiviral compounds by associating them with cytokines. Finally, gene therapy seems promising. Indeed it was shown that antisense oligo-deoxynucleotides inhibited viral replication in cell culture (Blum et al., 1991).

For the near future, it seems certain that a complete description of HBV replication strategy will be obtained. A better understanding of viral replication could is key to sign new strategies for anti-HBV therapy.

IV. NEW PERSPECTIVES IN ANTI-HBV CLINICAL TRIALS.

In chronic hepatitis B in patients, two different approaches have been evaluated namely nucleoside analogs and interferon, they were used initially separately and then, more recently in combination.

Among the nucleoside analogs, ara-A and its derivated ara-AMP, have proved efficacious, in inhibiting HBV replication in different models as well in therapy of chronic hepatitis patients. Different clinical studies have showed that they were able to clear HBV replication, trigger seroconversion from HBe to anti-HBe, normalise transaminases and improve the histological signs of necrosis and inflammation (Hoofnagle et al. 1984 ; Weller et al. 1985). The most significant results have been obtained in patients heterosexuals with recent chronic active hepatitis, serum ALT level > 3 x N and moderate viral replication. In addition, a second course of vidarabin can be advantageously administered to the patients who are still HBe Ag positive six months after the first course. A second course does increase efficacy on HBV replication without additional side effects. At last, in several preliminary studies, it appears that the combination of prednisolone and ara-A proved to be substantially more effective than either agent alone (Perillo et al. 1985 ; Miyakawa et al. 1984).

The second approach has taken advantage of recombinant alpha-interferon now readily available. Several controlled studies, randomised versus placebo, confirmed that doses of 5 to 10 million units/m^2 administered either daily or three times a week, were able to induce clinical, biochemical and histological remission in 30 to 40 % of the cases positive for HBV replication markers. For the non-responders, retreatment rarely leads to a response, even when higher doses and longer courses of interferon are used.

A more fruitful approach to increasing the response rate to interferon alpha alone has been pre-treatment with corticosteroids. Combination of interferon with short steroid therapy sequentially or more recently simultaneously may also increase the response rate, especially among patients with near normal transaminases (Perillo et al. 1989 ; Causse et al. 1990). Treatment of patients with chronic hepatitis with corticosteroids leads to an increase in serum levels of HBV DNA, associated with mild decreases in serum aminotransferase levels. Subsequent withdrawal of corticosteroids is followed by a flare in the hepatitis disease and is therefore hazardous in patients with cirrhosis.

Several studies have recently combined nucleoside analogs and interferon. This bi-therapy, generally well tolerated, may be superior to interferon alone in patients with high replication.

Altogether, when applied skilfully, antivirals are able to induce long lasting remissions, reduce infectivity and improve symptoms and activity of liver disease. Prevention of death from liver faiwre or hepatocellular carcinoma are the direct of benefit expected from a successful therapy.

V. PROMISES FOR THERAPY OF CHRONIC HEPATITIS C

Hepatitis C virus (HCV), only recently identified, has been shown to be the most common cause of non-A non-B chronic hepatitis. It is now possible to detect specifically the infection using ELISA to detect antibodies and PCR to demonstrate the presence of viral RNA in serum and liver. Hepatitis C is a common and often progressive viral liver disease. Chronic hepatitis develop in at least half the patients with acute hepatitis. Without therapy, this chronic infection will progress over 5 to 30 years towards cirrhosis and hepatocellular carcinoma (Dienstag, 1983 ; Koretz et al. 1985).

Corticosteroids and acyclovir have not proved effective (Pappas et al. 1985 ; Stokes et al. 1987). Prednisone may even be harmful in this disease. Several small, uncontrolled trials suggested that both interferon alpha and interferon beta may be useful in the patients with chronic hepatitis non-A non-B (Arima et al. 1986 ; Hoofnagle et al. 1986). The potential of interferon was discovered before the identification of HCV and avaisability of the above markers. On the basis of these early reports, randomised controlled trials have been conducted in the USA and Europe to assess the efficacy of interferon alpha. All studies proved that the efficacy of interferon is dose dependent. 3 million units, given for six months thrice weekly, appeared to be superior to 1 million units. Serum ALT levels became normal in 46 % and 28 % of patients receiving respectively 3 and 1 million units of interferon. Historical improvement is also dose dependent, more frequently (Davis et al. 1989) in patients treated with 3 million units of interferon, but no restricted to the patients who completely normalised ALT (Di Biscegli et al. 1990).

Possible predictive factors of response have not been discovered except for a few studies in which younger age, female sex and absence of cirrhosis appeared to be linked to better results. So far no virological parameters has been correlated with therapy response. The frequency of relapses have been a disapointing finding in all studies. Again 50 % of the patients relapsed shortly after stoping interferon. Studies in several centers including ours have documented the benefit of maintenance therapy. Subtained remission could be maintained by doses as low as 1 million units thrice weekly, given for 12 or 16 months, which are very well tolerated.

Finally the effects of interferon therapy on viral replication, infectivity, and the long term natural history of chronic hepatitis C remain to be defined. It is therefore crucial that adequate monitoring of HCV replication will be available in the future as for HBV or HDV and that a few models eventually similar to those described for HBV can be developed in the future.

REFERENCES

Arima, T., Shimomura, H. and Nakagawa, J. (1986): Treatment of non-A non-B hepatitis with human fibroblast interferon. Hepatology 6, 1117 (abstract)

Bichini, R., Capel, F., Dauguet, C., Dubanchet, S. and Petit, M.A. (1990): *In vitro* infection of human hepatoma (Hep G2) cells with hepatitis B virus. *J. Virol.* 64, 3025-3032.

Blum, H.E., Galun, E., Weizsäcker, F.V. and Wands, J.R. (1991): Inhibition of hepatitis B virus by antisense oligodeoxynucleotides. *Lancet.* 337, 1230.

Causse, X., Godinot, H., Zoulim, F., Chossegros, P., Fontanges, T., Zarski, J.P., Meschievitz, C., Albrecht, J. and Trépo, C. (1990): Remarkable improvment of chronic hepatitis B following simultaneous administration of interferon and short term prednisone therapy. J. Hepatol. 11 (suppl.2), S16

Chisari F.V. (1989): Hepatitis B virus gene expression in transgenic mice. *Mol. Biol. Med.* 6, 143-149.

Civitico, G., Wang Y.Y., Luscombe C., Bishop N., Tachedjian G., Gust I. and Locarnini S (1990): Antiviral stategies in chronic hepatitis B virus infection: II. Inhibition of duck hepatitis B virus in vitro using conventionnal antiviral agents and supercoiled-DNA active compounds. *J. Med. Virol.* 31, 90-97.

Davis, L., Balart, L.A., Schiff, E.R., Linsday, K., Bodenheimer, H.C., Perillo, R.P., Carey, W., Jacobson, J.M., Payne, J., Dienstal, J.L., Vanthiel, D.H., Tamburro, C., Lefkowitch, J., Albrecht, J., Carlton Meschievitz PH.D., Ortego, T.J., Gibas, A. and the Hepatitis Interventional Therapy Group. (1989): Treatment of chronic hepatitis C with recombinant interferon alpha. A multicenter randomised, controlled trial. N. Engl. J. Med. 321, 1501-1505

De Clercq, E. (1988): Recent advances in the search for selective antiviral agents. In "*Advances in drug research*" Academic Press Limited 17, 1-58.

Di Biscegli, A.M., Martin, P., Kassianides, C., Lisker-MacMan, M., Goodman, Z., Banks, S.M. and Hoofnagle, J.H. (1990): A randomized, double-blind, placebo-controlled trial of recombinant human alpha interferon therapy for chronic non-A non-B (type C) hepatitis. J. Hepatol. 11, S36-S42

Dienstag J.L. (1983): Non-A non-B hepatitis. I. Recognition, epidemiology and clinical features. Gastroenterology 85, 439-462

Fiume, L., Mattioli, A. and Spinoza, G. (1987): Distribution of a conjugate 9-β-D-arabinofuranosyladenine 5'-monophosphate (ara AMP) with lactosaminated albumin in parenchymal and sinusoidal cells of rat liver. *Cancer Drug Delivery.* 4, 11-16.

Fourel, I., Gripon, P., Hantz, O., Cova, L., Lambert, V., Jacquet, C., Watanabe, K., Fox, J., Guguen-Guillouzo, C. and Trépo C. (1989): Prolonged duck hepatitis B virus in duck hepatocytes cocultivated with rat epithelial cells : a useful system for antiviral testing. *Hepatology.* 10, 186-191.

Fourel, I., Hantz, O., Watanabe, K.A., Jacquet, C., Chomel, B., Fox, J.J. and Trépo, C. (1990): Inhibitory effects of 2'-fluorinated arabinosyl-pyrimidine nucleosides on woodchuck hepatitis virus replication in chronically infected woodchucks. *Antimicribial Agents Chemother.* 34, 473-475.

Freiman, J.S., Murray, S.M., Vickery, K., Lim, D and Cossart, Y.E. (1990): Postexposure treatment of exprimental DHBV infection : a new therapeutic strategy. *J. Med. Virol.* 30, 272-276.

Ganem, D. and Varmus, H.Z. (1987): The molecular biology of the hepatitis B viruses. *Ann. Rev. Biochem.* 56:651-693.

Gripon, P., Diot,, C., Thézé N., Fourel, I., Loréal, O., Bréchot, C. and Guguen-Guillouzo, C. (1988): Hepatitis B virus infection of adult human hepatocytes cultured in the presence of dimethylsulfoxide. *J. Virol.* 62, 4136-4143.

Haritani, H., Uchida, T., Okuda, Y. and Shikata, T. (1989): Effect of 3'-azido-3'-deoxythymidine on replication of duck hepatitis B virus *in vivo* and *in vitro*. *J. Med. Virol.* 29, 244-248.

Hirota, K., Sherker, A.H., Omata, M., Yokosuka, O and Okuda, K. (1987): Effects of adenine arabinoside on serum and intrahepatic replicative forms of duck hepatitis B virus in chronic infection. *Hepatology* . 7, 24-28.

Hoofnagle, J.H., Hanson, R.G., Minuk, G.Y. et coll. (1984): Randomised controlled trial of adenine arabinoside monophosphate in the treatment for chronic type B hepatitis. Gastroenterology 86, 150-157

Hoofnagle, J.H., Mullen, K.D., Jones, D.B. et al. (1986): Treatment of chronic non-A non-B hepatitis with recombinant human alpha interferon: a preliminary report. N. Engl. J. Med. 315, 1575-1578

Ishihara, H., Hayashi, Y., Hara, T., Aramaki, Y., Tsuchiya, S., Koike, K. (1991): Specific uptake of asialofetuin-tacked liposomes encapsulating interferon-γ by human hepatoma cells and its inhibitory effect on hepatitis B virus replication. *Biochem. Biophys. Res. Commun.* 174, 839-845.

Jacyna, M.R, and Thomas, H.C. (1990): Antiviral therapy : Hepatitis B. *Brit. Med. Bull.* 46, 368-382.

Kassianides, C., Hoofnagle, J.H., Miller, R.H., Doo, E., Ford, H., Broder, S. and Mitsuya, H. (1989): Inhibition of duck hepatitis B virus replication by 2', 3'-dideoxycytidine. *Gastroenterology.* 97, 1275-1280.

Koretz, R.L., Stone, O., Mousa, M. and Gitnick, G.L. (1985): Non-a non-B post transfusion hepatitis. A decade later. Gastroenterology 88, 1251-1254

Lampertico, P., Malter, J.S. and Gerber, M.A (1991): Development and application of an *in vitro* model for sreening anti-hepatitis B virus therapeutics. *Hepatology.* 13, 422-426.

Lee, B., Luo, W., Suzuki, S., Robins, M.J. and Tyrrell, D.L.J. (1989): *In vitro* and *in vivo* comparison of the abilities of purine and pyrimidine 2', 3'-dideoxynucleosides to inhibit duck hepadnavirus. *Antimicrob. Agents Chemother.* 33:336-339.

Mason, W.S. and Taylor, J. (1989): Experimental systems for the study of hepadnavirus and hepatitis delta infections. *Hepatology* . 9, 635-645

Matthes, E., Langen, P., von Janta-Lipinski, M., Will, H., Schröder, H.C., Merz, H., Weiler, B.E and Müller, W.E.G. (1990): Potent inhibition of hepatitis B virus production *in vitro* by modified pyrimidine nucleosides. *Antimicrobial Agents Chemother.* 34, 1986-1990.

Miyakawa, H., Hino, K., Kasuda, K., Iwasaki, M. and Takahashi, K. (1984): Combined therapy with prednisolone and adenine arabinoside available for chronic hepatitis. Gastroenterology 86, 1324 (abstract)

Nagahata, T., Ueda, K., Tsurimoto, T., Chisaka, O. and Matsubara, K. (1989): Anti-hepatitis B virus activities of purine derivatives of oxetanocin A. *J. Antibiot.* 62, 644-646.

Neurath, A.R., Kent, S.B.H., Strick, N. and Parker, K. (1986): Identification and chemical synthesis of a host cell receptor binding site on hepatitis B virus. *Cell.* 46, 429-436.

Niu, J., Wang, Y., Qiao, M., Gowans, E., Edwards, P., Thyagarajan, S.P., Gust, I. and Locarnini, S. (1990): Effect of *Phyllanthus amarus* on duck hepatitis B virus replication *in vivo*. *J. Med. Virol.* 32, 212-218.

Pappas, S.C., Hoofnagle, J.H., Young, M., Strauss, S.E. and Jones, E.A. (1985): Treatment of chronic non-A non-B hepatitis with acyclovir: pilot study. J. Med. Virol. 15, 1-9

Perillo, R., Schiff, E., Davis, G.L. et al. (1989): Multicenter randomized controlld trial of recombinant alpha interferon (r IFN Aa 2-b) alone and following prednisone withdrawal in chronic hepatitis. B. Hepatology 10, 579 (abstract)

Perillo, R.P., Regenstein, F.G., Bodicky, C.J. et coll. (1985): Comparative efficacy of adenine arabinoside 5'-monophosphate and prednisone withdrawal followed by arabinoside 5'-monophosphate in the treatment of chronic active hepatitis type B. Gastroenterology 88, 780-786

Petcu, D.J., Aldrich, C.E., Coates, L., Taylor, J.M. and Mason, W.S. (1990): Suramin inhibits *in vitro* infection by Duck hepatitis B virus, Rous sarcoma virus, and Hepatitis delta virus. *Virology* . 167, 385-392.

Popper, H., Shafritz, A. and Hoofnagle, J.H. (1987): Relation of the hepatitis B virus carrier state to hepatocellular carcinoma. *Hepatology.* 7:764-772.

Price, P.M., Banerjee, R. and Acs, G. (1989): Inhibition of the replication of hepatitis B virus by the carbocyclic analogue of 2'-deoxyguanosine. *Proc. Natl Acad. Sci. USA*. 86, 8541-8544.
Pugh, J.C. and Summers, J.W. (1989): Infection and uptake of duck hepatitis B virus by duck hepatocytes maintained in the presence of dimethyl sulfoxide. *Virology*. 172, 564-572.
Sherker, A.H., Hirota, K., Omata, K. and Okuda, K. (1986): Foscarnet decreases serum and liver duck heaptitis B virus DNA in chronically infected ducks. *Gastroenterology*. 91, 818-824.
Smee, D.F., Knight, S.S., Duke, A.E., Robinson, W.S., Matthes, T.R.and Marion, P.L. (1985): Activities of arabinosyladenine monophosphate and 9-(1,3-dihydroxy-2-propoxymethyl) guanine against ground squirrel hepatitis virus *in vivo* as determinated by reduction in serum virion associated DNA polymerase. *Antimicrobial Agents Chemother*. 27, 277-279.
Steinberg, H.N., Bouffard, P., Trépo, C. and Zeldis, J.B. (1990): *In vitro* inhibition of hemopoietic cell line growth by hepatitis B virus. *J. Virol*. 64, 2577-2581.
Stokes, P., Lopez, W.C. and Balart, L.A. (1987): Effects of short-term corticosteroid therapy in patients with chronic non-A non-B hepatitis (NANB). Gastroenterology 92, 1783 (abstract)
Summers, J. and Mason, W.S. (1982): Replication of the genome of a hepatitis B-like virus by reverse transcription of an RNA intermediate. *Cell*. 29, 403-415.
Summers, J., Smith, P.M. and Horwich, A.L. (1990): Hepadnavirus envelope proteins regulate covalently closed circular DNA amplification. *J. Virol*. 64, 2819-2824.
Thomas, H.C., Pignatelli, M., Goodall, A., Waters, J., Karrayiannis, P. and Brown, D. (1984): Immunologic mechanisms of cell lysis in hepatitis B virus infection. In: "*Viral Hepatitis and Liver Disease*". Grune & Stratton, Orlando, pp 167-177.
Tuttleman, J.S., Pugh, J.C. and Summers, J.W. (1986): *In vitro* experimental infection of primary duck hepatocyte cultures with duck hepatitis B virus. *J. Virol*. 58, 17-25.
Uchida, T., Suzuki, K., Okuda, Y. and Shigata, T. (1988): *In vitro* transmission of duck hepatitis B virus to primary duck hepatocytes cultures. *Hepatology*. 8, 760-765.
Ueda, K., Tsurimoto, T., Nagahata, T., Chisaka, O. and Matsubara, K. (1989): An *in vitro* system for screening anti-hepatitis B virus drugs. *Virology*. 169, 213-216.
Venkastewaran, P.S., Millman I. and Blumberg, B.S. (1987): Effect of an extract from *Phyllanthus niruri* on hepatitis B and woodchuck hepatitis viruses : *in vitro* and *in vivo* studies. *Proc. Natl. Acad. Sci. USA*. 84, 274-278.
Weller, U.D., Lok, A.S.F. et coll. (1985): Randomised controlled trial of adenine arabinoside 5'-monophosphate (Ara-AMP) in chronic hepatitis B virus infection. Gut 26, 745-751
Wu, T. T., Coates, C. E., Aldrich, C. E., Summers, J. and Mason, W. (1990): In hepatocytes infected with duck hepatits B virus, the template for viral RNA synthesis is amplified by an intracellular pathway. *Virology*. 175, 255-261.
Yokota, T., Konno, K., Chonan, E., Mochizuki, S., Kojima, K., Shigeta, S and De Clercq, E. (1990): Comparative avtivities of several nucleoside analogs against duck hepatitis B virus *in vitro*. *Antimicrobial Agents Chemother*. 34, 1326-1330.
Yokota, T., Mochizuki S., Konno, K., Mori, S., Shigeta, S. and De Clercq E. (1991: Inhibitory effects of selected antiviral compounds on human hepatitis B virus DNA synthesis. *Antimicrobial Agents Chemother*. 35-394-397.
Zhai, W.R., Vajta, G., Acs, G. and Paronetto, F. (1990): A nude mouse model for the *in vivo* production of hepatitis B virus. *Gastroenterology*. 98, 470-477.
Zuckerman, A.J. (1987): Screening of antiviral drugs for hepadna virus infection in Pekin ducks : a review. *J. Virol. Meth*. 17, 119-126.

Résumé

L'hépatite virale B (HVB) est cause d'infections aiguës et chroniques. Ces dernières constituent un risque majeur de développement d'un carcinome hépatocellulaire (CHC). Le but de la thérapie antivirale au cours de l'infection chronique à l'HVB est de prévenir la progression vers le CHC. Les protocoles antiviraux actuels manquent d'efficacité. Les problèmes que pose le développement de médicaments antiviraux sont la grande spécificité d'hôte et l'absence de modèles de cultures pour la propagation du virus. La découverte de virus semblables au virus B chez certains animaux et les progrès de la biologie moléculaire ont permis des avancées rapides. Plusieurs approches sont actuellement accessibles pour évaluer *in vitro* et *in vivo* les effets inhibiteurs de molécules antivirales potentielles. Elles incluent : a) la culture d'hépatocytes qui supporte la réplication complète du virus ; b) les lignées d'hépatome transfectés avec l'ADN viral qui supportent une réplication virale continue ; c) les modèles animaux tels que le canard et la marmotte. Dans cette revue, nous avons résumé les études récentes sur l'évaluation de molécules antivirales (inhibiteurs de l'ADN polymérase virale), à la fois *in vitro* et *in vivo* et au cours d'essais cliniques. D'autres travaux sont nécessaires dans ce domaine mais de nouvelles approches devraient bientôt apporter quelques éclaircissements. Pour l'instant, l'hépatite chronique HVC n'a été étudiée qu'en clinique.

Cellular and Molecular Aspects of Cirrhosis. Eds B. Clément, A. Guillouzo. Colloque INSERM/John Libbey Eurotext Ltd. © 1992, Vol. 216, pp. 369-372

Glutathione S transferase class μ in French cirrhotic (alcoholic and non alcoholic) patients

C. Coutelle [1], A. Groppi [2], B. Fleury [1], A. Iron [1], F. Dumas [3], L. Schouler [3], A. Cassaigne [1], J. Begueret [2] and P. Couzigou [1,3]

[1] Département de biochimie médicale et de biologie moléculaire, Université de Bordeaux II, 146, rue Léo Saignat, 33076 Bordeaux Cedex, France; [2] Laboratoire de génétique CNRS UA 542, avenue des Facultés, 33405 Talence Cedex, France; [3] Département d'hépatologie et de gastro-entérologie, de nutrition et d'alcoologie, Hôpital du Haut-Lévêque, avenue de Magellan, 33604, Pessac, France

INTRODUCTION

The glutathione S-transferases (GST; glutathione, S-transferase; EC (2.5.1.18.)) are a family of related iso-enzymes that catalyse the conjugation of reduced glutathione to a wide range of electrophilic substrates (Mannervik et al. 1985). These enzymes play a major role in detoxification processes in a variety of tissues.

These enzymes have been grouped intro three major classes designated, α μ and π(Mannervik et al. 1985). Three genetic loci encoding human liver glutathione S-transferase have been characterized : GST_1, GST_2, and GST_3. They code, respectively, for the class μ isoenzyme, the class α isoenzyme and the placental class π(Board 1981; Strange et al. 1984). Three other human loci have also been identified: GST_4, GST_5 (expressed in the brain) and GST_6 (Laisney et al. 1984; Suzuki et al. 1987).

The GST_1 locus exhibits some polymorphism . Three alleles were found at this locus : $GST_1{}^0$ (NULL), $GST_1{}^1$ and $GST_1{}^2$ (Laisney et al. 1984). The $GST_1{}^0$ allele corresonds to a gene deletion (Seidegard et al. 1988). Previous studies suggest that the absence of GST isoenzyme (homozygous deletion of the GST_1 gene) increases the risk of lung cancer (Seidegard et al.1990).

Only 12%-13% of all heavy drinkers develop cirrhosis. A previous study (Hrubec and Omenn 1981) provides evidence that this heterogeneous response is the result of heterogeneity in the genetic background. Considering the protective role of GST againts xenobiotics, the study of the lack of GST isoenzyme μ($GST_1{}^0$ homozygous) in individuals might reveal linkage between a specific genotype and the development of cirrhosis in heavy consumers of ethanol, as suggested by preliminary results from Harada. The lack of GSTμ isoenzyme may promote cirrhosis in alcoholic but possibly also in other cirrhotic condition as viral cirrhosis.

SUBJECTS AND METHODS

Blood samples

Human whole blood samples were stored at -20°C after addition of citrate. Genotyping was carried out in two groups.

Group I: Fourtyfive cirrhotic caucasians (>100 grams pure alcohol per day for more than 5 years), medium age 57 years, Ag HbS negative, with ascite and/or persistent oesophageal varices treated by sclerotherapy.

*Group II :*Fourty non alcoholic cirrhotic caucasians with ascite and/or persistent oesophageal varices treated by sclerotherapy and/or histologically proved cirrhosis, Ag HbS positive or anti HCV positive.

Group III: 45 healthy Caucasians (<40 grams pure alcohol per day), medium age 23 years.

PCR and southern blots were performed as previous described (Groppi et al. 1990; Groppi et al. in Press)

Enzyme - linked immunosorbent assay (ELISA)

The presence of GSTμ was determined by ELISA (Mukit, Medlabs, Dublin) in 10 samples randomly chosen from group I and group III. Perfect concordance of the results allow to test group II patients only by Elisa method.

RESULTS AND DISCUSSION

The location of the GST_1 deletion responsible for the null allele (GST_1^0) and its limits are not precisely known. Some authors have previously developed a method to determine the presence or the absence of this deletion by PCR (Comstock et al. 1990; Harada, personal communication). Because of the high degree of homology in the coding sequence between GST_1 and GST_4 (Board et al. 1988; Harada, personal communication), the location of the first primer was chosen in the fourth intron of the GST_1 gene (Comstock et al. 1990) to avoid any cross amplification . The second primer used hybridized in the 3' region of the fifth exon leading to a 165-bp amplification fragment. This 165-bp product was present in individuals heterozygous for the null allele, i.e., they did not have the gene deletion, and was absent if individuals were GST_1^0 homozygous, i.e. lacking the GSTμ enzyme.
The specificity of this detection was controlled by Southern Blot analysis. The probe was a 23-mer oligo nucleotide that specifically hybridizes within the fourth intron. Figure 1b shows the result of this analysis. The reliability of this method was verified by testing 10 samples from each group with ELISA. The results obtained with this method were identical to those obtained by PCR detection. We were then able to study group I and group III using PCR detection procedure and group II using Elisa method.

Table 1. Percentages of GSTμ deficiency in different healthy populations. GT-tSBO glutathione transferase activity on the substrate *trans*-stilbene oxide

Population	*n*	Presence of GSTμ		Absence of GSTμ		Methods	Authors
Caucasians (France)	56	32	57%	24	43%	Starch-gel electrophoresis	Laisney *et al.* (1984)
Caucasians (Europe)	49	29	59%	20	41%	Starch-gel electrophoresis	Strange *et al.* (1984)
Japanese	168	88	52,3%	80	47,7%	Starch-gel electrophoresis	Harada *et al.* (1987)
Caucasians (Scotland)	42	23	54,76%	19	45,24%	Radioimmunoassay	Hussey *et al.* (1987)
Caucasians (Sweden)	248	114	46%	134	54%	GT-tSBO	Seidegard *et al.* (1985)
Caucasians (France)	45	24	53,33%	21	46,67%	PCR detection	Present study

Table 2. Percentages of GSTμ deficiency in different cirrhotic populations.

Population	*n*	Presence of GSTμ		Absence of GSTμ		Methods	Authors
Japanese	8	2	25%	6	75%	Starch-gel electrophoresis	Harada et al. (1987)
Caucasians (France)	45	23	51,14%	22	48,89%	PCR detection	Present study

Odds ratio = 1.093
confidence interval [0.476 : 2.5]

$\chi 2$ (cirrhotic/heatly) = 0.0444
df = 1
Level of significance = 5% $\chi 2 < 3.84$

The results for healthy subjects (group III) are presented in table I. The percentage of samples lacking GSTμ in this healthy population is comparable with the results obtained by other authors (Table 1). However, the principal result of this study is the distribution obtained in the group I and III. Table 2 presented results in alcoholic cirrhotic patients (group I) with the preliminary data from Harada χ^2. These values are similar to those obtained in the group I, a conclusion confirmed by the value calculated with the homogeneity test performed between the two groups (table 2). This fact indicates that there is no difference between the two groups for the lack of GSTμ , and that there is no link between the lack of GSTμ (individuals $GST1^0$ homozygous) and the development of a cirrhosis in heavy consumers of ethanol.
In the group of fourty non alcoholic cirrhotic patients (groups II), GSTμ was present in 26 (65%) and absent in 14 (35%), with no significant difference when compared with control group. So, in non alcoholic viral cirrhosis, it can be conclude that lack of GSTμ does not seem to promote cirrhotic evolution in case of viral hepatitis B ou C.
We have previously compared the alcohol dehydrogenase genotype (ADH; alcohol : NAD^+ oxidoreductase, EC 1.1.1.1.) at two loci, ADH_2 and ADH_3, in the same two groups of subjects (cirrhotic caucasians/healthy caucasians). The conclusion was that there is no significant difference in the distribution of each genotype and in the frequencies of each allele between these two groups (Couzigou et al. 199O). Now we can also exclude the gene deletion at the GST_1 locus as a genetic factor that increases the risk of cirrhosis development in heavy consumers of ethanol. These two studies have allowed us to explore the hypothesis of the influence of genetic factors in the development of cirrhosis in heavy consumers of ethanol. It will be interesting to explore the potential influence of other genetic factors in the development of cirrhosis in chronic consumers of ethanol (>4O g and < 1OO g of pure alcohol per day). If the genetic background is not a preponderant factor in the heterogeneity of response in alcoholic cirrhosis, it could be masked in heavy consumers or ethanol. In further studies, it would thus be interesting to explore the effects of other factors, such as nutrition.
It will be interesting to test the same hypothesis of a link between lack of GSTμ and alcoholic cirrhosis according to sex. In unpublished data we observed a non significant trend for lack of GSTμ in women with alcoholic cirrhosis.

Acknowkedgement. This work supported by grants from Haut Comité d'Etude et d'Information sur l'Alcoolisme no. 1989-06 and from Conseil Régional d'Aquitaine.

REFERENCES

Board PG (1981) Biochemical genetics of glutathione S-transferase in man. Am J Hum Genetic 33:36-43

Board PG, Suzuki T et al. (1988) Human muscle glutathione S-transferase (GST_4) shows close homology to human liver. GST1 Biochim Biophys Acta 953:214-217

Comstock KE, Sanderson HS et al. (199O) GST1 gene deletion determined by polymerase chain reaction. Nucleic Acids Res 18: 367O

Couzigou P, Fleury B et al. (199O) Genotypic study of alcohol dehydrogenase class I polymorphism in French alcoholic cirrhosis patient. Alcohol Alcohol 25: 623-626

Groppi A, Begueret J et al. (199O) Improved methods for genotype determination of human alcohol dehydrogenase (ADH) at ADH_2 and ADH_3 loci by using PCR-directed mutagenesis. Clin Chem 36: 1765-1768

Groppi A, Coutelle C et al. (1991) Glutathion S-transferase in French alcoholic cirrhotic patients. Hum Genet. 87 : 628-630

Harada S, Abei M, et al. (1987) Liver glutathione S-transferase polymorphism in Japanese and its pharmacogenetic importance. Hum Genet 75: 322-325

Hrubec Z, Omenn GS (1981 Evidence of genetic predisposition to alcoholic cirrhosis and psychosis : twin concordances for alcoholism and its biological end points by zygosity among male veterans. Alcoholism (CNY). Alcohol clin Exp Res 5: 2O7-215.

Hussey AJ, Hayes JD et al. (1987) The polymorphic expression of neutral glutathione S-transferase in human mononuclear leukocytes as measured by specific radio immuno assay. Biochem Pharmacol 36:4O13-4O15.

Laisney V, Van Cong N, et al. (1984) Human genes for glutathione S-transferases. Hum Genet 68:221-227.

Seidegard J, Pero RW et al. (1990) Isoenzymes(s) of glutatione transferase (class mu) as a marker for the susceptibility to lung cancer: a follow up study. Carcinogenesis 11:33-36

Strange RC, Faulder CG et al. (1984) The human glutathione S-transferases : studies on the tissue distribution and genetic variation of the GST_1, GST_2 and GST_3 isozymes. Ann Hum Genet 48: 11-20

Suzuki T, Coggan M et al. (1987) Electrophoretic and immunological analysis of human glutatione S-transferase isozymes. Ann Hum Genet 51:95-106

Author index
Index des auteurs

List and address of speakers

Liste et adresse des orateurs

Arthur Michael J.P., Professorial Medical Unit, Room LD 68/Level D, South Laboratory and Pathology block, Southampton General Hospital, Tremona Road, Southampton SO9 4XY, United Kingdom

Bernuau Dominique, INSERM U 327, Faculté de Médecine Xavier Bichat 16, rue Henri Huchard, 75018 Paris, France

Bioulac-Sage Paulette, Université de Bordeaux II, Laboratoire des Interactions Cellulaires, 146, rue Léo Saignat, 33076 Bordeaux Cedex, France

Bissell D. Montgomery, Liver Center Laboratory, Building 40, Room 4102 San Francisco General Hospital, San Francisco, CA 94110, USA

Bréchot Christian, INSERM U 75, Faculté de Médecine Necker-Enfants Malades, 156, rue de Vaugirard, 75730 Paris Cedex 15, France

Brissot Pierre, Clinique de Médecine Interne et des Maladies du Foie et INSERM U 49, Hôpital Pontchaillou, 35033 Rennes Cedex, France

Burbelo Peter, National Institute of Dental Research, NIH, Laboratory of Developmental Biology, NIDR, Bldg 30, room 414, Bethesda, MD 20892, USA

Clément Bruno, INSERM U 49, Unité de Recherches Hépatologiques, Hôpital Pontchaillou, 35033 Rennes Cedex, France

Desmet Valer Julien, Universitaire Ziekenhuizen Leuven, Pathologische Ontleedkunde II, U.Z. Sint-Rafaël Kapucijnenvoer 33 , B-3000 Leuven, Belgium

Erlinger Serge, INSERM U 24, Hôpital Beaujon, Centre Abrami, 100, boulevard du Général Leclerc, 92118 Clichy Cedex, France

Fey Georg, Erlangen University, Standstrasse 5, D-852 Erlangen, Germany

Gressner Axel M., Klinikum der Philipps-Universität Marburg, Abteilung für Klinische Chemie und Zentrallaboratorium, Baldingerstrasse, Postfach 2360, D-3550 Marburg, Germany

Guguen-Guillouzo Christiane, INSERM U 49, Unité de Recherches Hépatologiques, Hôpital Pontchaillou, 35033 Rennes Cedex, France

Guillouzo André, INSERM U 49, Unité de Recherches Hépatologiques, Hôpital Pontchaillou, 35033 Rennes Cedex, France

Hahn Eckhart G., Medizinische Klinik I, Krankenhausstrasse 12, D-8520 Erlangen, Germany

Huet P. Michel, Département de Médecine, Hôpital St Luc, 1058, rue Saint-Denis, Montréal, Québec X2X 3J4, Canada

Israël Yedy, Department of Pharmacology, Primary Mechanisms Research and Development Department, Medical Sciences Building, University of Toronto, Toronto M5S 1A8, Canada

Klotman Paul E., Department of Health and Human Services, Public Health Service, Laboratory of Developmental Biology, National Institute of Dental Research, NIH, Bldg 30, room 433, Bethesda, MD 20892, USA

Laperche Yannick, INSERM U 99, Hôpital Henri Mondor, 51, avenue du Maréchal de Lattre de Tassigny, 94010 Créteil, France

Matsumoto Kunio, Faculty of Science, Kyushu University 33, Fukuoka 812, Japan

Phillips S. Michael, University of Pensylvania, Department of Medicine, Allergy and Immunology Section, 518 Johnson Pavilion, Philadelphia, PA 19104-6057, USA

Poupon Raoul, Hôpital Saint-Antoine, Unité d'Hépatologie et de Gastro-Entérologie, 184, rue du Faubourg Saint-Antoine, 75571 Paris Cedex 12, France

Ramadori Giuliano, Klinikum der Johannes Gutenberg-Universität, I. Medizinische Klinik und Poliklinik, Postfach 3960, Langenbeckstrasse 1, 6500 Mainz, Germany

Schuppan Detlef, Freie Universität Berlin, Universitätsklinikum Steglitz Medizinische Klnik und Poliklinik, Abteilung für Gastroenterologie und Hepatologie, Hindenburgdamm 30, 1000 Berlin 45, Germany

Thorgeirsson Snorri S., Department of Health and Human Services, Laboratory of Experimental Carcinogenesis , NCI, Building 37, Room 3B27, NIH, Bethesda, MD 20892, USA

Trépo Christian, INSERM U 271, 151, rue Albert Thomas, 69424 Lyon Cedex 03, France

Zarnegar Reza, Duke University Medical Center, Department of Pathology, PO Box 3432, Durham, NC 27710, USA

Zern Mark A., Brown University, Department of Medicine, Roger Williams General Hospital, 825 Chalkstone Avenue, Providence, RI 02908, USA

***Colloques* INSERM**
ISSN 0768-3154

Other *Colloques* published as co-editions by John Libbey Eurotext and INSERM

153 Hormones and Cell Regulation (11th European Symposium). *Hormones et Régulation Cellulaire (11e Symposium Européen).*
Edited by J. Nunez and J.E. Dumont.
ISBN : John Libbey Eurotext 0 86196 104 8
INSERM 2 85598 324 X

158 Biochemistry and Physiopathology of Platelet Membrane. *Biochimie et Physiopathologie de la Membrane Plaquettaire.*
Edited by G. Marguerie and R.F.A. Zwaal.
ISBN : John Libbey Eurotext 0 86196 114 5
INSERM 2 85598 345 2

162 The Inhibitors of Hematopoiesis. *Les Inhibiteurs de l'Hématopoïèse.*
Edited by A. Najman, M. Guignon, N.C. Gorin and J.Y. Mary.
ISBN : John Libbey Eurotext 0 86196 125 0
INSERM 2 85598 340 1

164 Liver Cells and Drugs. *Cellules Hépatiques et Médicaments.*
Edited by A. Guillouzo.
ISBN : John Libbey Eurotext 0 86196 128 5
INSERM 2 85598 341 X

165 Hormones and Cell Regulation (12th European Symposium). *Hormones et Régulation Cellulaire (12e Symposium Européen).*
Edited by J. Nunez, J.E. Dumont and E. Carafoli.
ISBN : John Libbey Eurotext 0 86196 133 1
INSERM 2 85598 347 9

167 Sleep Disorders and Respiration. *Les Evénements Respiratoires du Sommeil.*
Edited by P. Lévi-Valensi and D. Duron.
ISBN : John Libbey Eurotext 0 86196 127 7
INSERM 2 85598 344 4

169 Neo-Adjuvant Chemotherapy. *Chimiothérapie Néo-Adjuvante.*
Edited by C. Jacquillat, M. Weil, D. Khayat.
ISBN : John Libbey Eurotext 0 86196 150 1
INSERM 2 85598 349 5

171 Structure and Functions of the Cytoskeleton. *La Structure et les Fonctions du Cytosquelette.*
Edited by B.A.F. Rousset.
ISBN : John Libbey Eurotext 0 86196 149 8
INSERM 2 85598 351 7

Colloques INSERM
ISSN 0768-3154

172 The Langerhans Cell. *La Cellule de Langerhans.*
Edited by J. Thivolet, D. Schmitt.
ISBN : John Libbey Eurotext 0 86196 181 1
INSERM 2 85598 352 5

173 Cellular and Molecular Aspects of Glucuronidation. *Aspects Cellulaires et Moléculaires de la Glucuronoconjugaison.*
Edited by G. Siest, J. Magdalou, B. Burchell
ISBN : John Libbey Eurotext 0 86196 182 X
INSERM 2 85598 353 3

174 Second Forum on Peptides. *Deuxième Forum Peptides.*
Edited by A. Aubry, M. Marraud, B. Vitoux
ISBN : John Libbey Eurotext 0 86196 151 X
INSERM 2 85598 354 1

176 Hormones and Cell Regulation (13th European Symposium). *Hormones et Régulation Cellulaire (13e Symposium Européen).*
Edited by J. Nunez, J.E. Dumont, R. Denton
ISBN : John Libbey Eurotext 0 86196 183 8
INSERM 2 85598 356 8

179 Lymphokine Receptors Interactions. *Interactions Lymphokines-récepteurs.*
Edited by D. Fradelizi, J. Bertoglio
ISBN : John Libbey Eurotext 0 86196 148 X
INSERM 2 85598 359 2

191 Anticancer Drugs (1st International Interface of Clinical and Laboratory responses to anticancer drugs). *Médicaments anticancéreux (1re Confrontation internationale des réponses cliniques et expérimentales aux médicaments anticancéreux).*
Edited by H. Tapiero, J. Robert, T.J. Lampidis
ISBN : John Libbey Eurotext 0 86196 223 0
INSERM 2 85598 393 2

193 Living in the Cold (2nd International Symposium). *La Vie au Froid (2e Symposium International).*
Edited by A. Malan, B. Canguilhem
ISBN : John Libbey Eurotext 0 86196 234 9
INSERM 2 85598 395 9

Colloques INSERM
ISSN 0768-3154

194 Progress in Hepatitis B Immunization. *La Vaccination contre l'épatite B.*
Edited by P. Coursaget, M.J. Tong
ISBN : John Libbey Eurotext 0 86196 249 4
INSERM 2 85598 396 7

196 Treatment Strategy in Hodgkin's Disease. *Stratégie dans la maladie de Hodgkin.*
Edited by P. Sommers, M. Henry-Amar, J.H. Meezwaldt, P. Carde
ISBN : John Libbey Eurotext 0 86196 226 5
INSERM 2 85598 398 3

198 Hormones and Cell Regulation (14th European Symposium). *Hormones et Régulation Cellulaire (14e Symposium Européen).*
Edited by J. Nunez, J.E. Dumont
ISBN : John Libbey Eurotext 0 86196 229 X
INSERM 2 85598 400 9

199 Placental Communications : Biochemical, Morphological and Cellular Aspects. *Communications placentaires : aspects biochimique, morphologique et cellulaire.*
Edited by L. Cedard, E. Alsat, J.C. Challier, G. Chaouat, A. Malassiné
ISBN : John Libbey Eurotext 0 86196 227 3
INSERM 2 85598 401 7

204 Pharmacologie Clinique : Actualités et Perspectives. (6e Rencontres Nationales de Pharmacologie clinique).
Edited by J.P. Boissel, C. Caulin, M. Teule
ISBN : John Libbey Eurotext 0 86196 225 7
INSERM 2 85598 454 8

205 Recent Trends in Clinical Pharmacology (6th National Meeting of Clinical Pharmacology).
Edited by J.P. Boissel, C. Caulin, M. Teule
ISBN : John Libbey Eurotext 0 86196 256 7
INSERM 2 85598 455 6

206 Platelet Immunology : Fundamental and Clinical Aspects. *Immunologie plaquettaire : aspects fondamentaux et cliniques.*
Edited by C. Kaplan-Gouet, N. Schlegel, Ch. Salmon, J. McGregor
ISBN : John Libbey Eurotext 0 86196 285 0
INSERM 2 85598 439 4

Colloques INSERM
ISSN 0768-3154

207 Thyroperoxidase and Thyroid Autoimmunity. *Thyroperoxydase et auto-immunité thyroïdienne.*
Edited by P. Carayon, T. Ruf
ISBN : John Libbey Eurotext 0 86196 277 X
INSERM 2 85598 440 8

208 Vasopressin. *Vasopressine.*
Edited by S. Jard, R. Jamison
ISBN : John Libbey Eurotext 0 86196 288 5
INSERM 2 85598 441 6

210 Hormones and Cell Regulation (15th European Symposium). *Hormones et Régulation Cellulaire (15e Symposium Européen).*
Edited by J.E. Dumont, J. Nunez, R.J.B. King
ISBN : John Libbey Eurotext 0 86196 279 6
INSERM 2 85598 443 2

211 Medullary Thyroid Carcinoma. *Cancer Médullaire de la Thyroïde.*
Edited by C. Calmettes, J.M. Guliana
ISBN : John Libbey Eurotext 0 86196 287 7
INSERM 2 85598 440 0

212 Cellular and Molecular Biology of the Materno-Fetal Relationship. *Biologie cellulaire et moléculaire de la relation materno-fœtale.*
Edited by G. Chaouat, J. Mowbray
ISBN : John Libbey Eurotext 0 86196 909 1
INSERM 2 85598 445 9

215 Aldosterone. Fundamental Aspects.
Aspects fondamentaux.
Edited by J.P. Bonvalet, N. Farman, M. Lombes, M.E. Rafestin-Oblin
ISBN : John Libbey Eurotext 0 86196 302 4
INSERM 2 85598 482 3

217 Sleep and Cardiorespiratory Control. *Sommeil et contrôle cardio-respiratoire.*
Edited by C. Gaultier, P. Escourrou, L. Curzi-Dascalora
ISBN : John Libbey Eurotext 0 86196 307 5
INSERM 2 85598 484 X

219 Human Gene Transfer. *Transfert de gènes chez l'homme.*
Edited by O. Cohen-Haguenauer, M. Boiron
ISBN : John Libbey Eurotext 0 86196 301 6
INSERM 2 85598 497 1

L O U I S - J E A N
avenue d'Embrun, 05003 GAP cedex
Tél. : 92.53.17.00
Dépôt légal : 38 — Janvier 1992
Imprimé en France